T0383898

A HISTORY

OF

EPIDEMICS IN BRITAIN.

A HISTORY

OF

EPIDEMICS IN BRITAIN

BY

CHARLES CREIGHTON, M.A., M.D.,

FORMERLY DEMONSTRATOR OF ANATOMY IN THE UNIVERSITY OF CAMBRIDGE.

VOLUME II.

From the Extinction of Plague to the present time.

CAMBRIDGE:

AT THE UNIVERSITY PRESS.

1894

CAMBRIDGE UNIVERSITY PRESS
Cambridge, New York, Melbourne, Madrid, Cape Town,
Singapore, São Paulo, Delhi, Mexico City

Cambridge University Press
The Edinburgh Building, Cambridge CB2 8RU, UK

Published in the United States of America by Cambridge University Press, New York

www.cambridge.org
Information on this title: www.cambridge.org/9781107621954

First published 1894
First paperback edition 2013

A catalogue record for this publication is available from the British Library

ISBN 978-1-107-62195-4 Paperback

PREFACE.

THIS volume is the continuation of 'A History of Epidemics in Britain from A.D. 664 to the Extinction of Plague' (which was published three years ago), and is the completion of the history to the present time. The two volumes may be referred to conveniently as the first and second of a 'History of Epidemics in Britain.' In adhering to the plan of a systematic history instead of annals I have encountered more difficulties in the second volume than in the first. In the earlier period the predominant infection was Plague, which was not only of so uniform a type as to give no trouble, in the nosological sense, but was often so dramatic in its occasions and so enormous in its effects as to make a fitting historical theme. With its disappearance after 1666, the field is seen after a time to be occupied by a numerous brood of fevers, anginas and other infections, which are not always easy to identify according to modern definitions, and were recorded by writers of the time, for example Wintringham, in so dry or abstract a manner and with so little of human interest as to make but tedious reading in an almost obsolete phraseology. Descriptions of the fevers of those times, under the various names of *synochus, synocha,* nervous, putrid, miliary, remittent, comatose, and the like, have been introduced into the chapter on Continued Fevers so as to show their generic as well as their differential character; but a not less important purpose of the chapter has been to illustrate the condition of the working classes, the unwholesomeness of towns, London in particular, the state of the gaols and of the navy, the seasons of dearth, the

times of war-prices or of depressed trade, and all other vicissitudes of well-being, of which the amount of Typhus and Relapsing
Fever has always been a curiously correct index. It is in this
chapter that the epidemiology comes into closest contact with
social and economic history. In the special chapter for Ireland
the association is so close, and so uniform over a long period,
that the history may seem at times to lose its distinctively
medical character.

As the two first chapters are pervaded by social and economic
history, so each of the others will be found to have one or more
points of distinctive interest besides the strictly professional.
Smallpox is perhaps the most suitable of all the subjects in this
volume to be exhibited in a continuous view, from the epidemics
of it in London in the first Stuart reigns to the statistics of last
year. While it shares with Plague the merit, from a historical
point of view, of being always the same definite item in the bills
of mortality, it can be shown to have experienced, in the course
of two centuries and a half, changes in its incidence upon the
classes in the community, upon the several age-periods and upon
town and country, as well as a very marked change relatively
to measles and scarlatina among the infective scourges of infancy
and childhood. For certain reasons Smallpox has been the most
favoured infectious disease, having claimed an altogether disproportionate share of interest at one time with Inoculation, at
another time with Vaccination. The history of the former practice,
which is the precedent for, or source of, a whole new ambitious
scheme of prophylaxis in the infectious diseases of men and brutes,
has been given minutely. The latter practice, which is a radical
innovation inasmuch as it affects to prevent one disease by the
inoculation of another, has been assigned as much space in the
chapter on Smallpox as it seems to me to deserve. Measles and
Whooping-cough are historically interesting, in that they seem
to have become relatively more prominent among the infantile
causes of death in proportion as the public health has improved.
Whooping-cough is now left to head the list of its class by the
shrinkage of the others. It is in the statistics of Measles and

Whooping-cough that the principle of population comes most into view. The scientific interest of Scarlatina and Diphtheria is mainly that of new, or at least very intermittent, species. Towards the middle of the 18th century there emerges an epidemic sickness new to that age, in which were probably contained the two modern types of Scarlet Fever and Diphtheria more or less clearly differentiated. The subsequent history of each has been remarkable: for a whole generation Scarlatina could prove itself a mild infection causing relatively few deaths, to become in the generation next following the greatest scourge of childhood; for two whole generations Diphtheria had disappeared from the observation of all but a few medical men, to emerge suddenly in its modern form about the years 1856–59.

The history of Dysentery, as told by the younger Heberden, has been a favourite instance of the steady decrease of a disease in London during the 18th century. I have shown the error in this, and at the same time have proved from the London bills of mortality of the 17th and 18th centuries that Infantile Diarrhoea, which is now one of the most important causes of death in some of the great manufacturing and shipping towns, was formerly still more deadly to the infancy of the capital in a hot summer or autumn. Asiatic Cholera brings us back, at the end of the history, to the same great problem which the Black Death of the 14th century raised near the beginning of it, namely, the importation of the seeds of pestilence from some remote country, and their dependence for vitality or effectiveness in the new soil upon certain favouring conditions, which sanitary science has now happily in its power to withhold. I have left Influenza to be mentioned last. Its place is indeed unique among epidemic diseases; it is the oldest and most obdurate of all the problems in epidemiology. The only piece of speculation in this volume will be found in the five-and-twenty pages which follow the narrative of the various historical Influenzas; it is purely tentative, exhibiting rather the *disjecta membra* of a theory than a compact and finished hypothesis. If there is any new light thrown upon the subject, or new point of view opened, it is in bringing forward in the same context the strangely neglected history of Epidemic Agues.

Other subjects than those which occupy the nine chapters of this volume might have been brought into a history of epidemics, such as Mumps, Chickenpox and German Measles, Sibbens and Button Scurvy, together with certain ordinary maladies which become epidemical at times, such as Pneumonia, Erysipelas, Quinsy, Jaundice, Boils and some skin-diseases. While none of these are without pathological interest, they do not lend themselves readily to the plan of this book; they could hardly have been included except in an appendix of *miscellanea curiosa*, and I have preferred to leave them out altogether. It has been found necessary, also, to discontinue the history of Yellow Fever in the West Indian and North American colonies, which was begun in the former volume.

I have, unfortunately for my own labour, very few acknowledgements to make of help from the writings of earlier workers in the same field. My chief obligation is to the late Dr Murchison's historical introduction to his 'Continued Fevers of Great Britain.' I ought also to mention Dr Robert Willan's summary of the throat-distempers of the 18th century, in his 'Cutaneous Diseases' of 1808, and the miscellaneous extracts relating to Irish epidemics which are appended in a chronological table to Sir W. R. Wilde's report as Census Commissioner for Ireland. For the more recent history, much use has naturally been made of the medical reports compiled for the public service, especially the statistical.

September, 1894.

CONTENTS.

CHAPTER I.

TYPHUS AND OTHER CONTINUED FEVERS.

CHAPTER II.

FEVER AND DYSENTERY IN IRELAND.

CHAPTER III.

INFLUENZAS AND EPIDEMIC AGUES.

CHAPTER IV.

SMALLPOX.

CHAPTER V.

MEASLES.

CHAPTER VI.

WHOOPING-COUGH.

CHAPTER VII.

SCARLATINA AND DIPHTHERIA.

CHAPTER VIII.

INFANTILE DIARRHOEA, CHOLERA NOSTRAS, AND DYSENTERY.

CHAPTER IX.

ASIATIC CHOLERA.

CHAPTER I.

IT was remarked by Dr James Lind, in 1761, that a judicious synopsis of the writings on fevers, in a chronological sense, would be a valuable book: it would bring to light, he was fain to expect, treasures of knowledge; "and perhaps the influence of a favourite opinion, or of a preconceived fancy, on the writings of some even of our best instructors, such as Sydenham and Morton, would more clearly be perceived[1]." Lind himself was the person to have delivered such a history and criticism. He was near enough to the 17th century writers on fevers to have entered correctly into their points of view; while so far as concerned the detection of theoretical bias or preconceived fancies, he had shown himself a master of the art in his famous satire upon the "scorbutic constitution," a verbal or mythical construction which had been in great vogue for a century and a half, and was still current, at the moment when Lind destroyed it, in the writings of Boerhaave and Haller. A judicious historical view of the English writings on fevers, such as this 18th century critic desired to see, may now be thought superfluous. The theories, the indications for treatment, the medical terms, have passed away and become the mere objects of a learned curiosity. But the actual history of the old fevers, of their kinds, their epidemic prevalence, their incidence upon rich or poor, upon children or adults, their fatality, their contagiousness, their connexion with the seasons and other vicissitudes of the people—all this is something more than curious.

[1] James Lind, M.D., *Two Papers on Fevers and Infection*. Lond. 1763, p. 79.

1

Unfortunately for the historian of diseases, he has to look for the realities amidst the "favourite opinions" or the "preconceived fancies" of contemporary medical writers. Statements which at first sight appear to be observations of matters of fact are found to be merely the necessary truths or verbal constructions of some doctrine. One great doctrine of the 17th and 18th centuries was that of obstructions: in this doctrine, as applied to fevers, obstructions of the mesentery were made of central importance; the obstructions of the mesentery extended to its lymphatic glands; so that we come at length, in a mere theoretical inference, to something not unlike the real morbid anatomy of enteric fever. Another great doctrine of the time, specially applied by Willis to fevers, was that of fermentations and acrimonies. "This ferment," says a Lyons disciple of Willis in 1682, "has its seat in the glandules of the velvet coat of the stomach and intestines described by Monsieur Payer[1]." But the Lyons physician is writing all the while of the fevers that have always been common in the Dombes and Bresse, namely intermittents; the tertian, double tertian, quotidian, quartan, or double quartan paroxysm arises, he says, from the coagulation of the humours by the ferment which has its seat in the glandules described by M. Payer, even as acids cause a coagulation in milk, the paroxysm of ague continuing, "until this sharp chyle be dissipated and driven out by the sweat or insensible perspiration." The lymphatic follicles of the intestine known by the name of Payer, or Peyer, were then the latest anatomical and physiological novelty, and were chosen, on theoretical grounds, as the seat of fermentation or febrile action in agues. On the ground of actual observation they were found about a century and a half after to be the seat of morbid action in typhoid fever.

While there are such pitfalls for the historian in identifying the several species of fevers in former times, there are other difficulties of interpretation which concern the varieties of a continued fever, or its changes of type from generation to generation. Is change of type a reality or a fiction? And, if a reality, did it depend at all upon the use or abuse of a certain regimen or treatment, such as blooding and lowering, or heating and corroborating? A pupil of Cullen, who wrote his thesis in

---

[1] *Observations on Fevers and Febrifuges.* Made English from the French of M. Spon. London, 1682.

1782 upon the interesting topic of the change in fevers since the time of Sydenham[1], inferred that the great physician of the Restoration could not have had to treat the low, putrid or nervous fevers of the middle and latter part of the 18th century, otherwise he would not have resorted so regularly to blood-letting, a practice which was out of vogue in continued fevers at the time when the thesis was written, as well as for a good many years before and after. Fevers, it was argued, had undergone a radical change since the time of Sydenham, in correspondence with many changes in diet, beverages and creature comforts, such as the greatly increased use of tea, coffee and tobacco, and of potatoes or other vegetables in the diet, changes also in the proportion of urban to rural population, in the use of carriages, and in many other things incident to the progressive softening of manners. In due time the low, putrid, nervous type of typhus fever, which is so much in evidence in the second half of the 18th century, ceased to be recorded, an inflammatory type, or a fever of strong reaction, taking its place; so that Bateman, of London, writing in 1818, said : " The putrid pestilential fevers of the preceding age have been succeeded by the milder forms of infectious fever which we now witness"; while Armstrong, Clutterbuck, and others, who had revived the practice of blood-letting in fevers shortly before the epidemic of 1817–18, claimed the comparatively slight fatality and short duration of the common fever of the time as an effect of the treatment. After 1831, typhus again became low, depressed, spotted, not admitting of the lancet ; on which occasion the doctrine of " change of type" was debated in the form that the older generation of practitioners still remember.

Thus the task of the historian, whose first duty is to ascertain, if he can, the actual matters of fact, or the realities, in their sequence or chronological order, is made especially difficult, in the chapter on continued fevers, by the contemporary influence of theoretical pathology or "a preconceived fancy," by the ascription of modifying effects to treatment, whether cooling or heating, lowering or supporting, and, most of all, by the absence of that more exact method which distinguishes the records of fever in our own time. Nor can it be said that the work of historical research has been made easier in all respects, by the

---

[1] James Hutchinson, M.D., *De Mutatione Febrium e tempore Sydenhami, etc.* Edin. 1782. Thesis.

exact discrimination and perfected diagnosis to which we are accustomed in present-day fevers. In the years between 1840 and 1850, the three grand types of fever then existing in Britain, namely, spotted typhus, enteric, and relapsing fever, were at length so clearly distinguished, defined and described that no one remained in doubt or confusion. Thereupon arose the presumption that these had always been the forms of continued fever in Britain, and that the same fevers, presumably in the same relative proportions to each other, might have been left on record by the physicians of former generations, if they had used the modern exactness and minuteness in observing both clinical history and anatomical state, which were seen at their best in Sir William Jenner. It would simplify history, indeed it would make history superfluous, if that were really the case. There are many reasons for believing that it was not the case. As Sydenham looked forward to his successors having experiences that he never had, so we may credit Sydenham with having really seen things which we never see, not even those of us who saw the last epidemics of relapsing fever and typhus. It is due to him, and to his contemporaries and nearest successors, to reciprocate the spirit in which he concludes the general chapter on epidemics prefatory to his annual constitutions from 1661 to 1676:

> "I am far from taking upon myself the credit of exhausting my subject in the present observations. It is highly probable that I may fail even in the full enumeration of the epidemics. Still less do I warrant that the diseases which during the years in question have succeeded each other in the sequence about to be exhibited shall remain the same in all future years. One thing most especially do I aim at. It is my wish to state how things have gone lately ; how they have been in this country, and how they have been in this the city which we live in. The observations of some years form my ground-work. It is thus that I would add my mite, such as it is, towards the foundation of a work that, in my humble judgment, shall be beneficial to the human race. Posterity will complete it, since to them it shall be given to take the full view of the whole cycle of epidemics in their mutual sequences for years yet to come[1]."

The epidemic fever of 1661, according to Willis.

On the very threshold of the period at which the history is resumed in this volume, we find a minute account by Willis of an epidemic in the year 1661, which at once raises the question whether a certain species of infectious fever did really exist at

---

[1] *Observationes Medicae*, 3rd ed. 1676, I. 2. § 23. English by R. G. Latham, M.D.

that time which exists no longer, or whether Willis described as "a fever of the brain and nervous stock" what we now call enteric fever. Willis's fever corresponds in every respect to the worm fever, the comatose fever, the remittent fever of children, the acute fever with dumbness, the convulsive fever, which was often recorded by the medical annalists and other systematic observers as late as the beginning of the 19th century[1]. It ceased at length to be recorded or described, and it has been supposed that it was really the infantile or children's part of enteric fever, which had occurred in former times as now[2]. The epidemic fever which Willis saw in the summer of 1661, after a clear interval of two years from the great epidemics of agues, with influenzas, in 1657–59, is called by him "a certain irregular and unaccustomed fever[3]." It was not, however, new to him altogether; for he had seen the same type, and kept notes of the cases, in a particular household at Oxford in 1655, as well as on other occasions. It was an epidemical fever "chiefly infestous to the brain and nervous stock." It raged mostly among children and youths, and was wont to affect them with a long and, as it were, a chronical sickness. When it attacked the old or middle-aged, which was more rarely, it did sooner and more certainly kill. It ran through whole families, not only in Oxford and the neighbouring parts, "but in the countries at a great distance, as I heard from physicians dwelling in other places." Among those other witnesses, we shall call Sydenham; but meanwhile let us hear Willis, whose account is the fullest and least warped by theory.

Its approach was insidious and scarce perceived, with no immoderate heat or sharp thirst, but producing at length great debility and languishing, loss of appetite and loathing. Within eight days there were brain symptoms— heavy vertigo, tingling of the ears, often great tumult and perturbation of the brain. Instead of phrensy, there might be deep stupidity or insensibility; children lay sometimes a whole month without taking any notice of the bystanders, and with an involuntary flux of their excrements; or there might be frequent delirium, and constantly absurd and incongruous chimaeras in their sleep. But in men a fury, and often-times deadly phrensy, did succeed. If, however, neither stupidity nor great distraction did fall upon them, swimmings in the head, convulsive movements, with convulsions of the

---

[1] Reports of Whitehaven Dispensary (Dixon) and of Nottingham General Hospital (Clarke), cited in the sequel.

[2] Rilliet, *De la Fièvre Typhoïde chez les Enfants,* Thèse, Paris, 2 *Janv.* 1840, based on 61 cases; West, *Diseases of Infancy and Childhood,* 3rd ed. Lond. 1854.

[3] "Febris epidemicae cerebro et nervoso generi potissimum infestae, anno 1661 increbescentis descriptio," in *Pathologia Cerebri,* Cap. VIII, "De Spasmis universalibus qui in febribus malignis" etc., Eng. transl. p. 51.

members and leaping up of the tendons did grievously infest them. In almost all, there were loose and stinking motions, now yellow, now thin and serous ; vomiting was unusual ; the urine deep red. The sufferers in this prolonged sickness wasted to a skeleton, with no great heat or evacuations to account for the wasting. Some, at the end of the disease, had a severe catarrh. In others, with little infection of the head, soon after the beginning of the fever a cruel cough and a stinking spittle, with a consumptive disposition, grew upon them, and seemed to throw them suddenly into a phthisis, from which, however, they recovered often beyond hope. In some there were swellings of the glands near the hinder part of the neck, which ripened and broke, and gave out a thin stinking ictor for a long time. " I have also seen watery pustules excited in other parts of the body, which passed into hollow ulcers, and hardly curable. Sometimes little spots and *petechiales* appeared here and there." But none of the spots were broad and livid, nor were there many malignant spots.

Willis then gives several cases clinically, in his usual manner. The first is of a strong and lively young man, who was sick above two months and seemed near death, but began to mend and took six weeks to recover, sweating every night or every other night of his convalescent period. The second case, aged twelve, was restored to health in a month. Numbers three and four were children of a nobleman, who both died, the convulsive type being strongly marked ; one of the two was examined after death, and found to have several sections of the small intestine telescoped, but all the abdominal viscera free from disease[1], the lungs engorged, the vessels of the brain full, much water in the sub-arachnoid space, and more than half a pint in the lateral ventricles.

In farther illustration of this type of fever, epidemic in 1661, Willis goes back to his notes of a sporadic outbreak of what he thinks was the same disease in a certain family at Oxford in the winter of 1653-4[2]: "yea I remember that sometime past very many laboured with such a fever." In the family in question, five children took the fever one after another during a space of four months, two of the cases proving fatal ; the domestics also took it, and some strangers who came in to help them, "the evil being propagated by contagion." The cases in the children are fully recorded[3], the following being some of the symptoms :

In case 1, aged seven, the illness began at the end of December, 1653 (or 1655): there were contractions of the wrist tendons, red spots like flea-bites on his neck and other parts, drowsiness, and involuntary passage of the excrements. At the end of a fortnight, a flux set in and lasted for four days ; next, after that, a whitish crust or scurf, as it were chalky, began to spread over the whole cavity of his mouth and throat, which being often in a day wiped away, presently broke forth anew. He mended a little, but had paralysis of his throat and pharynx, was reduced to a living skeleton, but at length got well.

Case 2, a brother, aged nine, had frequent loose and highly putrid motions on the eleventh day; and next day, the flux having ceased, the most severe colic, so that he lay crying out day and night, his belly swollen and hard as a drum, until, on the 24th day, he died in an agony of convulsions.

Case 3, a brother, aged 11, was taken with similar symptoms on the 13th February, and died on the 13th day.

---

[1] " Itaque ventrem inferiorem primo aperiens, viscera omnia in eo contenta satis sana et sarte tecta inveni "—the small intestine being telescoped in several places.

[2] Elsewhere he says the first case of the series was " circa solstitium hyemale anno 1655."

[3] *De Febribus*, chapter " De febribus pestilentibus."

Case 4, a sister, was taken ill in March, with less marked symptoms, and recovered slowly, having had no manifest crisis.

Case 5, a boy of the same family, and the youngest, fell ill about the same time as No. 4, and after the like manner, "who yet, a looseness arising naturally of itself, for many days voiding choleric and greenish stuff, was easily cured."

Then comes a general reference to the domestics and visitors, who fell sick of the same and all recovered.

The prolonged series of cases in the household of this "venerable man" appears to have made a great impression upon Willis, as something new in his experience, as well as in the experience of several other physicians who gave their services. That it was malignant he considers proved "ex contagio, pernicie, macularum pulicularum apparentia, multisque aliis indiciis." He adds that he had seen the same disease sporadically at other times ; and again "I remember that formerly several laboured under such a fever." Those cases were all previous to the general prevalence of the fever which he identifies with them in the summer of 1661, under the name of a "fever of the brain and spinal cord."

The signs given by Willis are as nearly as may be the signs of infantile remittent fever, or worm fever, or febris synochus puerorum, or hectica infantilis, or febris lenta infantum, or an acute fever with dumbness, of which perhaps the first systematic account in this country was given by Dr William Butter of Lower Grosvenor Street, in 1782[1]. It is, he says, both a sporadical and an epidemical disease, "and when epidemical it is also contagious." The age for it is from birth up to puberty ; but "similar symptoms are often observed in the disorders of adults." Morton, writing in 1692–94, clearly points to the same fever under the name of worm fever (febris verminosa). He adds it at the very end of his scheme of fevers, as if in an appendix, having been unable to find a place for it in any of his categories owing to its varying forms—hectic, acute, intermittent, continued, συνεχής, inflammatory, but for the most part colliquative or σύνοχος, "and malignant according to the varying degrees of the venomous miasm causing it[2]." Butter also recognizes its varying types : it has many symptoms, but they seldom all occur in the same case ; there are three main varieties—the acute, lasting from eight to ten days up to two or three weeks ;

[1] *Treatise on the Infantile Remittent Fever.* London, 1782.
[2] *Pyretologia*, 2 vols. Lond. 1692—94, i. 68, at the end of "Synopsis Febrium" :—
"Febris verminosa, quae nulli e specibus memoratis praecisé determinari potest."

the slow, lasting two or three months; and the low, lasting a month or six weeks. The slow form, he says, is only sporadic; the low is only epidemic, and is never seen but when the acute is also epidemical; it is rare in comparison with the latter, and not observed at all except in certain of the epidemical seasons. Waiving the question whether the remittent fever of children, thus systematically described, was not a composite group of maladies, of which enteric fever of children was one, we can hardly doubt that Willis found a distinctive uniform type in the epidemic of 1661, in Oxford as he saw it himself, in other parts of England by report. It had symptoms which were not quite clearly those of enteric fever: spots, like fleabites, on the neck and other parts, swelling and suppuration of the glands in the hinder part of the neck, effusion of fluid on the brain and in the lateral ventricles, and the intestine free from disease[1].

Confirming Willis's account for Oxford, is the case of Roger North, when a boy at Bury St Edmunds Free School in 1661, as related by himself in his 'Autobiography[2].' Being then "very young and small," after a year at school he had "an acute fever, which endangered a consumption." Elsewhere he attributes his bad memory with "confusion and disorder of thought," to that "cruel fit of sickness I had when young, wherein, I am told, life was despaired of, and it was thought part of me was dead; and I can recollect that warm cloths were applied, which could be for no other reason, because I had not gripes which commonly calls for that application." That "great violence of nature," while it had impaired his mental faculties, had sapped his bodily vigour somewhat also, of which he gives a singular illustration.

This special prevalence of epidemic fevers in the summer and autumn of 1661 is noticed also by the London diarists.

Evelyn says that the autumn of 1661 was exceedingly sickly and wet[3]. Pepys has several entries of fever[4]. On 2 July, 1661: "Mr Saml. Crewe died of the spotted fever." On 16 August: "At the [Navy] Office all the morning, though little to do;

---

[1] Häser gives a reference to an essay in which Willis's fever of 1661 is compared to enteric fever: C. M. W. Rietschel, *Epidemia anni 1661 a Willisio et febris nervosa lenta ab Huxhamio descriptae, etc. cum typho abdominali nostro tempore obvio comparantur.* Lips. 1861. Not having found this essay, I cannot say on what grounds the comparison is made.

[2] *Lives of the Norths.* New ed. by Jessopp. 3 vols. 1890, iii. 8, 21.

[3] *Diary of John Evelyn, Esq., F.R.S.,* 1641—1706, under the date of 18 Sept.

[4] *Diary of Samuel Pepys, Esq., F.R.S.,* 1659—69.

because all our clerks are gone to the burial of Tom Whitton, one of our Controller's clerks, a very ingenious and a likely young man to live as any in the office. But it is suc h a sickly time both in the city and country everywhere (of a sort of fever) that never was heard of almost, unless it was in a plague-time. Among others the famous Tom Fuller [of the 'Worthies of England'] is dead of it ; and Dr Nichols [Nicholas], Dean of St Paul's ; and my Lord General Monk is very dangerously ill." On 31 August : " The season very sickly everywhere of strange and fatal fevers." On 15 January, 1662 : " Hitherto summer weather, both as to warmth and every other thing, just as if it were the middle of May or June, which do threaten a plague (as all men think) to follow ; for so it was almost the last winter, and the whole year after hath been a very sickly time to this day."

The great medical authority of the time is Sydenham. His accounts of the seasons and reigning diseases of London extend from 1661 to 1686, so that they begin with the year for which Willis described the epidemic fever "chiefly infestous to the brain and nervous stock," popularly called the new disease. But Sydenham did not describe the epidemic in the same objective way that Willis did. He records a series of "epidemic constitutions of the air," the particular constitution of each year being named from the epidemic malady that seemed to him to dominate it most. It was, perhaps, because it had to cohform to Sydenham's "preconceived fancy," as Lind said, that his account of the dominant type of fever in 1661 differs somewhat from that given by Willis.

Sydenham's epidemic Constitutions.

Sydenham adopted the epidemic constitutions from Hippocrates, as he did much else in his method and practice. In the first and third books of the 'Epidemics,' Hippocrates describes three successive seasons and their reigning diseases in the island of Thasos, as well as a fourth plague-constitution which agrees exactly with the facts of the plague of Athens as described by Thucydides. The Greek term translated "constitution" is κατάστασις, which means literally a settling, appointing, ordaining, and in the epidemiological sense means the type of reigning disease as settled by the season. The method of Hippocrates is first to give an account of the weather—the winds, the rains, the temperature and the like,—and then to describe the diseases of the seasons[1]. Sydenham followed his model with remarkable closeness. The great plague of London has almost the same place in his series of years that the plague-constitution, the fourth in order, has in that of Hippocrates. It looks, indeed, as if Sydenham had begun with the year 1661, more for the purpose of having several constitutions preceding that of the plague than because he had any full observations of his own to record previous to 1665. He is also much influenced by the example of Hippocrates in giving prominence to the intermittent type of fevers. It was remarked by one of our best 18th century epidemiologists, Rogers of Cork, and with special reference to Sydenham's "intermittent constitutions," that fevers proper to the climate of Thasos were not likely to be identified in or near London excepted by a forced construction.

Sydenham's Constitutions.

	Constitutions	Total deaths in London	Plague	Fever and Spotted Fever	Small-pox	Measles	Griping in the Guts
1661	"Intermittent" con-	16,665	20	3,490	1,246	188	1,061
1662	stitution: with a con-	13,664	12	2,601	768	20	835
1663	tinued fever through-	12,741	9	2,107	411	42	866
1664	out.	15,453	5	2,258	1,233	311	1,146
1665	Constitution of plague	97,306	68,596	5,257	655	7	1,288
1666	and pestilential fever.	12,738	1,998	741	·38	3	676
1667	Constitution of small-	15,842	35	916	1,196	83	2,108
1668	pox, with a continued	17,278	14	1,247	1,987	200	2,415
1669	"variolous" fever.						
1669	Constitution of dysen-	19,432	3	1,499	951	15	4,385
1670	tery and cholera nostras,	20,198	0	1,729	1,465	295	3,690
1671	with a continued fever.	15,729	5	1,343	696	17	2,537
1672	Measles in 1670.	18,230	5	1,615	1,116	118	2,645
1673	Constitution of "co-	17,504	5	1,804	853	15	2,624
1674	matose" fevers.	21,201	3	2,164	2,507	795	1,777
1675	Influenza in 1675.	17,244	1	2,154	997	1	3,321
1676		18,732	2	2,112	359	83	2,083
1677	Not recorded.	19,067	2	1,749	1,678	87	2,602
1678	Return of the "inter-	20,678	5	2,376	1,798	93	3,150
1679	mittent" constitution,	21,730	2	2,763	1,967	117	2,996
1680	absent since 1661–64.	21,053	0	3,324	689	49	3,271
1681	"Depuratory" fevers,	23,951	0	3,174	2,982	121	2,827
1682	or dregs of the inter-	20,691	0	2,696	1,408	50	2,631
1683	mittents.	20,587	0	2,250	2,096	39	2,438
1684		23,202	0	2,836	1,560	6	2,981
1685	Constitution of a	23,222	0	3,832	2,496	197	2,203
1686	"new" continued fever.	22,609	0	4,185	1,062	25	2,605

[1] An analysis of the four Hippocratic constitutions, with modern illustrative cases, is given by Alfred Haviland, *Climate, Weather, and Disease.* London, 1855.

The foregoing is a Table of Sydenham's epidemic constitutions from 1661 to 1686, compiled from his various writings, with the corresponding statistics from the London Bills of Mortality.

I give this Table both as a convenient outline and in deference to the great name of Sydenham. But we should be much at fault in interpreting the figures of the London Bills, or the history of epidemic diseases in the country at large, if we had no other sources of information than his writings. Only some of the figures in the Table concern us in this chapter; plague has been finished in the previous volume, smallpox, measles and "griping in the guts" are reserved each for a separate chapter, as well as the influenzas and epidemic agues which formed the chief part of the "strange" or "new" fevers. If this work had been the Annals of Epidemics in Britain, it would have been at once proper and easy to follow Sydenham's constitutions exactly, and to group under each year the information collected from all sources about all epidemic maladies. But as the work is a history, it proceeds, as other histories do, in sections, observing the chronological order and the mutual relations of epidemic types as far as possible; and in this section of it we have to cull out and reduce to order the facts relating to fevers, beginning with those of 1661.

Cases of fever, says Sydenham, began to be epidemic about the beginning of July 1661, being mostly tertians of a bad type, and became so frequent day by day that in August they were raging everywhere, and in many places made a great slaughter of people, whole families being seized. This was not an ordinary tertian intermittent; indeed no one but Sydenham calls it an intermittent at all, and he qualifies the intermittence as follows :

"Autumnal intermittents do not at once assume the genuine type, but in all respects so imitate continued fevers that unless you examine the two respectively with the closest scrutiny, they cannot be distinguished. But, when by degrees the impetus of the 'constitution' is repelled and its strength reined in, the fevers change into a regular type ; and as autumn goes out, they openly confess themselves, by casting their slough (*larva abjecta*) to be the intermittents that they really were from the first, whether quartans or tertians. If we do not attend to this diligently" etc. And again, in a paragraph which does not occur in the earlier editions, he writes as follows in the context of the "Intermittent Fevers of the years 1661–1664 :"

"It is also to be noted that in the beginning of intermittent fevers, especially those that are epidemic in autumn, it is not altogether easy to distinguish the type correctly within the first few days of their accession, since they arise at first with continued fever superadded. Nor is it always easy, unless you are intent upon it, to detect anything else than a slight remission of the disease, which, however, declines by degrees into a perfect intermission, with its type (third-day or fourth-day) corresponding fitly to the season of the year."

The intermittent character of these fevers seems to have struck Sydenham himself in a later work as forced and unreal. Writing in 1680, when the same kind of fevers were prevalent, after the epidemic agues of 1678 and 1679, he calls them "depuratory," and says that "doubtless those depuratory fevers which reigned in 1661–64 were as if the dregs of the intermittents which raged sometime before during a series of years," i.e. the agues of 1657–59[1].

Theory or names apart, Sydenham's account of the fatal epidemic fever of the summer and autumn of 1661, comes to nearly the same as Willis's. Without saying expressly, as Willis does, that the victims were mostly children or young people, he speaks in one place of those of more mature years lying much longer in the fever, even to three months, and he specially mentions the same sequelae of the fever in children that Willis mentions, and that Roger North remembered in his own case—namely that they sometimes became hectic, with bellies distended and hard, and often acquired a cough and other consumptive symptoms, "which clearly put one in mind of rickets." He refers also to pain and swelling of the tonsils and to difficulty of swallowing, which, if followed by hoarseness, hollow eyes, and the *facies Hippocratica*, portended speedy death. Among the numerous other *accidentia* of the fever, was a certain kind of mania. Among the symptoms were phrensy, and coma-vigil ; diarrhœa occurred in some owing, as he thought, to the omission of an emetic at the outset ; hiccup and bleeding at the nose were occasional.

But, although Sydenham must have had the same phenomena of fever before him that Willis had, the epidemic being general, according to the statements of both, one would hardly guess from his way of presenting the facts, that the fever was what Willis took it to be—a slow nervous fever, with convulsive and ataxic symptoms, specially affecting children and the young. Both Willis and Sydenham recognised something new in it ; the common people called it, once more, the "new disease," and Pepys calls it a "sort of fever," and "strange and fatal fevers."

---

[1] *Epist. I. Respons.* § 57.   Greenhill's ed. p. 298.

As Sydenham maintains that the same epidemic constitution continued until 1664 (although the fever-deaths in London are much fewer in 1662–3–4 than in the year 1661, which was the first of it), we may take in the same connexion Pepys's account of the Queen's attack of fever in 1663. The young princess Katharine of Portugal, married to Charles II. in 1662, had the beginning of a fever at Whitehall about the middle of October, 1663; Pepys enters on the 19th that her pulse beat twenty to eleven of the king's, that her head was shaved, and pigeons put to her feet, that extreme unction was given her (the priests so long about it that the doctors were angry). On the 20th he hears that the queen's sickness is a spotted fever, that she was as full of the spots as a leopard : " which is very strange that it should be no more known, but perhaps it is not so." On the 22nd the queen is worse, 23rd she slept, 24th she is in a good way to recovery, Sir Francis Prujean's cordial having given her rest; on the 26th " the delirium in her head continues still ; she talks idle, not by fits, but always, which in some lasts a week after so high a fever, in some more, and in some for ever." On the 27th she still raves and talks, especially about her imagined children ; on the 30th she continues " light-headed, but in hopes to recover." On 7th December, she is pretty well, and goes out of her chamber to her little chapel in the house ; on the 31st " the queen after a long and sore sickness is become well again."

Typhus fever perennial in London.

Sydenham says that a continued fever, the symptoms of which so far as he gives them suggest typhus, was mixed with the masked intermittent, (or the convulsive fever of children, as in Willis's account), in every one of the years 1661–4 ; and that statement raises a question which may be dealt with here once for all. Fever in the London bills is a steady item from year to year, seldom falling below a thousand deaths and in the year 1741, during a general epidemic of typhus, rising to 7500. The fevers were a composite group, as we have seen, and shall see more clearly. But the bulk of them perennially appears to have been typhus fever. Where the name of " spotted fever " is given there can be little doubt. Every year the bills have a small number of deaths from " spotted fever," and the number of them always rises in the weekly bills in proportion to the increase of "fever" in general, sometimes reaching twenty in the week when the other fevers reach a hundred.   It would be a mistake to suppose that only the fevers called spotted were typhus, the other and larger part being something else.   The more reasonable supposition is that the name of spotted was given by the searchers in cases where the spots, or vibices or petechiae of typhus were especially notable.   If a score, or a dozen or half-a-dozen deaths in a week are set down to spotted fever, it probably means that a large part of the remaining hundred, or seventy, or fifty cases of "fever" not called spotted were really of the same kind, namely typhus.   In the plague itself, the "tokens," which were of the same haemorrhagic nature as the larger or more defined spots of typhus, were exceedingly variable[1].   One of the synonyms of typhus (the common name in Germany) is spotted typhus; but the spots were of at least two kinds, a dusky mottling of the skin and more definite spots, sometimes large, sometimes like fleabites.

Assuming that the cases specially called "spotted" in the London Bills were only a part of all that might have been called by the same name in the wider acceptation of the term (as in Germany), it is a significant fact that there are few of the weekly bills for a long series of years in the 17th and 18th centuries without some of the former.   Such a case as that of Mr Samuel Crewe, brother of Lord Crewe, who died of the "spotted fever" on 2 July, 1661, probably means that there were more cases of the same kind in the poorer parts of the town, from which no account of the reigning sicknesses ever came unless it were the number of deaths in the bills.   The conditions of endemic typhus were there long before we have authentic accounts, towards the end of the 18th century, of that disease being ever present in the homes of the lower classes.   In the time of Sydenham, and even in the time of Huxham two generations after, there was no thought of the unwholesome domestic life graphically described by Willan and others, as a cause of typhus—the overcrowding, the want of ventilation, the foul bedding and the excremental effluvia.

If there had been any reason to suppose that the London of the Restoration, or of the time of Queen Anne, or of the first

---

[1] Tillison to Sancroft, 14 Sept. 1665.   Cited in former volume, p. 677: "One week full of spots and tokens, and perhaps the succeeding bill none at all."

Georges had enjoyed better public health in its crowded liberties and out-parishes than we know it to have done from the time when the authentic accounts of Lettsom and other dispensary physicians begin, then one might err in assuming the perennial existence of typhus fever and in assigning to that cause the bulk of the deaths under the heading of "fevers" in the Parish Clerks' bills. But the public health was undoubtedly worse in the earlier period. A writer as late as the year 1819, who is calling for that reform of the dwellings of the working classes in London which was soon after carried out, namely the construction of regular streets instead of mazes of courts and alleys, speaks of the "silent mortality" that went on in the latter[1]. It was still more silent in earlier times, when the west end of London knew nothing of what was passing in the east end[2].

In all matters of public health, after the somewhat romantic interest in plague had ceased, the poorer parts of London were for long an unexplored territory. Dr John Hunter, who had been an army physician and was afterwards in practice in Mayfair, began about the year 1780 to visit the homes of the poor in St Giles's or other parishes near him, and was surprised to find in them a fever not unlike the hospital typhus of his military experience. I quote at this stage only a sentence or two[3].

"It may be observed, that though the fever in the confined habitations of the poor does not rise to the same degree of violence as in jails and hospitals, yet the destruction of the human species occasioned by it must be much greater, from its being so widely spread among a class of people whose number bears a large proportion to that of the whole inhabitants. There are but few of the sick, so far as I have been able to learn, that find their way into the great hospitals in London." I shall defer the subject of the dwellings of the working class in London until a later stage.

The "constitution" in Sydenham's series which succeeded the febrile one of 1661–64 was "pestilential fever." It began in the end of 1664, lasted into the spring of 1665, and passed by an easy transition into the plague proper. The bills for those months have very large weekly totals of deaths from "fever," as well as a good many deaths from "spotted fever," before they begin to have more than an occasional death from plague. It is

[1] H. Clutterbuck, M.D., *Obs. on the Epidemic Fevers prevailing in the Metropolis.* Lond. 1819, pp. 58—60.
[2] Horace Walpole's *Letters* give two instances: he himself had never set foot in Southwark; a small tradesman in the City had never heard of Sir Robert Walpole.
[3] *Transactions of the College of Physicians*, iii. 366.

this particular form of typhus fever that Bateman had in mind when he wrote, in 1818, "We never see the pestilential fever of Sydenham and Huxham"; although Willan, who preceded him at the Carey Street dispensary, described in 1799 a fever of so fatal a type that it gave rise to the rumour that the plague was back in London. The term "pestilential" was technically applied to a kind of fever a degree worse than the "malignant."

Willis, the earliest of the Restoration authorities on fevers, had three names in an ascending scale of severity—putrid, malignant and pestilential. The putrid fevers were what we might call idiopathic, engendered within the body in some way personal to the individual from "putrefaction" or fermentation of the humours; all the intermittents were included in that class, and the theory of their cure by bark was that the drug corrected putridity. In the malignant and pestilential, an altogether new element came in—the τὸ θεῖον of Hippocrates, the mysterious something which we call infection; and of these two infectious fevers, the malignant was milder than the pestilential[1].

Morton drew out the scale of fevers in an elaborate classification, of which only the last section of continued contagious fevers concerns us at present[2]:

Synochus	Simple Malignant Fever	Fever mostly with sweats and other signs of malignity, but without buboes, carbuncles, petechiae or miliary rash.
	Pestilential Fever	Fever with petechiae, purple spots, miliaria, morbillous rash on the chest.
	Plague	With buboes, carbuncles and black spots.

The order in this Table was also the order in time: the fever of 1661, which Willis calls malignant, remained as the constitu-

---

[1] Willis, Op. ed. 1682, Amstelod. p. 110. "De febribus pestilentibus": "Etenim vulgo notum est febres interdum populariter regnare, quae pro symptomatum vehementia, summa aegrorum strage, et magna vi contagii, pestilentiae vix cedant; quae tamen, quia putridarum typos innotantur, nec adeo certo affectos interemunt aut alios inficiunt haud *pestis* sed diminutiori appellatione *febris pestilens* nomen merentur. Praeter has dantur alterius generis febres, quarum et pernicies et contagium se remissius habent, quia tamen supra putridarum vires infestae sunt, et in se aliquatenus τὸ θεῖον Hippocratis continere videntur, tenuiori adhuc vocabulo *febres malignae* appellantur."

The war-typhus of 1643, which was sometimes bubonic, and was succeeded by plague in 1644, is given as an example of *febris pestilens*; the epidemic of 1661 as an example of *maligna*.

[2] *Pyretologia*, i. 68.

tion of the years following until the end of 1664; then began the pestilential, which passed definitely in the spring of 1665 into the plague proper. Willis, Sydenham and Morton, differing as they did on many points of theory and treatment, all alike taught the scale of malignity in fevers and plague, and all used the language of "constitutions." The Great Plague of 1665 was, in their view, the climax of a succession of febrile constitutions of the air, being attended by much pestilential fever and followed by a fever which Morton places in the milder class of συνεχής.

The epidemic Constitutions following the Great Plague.

During the ten or twelve years following the Great Plague of London, the epidemic maladies which Sydenham dwelt most upon as the reigning types will appear on close scrutiny to have been on the whole proper to the earlier years of life. This cannot be shown in the simple way of figures; for the ages at death from the several maladies, although they were in the books of the Parish Clerks, were not published.

There was some continued fever every year, which we may take to have been chiefly the endemic typhus of a great city, and there were also deaths among adults due to those reigning epidemics which fell most on the young. In 1667 and 1668 the leading epidemic was smallpox, with a continued fever towards the end of the period which Sydenham called "variolous," for no other reason, apparently, than that it was part of a variolous constitution. In the autumn of 1669, and in the three years following, the epidemic mortality was peculiarly infantile, in the form of diarrhoea or "griping in the guts," with some dysentery of adults, and some measles in 1670. From 1673 to 1676, the constitution was a comatose fever, which chiefly affected children, with a sharp epidemic of measles in the first half of 1674, attended by a very high mortality from all causes, and a severe smallpox in the second half of 1674, attended by a much lower mortality from all causes. There was also an influenza for a few weeks in 1675. In 1678 the "intermittent" constitution returned, having been absent for thirteen years, and continued through 1779-80, until its "strength was broken." In 1681 smallpox was unusually mortal, the deaths being more than in any previous year. Most of these constitutions fall to be dealt with fully in other chapters: but as we are here specially concerned with the succession to the plague, it is to be noted how largely the epidemic mortality in London fell upon the age of childhood for a number of years after the Great Plague of 1665. It was observed both by English and foreign writers that the next epidemic following the Black Death of 1348–49, namely, that of 1361 in England and of 1359–60 in some other parts of Europe, fell mostly upon children and upon the upper classes of adults. There is doubtless some particular application of the population principle in the earlier instance as in the later, but not the same application in both. The conditions at the beginning of the three hundred years' reign of plague in Britain were different from those at the end of it. The increased prevalence of smallpox in the generation before the last great outburst of plague, and the infantile or puerile character of the epidemic fever of 1661, as described by Willis, show that the incidence of infectious mortality had already begun to shift towards the age of childhood. It looks as if the conditions of population, intricate and obscure as they must be confessed to be, were somehow determining what the reigning infectious maladies, with their special age-incidence, should be. Such a gradual change is the more probable for the reason that infectious mortality came in due time to be mostly an affair of childhood. The plague, which was the great infection of the later medieval and earlier modern period, was peculiarly fatal to adult lives; on the other hand, the mortality from infectious diseases in our own time falls in much the larger ratio upon infants and children. It looks as if this change, now so obvious, had begun before the end of plague in Britain, having become more marked in the generation following its extinction. The direct successor of plague, so far as concerns age-incidence and nosological affinity, was the pestilential or malignant typhus, which came into great prominence in 1685–86, in circumstances that seemed to contemporaries to forebode a return of the plague. But before we come to that, there remains a little to be said of some other fevers, especially of the comatose fever of 1673–76, which was largely an affair of childhood.

Pepys says that he went on 3 May, 1668, to Old Street (St Luke's) to see Admiral Sir Thomas Teddiman, "who is very ill in bed of a fever," and, in a later entry, that he "did die by a thrush in his mouth" on the 12th of May. Next year, 1669,

Pepys and his wife went on tour through several parts of Europe, and had hardly returned to their house in Seething Lane when the lady fell ill of a fever; on 2nd November, it was "so severe as to render her recovery desperate," and on 10th November she died in her 29th year,—a surprising sequel, as her husband felt, to a "voyage so full of health and content." These two years, for which we have a sample of the London fevers, were marked in the Netherlands by epidemics of fevers which are among the most extraordinary in the whole history. At Leyden in 1669 the fever reached such a height as to cut off 7000—a mortality which would not have been surprising if the disease had been plague; but it was not plague, it wanted the buboes, carbuncles &c., was longer in its course, and, strangest of all, affected the upper classes far more severely than the poor, so much so "that of seventy men administering the public affairs, scarcely two were left[1]," while, according to Fanois, who was the Leyden poor's doctor, the lower classes, "protected as it were by having survived the simpler forms of fever," suffered from this malignant epidemic far less than the rich[2]. The mortality is said to have risen as high as three-fourths of the attacks. At Haarlem the burials in a week rose to three or four hundred (which was a fair week's average for London itself in an ordinary season), the epidemic lasting four months and leaving hardly one family untouched. Among the symptoms were extreme praecordial anxiety, weight at the pit of the stomach, constant nausea and loathing, vomiting, in part bilious but chiefly "pituitous," thirst and restless tossing. It was attended by an affection of the throat and mouth—an angina with aphthae or thrush of the palate. The pools and other sources of water for domestic use were unusually stagnant that summer in Holland, and were commonly blamed for the epidemic; but Fanois points out that at Haarlem and Emden, where similar fevers raged, "salubriores non desunt aquae[3]."

---

[1] C. L. Morley, *De morbo epidemico, in* 1678—9, *narratio.* Lond. 1680.

[2] Guido Fanois, *De morbo epidemico hactenus inaudito, praeterita aestate anni* 1669 *Lugduni Batavorum vicinisque locis grassante.* Lugd. Bat. 1671.

[3] Brownrigg cites the Leyden epidemic of 1669, which he calls an intermitting fever, as an instance of the effects of changes in the ground water; it was "powerfully aggravated by the mixture of salt water with the stagnant water of the canals and ditches. This fever happened in the month of August, 1669, and continued to the end of January, 1670." "Observations on the Means of Preventing Epidemic Fevers." Printed in the *Literary Life of W. Brownrigg, M.D., F.R.S.* By Joshua Dixon, Whitehaven, 1801.

After such an instance as the Leyden fever of 1669, nothing is incredible in the records of fever subsequent to the extinction of plague. Turning to Sydenham's account of the continued fever which occurred in London during the same season, the latter half of 1669, as well as in the three years following, we find that it was characterized rarely by diarrhoea or sweats, commonly by pain in the head, by a moist white tongue which afterwards became covered by a dense skin, and by a greater tendency than Sydenham had ever seen to aphthae (the "thrush in the mouth" of Admiral Teddiman in 1668) when death threatened—the same being a "deposition from the blood of foul and acrid matter upon the mouth and throat." But London in 1668 and 1669 suffered little from fevers in comparison to Leyden, Haarlem and other Dutch towns, its high mortality in the summer and autumn of 1669 being from infantile diarrhoea, cholera nostras and dysentery.

Sydenham's continued fever from 1673 to 1676 (he was absent from his practice in 1677 owing to ill health) was a malady which affected adults as well as children, but, it would appear, the latter especially. The only characteristic case given is of a boy of nine who did not begin to mend until the thirtieth day. Many recovered in a fortnight, while others were not clear of the fever in a month. On account of the remarkable stupor which almost always attended it, Sydenham called the fever of this constitution a comatose fever. It began with sharp pains in the head and back, pains in the limbs, heats and chills, etc. His account of the comatose state is exactly like that given by Willis for the fever of children in 1661—profound stupor, sometimes for a week long, so profound in some as to pass into absolute aphonia (the "acute fever with dumbness" of later writers), while others would talk a few words in their sleep, or would seem to be angry or perturbed by something (the chimaeras mentioned by Willis) and would then become tranquil again; when roused to take physic or to drink they would open the eyes for a moment and then fall back into stupor. When they began to mend, they would crave for absurd things to eat or drink. During convalescence the head, through weakness, could not be kept straight but would incline first to one side and then to the other[1].

---

[1] *Obs. Med.* 3rd ed., v. 2.

The years 1678–1680 witnessed remarkable epidemics of ague, such as had occurred on several occasions before, the last in the years 1657–59. They engross so much of Sydenham's writing, especially in connexion with the Peruvian-bark controversy, that we hear little of any other fever until the great epidemic of continued fever, or typhus, in 1685–6. But he does mention briefly that the interval between the decline of the agues in 1680 and the beginning of the "new fever" of 1685, was occupied by "continued depuratory" fevers—depuratory of the dregs of the preceding intermittent constitution, and comparable in that respect to the fevers of 1661–64 which followed the agues of 1657–59[1].

Sydenham's term "depuratory" does not help us much; but we learn something from Morton as to what fevers were prevalent, besides the epidemical intermittents, in the years preceding the epidemic of 1685–86. Morton classes them as continued συνεχής (*Synocha*), by which he means something less malignant than *Synochus*. A fever which began in the milder form would often degenerate into the more malignant, the cause assigned, in the usual recriminatory manner of the time between rival schools, being mistaken treatment. But sometimes the fever was malignant from the outset, with purple spots, petechiae, morbillous efflorescence, watery vesicles on the neck and breast, buboes, and anthraceous boils. All these fevers, says Morton, whether they were spurious forms of synocha, or malignant from the outset, were sporadic, "neque contagione, ut in pestilentiali constitutione, sese propagabant[2]." This points to their having been part of that strange aguish epidemic of which an account is given in another chapter. In Short's abstracts of parish registers, the year 1680 seems to have been the most unhealthy of the series in country parishes, and that is borne out by one Lamport, or Lampard, an empiric who practised in Hampshire: "I will tell you somewhat concerning a malignant fever. In the year '80 or '81 there were great numbers of people died of such fevers, many whereby were taken with vomitings, etc., yet I had the good fortune to cure eighteen in the parish of Aldingbourn, not one dying, in that great compass, of that disease[3]." The moral is that the empiric recovered his

---

[1] *Epist. I. Respons.* §§ 56, 57.
[2] *Pyretologie*, i. 429.
[3] John Lamport *alias* Lampard, *A direct Method of ordering and curing People of that loathsome disease the Smallpox.* Lond. 1685, p. 28.

cases, whereas the regular faculty lost theirs; which means
that the fevers were of various degrees, some aguish, some
typhus, as in the exactly similar circumstances a century after,
1780–85.

In the London Bills from 1681 to 1684, the deaths from fever
were many, with some from "spotted fever" nearly every week,
while the annual mortalities from all causes were high.   It is
the more remarkable, therefore, that Sydenham should have
discovered, in the beginning of 1685, the outbreak of a new
fever, different from any that had prevailed for seven years
before.   The explanation seems to be that a malignant typhus
fever, such as might have been discovered in any year in the
crowded parishes where the working classes lived, broke out at
the Court end of the town, where Sydenham's practice lay.

The epidemic fever of 1685–86.

A letter of 12 March, 1685, says: "Sir R. Mason died this
morning in his lodging at Whitehall.   A fever rages that proves
very mortal, and gives great apprehensions of a plague[1]."
Sydenham also was reminded of the circumstances preceding
the Great Plague of London in 1665.   In his first account of
the epidemic of fever in 1685[2], which began with a thaw in
February, he points out that the thaw in March, 1665, had been
followed by pestilential fever and thereafter by the plague
proper.   In a later reference, when the epidemic of fever was
in its second year (1686) he says: "How long it may last I
shall not guess; nor do I quite know whether it may not be a
certain more spirituous, subtle beginning, and as if *primordium*,
of the former depuratory fever [1661–64] which was followed
by the most terrible plague.   There are some phenomena which
so far incline me to that belief[3]."   However, no plague followed
the malignant, if not pestilential, fever of 1685–86.   The reign
of plague, as the event showed, was over; the fever which had
been on former occasions its portent and satellite, came into the
place of reigning disease.   It is true that Sydenham does not
identify the fever of 1685–86 by name as pestilential fever; on

[1] *Hist. MSS. Com.* v. 186.   Duke of Sutherland's historical papers.
[2] *Schedula Monitoria I.*   "De novae febris ingressu."   §§ 2, 3.
[3] *Ibid.* § 46.

the contrary, he entitles his essay "De Novae Febris Ingressu." But the novelty of type was partly in contrast to the fevers immediately preceding, which admitted treatment by bark, and its principal difference from the pestilential fever of former occasions seems to have been that it was not followed by plague[1]. Its antecedents and circumstances were very much those of plague itself. Its mortality was greatest in the old plague-seasons of summer and autumn, it had slight relation to famine or scarcity, or to other obvious cause of domestic typhus. Sydenham can find no explanation of the new constitution but "some secret and recondite change in the bowels of the earth pervading the whole atmosphere, or some influence of the celestial bodies." He enlarges, however, on the character of the seasons preceding, which would have affected the surface, if not the bowels, of the earth, and the levels of the ground-water.

The winter of 1683–84 was one of intense frost; an ice-carnival was held on the Thames during the whole of January. The long dry frost of winter was followed by an excessively hot and dry summer, the drought being such as Evelyn did not remember, and as "no man in England had known." For eight or nine months there had not been above one or two considerable showers, which came in storms. The winter of 1684–85 set in early, and became "a long and cruel frost," more interrupted, however, than that of the year before. The spring was again dry, and it was not until the end of May 1685 that "we had plentiful rain after two years' excessive drought and severe winters[2]."

The two years of excessive drought, with severe winters, had their effect upon the public health, as will appear from Short's abstracts of parish registers in town and country[3]; the years 1683–85 being conspicuous for the excess of burials over baptisms:

---

[1] In the Belvoir Letters (*Hist. MSS. Com. Calendar*) Charles Bertie writes from London to the Countess of Rutland, 26 January, 1685, that "many are sick of pestilential fevers." Evelyn says that the winter of 1685-6 was extraordinarily wet and mild, but does not mention sickness until June, 1686, when the weather was hot and the camp at Hounslow Heath was broken up owing to sickness.

[2] Evelyn's *Diary*, which gives other particulars, including a description of the ice-carnival on the Thames.

[3] Thomas Short, M.D. of Sheffield, *New Observations on City, Town and Country Bills of Mortality*. London, 1750.

Country Parishes.

Year	Registers examined	Registers with excess of death	Deaths in them	Births in them
1683	140	37	923	685
1684	140	31	900	629
1685	140	19	574	478
1686	140	16	419	301
1687	143	19	522	427
1688	143	11	327	267

Towns.

Year	Registers examined	Registers with excess of death	Deaths in them	Births in them
1683	25	8	1398	1169
1684	25	8	1243	865
1685	25	4	1191	741
1686	25	2	555	418
1687	25	1	313	269
1688	25	2	191	146

There is no clue to the forms of sickness that caused the excessive mortality in country parishes and provincial towns. But in London it appears from the Bills that the one great cause of the unusual excess of deaths in 1684 was an enormous mortality from infantile diarrhoea, from the end of July to the middle of September, during the weather which Evelyn describes as excessively hot and dry with occasional storms of rain.

It was in the second year of the long drought, February, 1685, that Sydenham dated the beginning of his new febrile constitutions. The mortality of 1685 was just twenty deaths more than in 1684 (23,222); but fever (with spotted fever) and smallpox had each a thousand more out of the total than in the year before. Sydenham says that the fever did not spare children, which might be alleged of typhus at all times; but a fever of the kind, even if it ran through the children of a household, seldom cut off the very young, the mortality being in greatest part of adults and adolescents. Excepting smallpox for the year 1685, infantile and children's maladies were not prominent during the constitution of the "new fever;" the usual items of high infantile mortality, such as convulsions and "griping in the guts" or infantile diarrhoea, were moderate and even low. Hence, although the weekly fever-deaths in the following Table may not appear sufficient for the professional and other interest that they excited, it is to be kept in mind that they had been mostly of adult lives. It is probable also that a good many of them had been among the well-to-do, and perhaps at first in the

West End; for there is nothing in the height of the weekly bills for all London to bear out the remark of the letter of 12 March, already quoted, "A fever rages that proves very mortal and gives apprehensions of a plague."

Weekly Mortalities in London.

1685.

Week ending	Dead	Of fever	Of spotted fever	Of small-pox	Of griping in the guts
March 3	376	49	0	11	35
10	458	73	2	30	31
17	367	53	1	25	17
24	441	63	3	33	27
31	366	53	5	24	36
April 7	421	47	10	28	30
14	433	64	8	32	27
21	473	66	6	47	45
28	470	68	3	49	45
May 5	385	50	6	35	39
12	447	75	3	59	41
19	437	79	4	58	43
26	452	61	2	74	39
June 2	469	65	8	65	36
9	521	88	14	62	41
16	499	91	9	66	34
23	478	76	12	71	53
30	526	82	13	84	45
July 7	497	81	8	87	53
14	478	82	11	78	51
21	464	79	11	87	47
28	488	62	6	68	54
Aug. 4	493	82	5	86	51
11	529	109	13	89	47
18	580	74	13	99	71
25	536	91	7	67	85
Sept. 1	556	94	13	53	104
8	539	82	10	81	77
15	485	90	7	63	70
22	459	90	10	37	51
29	502	114	3	58	53
Oct. 6	444	108	11	40	54
13	445	89	13	61	38
20	369	86	5	40	28
27	379	73	7	29	45
Nov. 3	443	96	8	55	43
10	410	84	7	26	35
17	432	103	8	35	39
24	471	107	6	56	31
Dec. 1	384	87	4	36	24
8	452	98	8	49	24
15	403	69	3	29	47
22	438	99	2	34	27
29	432	80	9	28	28

Weekly Mortalities in London.

1686.

Week ending	Dead	Of fever	Of spotted fever	Of small-pox	Of griping in the guts
Jan. 5	394	80	5	28	29
12	400	80	3	27	48
19	396	67	5	36	32
26	366	76	2	21	30
Feb. 2	452	87	8	16	30
9	416	78	5	37	30
16	405	94	9	20	25
23	419	74	7	16	40
March 2	417	84	1	20	37
9	455	95	6	18	30
16	415	71	10	31	21
23	453	78	11	22	46
30	372	58	8	17	35
April 6	392	80	11	13	27
13	393	72	7	21	29
20	420	61	10	26	37
27	471	99	9	27	22
May 4	429	78	21	28	46
11	374	71	6	16	22
18	395	69	5	17	3 (sic)
25	395	66	11	24	36
June 1	383	63	4	15	49
8	404	66	6	26	38
15	523	88	9	43	64
22	503	99	9	25	73
29	473	90	10	31	62
July 6	430	71	6	18	62
13	401	76	2	19	56
20	464	87	14	24	74
27	508	99	3	23	76
Aug. 3	506	86	9	14	90
10	493	74	7	14	104
17	522	99	7	26	101
24	536	115	5	18	104
31	520	90	8	22	93
Sept. 7	531	94	4	21	104
14	498	84	6	18	110
21	540	100	3	17	101
28	443	90	5	13	67
Oct. 5	425	81	4	13	60
12	432	96	2	9	56
19	391	73	1	9	33
26	402	79	3	11	43
Nov. 2	373	64	1	23	39
9	456	85	1	19	31
16	401	73	2	9	23
23	359	61	4	10	54
30	397	68	1	7	34
Dec. 7	359	76	0	9	21
14	438	60	0	8	46
21	354	49	1	8	39
28	356	53	2	9	32

Sydenham says that he regarded the new fever at first as nothing more than the "bastard peripneumony" which he had described for previous seasons; but he had soon cause to see that it wanted the violent cough, the racking pain in the head during coughing, the giddiness caused by the slightest movement, and the excessive dyspnoea of the latter (Huxham likewise distinguished typhus from "bastard peripneumony"). The early symptoms of the "new fever" were alternating chills and flushings, pain in the head and limbs, a cough, which might go off soon, with pain in the neck and throat. The fever was a continued one, with exacerbation towards evening; it was apt to change into a phrensy, with tranquil or muttering delirium; petechiae and livid blotches were brought out in some cases (Sydenham thought they were caused by cordials and a heating regimen), and there were occasional eruptions of miliary vesicles. The tongue might be moist and white at the edges for a time, latterly brown and dry. Clammy sweats were apt to break out, especially from the head. If the brain became the organ most touched, the fever-heat declined, the pulse became irregular, and jerking of the limbs came on before death.

Later writers, for example those who described the great epidemic fever of 1741, have identified the fever of 1685–86 with the contagious malignant fever afterwards called typhus, and Murchison, in his brief retrospect of typhus in Britain, has included it under that name. Sydenham mentions petechiae and livid blotches in some cases, and the Bills give a good many of the deaths in the worst weeks of the epidemic under the head of "spotted fever." It is not at first easy to understand why Sydenham should have written an essay specially upon itt in September, 1686, to claim it as a new fever[1] and not rather as the old pestilential fever—" populares meos admonens de subingressu novae cujusdam Constitutionis, a qua pendet Febris nova species, a nuper grassantibus multum abludens." It should be kept in mind that his motive was correct treatment,

---

[1] Freind (*Nine Commentaries upon Fever, &c.*, engl. by Dale, Lond. 1730, p. 4) has the following general criticism upon Sydenham's varying constitutions of fevers: " I believe also I may truly affirm that those very fevers which Sydenham explains as distinct species, according to the various temperature of the seasons, do not differ much from one another. For, if perhaps you should except the *Petechiae*, they differ rather in degree than in kind. There hardly ever appeared a fever in any season where the signs so constantly answered one another, that those which you found collected in one person should unite after the same manner in another; however upon this account you would not deny their labouring under the same distemper."

and that the fashionable treatment of the day by Peruvian bark was, in his judgment, unsuited to this fever, however much it may have suited the epidemical intermittents of 1678–79 and the "depuratory" dregs of them for several years after. Physicians, he says, had learned to drive off by bark the fevers of the former constitution, from 1677 to the beginning of 1685, even when the fever intermitted little and sometimes when it intermitted not at all; and they saw an indication for bark in the nocturnal exacerbations of the new fever. Sydenham found that even large doses of bark did not free the patient from fever, and that restoration to health under treatment with the bark was due "magis fortunato alicui morbi eventu quam corticis viribus." He seeks to establish the indications for another treatment by setting forth the symptoms minutely; and as the question of bark in fevers was the great medical question of the time, this may well have been Sydenham's motive for discovering in the epidemic of 1685–6 a "new fever" although he does not say so in as many words. We have a good instance of how the bark-craze was at this time influencing the very highest circles of practice in the case of Lord Keeper Guildford, in July, 1685, as related in another chapter.

It will be seen from the table of weekly deaths that the second of the two hard winters was over before the fever began to attract notice. Sydenham compares its beginning after the thaw in February, 1685, to the beginning of the plague when the frost broke in March, 1665.

If it had been merely the typhus of a hard winter, of overcrowding indoors, of work and wages stopped by the frost, and of want of fuel (which things Evelyn mentions as matters of fact), it would have come sooner than the spring of 1685. The Bills for years before have regularly a good many deaths from fever, and always some from spotted fever; but these may have come from parishes wholly beyond the range of Sydenham's practice. The fever began definitely for him in February, 1685, and was at its worst in the old plague-seasons of summer and autumn. If the seasons had any relation at all to it, the epidemic was a late effect of the long drought, an effect which was manifested most when the rain came, in the summer of 1685 and throughout the mild winter and normal summer of 1685–86. It must have been for that reason that Sydenham traced the source of it to "some secret and recondite change in the bowels of the earth," rather than to a change in the sensible qualities of the air. One must ever bear in mind that the physicians of the Restoration gave no thought to insanitary conditions of living; in that respect the later Stuart period seems to have been behind the Elizabethan or even the medieval; we cannot err in assuming, behind all Sydenham's speculative causes, a great deal of unwholesomeness indoors. Sydenham's fullest reference to the subterranean sources of poisonous miasmata occurs in his tractate on Gout:

"Whether it be that the bowels of the earth, if one may so speak, undergo various changes, so that by the accession of vapours exhaled therefrom the air is disturbed, or that the whole atmosphere is infected by a change which some peculiar conjunction of certain of the heavenly bodies induces in it;—the matter so falls out that at this or that time the air is furnished with particles that are adverse to the economy of the human body, just as at another time it is impregnated with particles of a like kind that agree ill with the bodies of some species of brute animals. At these times, as often as by inspiration we draw into the naked blood miasmata of this kind, noxious and inimical to nature, and we fall into those epidemical diseases which they are apt to produce, Nature raises a fever,— her accustomed means of vindicating the blood from some hostile matter. And such diseases are commonly called *epidemical;* and they are short and sharp because they have thus a quick and violent movement[1]."

It was Sydenham's intimate friend Robert Boyle who worked out the hypothesis of subterraneous miasmata as a cause of epidemic (and endemic) diseases. An account of his theory will be found in the chapter on Influenzas and Epidemic Agues. It may be said here that it needs only a few changes, especially the substitution of organic for inorganic matters in the soil, to bring it into line with the modern doctrine of miasmatic infective disease as expounded by the Munich school.

It has not been usual to think of spotted fever, (or of influenzas), in that connexion; but a telluric source of the epidemic constitution of 1685–86 was clearly Sydenham's view; and as the fever came in circumstances like those of the last great plague, and was thought at the time to be the forerunner of another great plague, its connexion with recondite decompositions in the soil, dependent on the phenomenal drought of two whole years before, cannot be set aside as a possibility, the less so that the fever, although of the type of typhus, was not a fever of cold, hunger, and domestic distress, but mainly of the warm, or mild, or soft weather following the long drought, and of many well-to-do-people, as in the great Netherlands fever of 1669.

[1] *Tractatus de Podagra*, § 35. Greenhill's edition, p. 428.

My view of it is that it was the modified successor of plague, the *pestis mitior*, which used to precede and accompany the plague, now become the dominant constitution.   The authentic figures of its mortality come from London ; but Sydenham says that its " effects were felt far more in other places " ; although Short's abstracts of parish registers, given above, do not indicate excessive mortality throughout England.

Retrospect of the great Fever of 1623–25.

The most instructive instance of *pestis mitior* in Britain is not the pestilential fever which led up to the last plague (1665–6), but the great epidemic of fever all over England and Scotland which reigned for two or three years before the great outburst of plague in 1625.   I go back to this because it was not wholly or even mainly a famine fever (although it was as general as one of the medieval famine-fevers), and because in that respect it furnishes a close parallel to the fever of 1685–86, which I regard as the successor of the plague.   After this interlude in the history, we shall proceed to consider the question of the final extinction of plague.

In Scotland the fever of 1622–23 was directly connected with famine, but in England it was not obviously so according to the records that remain. The dearth in Scotland began as early as the autumn of 1621 : " Great skarsitie of cornes throw all the kingdome," the harvest having been spoiled by wet weather and unheard-of river floods ; however, abundance of foreign victual came in, and the scarcity was got over[1].   In England the same harvest of oats was abundant, and probably yielded the "foreign victual" which relieved the Scots ; but the price of wheat rose greatly[2].   It was the year following, 1622, that really brought famine and famine-sickness to Scotland, as the second of two bad harvests had always done.   On 21 July, 1622, a fast was proclaimed at Aberdeen for "the present plague of dearth and famine, and the continuance thereof threatened by tempests, inundations and weets likely to rot the fruit on the ground[3]."

In an entry of the Chronicle of Perth, subsequent to July, 1622, it is said : " In this yeir about the harvest and efter, thair wes suche ane universall seiknes in all the countrie as the ellyke hes not bene hard of.   But speciallie in this burgh, that no familie in all the citie was frie of this visitation.   Thair was also great mortalitie amonge the poore."   From which it appears that the autumnal fever of 1622 was among all classes in Scotland.   The famine in Scotland became more acute in the spring and summer of 1623 ; the country swarmed with beggars, and in July, says Calderwood, the famine increased daily until "many, both in burgh and land, died of hunger."   At Perth ten or twelve died every day from Mid-

[1] *Chronicle of Perth* (Maitland Club) under date 14 Oct. 1621.
[2] Thorold Rogers, *Hist. of Agric. and Prices*, sub anno.
[3] *Extracts from Kirk Session Records*.   Spalding Club, 1846.

summer to Michaelmas ; the disease was not the plague, but a fever[1]. At Dumfries 492 died during the first ten months of 1623, perhaps a ninth part of the inhabitants. about one hundred of the deaths being specially marked as of "poor[2]." The "malignant spotted fever" which caused numerous deaths in 1623 in Wigton, Penrith and Kendal is clearly part of the famine-fever of Scotland extending to the Borders and crossing them. This is a famine-fever of the old medieval type, like that of 1196 which, according to William of Newburgh "crept about everywhere," always the same acute fever, putting an end to the miseries of the starving, but attacking also those who had food.

The same spotted fever was all over England in 1623, but it did not, as in Scotland, come in the wake of famine. It is true that the English harvest of 1622 was a good deal spoiled ; a letter of 25 September says[3]: "Though the latter part of this summer proved so far seasonable, yet the harvest is scant, and corn at a great price by reason of the mildews and blasting generally over the whole realm," rye being quoted a few weeks later at 7/- the bushel and wheat at 10/-, although the average of wheat for the year, in Rogers's tables, is not more than 51/1*d.* per quarter. while the average of next year falls to 37/8*d.* These were not famine-prices in England, and there is no evidence of general sickness directly after the harvest of 1622, when corn was dearest. Also, although the autumn of 1623 was a time of "continual wet" in England[4], the price of wheat remained moderate, and even low as compared with the rather stiff price of the winter of 1622-23. But it was not until the summer and autumn of 1623 that the spotted fever became epidemic in England. Short's abstracts of the registers of market towns show how sickly that year was :

Year.	No. of registers examined.	No. with excess of burials.	Buried in the same.	Baptised in the same.
1622	25	4	442	345
1623	25	16	2254	439 (sic)
1624	25	9	978	714
1625	25	9	666	563

In September, 1623, the corporation of Stamford made a collection "in this dangerous time of visitation," and sent £10 of it to Grantham, the rest to go "to London or some other town, as occasion offered." A London letter of 6 December, 1623, from Chamberlain to Carleton says[5]:—

"Here is a contagious spotted or purple fever that reigns much, which, together with the smallpox, hath taken away many of good sort, as well as meaner people." He then gives the names of notables dead of it, and adds : "Yet many escape, as the dean of St Paul's [Dr Donne, who used the occasion to compile a manual of devotion] is like to do, though he were in great danger." One of the Coke family writes early in January, 1624, from London[6]: "Having two sons at Cambridge, we sent for them to keep Christmas with us, and not many days after their coming my eldest son Joseph fell suddenly into the sickness of the time which they call the spotted fever, and which after two days' extremity took away his life." From another letter it appears that one of his symptoms was "not being able to sleep," the unmistakable vigil of typhus. Although there is no word of the epidemic continuing in Scotland in 1624, it was undoubtedly as prevalent in England in that year as the year before, and prevalent in country houses as

[1] *Chronicle of Perth.*
[2] *History of the Burgh of Dumfries.* By W. MacDowall. 2nd ed. Edin. 1873, p. 381.
[3] *Court and Times of James I.*, ii. 331.
[4] *Ibid.*, under date 25 Oct. 1423.
[5] *Ibid.* ii. 439.   [6] *Cal. Coke MSS.* (Hist. MSS. Com.) i. 158.

well as in towns and cities. Thus, on 7 August, 1624, Chamberlain writes :
"The [king's] progress is now so far off that we hear little thence, but only
that there be many sick of the spotted ague, which took away the Duke of
Lennox in a few days. He died at Kirby," a country house in Northamptonshire[1]. On 21 August he writes again : "This spotted fever is cousin-
german to it [the plague] at least, and makes as quick riddance almost.
·The Lady Hatton hath two or three of her children sick of it at her brother
Fanshaw's in Essex, and hath lost her younger daughter, that was buried at
Westminster on Wednesday night by her father ; a pretty gentlewoman,
much lamented." A letter of 4 September says there was excessive mortality
in London, in great part among children (doubtless from the usual infantile
trouble of a hot autumn, diarrhoea), while "most of the rest are carried
away by this spotted fever, which reigns almost everywhere, in the country
as ill as here." Sir Theodore Mayerne, the king's physician, confirms this,
under date 20 August, 1624 : the purple fever, he says, was "not so much
contagious as common through a universal disposing cause," seizing upon
many in the same house, and destroying numbers, being most full of
malignity[2]. It was clearly an inexplicable visitation. The summer was hot
and dry, from which character of the season, says Chamberlain, "some
have found out a far-fetched speculation, which yet runs current, and would
ascribe it [the spotted fever] to the extraordinary quantity of cucumbers this
year, which the gardeners, to hasten and bring forward, used to water out of
the next ditches, which this dry time growing low, noisome and stinking,
poisoned the fruit. But," adds Chamberlain, "that reason will reach no
farther than this [London] town, whereas the mortality is spread far and
near, and takes hold of whole households in many places." He then gives
the names of several eminent persons dead of it, and speaks of others who
were "still in the balance[3]." On 9 October, "the town continues sickly
still," and Parliament had been put off, "in consideration of the danger,"
from 2 November, 1624, to 15 February, 1625. On Ash Wednesday, 1625,
the Marquis of Hamilton died of the pestilent fever at Moor Park,
Rickmansworth. Thus far there had been no plague ; and if the spotted
fever were cousin-german to the plague, as Chamberlain said, it was remarkable in this that it prevailed in the mansions of the rich in town and
country and took off more victims among the upper classes than the
plague itself even in its most terrific outbursts. However, a plague of the
first rank followed in London and elsewhere in the summer and autumn
of 1625.

The cucumber-theory, above mentioned, shows how puzzled people must
have been to account for the spotted fever, or "spotted ague" as it was also
called, in 1624. Sir Theodore Mayerne did not think contagion from person
to person could explain it, but referred it to "some universal disposing
cause." It is conceivable that the famine-fever of 1622 and 1623 in Scotland
and the Marches may have spread by contagion into England in the latter
year ; but in 1624 there is nothing said of fever in Scotland or of scarcity as
a primary cause in England.

Besides the famine-fever of Scotland in 1622–23, there was another
associated thing which should not be left out of account. Before the famine
and fever had begun in that country, the notorious Hungarian fever was
raging in the Palatinate, and continued to rage for four years. "Hungarian
fever" had become the dreaded name for war-typhus of a peculiar malignity
and diffusive power. It had been so often engendered since the 16th
century in campaigns upon Hungarian soil as to have become known
everywhere under the name of that country. Its infection spread, also,
everywhere through Europe ; thus it is said to have even reached England

---

[1] *C. and T. James I.*, ii. 469.
[2] Mayerne, *Opera Medica*, Lond. 1700.   [3] *Ibid.* ii. 473.

in 1566, and again in 1589, although it is not easy to find English evidence of it for either year. It was this type of fever which broke out in the Upper Palatinate, occupied by troops of the Catholic powers, in 1620, and continued through the years 1621, 1622 and 1623; as the title of one of the essays upon this outbreak somewhat fantastically declares, it spread "ex castris ad rastra, ex rastris ad rostra, ab his ad aras et focos[1]." Was the epidemic constitution of "spotted ague" in England in 1623 and 1624 derived from the centre of famine-fever in Scotland, or from the centre of camp-fever in the Palatinate? In the last years of James I. communications were frequent with the latter country, and there was of course much intercourse with Scotland.

The spotted fever or spotted ague of 1623–24, the plague of 1625, and the country agues of the same autumn make really a more instructive series of epidemic constitutions than any that fell under Sydenham's observation, so instructive, indeed, that it has seemed worth while to revert to it for the sake of illustrating the doctrine of epidemics then in vogue. That doctrine made little of contagion from person to person; yet the idea of contagion was familiar, and had been so since medieval times. If we might assume contagion to explain such cases as those that occurred in the houses of squires and nobles, we might find a source of it either in the famine-fever of Scotland or in the war-fever of the Palatinate. But the teaching of the time was that it was in the air; and if the infective principle had been generated either in Scotland or on the upper Rhine it had diffused itself in some inscrutable way. The doctrine of epidemic constitutions seems strange to us; but some of the facts that it was meant to embrace are also strange to us. Were it not for an occasional reminder from influenza, we should hardly believe that any fevers could have travelled as the Hungarian fevers, the spotted fevers or "spotted agues" of former times are said to have done.

On the other hand, we have now a scientific doctrine of the effects of great fluctuations of the ground-water upon the production of telluric miasmata, which may be used to rationalize the theory of emanations adopted by Sydenham and Boyle. From this modern point of view the remarkable droughts preceding the pestilential fevers and plagues of 1624–25 and 1665, and preceding the fever of 1685–86, which is the one that immediately concerns us, may be not without significance.

The London fever of 1685–86 having been suspected at the time to be the forerunner of a plague, as other such fevers in

[1] Janus Chunradus Rhumelius, *Historia morbi, qui etc.* Norimb. 1625.

the earlier part of the century had been, and no plague having ensued, the question arises most naturally at this stage, why the plague should have never come back in London or elsewhere in Britain after the great outbreak of 1665–66.

The extinction of Plague in Britain.

Plague had been the grand infective disease of Britain from the year of the Black Death, 1348–9, for more than three centuries, down to 1666. The last of plague in Scotland was in 1647–8, in the west and north-west of England about 1650 (in Wales probably in 1636–8), in Ireland in 1650, and in all other parts of the kingdom including London in 1666, the absolute last of its provincial prevalence having been at Peterborough in the first months of 1667[1], while two or three occasional deaths continued to occur annually in London down to 1679. False reports of plague, contradicted by public advertisement, were circulated for Bath in 1675[2], and for Newcastle in 1710[3]; while in London as late as 1799, during a bad time of typhus fever, the occurrence of plague was alleged[4].

It is not easy to say why the plague should have died out. It had been continuous in England from 1348, at first in general epidemics, all over the country in certain years, thereafter mostly in the towns, either in great explosions at long intervals or at a moderate level for years together. The final outburst in 1665, which was one of the most severe in its whole history, had followed an unusually long period of freedom from plague in London, and was followed, as it were, by a still longer period of freedom until at last it could be said that the plague was extinct. In some large towns it had been extinct, as the event showed, at a much earlier date; thus at York the last known epidemic was in 1604, and it can hardly be doubted that many

[1] W. D. Cooper, *Archæologia*, XXXVII. (1857) p. 1. I had overlooked this important paper on English plagues in my former volume. The chief additional facts that it contains are the very severe plague at Cambridge in the summer of 1666, the deaths of 417 by plague at Peterborough in 1666, and of 8 more in the first quarter of 1667, and the slightness of the Nottingham outbreak, which was in August, 1666 (p. 22).

[2] *London Gazette*, 17–21 June, 1675, repeated in the number for 28 June–1 July.

[3] Brand, *Hist. of Newcastle*, II. 509. Report contradicted on 18 Dec.

[4] "The habitations of the poor within or adjoining to the City," says Willan, "have suffered greatly; and some, I am informed, have been almost depopulated, the infection having extended to every inmate. The rumour of a plague was totally devoid of foundation."

other towns in England, Scotland and Ireland would have closed their records of plague earlier than they did had not the sieges and military occupations of the Civil Wars given especial occasion for the seeds of the infection to spring into life. Plague seemed to be dying out all over England and Scotland (in Ireland it is little heard of except in connexion with the Elizabethan and Cromwellian conquests) for some time before its final grand explosion in London in 1665.

In seeking for the causes of its decline and extinction we must keep prominently in view the fact that the virus was brought into the country from abroad as the Black Death of 1348–9. But for that importation it is conceivable that there would have been no signal history of plague in Britain. Its original prevalence was on a great scale, and there were several other widespread epidemics throughout the rest of the 14th century. In the first volume of this history I have collected evidence that plague was endemic or steady for long periods of the 15th and 16th centuries in London, with greater outbursts at intervals, and that in the 17th century it came chiefly in great explosions. Something must have served to keep the virus in the country, and more especially in the towns, until at length it was exhausted. An exotic infection, or one that had not arisen from indigenous conditions, and would probably never have so arisen, does not remain indefinitely in the country to which it is imported. Thus Asiatic cholera, imported into Europe on six, or perhaps five, occasions in the 19th century, has never become domesticated; and yellow fever had a career in the southern provinces of Spain during some twenty years only. Plague did become domesticated for about three centuries in England, and for longer in some other countries of Europe; but it died out at length, and it would almost certainly have died out sooner had it not found in all European countries some conditions not altogether unsuited to it. What were the favouring conditions?

If, as I believe, the virus of plague had its habitat in the soil, from which it rose in emanations, and if it depended therein, both remotely for its origin in some distant country, as well as immediately for its continuance in all countries, upon the decomposition of human bodies, then it is easy to understand that the immense mortalities caused by each epidemic would preserve the seeds of the disease, or the crude matters of the disease, in the soil. Buried plague-bodies would be the most obvious

3—2

sources of future plagues.   But if the theory given of the Black
Death be correct, bodies dead of famine or famine-fever would
also favour in an especial way the continuance of the plague-
virus in certain spots of ground, although they would probably
never have originated it in this country.   Moreover, the products
of ordinary cadaveric decomposition would be so much pabulum
or nutriment for the continuance of the virus.   But all those
things being constant, the continuance of plague would largely
depend upon the manner in which the dead, after plague, or
after famine and fever, or in general, were disposed of.   The
soil of all England in 1348-9 was filled with multitudes of the
dead laid in trenches, and there were several general revivals of
plague in the fifty or sixty years following.   In London there
were plague-pits opened in the suburbs in many great epidemics
during three centuries.   Even when there was no epidemic the
dead were laid in the ground in such a manner that their resolution
was speedy, and the diffusion of the products unchecked.   But
it is undoubted that greater care in the disposal of the dead did
at length come into vogue.   Thus, in the Black Book of the
Corporation of Tewkesbury there is an entry under the year
1603, that all those dead of plague, "to avoid the perill, were
buried in coffins of bourde," the disease having carried off no
fewer than 560 the year before (1602) and being then in its
second season[1].   The reason given is "to avoid the peril," and
it is beyond question that burial in a coffin did in fact delay
decomposition (unless in peculiar circumstances which need not
be particularized), and kept the cadaveric products from passing
quickly and freely into the pores of the ground.   Again, if the
burial were in such coffins as the Chinese commonly use, the
decomposition would proceed almost as slowly as if the body
had been embalmed, and with as little risk of befouling the soil.
For a long time in England such burials were the privilege only
of the rich ; but as wealth increased by commerce they became
the privilege of all classes; and in the last great plague of London,
as I said in my former volume, " even at the worst time coffins
would seem to have been got for most."   Defoe's account of the
burials in heaps in plague-pits is so exactly like that of Dekker
for the plague of 1603, and of other contemporaries for the
plague of 1625, that one may reasonably suspect him to
have used these earlier accounts as his authority for the practice

[1] Rudder, *A New History of Gloucestershire*, 1779, p. 737.

in 1665, which he had no direct knowledge of. However, I do not contend that there were no such burials in 1665; just as one learns from Dekker that the coffin-makers in 1603 were busily employed and grew rich, although he also describes how a husband "saw his wife and his deadly enemy whom he hated" launched into the pit "within a pair of sheets." In ordinary times, as we learn from the tables of burial-dues, there were poorer interments without coffins as late as 1628, according to a document printed by Spelman, the name of the parish being withheld, and even as late as 1672 in the parish of St Giles's, Cripplegate. Spelman's object in writing in 1641 was to protest against the mercenary practices of the clergy in the matter of burial, recalling the numerous canons of the medieval Church directed against all such forms of simony; and incidentally he mentions that it was testified before the Commissioners that a certain parson "had made forty pound of one grave in ten yeeres, by ten pounds at a time"[1]—a "tenancy of the soil" short enough to satisfy even the so-called Church of England Burial Reform Association. The use of coffins in the burial of the very poorest is now so universal that we hardly realize how gradually it was introduced. I am unable to say when burial in a sheet or cerecloth ceased; but it became less and less the rule for the poorer classes throughout the 17th century. In 1666 was passed the Act for burial in woollen, which was re-enacted more strictly in 1678[2]. The motive of it was to encourage the native woollen manufactures, or to prevent the money of the country from being expended on foreign-made linen; and its clauses ordained that woollen should be substituted for linen in the lining of the coffin and in the shrouding of the corpse, but that no penalty should be exacted for burying in linen any that shall die of the plague. Whether it prohibited in effect the use of linen cerecloths to enshroud corpses where no coffin was used does not appear clearly from the terms of the Act; but, as the intention was to discourage the use of linen, and to bring in the use of woollen, for all purposes of burial, it is probable that it served to put an end to coffinless burials altogether, wherever it was

---

[1] Spelman, *De Sepultura.* English ed. 1641, p. 28. He cites the burial fees paid to the parson as twice as much for coffined as for uncoffined corpses. This agrees on the whole with the evidence adduced in the former volume of this history, p. 335.

[2] 18 and 19 Car. II. cap. 4; 30 Car. II. (1), cap. 3. These Acts were repealed by 54 Geo. III., cap. 108.

enforced, inasmuch as the prescribed material was wholly un-suited for the purpose of a cerecloth.

The history of the London plague-pit between Soho and the present Regent Street shows that, after the last great plague of 1665–66, more caution was used against infection from the buried plague-bodies. Macaulay says it was popularly believed that the earth was deeply tainted with infection, and could not be disturbed without imminent risk to human life ; and he asserts that no foundations were laid in the pest-field till two generations had passed and till the spot had long been sur-rounded with buildings, the space being left blank in maps of London as late as the end of George I.'s reign[1].

After 1666 the old churchyards were not less crowded than before, but more crowded, perhaps because coffined corpses occupied more space and decayed more slowly. On 17 October, 1672, Evelyn paid a visit to Norwich : " I observed that most of the churchyards (tho' some of them large enough) were filled up with earth, or rather the congestion of dead bodys one upon another, for want of earth, even to the very top of the walls, and some above the walls, so as the churches seemed to be built in pitts." The same day he had visited Sir Thomas Browne, the author of the famous essay on urn burial or cremation, (suggested to him by the digging up of forty or fifty funeral urns in a field at Old Walsingham). The essay is full of curious learning and equally curious moralizing. But Sir Thomas, though a physician, has not a word to say on so proximate a topic as the state of the Norwich churchyards, which came under his eyes and perhaps under his nose every day of his life[2].

The practice of burying in coffins, which came at length within the means of all classes, may seem too paltry a cause to assign, even in part, for so remarkable an effect as the absolute disappearance of plague after a duration of more than three

[1] *History of England*, I. 359.
[2] He has one or two relevant remarks : " But while we suppose common worms in graves, 'tis not easy to find any there; few in churchyards above a foot deep, fewer or none in churches, though in fresh-decayed bodies. Teeth, bones, and hair give the most lasting defiance to corruption. In an hydropsical body, ten years buried in the churchyard, we met with a fat concretion [adipocere] where the nitre of the earth and the salt and lixivious liquor of the body had coagulated large lumps of fat into the consistence of the hardest Castille soap, whereof part remaineth with us. The body of the Marquis of Dorset seemed sound and handsomely cerecloth ed, that after seventy-eight years was found uncorrupted. Common tombs preserve not beyond powder : a firmer consistence and compage of parts might be expected from arefaction, deep burial, or charcoal."

centuries. My view of the matter is that the virus would have died out of itself had it not been continually augmented, or fed by its appropriate pabulum, and that the gradual change in the mode of interment helped to check such augmentation or feeding.

But the more elaborate interment of the dead was itself an index of the greater spending power of the community, and it may be said that it was the better condition of the people, and not this one particular thing in it, which put an end to the periodical recurrences of plague. In all but its earliest outbursts in the fourteenth, and perhaps the fifteenth century, plague had been peculiarly an infection of the poor, being known as "the poor's plague." Perhaps the chief reason why the richer classes usually escaped it was that they fled from the plague-tainted place, leaving the poorer classes unable to stir from their homes, exposed to the infectious air, and all the more exposed that their habitual employments and wages would cease, their sustenance become precarious, their condition lowered, and their manners reckless. Again, it was not unusual for the plague to break out in a season of famine or scarcity, during which the ordinary risks of the labouring class would be aggravated. Famines ceased (except in Ireland, where there had been comparatively little plague), and scarcities became less common. The sieges and occupations of the Civil Wars in the middle of the 17th century, which undoubtedly were the occasion of the last outbursts of plague in many of the towns, were a brief experience, followed by unbroken tranquillity. Whatever things were tending to the removal of plague in all its old seats had free course thereafter.

On the other hand, one may make too much of the increase of well-being among the labouring class which coincided with the cessation of plague. As a check upon population plague worked in a very remarkable way. In London, as well as in towns like Newcastle and Chester, plague towards the end of its reign arose perhaps once in a generation and made a clean sweep of a fifth or a fourth part of the inhabitants, including hardly any of the well-to-do. It destroyed, of course, many bread-winners and many that were not absolutely sunk in poverty; but its broad effect was to cut off the margin of poverty as if by a periodical process of pruning. The Lord Mayor of London wrote to the Privy Council at the end of the great plague of 1625: "The great mortality, although it had taken many poor people away, yet had made more poverty by decay of tradesmen "—a decay of trade which they might reasonably expect to recover from before long. No such ruthless shears was ever applied at intervals to the growing fringe of poverty in after times. The poor were a more permanent residue, pressing more upon each other; but they did not press more upon the rich, except through the poor rate; on the contrary, the separation of classes became more marked.

Perhaps I ought to give an illustration of this, so as not to leave so radical a change in the vague and disputable form of a generality. I shall take the instance of Chester; its circuit of walls, remaining from the Roman conquest, is something fixed for the imagination to rest upon amidst changes within and without them.

Passing over its medieval and its not infrequent Tudor experiences of epidemic sickness, let us come to the beginning of the 17th century. In two or three successive seasons from 1602 to 1605 it lost 1,313 persons by plague, as well as about 250 from other causes. The population was then mostly within the walls, and probably did not exceed 5000. There was a shipping quarter on the west side, with egress by the Water-gate to the landing-places on the Dee; a millers' quarter, with corn-market and hostelries, on the south, connecting by the South gate and bridge with a hamlet across the river along the road to Wales; a Liberty or Freedom of the city outside the walls on the east, along the road to Warrington and Manchester, with a Bar, a short distance out, as in London, to mark the limit of the mayor's jurisdiction; and on the north side, within the walls, the cattle-market and shambles, with the market for country produce, and a few straggling houses without the gate on the road leading to Liverpool. Chester was a characteristic county town, with its cathedral clergy, its garrison, its resident nobility and gentry, its professional classes, its tradesmen, market people and populace, with the addition of a shipping trade to Ireland and afterwards to foreign and colonial ports. Plague continuing from 1602 to 1605 cut off a fourth or a fifth of its population, and these the poorest. The gaps in the population would gradually have filled up, and the fringe of poverty grown again[1].

The plague came again in 1647, and cut off 2053 in the short space of twenty-three weeks from 22 June to 30 November. The bills of it are extant[2], and show on what parishes the plague fell most. All the parishes were originally within the walls but one, St John's, the ancient collegiate church of Mercia, built upon a rocky knoll in the south-east angle made by the walls with the river. The other nine parish churches and their graveyards were within the walls; but the parishes of three of them extended beyond the gates, just as the three parishes dedicated to St Botolph at the gates of London did. These three were St Oswald's, which included the Liberty on the east side, Trinity, which included the shipping quarter on the

---

[1] One may allege poverty on general grounds, as well as on particular. Thus, in 1636, the mayor was unpopular: "He was a stout man and had not the love of the commons. He was cruel, and not pitying the poor, he caused many dunghills to be carried away; but the cost was on the poor—it being so hard times might well have been spared." Ormerod, I. 203.

[2] Printed plague-bill, with MS. additions, Harl. MS. 1929.

west as well as the houses along the Liverpool road on the north, and
St Mary's, which included the millers' suburb across the Dee on the south.
Hollar's map, made a few years after the plague of 1647, shows very few
houses beyond the walls, except in the ancient Liberty on the east. But it
will appear from the following table that the parishes which had extended
beyond the walls must either have been very crowded close up to the walls
(as the Gate parishes were always apt to be), or there must have actually
been a greater population outside the gates than the contemporary map
shows :

*Burials from Plague in the several Parishes of Chester in 23 weeks,
June 22—Nov. 30, 1647.*

5 parishes wholly within the walls.

	Total.	First week.	Worst (7th) week.
St Peter	75	0	14
St Bridget	85	7	9
St Martin	173	9	23
St Michael	133	26	9
St Olave	59	3	5

3 parishes extending beyond the walls.

St Oswald	396	11	37
St Mary	314	5	20
Trinity	232	1	32

1 parish wholly without the walls.

St John	358	2	26
Pesthouse	228	0	34
	2053	64	209

This was the last plague of Chester, but for a small outbreak in 1654.
The next vital statistics that we get for the city are more than a century
after, in 1774[1]. The population of 14,713 was then divided into two almost
distinct parts, separated by the wall. The old city was being rebuilt, all
but some ancient blocks of buildings held in the dead hand of the cathedral
chapter ; it was becoming a model 18th century place of residence for a
wealthy and refined class, who were remarkably healthy and not very
prolific, the parishes wholly within the walls having 3502 inhabitants. The
poorer class had gone to live mostly outside the walls in new and mean
suburbs, the three parishes at the Gates and extending now far beyond the
walls, together with the original extramural parish of St John's, having a
population of 11,211. There was no town in Britain where the separation of
the rich from the poor was more complete ; there was hardly another town
of the size where the health of the rich was better ; and although the health
of the populace was not so bad as in the manufacturing towns of Lancashire
and Cumberland, close at hand, yet it is hardly possible to find so great a
contrast as that between the clean and wholesome residential quarter
within the walls and the mean fever-stricken suburbs as described by Haygarth in 1774 :

"The inhabitants of the suburbs," he says, "are generally of the lowest
rank ; they want most of the conveniences and comforts of life ; their houses
are small, close, crowded and dirty ; their diet affords very bad nourishment,
and their cloaths are seldom changed or washed...These miserable wretches,
even when they go abroad, carry a poisonous atmosphere round their
bodies that is distinguished by a noisome and offensive smell, which is
peculiarly disgustful even to the healthy and vigorous, exciting sickness and
a sense of general debility. It cannot therefore be wondered that diseases
should be produced where such poison is inspired with every breath."

[1] Haygarth, *Phil. Trans.*, LXVIII. 139.

The case of Chester shows by broader contrasts than anywhere else the change from the public health of plague-times to that of more modern times. But it can hardly be said to show the populace better off than before; it shows them changed into a proletariat, and separated from the richer classes by walls several feet thick. Such, at least, was the result after four generations of immunity from plague, a result which indicates, as I have said, that we may easily make too much of the improved well-being of the poorer classes as a cause of the cessation of plague.

An easy explanation of plague ceasing in London has long been current, and just because it is an easy explanation it will probably hold the field for many years to come. It is that the fire of 1666 burnt out the seeds of plague. Defoe, writing in 1723, ascribed this opinion to certain "quacking philosophers," but he would hardly have said so if he could have foreseen the respectable authority for it in after times. The plague had ceased in most of its provincial centres after the Civil Wars, and in some of them, such as York, from as early a date as 1604. It ceased in all the principal cities of Western Europe within a few years of its cessation in London. In London itself it ceased after 1666, not only in the City which was the part burned down in September of that year, but in St Giles's, where the Great Plague began, in Cripplegate, Whitechapel and Stepney, where it was always worst, in Southwark, Bermondsey and Newington, in Lambeth and Westminster. Nor can it be said that the City was the source from which the infection used to spread to the Liberties and out-parishes. All the later plagues of London, perhaps even that of 1563, began in the Liberties or out-parishes and at length invaded the City. The part of London that was rebuilt after 1666 contained many finer dwelling-houses than before, built of stone, with substantial carpentry, and elegantly finished in fine and rare woods. The fronts of the new houses did not overhang so as to obstruct the ventilation of the streets and lanes; but the streets, lanes, alleys and courts were somewhat closely reproduced on the old foundations. A side walk in some streets was secured for foot-passengers by means of massive posts, which, with the projecting signs of houses and shops, were at length removed in 1766. The improvements in the City after the fire were mostly in the houses of the richer citizens. The City was the place of residence of the rich, with perhaps as many poorer purlieus in close proximity as the residential districts of London now have. But four-fifths of London at the time of the fire were beyond the walls of the City. It is in these extramural regions that the interest mostly lies for epidemical diseases. They remain, says Defoe in 1723, "still in the same condition they were in before." Unfortunately we know little of their condition, whether in the 17th centnry or in the 18th. But there must have been something in it most unfavourable to health; for we find from the Bills of Mortality that the cessation of plague made hardly any difference to the annual average of deaths, the increase of population being allowed for. This fact makes the disappearance of plague all the more remarkable.

Fevers to the end of the 17th century.

The epidemical seasons of 1685–86 were the last that Sydenham recorded; he was shortly after laid aside from active work by gout, and died in 1689. Morton, who made notes of fevers and smallpox until 1694, is more a clinical observer than a student of "epidemic constitutions"; and although his writings are of value to the epidemiologist, he does not help us to understand the circumstances in which epidemic diseases prevailed more at one time than another. To the end of the century there is no other medical source of information, and little besides generalities to be collected from any source. It is known that the years from 1693 to 1699 were years of scarcity all over the kingdom, that the fever-deaths in London reached the high figure of 5036 in 1694, and that there was a high mortality in many country parishes and market towns during the scarcity. But there are few particular illustrations of the type of epidemic sickness. There is, therefore, little left to do but to give the figures, and to add some remarks.

Fever Deaths in the London Bills, 1687—1700.

Year	Fever deaths	Spotted fever deaths	Deaths from all causes	Year	Fever deaths	Spotted fever deaths	Deaths from all causes
1687	2847	144	21460	1694	5036	423	24109
1688	3196	139	22921	1695	3019	105	19047
1689	3313	129	23502	1696	2775	102	18638
1690	3350	203	21461	1697	3111	137	20292
1691	3490	193	22691	1698	3343	274	20183
1692	3205	161	20874	1699	3505	306	20795
1693	3211	199	20959	1700	3675	189	19443

Tables from Short's Abstracts of Parish Registers.

Year	Registers examined	Registers with excess of death	Deaths in them	Births in them
		Country Parishes.		
1689	144	27	828	692
1690	146	17	532	324
1691	147	16	336	180
1692	147	10	207	146
1693	146	27	650	426
1694	148	18	465	348
1695	149	23	649	492
1696	150	19	503	344
1697	150	21	559	409
1698	152	12	397	289
1699	151	20	433	318
1700	160	29	890	739
		Market Towns.		
1689	25	12	1965	1415
1693	25	5	417	338
1694	25	6	1307	681
1695	25	3	309	246
1696	26	4	1020	708
1697	26	2	109	80
1698	26	4	575	423
1699	26	7	1181	867
1700	27	4	726	587

In the London figures the year 1694 stands out conspicuous by its deaths from all causes, and by its high total of fevers. The fever-deaths began to rise from their steady weekly level a little before Christmas, 1693, and remained high all through the year 1694, with a good many deaths from "spotted fever" in the worst weeks. Among the victims in London in February was Sir William Phipps, Governor of New England: his illness appeared at first to be a cold, which obliged him to keep his chamber; but it proved "a sort of malignant fever, whereof many about this time died in the city[1]." Pepys, writing to Evelyn on 10 August, 1694, calls it "the fever of the season," three being down with it at his house, but well advanced in their recovery. In that week and in the week following, the deaths in London from all causes touched the highest points of the year, the deaths from fever and spotted fever being a full quarter of them. Fever at its worst in London never made more than a quarter of the annual deaths from all causes; so that, if

---

[1] Cotton Mather's *Magnalia.* Ed. of 1853, I. 227.

we take it to have been the successor of the plague, it operated in a very different way—with a greatly lessened fatality of all that were attacked, with only a reminder of the old special incidence upon the summer and autumn seasons, but with a steadiness from year to year, and throughout each year, that made the fever-deaths of a generation little short of one of those enormous totals of plague-deaths that were rapidly piled up during a few months, perhaps once or twice in a generation.

The following table from the London weekly Bills shows the progress of the fever from the end of April, 1694, with the number of deaths specially assigned to " spotted fever":—

London : Weekly Mortalities from fever and all causes, epidemic of 1694.

Week ending	Fever	Spotted fever	All deaths	Week ending	Fever	Spotted fever	All deaths
April 24	90	15	427	Aug. 28	111	20	510
May 1	77	10	369	Sept. 5	115	16	505
8	89	9	413	12	112	12	462
15	80	5	395	18	98	9	504
22	101	3	428	25	106	4	490
29	72	8	430	Oct. 2	124	8	533
June 5	112	12	469	9	125	10	553
12	113	12	434	16	114	9	552
19	113	11	430	23	104	3	511
26	99	14	396	30	118	3	528
July 3	94	11	423	Nov. 6	70	3	439
10	89	7	453	13	106	2	471
17	86	10	445	20	117	13	538
24	115	13	507	27	79	6	456
31	84	13	484	Dec. 4	87	6	475
Aug. 7	99	10	462	11	87	3	407
14	110	20	530	18	78	4	445
21	135	19	583	25	66	3	394

The year 1694, to which the epidemic of malignant fever (as well as malignant smallpox) belongs, was one of the series of " seven ill years" at the end of the 17th century (1693-99). They were long noted, says Thorold Rogers, "for the distress of the people and for the exalted profits of the farmer." The price of wheat in the autumn and winter of 1693 was the highest since the famine of 1661. In 1697–8 corn was again dear and much of it was spoilt. At Norwich in 1698 wheat was sold at 44s. a comb.

Harvests spoiled by wet weather or unseasonable cold appear to have been the most general cause of the high prices of food. In London there was no unusual sickness except in 1694; indeed the other years to the end of the century show a somewhat low mortality, the year 1696, which Macaulay marks as a time of severe distress among the common people owing to the calling in of the debased coinage[1], had the smallest number of deaths from all causes (18,638) since many years before, and for a century after allowing for the increase of population. But the deaths from "fever" were some three thousand every year, and the births, so far as registered, were, as usual, far below the deaths.

It was in the country at large that the effects of the "seven ill years" were chiefly felt. According to Short's abstracts of parish registers, there was unusual mortality at the beginning of the period and at the end of it; in his Chronology he mentions spotted fever, bloody flux and agues in 1693 (besides an influenza or universal slight fever recorded by Molyneux of Dublin), and again in 1697 and 1698 "purples, quinsies, Hungarian and spotted fever, universal pestilential spotted fever," from famine and bad food.

When we look for the evidence of this in England we shall have difficulty in finding it. Short's own abstracts give almost no colour to it; but there are other figures from the parish registers, scattered through the county histories and statistical works, which prove that the seven ill years must have checked population. Thus at Sheffield in the ten years 1691–1700 there was the greatest excess of burials over baptisms in the whole history of the town from 1561—namely, 2856 burials to 2221 baptisms (688 marriages). At Minehead, Somerset, a parish of some 1200 people occupied in weaving, the deaths and births were as follows in four years of the decennium:

	Baptised.	Buried.		Baptised.	Buried.
1691	57	75	1695	47	48
1694	34	55	1697	35	65

A glimpse of spotted or pestilential fever in Bristol during the years of distress at the end of the 17th century comes from Dr Dover, a man of no academical repute, but at all events an articulate voice. Passing from an account of the spotted pestilential fever at Guayaquil, "when I took it by storm," he goes on[2]:

[1] *History of England &c.,* IV. 707. Evelyn (*Diary,* 21 *May,* 1696) says the city was "very healthy," although the summer was exceeding rainy, cold and unseasonable.
[2] Thomas Dover, M.B., *The Ancient Physician's Legacy.* London, 1732, p. 98.

"About thirty-seven years since [written in 1732], this fever raged much in Bristol, so that I visited from twenty-five to thirty patients a day for a considerable time, besides their poor children taken into their workhouse, where I engaged myself, for the encouragement of so good and charitable an undertaking, to find them physick and give them advice at my own expense and trouble for the two first years. All these poor children in general had this fever, yet no more than one of them died of it of the whole number, which was near two hundred."

—an experience of typhus in children which was strictly according to rule. This had clearly been the occasion of a memorial addressed to the Mayor and Aldermen of Bristol, in 1696, praying that a capacious workhouse should be erected for children and the aged, which "will prevent children from being smothered or starved by the neglect of the parish officers and poverty of their parents, which is now a great loss to the nation[1]."

The year 1698 was the climax of the seven ill years. The spring was the most backward for forty-seven years, the first wheat in the ear being seen near London on 16th June. For four months to the end of August the days were almost all rainy, except from the 18th to the 26th July. Whole fields of corn were spoilt. In Kent there was barley standing uncut on 29th September, and some lay in the swathe until December. Much of the corn in the north of England was not got in until Christmas, and in Scotland they were reaping the green empty corn in January[2].

Fevers of the seven ill years in Scotland.

It is from Scotland that we hear most of the effects of the seven ill years in the way of famine and fever. Scotland was then in a backward state compared with England; and its northern climate, making the harvest always a few weeks later than in England, told especially against it in the ill years. Fynes Morryson, in the beginning of the 17th century, contrasts the Scotch manner of life unfavourably with the English, and Sir Robert Sibbald's account towards the end of that century is little better. Morryson says, "the excess of drinking was then farre greater in generall among the Scots than the English." Sibbald remarks[3] on the drinking habits of the Scots common

---

[1] Broadsheet in the British Museum Library.
[2] Tooke, *Hist. of Prices*, Introd.
[3] *Scotia Illustrata.* Edin. 1684. Lib. II. p. 52.

people : their potations of ale or spirits on an empty stomach, especially in the morning, relaxed the fibres and induced "erratic fevers of a bad type, bastard pleurisies,...dropsies, stupors, lethargies and apoplexies." Morryson says: "Their bedsteads were then like cubbards in the wall, with doores to be opened and shut at pleasure, so as we climbed up to our beds. They used but one sheete, open at the sides and top, but close at the feete, and so doubled[1]." Sibbald says the peasantry had poor food and hard work, and were subject to many diseases —" heartburn, sleeplessness, ravings, hypochondriac affections, mania, dysentery, scrophula, cancer, and a dire troop of diseases which everywhere now invades the husbandmen that were formerly free from diseases." *Causa a victu est.* Therefore consumption was common enough. He has much to say of fevers,—of intermittents, especially in spring and autumn, catarrhal fevers, nervous fevers, comatose fevers, with delirium, spasms and the like symptoms, malignant, spotted, pestilential, hectic, &c. The continued fevers ranged in duration from fifteen to thirty-one days, recovery being ushered in with sweats, alvine flux and salivation. Purple fevers had sometimes livid or black spots mixed with the purple (mottling); in a case given, there were suppurations which appear to have been bubonic. There had been no plague in Scotland since 1647–48 ; but fevers, unless Sibbald has given undue prominence to them, would appear to have filled its place among the adults.

Another writer of this period, from whom some information is got as to fevers, was Dr Andrew Brown of Edinburgh. He is mainly a controversialist, and is on the whole of little use save for the history of the treatment of fevers. He came to London on a visit in 1687, attracted by the fame of Sydenham's method of curing fevers by antimonial emetics and by purgation : " Returning home as much overjoyed as I had gotten a treasure, I presently set myself to that practice "—of which he gave an account in his 'Vindicatory Schedule concerning the New Cure of Fever[2].' Continual fever, he says, takes up, with its pendicles, the half of all the diseases that men are afflicted with ; and some part of what he calls continual fever must have been spotted : " As concerning the eruption of spots in fevers, these altogether resemble the marks made by stroaks on the skin, and these

---

[1] Fynes Morryson, *Itinerary*, 1614. Pt. III. p. 156.
[2] Edinburgh, 1691, p. 67.

marks are also made by the stagnation and coagulation of the blood in the small channels [according to the doctrine of obstructions]......They tinge the skin with blewness or redness."

The bitter controversy as to the treatment of fevers led Brown into another writing in 1699[1].

"The fevers that reign at this time [it was towards the end of the seven ill years] are for the most part quick and peracute, and cut off in a few days persons of impure bodies. And as I have used this method by vomiting and purging in many, and most successfully at this time, so I have had lately considerable experience thereof in my own family: wherein four of my children and ten servants had the fever, and blessed be God, are all recovered, by repeated vomiting with antimonial vomits and frequent purgings, except two servants, the one having gotten a great stress at work, who bragging of his strength did contend with his neighbour at the mowing of hay, and presently sickened and died the sixth day, and whom I saw not till the day before he died, and found him in such a condition that I could not give him either vomit or purge: and the other was his neighbour who strove with him, being a man of most impure and emaciate body, who had endured want and stress before he came to my service, and who got not all was necessary because he had not the occasion of due attendance, all my servants being sick at the time[2]."

This account of the experience which Dr Andrew Brown had lately had among his children and domestics in or near Edinburgh was written in 1699, and may be taken as relating to part of the wide-spread sickliness of the seven ill years in Scotland. Fletcher of Saltoun gives us a general view of the deplorable state of Scotland at the end of the 17th century, which was intensified by the succession of bad harvests[3]. The rents of cultivated farms were paid, not in money, but in corn, which gave occasion to many inequalities, to the traditional fraudulent practices of millers and to usury. The pasture lands for sheep and black cattle had no shelters from the weather, and no winter provision of hay or straw (roots were unheard of until long after), "so that the beasts are in a dying condition." The country swarmed with vagrants (a hundred thousand, he estimates, in ordinary times, but doubled in the dear years), who lived and multiplied in incest, rioted in swarms in the nearest hills in times of plenty, and in times of distress fell upon farmhouses in gangs

---

[1] *The Epilogue to the Five Papers, etc.* Edin. 1699, p. 22. This title refers to a controversy on the use of antimonial emetics in fevers. See Dr John Brown's essay on Dr Andrew Brown, in his *Locke and Sydenham*, new ed. Edinb., 1866.

[2] He adds that "the fever has several times before been in my family and among my servants and children." In mentioning the case of the Master of Forbes in August, 1691, whom he cured, he remarks that "the malicious said he was under no fever"; to disprove which Dr Brown refers to the symptoms of frequent pulse, watching and raving, continual vomiting, frequent fainting, and extreme weakness.

[3] Andrew Fletcher, *Two Discourses.* 1699.

of forty or more, demanding food.   Besides these there were a
great many poor families very meanly provided for by the
Church boxes, who lived wholly upon bad food and fell into
various diseases.   He had been credibly informed that some
families in the years of mere scarcity preceding the climax of
1698–99 had eaten grains, for want of bread.   " In the worst time,
from unwholesome food diseases are so multiplied among poor
people that, if some course be not taken, the famine may very
probably be followed by a plague[1]."

We owe some details of these calamities in Scotland to
Patrick Walker, the Covenanter, who records them to show
how the prophecies of Divine vengeance on the land, uttered
during the Stuart persecutions by Cargill and Peden, had been
in due time fulfilled[2]:

" In the year 1694, in the month of August, that crop got such a stroke
in one night by east mist or fog standing like mountains (and where it
remained longest and thickest the badder were the effects, which all our old
men, that had seen frost, blasting and mildewing, had never seen the like) that
it got little more good of the ground.   In November that winter many were
smitten with wasting sore fluxes and strange fevers (which carried many
off the stage) of such a nature and manner that all our old physicians had
never seen the like and could make no help ; for all things that used to be
proper remedies proved destructive.   And this was not to be imputed to
bad unwholesome victual ; for severals who had plenty of old victual did
send to Glasgow for Irish meal, and yet were smitten with fluxes and fevers
in a more violent and infectious nature and manner than the poorest in the
land, whose names and places where they dwelt I could instance.

"These unheard-of manifold judgments continued seven years, not
always alike, but the seasons, summer and winter, so cold and barren,
and the wonted heat of the sun so much withholden, that it was discernible
upon the cattle, flying fowls and insects decaying, that seldom a fly or gleg
was to be seen.   Our harvests not in the ordinary months, many shearing in
November and December, yea some in January and February ; the names
of the places I can instruct.   Many contracting their deaths, and losing the
use of their feet and hands, shearing and working amongst it in frost and
snow ; and after all some of it standing still, and rotting upon the ground,
and much of it for little use either to man or beast, and which had no taste
or colour of meal.   Meal became so scarce that it was at two shillings a
peck, and many could not get it.

"Through the long continuance of these manifold judgments deaths and
burials were so many and common that the living were wearied with
burying of the dead.   I have seen corpses drawn in sleds.   Many got neither
coffins nor winding-sheet.

" I was one of four who carried the corpse of a young woman a mile
of way ; and when we came to the grave, an honest poor man came and
said, 'You must go and help me to bury my son, he is lien dead this

[1] The English Government took off the Customs duty upon victual imported from
England to Scotland, and placed a bounty of 20d. per boll upon it.
[2] Patrick Walker, *Some Remarkable Passages in the Life and Death of Mr Daniel
Cargill, &c.*   Edinb. 1732.   (Reprinted in *Biographia Presbyteriana.*   Edinb. 1827,
II. 25.)

two days ; otherwise I will be obliged to bury him in my own yard.' We went, and there were eight of us had two miles to carry the corpse of that young man, many neighbours looking on us, but none to help us. I was credibly informed, that in the North, two sisters on a Monday's morning were found carrying the corpse of their brother on a barrow with bearing-ropes, resting themselves many times, and none offering to help them.

"I have seen some walking about at sunsetting, and next day at six o'clock in the summer morning found dead in their houses, without making any stir at their death, their head lying upon their hand, with as great a smell as if they had been four days dead ; the mice or rats having eaten a great part of their hands and arms.

"The nearer and sorer these plagues seized, the sadder were their effects, that took away all natural and relative affections, so that husbands had no sympathy with their wives, nor wives with their husbands, parents with their children, nor children with their parents. These and other things have made me to doubt if ever any of Adam's race were in a more deplorable condition, their bodies and spirits more low, than many were in these years."

In the parish of West Calder, 300 out of 900 "examinable" persons wasted away.

Some facts and traditions of the Seven Ill Years were recorded nearly a century after in the Statistical Account of Scotland. From the Kirk Session records of the parish of Fordyce, Banffshire, it did not appear "that any public measures were pursued for the supply of the poor, nor anything uncommon done by the Session except towards the end. The common distribution of the collections of the church amounted only to about 1*s*. 2*d*. or 1*s*. 4*d*. weekly." The Kirk Session records bore witness to the numerous cases of immorality in the years before the famine that had been dealt with ecclesiastically, and to the entire and speedy cessation of such cases thereafter[1].

The account for the parish of Keithhall and Kinkell, Aberdeenshire, says that "many died of want, in particular ten Highlanders in a neighbouring parish, that of Kemnay ; so that the Session got a bier made to carry them to the grave, not being able to afford coffins for such a number[2]." In the upland parish of Montquhitter, in the same county, the dear years reduced the population by one half or more. Until 1709 many farms were waste. Of sixteen families that resided on the estate of Lettertie, thirteen were extinguished. The account of this parish contains several stories of the distress, with the names of individuals[3]. It is clear, however, that all the parishes of Scotland were not equally distressed. The county of Moray and "some of the best land along the east coast of Buchan and Formartine [Aberdeenshire] abounded with seed and bread ;" but transport to the upland parishes was difficult[4].

[1] Sir John Sinclair's *Statistical Account of Scotland*. 1st ed. III. 62.
[2] *Ibid*. II. 544.   [3] *Ibid*. VI. 122.
[4] In the remote parish of Kilmuir, Skye, the famine is referred to the year 1688, "when the poor actually perished on the highways for want of aliment." (*Ibid*. II. 551.) In Duthil and Rothimurchus, Invernessshire, the famine is referred to 1680, "as nearly as can be recollected:" "A famine in this and the neighbouring counties, of the most fatal consequence. The poorer sort of people frequented the churchyard to pull a mess of nettles, and frequently struggled about the prey, being the earliest spring greens....So many families perished from want that for six miles in a well-inhabited extent, within the year there was not a smoke remaining." (*Ibid*. IV. 316.) In the Kirk session records of the parish of Kiltearn, Rossshire, which I have seen in MS., there are various entries in the year 1697 relating to badges of lead to be worn by those licensed to beg from door to door: on 12 April, 34 such persons are named, and on 19 April, Robert Douglas was reimbursed for the cost of 35 badges. On 2 Aug., the number of poor who were to receive each from the heritors ten shillings Scots reads like "nighentie foure."

4—2

We may take it that these experiences in the reign of William III. were peculiar to Scotland; even Ireland, which had troubles enough of the same kind in the 18th and 19th centuries, was at that time resorted to as a place of refuge by the distressed Scots. Among the special and temporary causes in Scotland were antiquated agricultural usage, an almost incredible proportion of the people in a state of lawless vagrancy, such as Henry VIII. and Elizabeth had to deal with a century and a half before, a low state of morals, both commercial and private, a tyrannical disposition of the employers, a sullen attitude of the labourers, and a total decay of the spirit of charity. An ancient elder of the parish of Fordyce, who kept some traditions of the dear years, remarked to the minister: "If the same precautions had been taken at that time which he had seen taken more lately in times of scarcity, the famine would not have done so much hurt, nor would so many have perished."

The evil of vagrancy, for which Fletcher of Saltoun saw no remedy but a state of slavery not unlike that which Protector Somerset had actually made the law of England for a couple of years, 1547–49, in somewhat similar circumstances, gradually cured itself without a resort to the practices of antiquity or of barbarism.

The union with England in 1707, by removing the customs duties and opening the Colonial trade to Scots shipping (they had a share in the East India trade already) gave a remarkable impulse to the manufacture of linen and to commerce. Such was the demand for Scots linen that, it seemed to De Foe, "the poor could want no employment"; and it may certainly be taken as a fact that the establishment on a free basis of industries and foreign markets gave Scotland relief from the pauperism and vagrancy, like those of Ireland in the 18th and 19th centuries, that threatened for a time, and especially in the Seven Ill Years, to retard the developement of the nation.

For several years after the period of scarcity or famine from 1693 to 1699, the history of fever in Britain presents little for special remark.

A book of the time was Dr George Cheyne's *New Theory of Continual Fever*, London, 1701. His theory is that of Bellini and Borelli, which accounted for everything in fevers on mechanical principles, and ignored the infective element in them. Cheyne does not even describe what the fevers were; but in showing how the theory applies, he mentions incidentally the symptoms—quick pulse, pain in the head, burning heat, want of sleep, raving, clear or flame-coloured urine, and morbid strength. Equally theoretical is the handling of the subject by Pitcairn. Freind, in his essays on fevers[1], is mainly occupied with controversial matters of treatment, except in connexion with Lord Peterborough's expedition to Spain in 1705, as we shall see in a section on sickness of camps and fleets.

In the absence of clinical details from the medical profession, the following from letters of the time will serve a purpose:

On 18 September, 1700, Thomas Bennett writes to Thomas Coke from Paris giving an account of the fever of Coke's brother: His fever is very violent upon him, and he has a hickup and twitchings in his face; he is especially ill in the night, and has now and then violent sweats. He raved for eight days together and in all that time did not get an hour's sleep. He was attended by Dr Helvetius and other physicians. Lady Eastes, her son, and most of her servants are sick, but they are all on the mending hand; her steward is dead of a high fever, having been sick but five days[2]. These are Paris fevers, the symptoms suggesting typhus, especially the prolonged vigil in one of the cases. It is to be remarked that they occurred among the upper classes; and it appears that the universal fevers "of a bad type" in France in 1712 did not spare noble houses nor even the palace of Louis the Great[3].

The following from the London Bills will show the prevalence of fever from year to year[4].

---

[1] John Freind, M.D., *Nine Commentaries on Fevers*, transl. by T. Dale. London, 1730.

[2] *Cal. Coke MSS.* II. 405.

[3] Joannes Turner, *De Febre Britannica Anni* 1712. Lond. 1713, p. 3. " Vere proximè elapso, per Gallias passim ingravescere coeperunt febres mali moris in nobiles domos, et regiam praecipue infestae; quò Ludovicum Magnum ipsa infortunia ostenderent Majorem, et patientia Christianissima Maximum."

[4] From London, on 25 February, 1701, we hear of the illness from a violent fever of Mr Brotherton, at his house in Chancery Lane; he was member for Newton, and Mr Coke was advised to look after his seat. A letter of 18 April, 1701, from Chilcote, in Derbyshire, says that it has been a sickly time in these parts and that a certain lady and her daughter were both dead and to be buried the same day. In the same correspondence, cases of fever in London are mentioned on 18 June and 4 December the same year (1701). *Cal. Coke MSS.* II. 421, 424, 429, 441.

Year	Dead of Fever	Dead of Spotted Fever	Dead of all diseases
1701	2902	68	20,471
1702	2682	53	19,481
1703	3162	74	20,720
1704	3243	61	22,684
1705	3290	41	22,097
1706	2662	54	19,847
1707	2947	42	21,600
1708	2738	62	21,291
1709	3140	118	21,800
1710	4397	343	24,620
1711	3461	142	19,833
1712	3131	96	21,198
1713	3039	102	21,057
1714	4631	150	26,569
1715	3588	161	22,232
1716	3078	100	24,436
1717	2940	137	23,446
1718	3475	132	26,523
1719	3803	124	28,347
1720	3910	66	25,454

The London fever of 1709–10.

The "seven ill years" were followed by the fine summer and abundant harvest (although hardly more than half the breadth was sown) of 1699. Scarcity was not a cause of excessive sickness again until 1709–10; although the harvest of 1703 was unfavourable. The price of wheat in 1702 was 25s. 6d. per quarter, and continued low for a number of years, notwithstanding the war with France. In Marlborough's wars there were no war-prices for farmers, as in the corresponding circumstances a century after; on the contrary, corn and produce of all kinds were so cheap that farmers had difficulty in paying their rents. The bounty of five shillings per quarter on exported wheat had given a great impulse to corn-growing, so that the acreage of wheat sown was much more than the country in an ordinary year required, partly, no doubt, because the bread of the poorer classes was largely made from the coarser cereals. The period of abundance was broken by the excessively severe winter of 1708–9, one of three memorable winters in the 18th century. The frost lasted all over Europe from October to March, and was followed by a greatly deficient crop in 1709. The following shows the rise of the price of the quarter of wheat in England:

		s.	d.
1708	Lady-day	27	3
„	Michaelmas	46	3
1709	Lady-day	57	6
„	Michaelmas	81	9
1710	Lady-day	81	9

The export of corn was prohibited in 1709 and again in 1710.

An epidemic of fever began in London in the autumn of 1709 and continued throughout 1710, in which year the fever-deaths reached the highest total since 1694. But it was not altogether a fever of starvation or distress among the poor, and perhaps not mainly so. There is always the dual question in connexion with fever following bad seasons and high prices : how much of it was due to the scarcity, and how much to those states of soil and atmosphere upon which the failure of the crop itself depended. An authentic case of the malignant fever which began to rage in London in the autumn of 1709 will both serve to show the remarkable type of at least a portion, if not the whole of the epidemic, and to prove its incidence upon the houses of the rich.

The case is recorded by Sir David Hamilton[1]:

"About the 5th of October, 1709, the son of that worthy gentleman, William Morison, esquire, was seized with a fever ; at which time, and for some weeks before, a malignant fever raged in London." He had a quick and weak pulse, great difficulty or hindrance of speech, and a stupidity ; "whereto were added tremors, and startings of the tendons, a dry and blackish tongue, a high-coloured but transparent urine and coming away for the most part involuntarily, and a hot and dry skin." Dr Grew was called in, and prescribed alexipharmac remedies (cordials, sudorifics, etc.) "A few days after the patient's skin was stained or marked with red and purple spots, and especially upon his breast, legs and thighs. These symptoms, although a little milder now and then, prevailed for fourteen days ; after that the spots vanished, and the convulsive motions so increased that the young gentleman seemed ready to sink under them for several days together." He was treated with the application of blisters, and with doses of bark. His strength and flesh were so wasted that the hip whereon he lay was seized with a gangrene. For ten or twelve days before his death, "he breathed and perspired so offensive a smell that they were obliged to smoke his chamber with perfumes ; and even myself, whilst I inclined my body a little too near him, was, by receiving his breath into my mouth, seized all on a sudden with such a sickness and faintness that I was obliged to take the air in the open fields, and returning thence to drink plentifully of *mountain* wine at dinner." The examination after death was made by the celebrated anatomist Dr Douglas. There was still a heap of brown-coloured spots visible on the breast ; "there was nothing contained in the more conspicuous vessels of the abdomen but grumes or clots of blackish blood, without any serum in the interstices." Hamilton adds : "We too seldom dissect the bodies of those dying in fevers."

[1] *Tractatus Duplex.* Lond. 1710. Engl. transl. 1737, p. 253.

The tremors, offensive sweats and offensive breath are distinctive of a form of typhus that became common towards the middle of the century, and was called putrid fever (not in the sense of Willis) or miliary fever from the watery vesicles of the skin that often attended it. But although Hamilton was writing on miliary fever (of the factitious variety) this case is not given as an example, but is appended to his sixteen cases of the latter, as an example of "a deadly fever with loss of speech from the beginning." Among earlier cases, those belonging to the epidemic of 1661 as described by Willis correspond closely with this case, which we may take as representing part of the malignant fever that then raged in London. We have an anatomical record from each; but in neither was there sloughing of the lymph-follicles of the intestine, or of the mesenteric glands, as in the enteric fever of our own time; while in both there were red or purple spots on the breast or neck, and on the limbs. The "loss of speech from the beginning" suggests Sydenham's "absolute aphonia" in the comatose fever of 1673–76, which resembled in other respects Willis's fever of the brain and nervous stock (mostly of children) in 1661. One of the synonyms of "infantile remittent" was "an acute fever with dumbness[1]." This seems to have been a common type of fever in the latter part of the 17th century and early part of the 18th. Some likeness to enteric fever may be found in it, but there is no warrant for identifying it with that fever. Its main features may be said to have been its incidence upon the earlier years of life, but not to the exclusion of adult cases, its remarkable ataxic symptoms, which led Willis to refer it to "the brain and nervous stock" (spinal cord), its comatose character, its spots, occasional miliary eruption, ill-smelling sweats and other foetid evacuations, its protracted course, and its hectic sequelae.

The weekly bills of mortality in London bear little evidence of unusual prevalence of fever in 1709, except in the weeks ending 13 and 20 September, when the fever-deaths were 96 and 75 (including "spotted fever"). But the unusual entry of "malignant fever" appears in three weekly bills, 19 July, 9 August and 23 August, one death being referred to it on each occasion. It was in the summer and autumn of 1710 that the fever reached a height in London, being attended with a very

---

[1] W. Butter, M.D., *A Treatise on the Infantile Remittent Fever.* Lond. 1782.

fatal smallpox. An essay on the London epidemic of 1710[1] is interesting chiefly for recording a probable case of relapsing fever, a form which was almost certainly part of the great febrile epidemic in London in 1727–29.

Mrs Simon, aged 20, had a burning fever, stifling of her breath, frequent vomiting and looseness, foul tongue, loss of sleep, restlessness, intermitting, low and irregular pulse. This terrible fever disappeared on the fourth day, and she thought herself recovered. But on the seventh day from her being taken ill the fever returned, she was light-headed, did not know her relatives, and was fevered in the highest degree. It looked like a malignant fever, but there were no spots.

The following table shows the very high mortality from fever (as well as from smallpox) in the epidemic to which the above case belonged.

London: Weekly deaths from fever, smallpox and all causes.

1710.

Week ending	Dead of fever	Dead of spotted fever	Dead of smallpox	Dead of all diseases
May 2	103	[illegible]	99	571
9	90	6	60	517
16	84	7	71	502
23	93	15	71	503
30	106	11	83	550
June 6	93	2	98	508
13	79	8	84	509
20	106	12	99	574
27	105	15	86	503
July 4	106	7	99	482
11	107	13	97	467
18	126	16	89	509
25	109	13	105	562
Aug. 1	91	12	79	444
8	92	11	72	463
15	98	10	58	459
22	105	10	63	463
29	111	16	71	495
Sept. 5	76	4	63	414
12[2]	107	12	57	520
19	115	9	83	548
26	81	11	46	456
Oct. 3	98	9	45	469
10	79	10	49	480
17	90	5	41	477
24	107	5	45	470
31	106	14	51	421
Nov. 7	71	6	55	425
14	92	2	41	390
21	70	4	25	345

[1] Philip Guide, M.D., *A Kind Warning to a Multitude of Patients daily afflicted with different sorts of Fevers.* Lond. 1710.

[2] One death from "malignant fever," two from scarlet fever.

Throughout England, in country parishes and in towns, the
first ten years of the 18th century were on the whole a period of
good public health.   In Short's abstracts of the parish registers
to show the excess of deaths over the births, those years are as
little conspicuous as any in the long series.   It was a time when
there was a great lull in smallpox, and probably also in fevers.
The figures for Sheffield may serve as an example[1].   It will be
seen from the Table that the burials exceeded the baptisms in
every decade from the Restoration to the end of the century;
after that for twenty years the baptisms exceeded the burials,
the marriages having increased greatly.

Vital Statistics of Sheffield.

Ten-year periods	Marriages	Baptisms	Burials
1661—70	585	2086	2266
1671—80	537	2240	2387
1681—90	540	2595	2856
1691—1700	688	2221	2856
1701—10	942	3033	2613
1711—20	991	3304	2765

Of particular epidemics, we hear of a malignant fever at
Harwich in 1709.   Harwich was then an important naval
station, and the fever may have arisen in connexion with
the transport of troops to and from the seat of war, just as
camp- and war-fevers appeared at various ports in the next war,
1742–48.

There were rumours of a plague at Newcastle in 1710,
which were contradicted by advertisement in the *London Gazette*[2].
But, as there was so much plague in the Baltic ports in 1710
it is possible that the Newcastle rumour may have been one of
plague imported, and not a rumour suggested by the mortality
from some other disease.

[1] Hunter's *Hallamshire*, ed. Gatty.

[2] Brand, *Hist. of Newcastle*, II. 308. Swift writes to Stella on 8 December, 1710:
"We are terribly afraid of the plague; they say it is at Newcastle.   I begged Mr
Harley [the Lord President] for the love of God to take some care about it, or we are
all ruined.   There have been orders for all ships from the Baltic to pass their
quarantine before they land; but they neglect it.   You remember I have been afraid
these two years."   The orders referred to were probably the Order of Council of
9 Nov. 1710.   Parliament met on the 25th Nov. and passed the first Quarantine Act
(9 Anne, cap. II.).   Swift had a good deal to say with Ministers on many subjects, and
it is not impossible, however absurd, that his had been the first suggestion to Harley
of a quarantine law.   I had purposed including a history of quarantine in Britain,
but can find no convenient context for it.   I shall therefore refer the reader to the
historical sketch which I have appended to the Article "Quarantine" in the
Encyclopaedia Britannica, 9th ed.

To the same period of epidemic fever in London, about 1709–10, belongs also a curiously localized epidemic in an Oxford college, which reminds one somewhat of the circumstances of enteric fever in our time. It was told to Dr Rogers of Cork twenty-five or twenty-six years before the date of his writing (1734), by one who was a student at Oxford then : "There broke out amongst the scholars of Wadham College a fever very malignant, that swept away great numbers, whilst the rest of the colleges remained unvisited. All agreed that the contagious infection arose from the putrefaction of a vast quantity of cabbages thrown into a heap out of the several gardens near Wadham College[1]."

The next epidemic of fever in London was in 1714. Like that of 1710, it followed a great rise in the price of wheat, or perhaps it followed the unseasonable weather which caused the deficient harvest. Before the Peace of Utrecht wheat in England was as low as 33s. 9d. per quarter, in 1712, the peace next year sending it no lower than 30s. But at Michaelmas, 1713, it rose with a bound to 56s. 11d., doubtless owing to a bad harvest. The fever-deaths in London began to rise in the spring of 1714, reaching a weekly total of 103 in the week ending 20 April. All through the summer and autumn they continued very high, the weekly totals exceeding, on an average, those of the year 1710, as in the foregoing table, and having corresponding large additions of "spotted fever." The deaths from all causes in 1714 were a quarter more than those of the year before, the epidemic of fever being the chief contributor to the rise. This happened to be a very slack time in medical writing[2]; but, even in the absence of such testimony as we have for earlier and later epidemics of fever in London, we may safely conclude that the fever of 1714 was of the type of pestilential or malignant typhus, beginning in early summer and reaching a height in the old plague season of autumn.

A singular instance of what may be considered war-typhus

---

[1] *Essay on Epidemic Diseases.* Dublin, 1734, p. 34.
[2] Dr Guide, a Frenchman, who had been in practice in London for many years, says in his *Kind Warning to a Multitude of Patients daily afflicted with different sorts of Fevers* (1710) "the British physicians and surgeons are lately fallen into an unhappy and terrible confusion and mixture of honest and fraudulent pretenders." Another writer of 1710, Dr Lynn, quoted in the chapter on Smallpox, implies that physicians were taking an unusually cynical view of their business. The most interesting essay of the time on fevers is by J. White, M.D. (*De recta Sanguinis Missione &c.* Lond. 1712), a Scot who had been in the Navy and afterwards in practice at Lisbon ; but it throws no light upon the London fevers.

belongs to the winter of 1715–16. The political intrigues preceding and following the death of Queen Anne in 1714 culminated in the Jacobite rising in Scotland and the North of England in 1715. The Jacobites having been defeated at Preston on 13 November, prisoners to the number of 450 were brought to Chester Castle on the Sunday night before December 1st. A fortnight later (December 15th), Lady Otway writes of the 450 prisoners in the Castle:

"They all lie upon straw, the better and the worse alike. The king's allowance is a groat a day for each man for meat, but they are almost starved for want of some covering, though many persons are charitable to the sick." The winter was unusually severe, the snow lying "a yard deep." Many prisoners died in the Castle by "the severity of the season," many were carried off by "a very malignant fever." On February 16th Lady Otway writes again :—"So much sickness now in our Castle that they dye in droves like rotten sheep, and be 4 or 5 in a night throne into the Castle ditch ffor ther graves. The feavour and sickness increaseth dayly, is begun to spread much into the citty, and many of the guard solidyers is sick, it is thought by inffection. The Lord preserve us ffrom plague and pestilence[1]!"

Prosperity of Britain, 1715–65.

The fifty years from 1715 to 1765 were, with two or three exceptions, marked by abundant harvests, low prices and heavy exports of corn. This was undoubtedly a great time in the expansion of England, a time of fortune-making for the monied class, and of cheapness of the necessaries of life.

The well-being and comfort of the middle class were undoubtedly great; also there was something peculiar to England in the prosperity of towns and villages throughout all classes. In the very worst year of the period, the year 1741, Horace Walpole landed at Dover on the 13th September, having completed the grand tour of Europe. Like many others, he was delighted with the pleasant county of Kent as he posted towards London; and on stopping for the night at Sittingbourne, he wrote as follows in a letter :

"The country town delights me : the populousness, the ease, the gaiety, and well-dressed everybody, amaze me. Canterbury, which on my setting out I thought deplorable, is a paradise to Modena, Reggio, Parma, etc. I had before discovered that there was nowhere but in England the distinction of *middling people.* I perceive now that there is peculiar to us *middling houses :* how snug they are[2]!"

[1] Elizabeth, Lady Otway, to Benj. Browne, Dec. 1st and 15th, 1715, and Feb. 16, 1716. *Hist. MSS. Com.* x. pt. 4, p. 352; Hemingway's *Hist. of Chester*, ii. 244.
[2] *Letters,* ed. Cunningham, i. 72.

Our history henceforth has little to record of malignant typhus fevers, or of smallpox, in these snug houses of the middle class, although not only the middle class, but also the highest class had a considerable share of those troubles all through the 17th century. But the 18th century, even the most prosperous part of it, from the accession of George I. to the beginning of the Industrial Revolution in the last quarter or third of it, was none the less a most unwholesome period in the history of England. The health of London was never worse than in those years, and the vital statistics of some other towns, such as Norwich, are little more satisfactory. This was the time which gave us the saying, that God made the country and man made the town. Praise of rural felicity was a common theme in the poetry of the time, as in Johnson's *London :*

> "There every bush with nature's music rings,
> There every breeze bears health upon its wings."

Both for the country and the town the history of the public health does not harmonize well with the optimist views of the 18th century. The historians are agreed that, under the two first Georges, during the ministries of Walpole, the Pelhams and Pitt, the prosperity of Britain was general. Adam Smith speaks of "the peculiarly happy circumstances of the country" during the reign of George II. (1727–60). Hallam characterizes the same reign as "the most prosperous that England had ever experienced." The most recent historian of England in the 18th century is of the same opinion[1]. The novels of Fielding give us the concrete picture of the period with epic fidelity, and the picture is of abundance and prodigality. Agriculture and commerce with the Colonies, India and the continent of Europe, were the sources of the country's wealth. Farming and stock-raising had been greatly improved by the introduction of roots and sown grasses.

---

[1] Lecky, *History of England in the Eighteenth Century*, VI. 204 :—"All the evidence we possess concurs in showing that during the first three-quarters of the century the position of the poorer agricultural classes in England was singularly favourable. The price of wheat was both low and steady. Wages, if they advanced slowly, appear to have commanded an increased proportion of the necessaries of life, and there were all the signs of growing material well-being. It was noticed that wheat bread, and that made of the finest flour, which at the beginning of the period had been confined to the upper and middle classes, had become before the close of it over the greater part of England the universal food, and that the consumption of cheese and butter in proportion to the population in many districts almost trebled. Beef and mutton were eaten almost daily in villages."

In some country parishes the baptisms were three times the burials. But the public health during this period will not appear in a favourable light from what follows. More particularly there were three occasions, about the years 1718, 1728 and 1741, when a single bad harvest in the midst of many abundant ones brought wide-spread distress, with epidemics of typhus and relapsing fever; from which fact it would appear that the common people had little in hand. Thorold Rogers, among economists, was of the opinion that the prosperity was all on the side of the governing and capitalist classes, that the labourers were in "irremediable poverty" and "without hope," and that the law of parochial settlement, with the artificial fixing of wages by the Quarter Sessions and the bonuses out of the poor-rates, had the effect of keeping the mass of the people on the land "in a condition wherein existence could just be maintained[1]." I shall not attempt an independent judgment in economics, but proceed to those illustrations of national well-being which belong to my subject, leaving the latter to have their due weight on the one side of economical opinion or on the other. Besides the economical question there is of course also an ethical one. When the pinch came about 1766, there was the usual diversity of opinion expressed on the "condition of England" problem, one holding that the labourers were unfairly paid, another that the nation had been made "splendid and flourishing by keeping wages low," and that the distress was due to "want of industry, want of frugality, want of sobriety, want of principle" among the common people at large. "If in a time of plenty," wrote one austere moralist, "the labourers would abate of their drunkenness, sloth, and bad economy, and make a reserve against times of scarcity, they would have no reason to complain of want or distress at any time[2]." But there must have been something wrong in the economics and morals of their betters if it were the case that the working class as a whole, and not merely a certain number of individuals in it, was drunken, thriftless and slothful. The familiar proof of this is the apathy of the Church, broken by the Methodist revival of religion.

[1] *Six Centuries of Work and Wages*, pp. 398—415.
[2] *Gentleman's Magazine*, 1766.

The epidemic fevers of 1718–19.

In the fifty years from 1715 to 1765, the three worst periods of epidemic fever in England and Scotland correspond closely to the three periods of actual famine and its attendant train of sicknesses in Ireland, namely, the years 1718–19, 1727–29, and 1740–42. The three divisions of the kingdom suffered in common, Ireland suffering most. The first period, 1718–19, was an extremely slack tide in medical writing, insomuch that hardly any accounts of the reigning maladies remain, except those by Wintringham, of York, and Rogers, of Cork. The whole of the Irish history of fevers and the allied maladies is dealt with in a chapter apart. Of the Scots history, little is known for the first of the three periods beyond a statement that there was a malignant fever and dysentery in Lorn, Argyllshire, in January and February, 1717[1].

Wintringham gives the following account of the *synochus*, afterwards called typhus, which attracted notice in the summer of 1718 and became more common in the warm season of 1719: in each year it began about May, reached its height in July and lasted all August, carrying off many of those who fell into it.

It began with rigors, nausea and bilious vomiting, followed by alternate heats and chills, with great lassitude and a feeling of heaviness : then thirst and pungent heat, a dry and brown tongue, sometimes black. The patient slept little, did not sweat, and was mostly delirious, or anxious and restless, tossing continually in bed. About the 12th day it was not unusual for profuse and exhausting diarrhœa to come on. In a favourable case the fever ended in a crisis of sweating about the 16th day. Those who were of lax habit, unhealthy, hysteric, or cachectic, were apt to have tremors, spasms and delirium, while others were so prostrated as to have no control over their evacuations, lying in a stupor and raving when roused out of it. In these the fever would continue to the 20th day ; in some few it ended without a manifest crisis, and with a slow convalescence[2].

This applies to the city of York, but in what special circumstances we are not told. However, it happens that a physician of York, two generations after, in giving an account of the great improvement that had taken place in its public health, throws some light on its old-world state : " The streets

---

[1] Short.
[2] Clifton Wintringham, M.D., *Commentarium nosologicum, morbos epidemicos et aeris variationes in urbe Eboracensi locisque vicinis ab anno* 1715 *usque ad finem anni* 1725 *grassantes, complectens.* Londini, 1727.

have been widened in many places by taking down a number of old houses built in such a manner as almost to meet in the upper stories, by which the sun and air were almost excluded in the streets and inferior apartments[1]."

In London the fever-deaths, with the deaths from all causes, rose decidedly in 1718, and reached a very high figure in 1719, of which the summer was excessively hot. One cause, at least, was want of employment, especially among weavers in the East End[2]. But the epidemic fever of 1718–19 was not limited to the distressed classes; we have a glimpse of it, under the name of "spotted fever," in the family of the archbishop of Canterbury:

"On Friday night the archbishop of Canterbury's sixth daughter was interred in our chancel, with four others preceding, she dying on Monday after three days of the spotted fever. The fourth and seventh are recovered, and hoped past danger[3]."

The following table shows the fever-mortalities for London, from 1718 onwards, and, for comparison, the excessive mortalities in the epidemics of 1710 and 1714:

---

[1] W. White, M.D., *Phil. Trans.* LXXII. (1782), p. 35. The annual deaths under the old *régime* exceeded by a good deal the annual births: in the seven years 1728—35, according to the figures from the parish registers in Drake's *Eboracum*, the burials from all causes were 3488, and the baptisms 2803, an annual excess of 98 deaths over the births in an estimated population of 10,800 (birth-rate 37 per 1000, death-rate 46 per 1000). But in the seven years, 1770—76, the balance was the other way: the population had increased by two thousand (to 12,800), and the births were on an average 20 in the year more than the deaths (474 births, 454 deaths), the birth-rate being still 37 per 1000, and the death-rate fallen to 35 per 1000. But the correctness of these rates depends on the population being exactly given.

[2] "There has been very great mobbing by the weavers of this town, as they pretend, because they are starved for want of trade; and they pull the calico cloaths off women's backs wherever they see them. The Trainbands have been up since last Friday, and they were forced to fire at the mobb in Moor Fields before they would disperse, and four or five were shott and as many wounded." (Benjamin Browne to his father, 16 June, 1719: Mr Browne's MSS. *Hist. MSS. Com.* X. pt. 4, p. 351.) The calicoes which the London weavers tore from the backs of women were doubtless the Indian fabrics brought home by the ships of the East India Company. These imports were so injurious to home manufactures that an Act had been passed in 1700 prohibiting (with some exceptions) the use in England of printed or dyed calicoes or any other printed or dyed cotton goods. This prohibition was re-enacted in 1721, two years after the rioting at Moorfields. (7 Geo. I. cap. 7). Blomefield (*Hist. of Norfolk,* III. 437) says that at Norwich also there was tearing of calicoes, "as pernicious to the trade" of that city. On the 20th of September, 1720, a great riot arose there, the rabble cutting several gowns in pieces on women's backs, entering shops to seize all calicoes found there, beating the constables, and opposing the sheriff's power to such a degree that the company of artillery had to be called out.

[3] Ambrose Warren to Sir P. Gell, 16 Sept. 1718, *Hist. MSS. Com.* IX. pt. 2, p. 400 *b*.

London Mortalities from Fever, &c.

Year	Fevers	Spotted fevers	Smallpox	All causes
1710	4397	343	3138	24620
1714	4631	150	2810	26569
1718	3475	132	1884	26523
1719	3803	124	3229	28347
1720	3910	46	1442	25454
1721	3331	84	2375	26142
1722	3088	22	2167	25750
1723	3321	51	3271	29197
1724	3262	84	1227	25952
1725	3277	59	3188	25523
1726	4666	84	1569	29647
1727	4728	102	2379	28418
1728	4716	94	2105	27810
1729	5235	[The entry	2849	29722
1730	4011	ends.]	1914	26761
1731	3225		2640	25262
1732	2939		1197	23358
1733	3831		1370	29233
1734	3116		2688	26062
1735	2544		1594	23538
1736	3361		3014	27581
1737	4580		2084	27823
1738	3890		1590	25825
1739	3334		1690	25432
1740	4003		2725	30811

In country parishes, according to Short's abstracts of registers, there was no unusual sickness in 1718 and 1719. But in market towns the mortality rose greatly in 1719, which had an excessively hot summer; and that was the year when the *synochus* or typhus described by Wintringham reached its worst at York. The mortality kept high for several years after 1719.

Market Towns.

Year	Registers examined	Registers with excess of deaths	Deaths in same	Births in same
1716	30	8	1060	845
1717	30	9	1485	1290
1718	30	3	249	169
1719	30	6	1737	1320
1720	30	10	2186	1461
1721	33	9	1294	952
1722	33	11	1664	1345
1723	33	14	2532	2176

The high mortalities in 1721–23 were mostly from smallpox, exact figures of many of the epidemics in Yorkshire and elsewhere being given in the chapter on that disease. The country parishes shared in its prevalence:

Country Parishes.

Year	Registers examined	Registers with excess of deaths	Deaths in same	Births in same
1721	174	35	793	586
1722	175	35	1015	775
1723	174	63	2021	1583

Besides smallpox, diarrhoeas and dysenteries in the autumn are given by Wintringham as the reigning maladies, fever not being mentioned.

The Epidemic Fevers of 1726–29 : evidence of Relapsing Fever.

The four years 1726–29 were a great fever-period in London, the deaths having been as follows :

Year	Fever deaths	All deaths
1726	4666	29,647
1727	4728	28,418
1728	4716	27,810
1729	5335	29,722

In the last of those years the entry in the annual bills becomes " fever, malignant fever, spotted fever and purples."

The following are the weekly maxima of fever deaths and deaths from all causes during the four years, 1726–29; in nearly all the weeks the deaths from "convulsions" (generic name for most of the maladies of infants) contribute from a fourth to a third, or even more, of the whole mortality.

Week ending		Fever deaths	All deaths
1726			
Jan.	18	71	633
March	15	81	678
May	31	103	611
June	7	106	607
Aug.	30	102	711
Sept.	6	116	680
	13	109	643
	20	109	648
1727			
Aug.	8	103	577
	15	123	698
	22	132	730
	29	130	789
Sept.	5	150	764
	12	134	795
	19	165	798
	26	163	715
Oct.	3	150	684

Week ending		Fever deaths	All deaths
1728			
Feb.	6	112	748
	13	131	889
	20	121	850
	27	145	927
March	5	93	733
Aug.	27	138	525
Sept.	3	131	562
Dec.	10	122	734
1729			
Sept.	9	109	676
Nov.	4	213	908*
	11	267	993*
	18	166	783
Dec.	9	132	779

* The sudden rise was due to influenza; but the fever mortality was high for weeks before and after.

These are high mortalities, whatever were the types of fever that caused them. That the old pestilential fever of London was one of them we need have no doubt. Dr John Arbuthnot, writing two or three years after, said, " I believe one may safely affirm that there is hardly any year in which there are not in London fevers with buboes and carbuncles [the distinctive pestilential marks]; and that there are many petechial or spotted fevers is certain[1]."

The essay of Strother also has a reference to "spotted fever" in its title, although the text throws very little light upon it[2]. But, for the rest, the " constitution " of 1727–29 is more than usually perplexing. There was an influenza at the end of 1729, which can be separated from the rest easily enough by the help of the London weekly bills of mortality ; and it is probable, unless Arbuthnot, Huxham and Rutty have erred in their dates, that one or more epidemics of catarrhal fever had occurred before that, in the years 1727 and 1728. The greatest difficulty is with a certain " little fever," or "hysteric fever," or "febricula," which gave rise to some writing and a good deal of talk. Strother does not specially treat of it, at least under that name, although he says that " many, especially women, have been subject to fits of vapours, cold sweats, apprehensions, and unaccountable fears of death; every small disappointment dejected them, tremblings and weakness attended them," etc. (p. 116) ; and again, " never was a season when apoplexies, palsies and other obstructions of the nerves did prevail so much as they do at present, and have done for some time past " (p. 102) ; while he had frequently seen hysterical and hypochondriacal symptoms, dejection of spirits and the like remaining behind the fever (p. 109). For some years before this, much had been heard in London of the vapours, the " hypo," the spleen, and the like, an essay by Dr Mandeville, better known by his 'Fable of the Bees,' having first made these maladies fashionable in the year 1711[3].

---

[1] John Arbuthnot, M.D., *Essay concerning the Effects of Air on Human Bodies.* Lond. 1733, p. 187.

[2] Edward Strother, M.D., *Practical Observations on the Epidemical Fever which hath reigned so violently these two years past and still rages at the present time, with some incidental remarks shewing wherein this fatal Distemper differs from Common fevers ; and more particularly why the Bark has so often failed : and methods prescribed to render its use more effectual. In which is contained a very remarkable History of a Spotted Fever.* London, 1729. This book was written before the influenza of the end of 1729. At p. 126 the author was writing on the 24th of May, 1728. The preface is undated.

[3] Bernard de Mandeville, M.D., *A Treatise of the Hypochondriack and Hysteric Diseases*, 3rd ed. 1730, 1st ed. 1711. It contains nothing about the " little fever."

In due time it began to be noticed that symptoms which many physicians made light of as a "fit of vapours" were really the beginning of a fever. Dr Blackmore, in an essay on the Plague written in 1721, admitted the ambiguity :

> "For several days a malignant fever has so near a resemblance to one that is only hysterick, that many physicians and standers by, I am apt to believe, mistake the first for the last, and look upon a great and dangerous disease to be only the spleen, or a fit of the vapors, to the great hazard of the patient[1]."

In 1730, Dr William Cockburn, in a polemic against the physicians whom he styles "the academical cabal" (because they objected to his secret electuary for dysentery), professes to give a history of the mistakes of the faculty in London over this "little fever," or "hysteric fever," which often became dangerous[2] :

> "The present fever, with a variation in some of its symptoms, has now subsisted twelve years [or since 1718] not in England only, but all over Europe [Manningham says it was peculiarly English]. Few or no physicians suspected the reigning and popular disease to be a fever. Vapours, a nervous disease, and such general appellations it had from sundry physicians. Others, who discovered the fever, knew it was the low or slow fever, first mentioned by Hippocrates....The last were represented as ignorant for calling the distemper a fever, and affixing to it the name 'low' or 'slow,' a slow fever being, in their adversaries' opinion, altogether unheard of among physicians and never recorded in their books. Nothing was more monstrous than calling this distemper a fever, or confining persons afflicted with it to their bed, and dieting them with broth, or other liquid food of good nourishment, and what is easily concocted....'You are not hot, you are not dry ; you are in good temper ; and therefore you have no fever' was the common language of the town....They might have seen physicians practising for a destroying distemper, and yet, after seven years, they confess themselves ignorant of its very name."

At length, he continues, Blackmore admitted the ambiguity of diagnosis, while Mead, Freind and others, recognized that there was really such a thing as a slow, nervous fever, by no means free from danger to life. It is probably to this insidious fever that Strother refers :

> "Thus, having gone on for six or seven days in a train of indolence, they have been surprized on the seventh day, and have died on the eighth lethargick or delirious, whereas, if they had taken due care, the fever would have run its course in fifteen days or more." It was the remissions, or inter-missions, he explains, that often misled patients, by which he seems to mean the clear intervals between relapses. "Others, wearied out with relapses, have hoped their recovery would as certainly ensue as it had hitherto, and

---

[1] Richard Blackmore, M.D., *A Discourse upon the Plague, with a prefatory account of Malignant Fever.* London, 1721, p. 17.
[2] W. Cockburn, M.D., *Danger of improving Physick, with a brief account of the present Epidemick Fever.* London, 1730.

have deferred asking advice until it was too late." These relapses, he thought, were brought on by venturing too soon into the air : "it is too well known that the fever has been cured, and patients have soon, after they have ventured into the air, relapsed and have again run the same circle of ill symptoms, if not worse than before." Bark failed conspicuously in these "remittents :" "it is therefore incumbent on me to examine into the reason of this *new phenomenon.* I call it *new,*" he explains, because bark had hitherto succeeded. "Perhaps we may find reason to lay some blame on the air for the frequent relapses....Periodical comas have of late been common ; so soon as the fit was over, the drowsiness abated till the fit returned."

Elsewhere he speaks of the frequent relapses as belonging to a "quartan," under which diagnosis bark had been tried. The fevers were less apt to "relapse" when treated by mild cathartics. Another symptom of this fever was jaundice : "If jaundice breaks forth on the fourth day of a fever, it is much better than if it comes at the conclusion of a fever....Jaundices are now very common after the cure of these fevers."

These indications, dispersed throughout the rambling essay of Strother, point somewhat plainly to relapsing fever[1]. But his theoretical pathology comes in to obscure the whole matter. He explains everything by obstructions. The jaundice was due to obstruction of the liver by "styptics," the hysteric symptoms to obstructions of the nerves; there were also theoretical obstructions of the mesentery, part of the matter being sometimes "thrown off into the mesenteric glands"; also "congestions" or phlegmons of the liver, spleen and pancreas. But it is when he comes to the bowels that his subjective morbid anatomy becomes truly misleading. There is nothing to show that Strother examined a single body dead of this fever. He says, however, in his *à priori* way : "The crisis of these slow fevers is generally deposited on the bowels...The lent fever is a symptomatical fever, arising from an inflammation, or an ulcer fixed on some of the bowels. A lent fever, depending on some fixed cause of the bowels, must be cured by having regard to those causes some of which I shall enumerate" :—the first supposition being that the fever depends on phlegmons by congestion of "the liver, spleen, pancreas, or the mesentery"; the second, if it depends on extravasations in an equally comprehensive range of viscera ; the third, "if it depends on an ulcer, then all vulneraries must be administered internally; but to speak truth, when the viscera are ulcerated, there remains but small hope of life"; the fourth supposition is worms, the fifth

[1] I am the more persuaded of the identity with relapsing fever of much that was called remittent in Britain, and even intermittent, after reading the highly original treatise by R. T. Lyons on *Relapsing or Famine Fever*, London, 1872, relating to the epidemics of it in India.

corruption of the humours. All this is paper pathology. There is not a single precise fact relating to ulcerated Peyer's patches, or to swollen mesenteric glands, or to enlarged spleen, which last would have been equally distinctive of relapsing as of enteric fever; it is "the viscera" that are ulcerated, or congested, or extravasated, or it is "some of the bowels," or the pancreas and liver obstructed as well as the spleen, the obstruction of the liver being invoked to explain the highly significant jaundice.

It is not quite clear whether Strother's fever with relapses and jaundice corresponded exactly to the little fever, hysteric fever, or nervous fever of the same years; but it is worthy of note that relapsing fever in Ireland a century later was called febricula or the "short fever." It was not until 1746 that the excellent essay upon it by Sir Richard Manningham was written. By that time a good deal was being said in various parts of Britain of a slow, nervous, or putrid fever, Huxham, in particular, identifying the nervous fever with Manningham's febricula or little fever[1]. Some have supposed that the nervous fever of the 18th century included cases of enteric fever, if it did not stand for that disease exclusively. Murchison takes Manningham's essay to be "an excellent description of enteric fever, under the title of febricula or little fever, etc.[2]" The following are brief extracts from his description, by which the reader will be able to form his own opinion on the question of identity[3].

At the beginning patients feel merely languid or uneasy, with flying pains, dryness of the lips and tongue but no thirst; in a day or two they find themselves often giddy, dispirited and anxious without apparent reason, and passing pale urine. They have transient fits of chilliness, a low, quick and unequal pulse, sometimes cold clammy sweats and risings in the throat. They go about until more violent symptoms come on, simulating those of quotidian, tertian or quartan fever; sometimes the malady simulates pleurisy. There may be attacks of dyspnoea, nausea and haemorrhage; the menses in women are checked. A loss of memory and a delirium occur at intervals for short periods. The malady is very difficult to cure and too often becomes fatal in the end. It will last thirty or forty days, unless it end fatally in stupor or syncope. A form of mania is a consequence of it, where it has been neglected or badly treated; "of late years this species of madness has been more than ordinarily frequent." All sorts were liable to it, but mostly valetudinarians, delicate persons, and those in the decline of life; the

[1] Huxham, *On Fevers*, chap. VIII.
[2] Murchison, *Continued Fevers of Great Britain*, 2nd ed. Lond. 1873, p. 423.
[3] Sir Richard Manningham, Kt., M.D. *Febricula or Little Fever, commonly called the Nervous or Hysteric Fever, the Fever on the Spirits, Vapours, Hypo, or Spleen.* 1746.

fatalities were "especially among the opulent families of this great metropolis[1]."

This fever-period in London corresponds on the whole closely with a series of unhealthy years in Short's tables from the registers of market towns and country parishes, and with high mortalities in the Norwich register. It was not specially a smallpox period, as the last unhealthy year, 1723, was. On the other hand the epidemiographists in Yorkshire, Devonshire and Ireland dwell most upon fevers of the nature of typhus, some of which were due to famine or dearth, and upon "agues."

Market Towns.

Year	Registers examined	No. with excess of deaths	Deaths in same	Births in same
1727	33	19	3606	2441
1728	34	23	4972	2355
1729	36	27	6673	3494
1730	36	16	3445	2529

Norwich.

Year	Buried	Baptized
1728	1417	774
1729	1731	843

Country Parishes.

Year	Registers examined	With excess of burials	Burials in same	Baptisms in same
1726	181	22	542	495
1727	180	55	1368	1091
1728	180	80	2429	1536
1729	178	62	2015	1442
1730	176	39	1302	1022
1731	175	24	700	614

The best epidemiologists of the time were not in London, but at York, Ripon, Plymouth, Cork and Dublin. Leaving the Irish history to a separate chapter, we shall find in the annals of Wintringham, Hillary and Huxham a somewhat detailed account of the fevers which caused the very high mortalities of the years 1727–29, with an occasional glimpse of the circumstances in which the fevers arose. Much of what follows relates to the same nervous, hysteric or "putrid" fever, with or without relapses, that has been described for London. Going back a

---

[1] It is clear that the nervous fever established itself as a distinct type in England in the earlier part of the 18th century, both in medical opinion and in common acceptation: thus Horace Walpole, writing from Arlington Street on 28 January, 1760, says: "I have had a nervous fever these six or seven weeks every night, and have taken bark enough to have made a rind for Daphne: nay, have even stayed at home two days." *Letters of Horace Walpole*, ed. Cunningham, iii. 281.

little, Wintringham says[1] that the continued fevers of 1720 were milder than those of the year before (which were synochus or typhus) and were often languid or nervous, with giddiness, stupor and nervous tremblings, a quick pulse, a whitish tongue, no thirst, and sweats of the head, neck and chest: this fever lasted twenty days or more, and ended in a general sweat. He had mentioned the "languid nervous fevers" first in the years 1716 and 1717, and he mentions them again as mixed with or following the synochus or typhus of 1727–28.

In April, 1727, there were fevers prevalent, remitting and intermitting, but with uncertain paroxysms; in May, a fever with pleuritic pains; in July, a putrid fever in some, but the chief diseases of that month were "remittents and intermittents," which were often attended by cutaneous eruptions, sometimes of dusky colour and dry, at other times full of clear serum; which, "as they depended upon a scorbutic taint, tormented the sick with pruritus." The sick persons in these remittents were for the most part drowsy and stupid, especially during the paroxysm; the fevers were followed by lassitude, debility, languor of spirits and hysteric symptoms.

Hillary[2], who practised at Ripon, not far from Wintringham, at York, records in 1726 the prevalence of remittents and intermittents : "some had exanthematous eruptions towards the latter end of the disease, filled with a clear or yellowish water, which went or dried away without any other inconvenience to the sick but an uneasy itching for a few days"—just as Wintringham had described a miliary fever for 1727. It is also under 1726 that he describes the same drowsy and nervous symptoms of Wintringham's summer fever of 1727 :

"Ancient and weak hysterical people had nervous twitchings and catchings, and were comatous and delirious ; some were very languid, sick and faint, and had tremors ; the young and robust, who had more full pulses, were generally delirious, unless it was prevented or taken off by proper evacuations and cooling medicines. I found blistering to be of very great service in this fever, and the sick were more relieved by it than ever I observed in any other fever whatever. People of lax, weak constitutions were very low and faint, and had frequent, profuse, partial sweatings, which most commonly were cold and clammy." Huxham also, at the other end of England, says that in October and November, 1727, a slow nervous fever attacked not a few ; and under the date of January, 1728, he confirms the Yorkshire experiences of the prevalence of angina.

[1] *Commentar. Nosol.* u. s.
[2] William Hillary, M.D., "An Account of the principal variations of the Weather and the concomitant Epidemical Diseases from 1726 to 1734 at Ripon." App. to *Essay on the Smallpox*, Lond. 1740.

There can be little doubt that England in 1727 was already suffering in a measure from the distress that was acutely felt in Ireland; it was much aggravated by the hard winter of 1728–29[1], but it had begun before that and was doubtless the indirect cause of the great prevalence of sickness. The exports of corn under the bounty system used to bring two or three millions of money into the country in a year. But in 1727 there was a debt balance of 70,757 quarters of wheat imported, and in 1728 the import exceeded the export by 21,322 quarters, the price rising at the same time from 4*s.* to 8*s.* per bushel[2]. Under the year 1727 Hillary says:

"Many of the labouring and poor people, who used a low diet, and were much exposed to the injuries and changes of the weather, died; many of whom probably wanted the necessary assistance of diet and medicines." And after referring, under the winter of 1727–28, to the prevalence of a fatal suffocative angina, which fell, by a kind of metastasis, on the diaphragm or pleura, and sometimes on the peritoneum, he proceeds (p. 16):—

"Nor did any other method, which art could afford, relieve them: insomuch that many of the little country towns and villages were almost stripped of their poor people, not only in the country adjacent to Ripon, but all over the northern parts of the kingdom: indeed I had no certain account of what distempers those who were at a distance died of, but suppose they were the same as those which I have mentioned, which were nearer to us. Bleeding, pectorals with volatiles, and antiphlogistic diluters and blistering, were the most successful. I observed that very few of the richer people, who used a more generous way of living, and were not exposed to the inclemencies of the weather, were seized with any of these diseases at this time....The quartans were very subject to turn into quotidians, and sometimes to continual, in which the sick were frequently delirious."

The Yorkshire accounts by Wintringham and Hillary for the second year of this epidemic period, the year 1728, are very full, as regards the symptoms or types of the fevers; but it would be tedious to cite them at length, and unnecessary to do so unless to answer the not inconceivable cavil that the fevers were not of the nature of typhus in one or other of its forms. The chief point is that the second year, towards Midsummer, brought a fever with the symptoms of *synochus*, and not rarely marked with small red spots like fleabites or with purple petechiae. In the autumn of 1729, Hillary noticed a fever of a slow type, which might go on as long as thirty days and end without a perfect crisis—the nearest approach to enteric fever in any of the descriptions. For the same years, 1727–29, Huxham, of

---

[1] Brand, *History of Newcastle*, ii. 517, says that the magistrates of that town made a collection for the relief of poor housekeepers in the remarkably severe winter of 1728–29, the sum raised being £362. 18*s.*

[2] Tooke, *History of Prices from* 1793 *to* 1837. Introd. chap. p. 40.

Plymouth, describes languid fevers of the "putrid" type, with profuse sweating, followed by typhus of a more spotted type. Like the Yorkshire observer, Huxham mentions also "intermittents" as mixed with the continued fevers.

The great prevalence of these fevers, "intermittents and other fevers," in the west of England in 1728–29 was known to Dr Rutty of Dublin, who speaks especially of "the neighbourhoods of Gloucester and London, and very mortal in the country places, but less in the cities." This is confirmed by Dover:

"I happened to live in Gloucestershire in the years 1728 and 1729, when a very fatal epidemical fever raged to such a degree as to sweep off whole families, nay almost whole villages. I was called to several houses where eight or nine persons were down at a time ; and yet did not so much as lose one patient where I was concerned[1]."

Some of the cases of nervous or putrid fever in the epidemics of 1727–29 appear to have been marked by relapses in the country districts as well as in London. Huxham says under date of April, 1728, that those who had wholly got rid of the putrid fever were exceedingly apt to have relapses. Hillary does not mention relapses until March, 1733, when a fever, with many hysterical symptoms, which succeeded the influenza of that year, relapsed in several, "though seemingly perfectly recovered before." But he seems really to be contrasting relapsing fever and typhus when he points out that, whereas the inflammatory type of fever in the first year of the epidemic (1727) was greatly benefited by enormous phlebotomies, the fever patients in the two seasons following, when the fever was more of the nature of spotted typhus, could not stand the loss of so much blood, or, it might be, the loss of any blood[2]. This was precisely the remark made by Christison and others a century later, when the inflammatory synocha, which often had the relapsing type very marked, changed to the spotted typhus.

[1] *Ancient Physician's Legacy.* Lond. 1733, p. 144.

[2] "In the year 1727," says Hillary, "I ordered several persons to lose 120 to 140 ounces of blood at several times in these inflammatory distempers, with great relief and success ; whereas, in this winter [1728] I met with few, and even the strong and robust, who could bear the loss of above 40 or 50 ounces of blood, at three or four times ; but, in general, most of the sick could not bear bleeding oftener than twice, and then not to exceed 30 or 34 oz. at most, at two or three times ; and especially those who had been afflicted with, and debilitated by, the intermitting fever in the autumn before,—these could not bear blooding oftener than once, or twice at most, and in very small quantities too, though the acuteness of the pain, and the other symptoms in all, seemed at first to indicate much larger evacuations that way; but the first bleeding often sunk the pulse and strength of the patient so much that I durst not repeat it more than once, and in some not at all." Hillary, u. s. p. 26.

From the year 1731 we begin to have annual accounts (soon discontinued) of the reigning maladies in Edinburgh, on the same plan as Wintringham's, Hillary's and Huxham's, with which, indeed, they are sometimes collated and compared[1]. The fevers of Edinburgh and the villages near were as various as those of Plymouth, according to Huxham, and singularly like the latter. Thus, in the winter of 1731–32, there was much worm fever, comatose fever, or convulsive fever among children, but not limited to children, marked by intense pain in the head, raving in some, stupor in others, tremulous movements, leaping of the tendons, and all the other symptoms described by Willis for the fever of 1661, a fatal case of October, 1732, in a boy of ten, recorded by St Clair one of the Edinburgh professors, reading exactly like the cases of Willis already given[2]. St Clair's case, which was soon fatal, had no worms; but in the general accounts, both for the winter of 1731–32 and the autumn of 1732, it is said that many of the younger sort passed worms, both *teretes* and *ascarides*, and recovered, the fatalities among children being, as usual, few. In March and April, 1735, there were again "very irregular fevers of children." Huxham records exactly the same "worm-fever" of children at Plymouth in the spring of 1734—a fever with pains in the head, languor, anxiety, oppression of the breast, vomiting, diarrhoea, and a comatose state (*affectus soporosus*), which attacked the young mostly, and was often attended by the passage of worms. He gives the same account of the seasons as Gilchrist—the years 1734 and 1735 marked by almost continual rains, the country more squalid than had been known for some years[3].

But it is the nervous fever that chiefly engrosses attention both in Scotland and in England. In 1735, Dr Gilchrist, of Dumfries, made it the subject of an essay, returning to the subject a few years after[4]. "As *our* fever," he says, "seems to be peculiar to this age, it is not a little surprising that much more has not been said upon it." He is not sure whether its frequency of late years may not be owing to the manner of living (it was the time of the great drink-craze, which Huxham

[1] *Edin. Med. Essays and Obs.* I–VI. This annual publication was the original of the *Transactions* of the Royal Society of Edinburgh.
[2] *Ibid.* I. 40; II. 27; II. 287 (St Clair's case); IV.
[3] Huxham, *De aere et morbis.*
[4] Ebenezer Gilchrist, M.D., "Essay on Nervous Fevers." *Edin. Med. Essays and Obs.* IV. 347, and VI. (or V. pt. 2), p. 505.

also connects with the reigning maladies) and to a long course of warm, rainy seasons; the winters for some years had been warm and open, and the summers and harvests rainy. It was only the poorer sort and those a degree above them who were subject to this fever; he knew but few instances of it amongst those who lived well, and none amongst wine-drinkers. It was in some insidious in its approach; those who seemed to be in no danger the first days for the most part died. In others the onset was violent, with nausea, heat, thirst and delirium. Among the symptoms were looseness, pains in the belly, local sweating, tickling cough, leaping of the tendons. Sometimes they were in continual cold clammy sweats; at other times profuse sweats ran from them, as if water were sprinkled upon them, the skin feeling death cold.

At Edinburgh, from October, 1735, to February, 1736, the fever became very common, and was often a relapsing fever.

"The sick had generally a low pulse on the first two or three days, with great anxiety and uneasiness, and thin, crude urine. Delirium began about the fourth day, and continued until the fever went off on the seventh day. Sometimes the disease was lengthened to the fourteenth day. The approach of the delirium could always be foretold by the urine becoming more limpid, and without sediment....A large plentiful sweat was the crisis in some. Others were exposed to relapses, which were very frequent, and rather more dangerous than the former fever[1]."

These evidences, beginning with Strother's for London in 1728 and extending to the Edinburgh record of 1735, must suffice to identify true relapsing fever. In the chapter on Irish fevers we shall find clear evidence of relapsing fever in Dublin in 1739, before the great famine had begun.

Huxham's account of the fevers at Plymouth, in Devonshire generally, and in Cornwall about the years 1734–36 is of the first importance. It is highly complex, owing to the prevalence of an affection of the throat, so that one part of the constitution is "anginose fever." This has been dealt with in the chapter on Scarlatina and Diphtheria. Another part was true typhus. In his account of the nervous fever we are introduced, as in the Yorkshire annals, 1726–27, to a phenomenon that was almost distinctive of the low, nervous or putrid fever from about 1750 to 1760 or longer, namely, the eruption of red, or purple, or white watery vesicles, from which it got the name of miliary fever. Huxham's annals are full of this phenomenon about the

[1] *Ibid.* v. pt. 1, p. 30.

years 1734–36[1]. The red pustules, or white pustules, with attendant ill-smelling sweats, are mentioned over and over again. He thought them critical or relieving: "Happy was then the patient who broke out in sweats or in red pustules." These fevers are said to have extended to the country parts of Devonshire, after they had ceased in Plymouth, and to Cornwall in August, 1736. In Plymouth itself the type of fever changed after a time to malignant spotted fever, synochus, or true typhus.

The malignant epidemic seemed to have been brought in by the fleet; it had raged for a long time among the sailors of the fleet lying at Portsmouth, and had destroyed many of them. In March, 1735, it was raging among the lower classes of Plymouth. About the 10th day of the fever, previously marked by various head symptoms, there appeared petechiae, red or purple, or livid or black, up to the size of vibices or blotches, or the eruption might be more minute, like fleabites. A profuse, clammy, stinking sweat, or a most foetid diarrhoea wasted the miserable patients. A black tongue, spasms, hiccup, and livid hands presaged death about the 11th to 14th day. So extensive and rapid was the putrefaction of the bodies that they had to be buried at once or within twenty-four hours. It was fortunate for many to have had a mild sweat and a red miliary eruption about the 4th or 5th day; but for others the course of the disease was attended with great risk. In April the type became worse, and the disease more general. There was rarely now any constriction of the throat. Few pustules broke out; but in place of them there were dusky or purple and black petechiae, and too often livid blotches, with which symptoms very many died both in April and May. In July this contagious fever had decreased much in Plymouth, and in September it was only sporadic there. With a mere reference to Hillary's account of somewhat similar fevers at Ripon in 1734–5 (with profuse sweats, sometimes foetid, great fainting and sinking of spirits, starting of the limbs and beating of the tendons, hiccup for days, etc.[2]) we may pass to a more signal historical event, the great epidemic of fever in 1741–42, of which the Irish part alone has hitherto received sufficient notice[3].

[1] *Obs. de aere et morbis;* also his essay *On Fevers.*
[2] Hillary, App. to *Smallpox*, 1740, pp. 57, 66.
[3] Mr. Lecky (*History of England in the* 18th *Century*, II.), says that the famine and fever of 1740–41, which he describes as an important event in the history of

The epidemic fever of 1741–42.

The harvest of 1739 had been an abundant one, and the export of grain had been large. At Lady-day the price of wheat had been 31*s.* 6*d.* per quarter, and it rose 10*s.* before Lady-day, 1740. An extremely severe winter had intervened, one of the three memorable winters of the 18th century. The autumn-sown wheat was destroyed by the prolonged and intense frost, and the price at Michaelmas, 1740, rose to 56*s.* per quarter, the exportation being at the same time prohibited, but not until every available bushel had been sold to the foreigners. The long cold of the winter of 1739–40 had produced much distress and want in London, Norwich, Edinburgh and other towns. In London the mortality for 1740 rose to a very high figure, 30,811, of which 4003 deaths were from fever and 2725 from smallpox. In mid-winter, 1739–40, coals rose to £3. 10*s.* per chaldron, owing to the navigation of the Thames being closed by ice ; the streets were impassable by snow, there was a "frost-fair" on the Thames, and in other respects a repetition of the events preceding the London typhus of 1685–86. The *Gentleman's Magazine* of January, 1740, tells in verse how the poor were "unable to sustain oppressive want and hunger's urgent pain," and reproaches the rich,—"colder their hearts than snow, and harder than the frost" ; while in its prose columns it announces that "the hearts of the rich have been opened in consideration of the hard fate of the poor[1]." The long, hard winter was followed by the dry spring and hot summer of 1740, during which the sickness (in Ireland at least) was of the dysenteric type. In the autumn of 1740 the epidemic is said to have taken origin both at Plymouth and Bristol from ships arriving with infection among the men—at the former port the king's ships 'Panther' and 'Canterbury,' at the latter a merchant ship. At Plymouth it was certainly raging enormously from June to the end of the year—"febris nautica pestilentialis jam saevit maxime," says Huxham; it continued

---

Ireland, "hardly excited any attention in England." It was severely felt, however, in England ; and if it excited hardly any attention, that must have been because there were so many superior interests which were more engrossing than the state of the poor.

[1] *Gent. Magaz.* x. (1740), 32, 35. Blomefield, for Norwich, says that many there would have perished in the winter of 1739–40 but for help from their richer neighbours.

there all through the first half of 1741, "when it seemed to become lost in a fever of the bilious kind." It was in the dry spring and very hot summer of 1741 that the fever became general over England. Wall says that it appeared at Worcester at the Spring Assizes among a few; at Exeter also it was traced to the gaol delivery; and it was commonly said that the turmoil of the General Election (which resulted in driving Walpole from his long term of power) helped its diffusion. But undoubtedly the great occasion of its universality was a widely felt scarcity. The rise in the price of wheat was small beside the enormous leaps that prices used to take in the medieval period, having been at no time double the average low price of that generation. It was rather the want of employment that made the pinch so sharp in 1741. The weaving towns of the west of England were losing their trade; of " most trades," also, it was said that they were in apparent decay, "except those which supply luxury[1]." Dr Barker, of Sarum, the best medical writer upon the epidemic, says:

"The general poverty which has of late prevailed over a great part of this nation, and particularly amongst the woollen manufacturers in the west, where the fever has raged and still continues to rage with the greatest violence, affords but too great reason to believe that this has been one principal source of the disease[2]."

He explains that the price of wheat had driven the poor to live on bad bread. This is borne out by a letter from Wolverhampton, 27 November, 1741[3]. The writer speaks of the extraordinary havoc made among the poorer sort by the terrible fever that has for some time raged in most parts of England and Ireland. At first it seldom fixed on any but the poor people, and especially such as lived in large towns, workhouses, or prisons. Country people and farmers seemed for the most part exempt from it, "though we have observed it frequently in villages near market towns"; whereas, says the writer, the epidemic fevers of 1727, 1728 and 1729 were first observed to begin among the country people, and to be some time in advancing to large towns. This writer's theory was that the fever was caused by bad bread, and he alleges that

[1] W. Allen, *Landholder's Companion*, 1734. Cited by Tooke.
[2] *An Inquiry into the Nature, Cause and Cure of the present Epidemic Fever...with the difference betwixt Nervous and Inflammatory Fevers, and the Method of treating each*, 1742, p. 54.
[3] John Altree, *Gent. Magaz.* Dec. 1741, p. 655.

horse-beans, pease and coarse unsound barley were almost the only food of the poor. To this a Birmingham surgeon took exception[1]. Great numbers of the poor had, to his knowledge, lived almost entirely upon bean-bread, but had been very little afflicted with the fever. Besides, every practitioner knew that the fever was not confined to the poor. He pointed out that in Wolverhampton, whence the bad-bread theory emanated, the proportion of poor to those in easier circumstances was as six to one, poverty having increased so much by decay of trade that many wanted even the necessaries of life. The Birmingham surgeon was on the whole inclined to the theory of "the ingenious Sydenham, that the disease may be ascribed to a contagious quality in the air, arising from some secret and hidden alterations in the bowels of the earth, passing through the whole atmosphere, or to some malign influence in the heavenly bodies"—these being Sydenham's words as applied to the fever of 1685–6.

Barker, also, draws a parallel between the epidemic of 1741 and that of 1685–86: the Thames was frozen in each of the two winters preceding the respective epidemics, and the spring and summer of 1740 and 1741 were as remarkable for drought and heat as those of 1684 and 1685.

In London the deaths from fever in 1741 reached the enormous figure of 7528, the highest total in the bills of mortality from first to last, while the deaths from all causes were 32,119, in a population of some 700,000, also the highest total from the year of the great plague until the new registration of the whole metropolitan area in 1838. It will be seen from the following table (on p. 81) of the weekly mortalities that the fever-deaths rose greatly in the autumn, but, unlike the old plague, reached a maximum in the winter.

The effects of the epidemic of typhus upon the weaving towns of the west of England, in which the fever lasted, as in London, into the spring of 1742, were seen at their worst in the instance of Tiverton. It was then a town of about 8000 inhabitants, having increased little during the last hundred years. Judged by the burials and baptisms in the parish register it was a more unhealthy place since the extinction of plague than it had been before that. It was mostly a community of weavers, who had not been in prosperous circum-

---

[1] White, *ibid.* 1742, p. 43.

Mortality by Fever in London, 1741—42.

1741 Week ending	Fever	All causes		Week ending	Fever	All causes
				Sept. 1	171	675
March 10	123	660		8	190	691
17	103	564		15	182	760
24	112	624		22	199	748
31	105	573		29	189	733
April 7	123	670		Oct. 6	207	784
14	128	687		13	192	787
21	89	580		20	232	793
28	123	622		27	234	850
May 5	104	495		Nov. 3	250	835
12	141	587		10	228	772
19	129	573		17	182	670
26	153	600		24	214	806
June 2	138	512		Dec. 1	224	768
9	138	483		8	203	748
16	115	536		15	191	761
23	127	494		22	179	775
30	154	513		29	180	702
July 7	149	523	1742			
14	162	551		Jan. 5	221	893
21	130	485		12	184	760
28	151	621		19	184	826
Aug. 4	128	512		26	151	724
11	142	541		Feb. 2	132	675
18	172	636		9	103	533
25	192	665		16	108	675
				25	103	641

Effects of the Epidemic of 1741-42 *on Provincial Towns.*
(*Short's Abstracts of Parish Registers.*)

Year	Registers examined	With burials more than baptisms	Baptisms in the same	Burials in the same
1740	27	6	1409	1940
1741	27	14	3787	6205
1742	26	6	1721	3345

stances for sometime past. In 1735 the town had been burned down, and in 1738 it was the scene of riots. The hard winter of 1739–40 brought acute distress, and in 1741 spotted fever was so prevalent that 636 persons were buried in that year, being 1 in 12 of the inhabitants. At the height of the epidemic ten or eleven funerals were seen at one time in St Peter's churchyard. Its population twenty years after is estimated to have declined by two thousand, and at the end of the 18th century it was a less populous place than at the beginning[1].

[1] Dunsford, *Historical Memorials of Tiverton*. The accounts of the great weaving towns of the South-west are not unpleasing until we come to the time when they

Other parts of the kingdom may be represented by Norwich, Newcastle and Edinburgh. The record of baptisms in Norwich is almost certainly defective; in only two years from 1719 to 1741, is a small excess of baptisms over burials recorded, namely, in 1722 and 1726, while in a third year, 1736, the figures are exactly equal. In 1740 there are 916 baptisms to 1173 burials, and in 1741, 851 baptisms to 1456 burials; while in 1742, owing to an epidemic of smallpox, the deaths rose to 1953, or to more than double the recorded births[1]. The distress was felt most in East Anglia in 1740. Blomefield, who ends his history in that year, says there was much rioting throughout the kingdom, "on the pretence of the scarcity and dearness of grain." At Wisbech Assizes fourteen were found guilty, but were not all executed. In Norfolk two were convicted and executed accordingly. At Norwich the military fired upon the mob and killed seven persons, of whom only one was truly a rioter[2]. It was also in the severe winter of 1739–40 that the distress began in Edinburgh. The mills were stopped by ice and snow, causing a scarcity of meal; the harvest of 1740 was bad, riots took place in October, and granaries were plundered[3]. The deaths from fever were many in 1740, but were nearly doubled in 1741, with a significant accompaniment of fatal dysentery[4]:

Edinburgh Mortalities, 1740–41.
(Population in 1732, estimated at 32,000.)[5]

	1740	1741
All causes	1237	1611
Consumption	278	349
Fever	161	304
Flux	3	36
Smallpox	274	206
Measles	100	112
Chincough	26	101
Convulsions	22	16

were overtaken by decay of work and distress, from about 1720 onwards. The district, says Defoe, was "a rich enclosed country, full of rivers and towns, and infinitely populous, in so much that some of the market towns are equal to cities in bigness, and superior to many of them in numbers of people." Taunton had 1100 looms. Tiverton in the seven years 1700–1706 had 331 marriages, 1116 baptisms, 1175 burials (a slight excess), and an estimated population of 8693, which kept nearly at that level for about twenty years longer (from 1720 to 1726 the marriages were 284, the baptisms 1070 and the burials 1175).

[1] *Gent. Magaz.* XI. (1742), p. 704.
[2] Blomefield, *History of Norfolk*, III. 449.
[3] Arnot, *History of Edinburgh*, 1779, p. 211.
[4] *Gent. Magaz.* 1741, p. 705.   [5] *Edin. Med. Essays and Obs.* I. Art. I.

The last four items are of children's maladies, for which Edinburgh was worse reputed even than London.

At Newcastle the deaths in the register in 1741 were 320 more than in 1740, in which year they were doubtless excessive, as elsewhere. But there is a significant addition: "There have also been buried upwards of 400 upon the Ballast Hills near this town[1]."

The symptoms of the epidemic fever of 1741–42 are described by Barker, of Salisbury, and Wall, of Worcester[2]. It began like a common cold, as was remarked also in Ireland. On the seventh day spots appeared like fleabites on the breast and arms; in some there were broad purple spots like those of scurvy. Miliary eruptions were apt to come out about the eleventh day, especially in women. In most, after the first six or seven days, there was a wonderful propensity to diarrhoea, which might end in dysentery. The cough, which had appeared at the outset, went off about the ninth day, when stupor and delirium came on. Gilchrist, of Dumfries, describes the fever there in November, 1741, as more malignant than the "nervous fever" which he had described in 1735. It came to an end about the fourteenth day; the sick were almost constantly under a coma or raving, and they died of an absolute oppression of the brain; a profuse sweat about the seventh day was followed by an aggravation of all the symptoms[3]. An anonymous writer, dating from Sherborne, uses the occasion to make an onslaught upon blood-letting[4].

---

[1] *Gent. Magaz.* 1742, p. 186.

[2] John Wall, M.D., *Medical Tracts*, Oxford, 1780, p. 337. See also *Obs. on the Epid. Fever of* 1741, 3rd ed., by Daniel Cox, apothecary, with cases.

[3] *Edin. Med. Essays and Obs.* VI. 539.

[4] "And here I cannot but observe how many ignorant conceited coxcombs ride out, under a shew of business, with their lancet in their pocket, and make diseases instead of curing them, drawing their weapon upon every occasion, right or wrong, and upon every complaint cry out, 'Egad! I must have some of your blood,' give the poor wretches a disease they never might have had, drawing the blood and the purse, torment them in this world," etc.—*An Essay on the present Epidemic Fever*, Sherborne, 1741. The practice of blood-letting in continued fevers received a check in the second half of the 18th century, but it was still kept up in inflammatory diseases or injuries. Even in the latter it was freely satirized by the laity. When the surgeon in *Tom Jones* complained bitterly that the wounded hero would not be blooded though he was in a fever, the landlady of the inn answered: "It is an eating fever, then, for he hath devoured two swingeing buttered toasts this morning for breakfast." "Very likely," says the doctor, "I have known people eat in a fever; and it is very easily accounted for; because the acidity occasioned by the febrile matter may stimulate the nerves of the diaphragm, and thereby occasion a craving which will not be easily distinguishable from a natural appetite....Indeed I think the gentleman in a very dangerous way, and, if he is not blooded, I am afraid will die."

6—2

Sanitary Condition of London under George II.

The great epidemic of fever in 1741–42 was the climax of a series of years in London all marked by high fever mortalities. If there had not been something peculiarly favourable to contagious fever in the then state of the capital, it is not likely that a temporary distress caused by a hard winter and a deficient harvest following should have had such effects. This was the time when the population is supposed to have stood still or even declined in London. Drunkenness was so prevalent that the College of Physicians on 19 January, 1726, made a representation on it to the House of Commons through Dr Freind, one of their fellows and member for Launceston:

"We have with concern observed for some years past the fatal effects of the frequent use of several sorts of distilled spirituous liquor upon great numbers of both sexes, rendering them diseased, not fit for business, poor, a burthen to themselves and neighbours, and too often the cause of weak, feeble and distempered children, who must be, instead of an advantage and strength, a charge to their country[1]."

"This state of things," said the College, "doth every year increase." Fielding guessed that a hundred thousand in London lived upon drink alone; six gallons per head of the population per annum is an estimate for this period, against one gallon at present. The enormous duty of 20s. per gallon served only to develope the trade in smuggled Hollands gin and Nantes brandy. In the harvest of 1733 farmers in several parts of Kent were obliged to offer higher wages, although the price of grain was low, and could hardly get hands on any terms, "which is attributed to the great numbers who employ themselves in smuggling along the coast[2]."

The mean annual deaths were never higher in London, not even in plague times over a series of years, the fever deaths keeping pace with the mortality from all causes, and, in the great epidemic of typhus in 1741, making about a fourth part of the whole. The populace lived in a bad atmosphere, physical and moral. As Arbuthnot said in 1733, they "breathed their own steams"; and he works out the following curious sum:

"The perspiration of a man is about $\frac{1}{34}$ of an inch in 24 hours, consequently one inch in 34 days. The surface of the skin of a middle-sized man is about 15 square feet; consequently the surface of the skin of 2904 such

[1] Munk, *Roll of the College of Physicians,* II. 53.
[2] *Gentleman's Magaz.* III. 1733, Sept., p. 492.

men would cover an acre of ground, and the perspir'd matter would cover an acre of ground 1 inch deep in 34 days, which, rarefi'd into air, would make over that acre an atmosphere of the steams of their bodies near 71 foot high." This, he explains, would turn pestiferous unless carried away by the wind; "from whence it may be inferred that the very first consideration in building of cities is to make them open, airy, and well perflated[1]."

In the growth of London from a medieval walled city of some forty or sixty thousand inhabitants to the " great wen " of Cobbett's time, these considerations had been little attended to so far as concerned the quarters of the populace. The Liberties of the City and the out-parishes were covered with aggregates of houses all on the same plan, or rather want of plan. In the medieval period the extramural population built rude shelters against the town walls or in the fosse, if it were dry, or along the side of the ditch. The same process of squatting at length extended farther afield, with more regular building along the sides of the great highways leading from the gates. Queen Elizabeth's proclamation of 1580 was designed to check the growth of London after this irregular fashion; but as neither the original edict nor the numerous copies of it, reissued for near a hundred years, made any provision for an orderly expansion of the capital, these prohibitions had merely the effect of adding to the hugger-mugger of building, " in odd corners and over stables." The outparishes were covered with houses and tenements of all kinds, to which access was got by an endless maze of narrow passages or alleys; regular streets were few in them, and it would appear from the account given by John Stow in 1598 of the parish of Whitechapel that even the old country highway, one of the great roads into Essex and the eastern counties, had been " pestered[2]." The " pestering " of the field lanes in the suburban parishes with poor cottages is Stow's frequent theme[3].

[1] *Effects of Air on Human Bodies*, 1733, pp. 11, 17. His excellent remarks on the need of fresh air in the treatment of fevers, two generations before Lettsom carried out the practice, are at p. 54. The curious calculation above cited was copied by Langrish, and usually passes as his.

[2] " Also without the bars both sides of the street be pestered with cottages and alleys even up to Whitechapel Church, and almost half a mile beyond it, into the common field: all which ought to be open and free for all men. But this common field, I say, being sometime the beauty of this city on that part, is so encroached upon by building of filthy cottages, and with other purprestures, enclosures and laystalls (notwithstanding all proclamations and Acts of Parliament made to the contrary) that in some places it scarce remaineth a sufficient highway for the meeting of carriages and droves of cattle. Much less is there any fair, pleasant or wholesome way for people to walk on foot, which is no small blemish to so famous a city to have so unsavoury and unseemly an entrance or passage thereunto." Stow's *Survey of London*, section on " Suburbs without the Walls."

[3] The line of an old field walk can still be followed from Aldermanbury Postern to Hackney, Goldsmiths' Row being one of the wider sections of it.

The borough of Southwark, as part of the City, may have been better than most: "Then from the Bridge straight towards the south a continual street called Long Southwark, built on both sides with divers lanes and alleys up to St George's Church, and beyond it through Blackman Street towards New Town or Newington"—the mazes of courts and alleys on either side of the Borough Road which may be traced in the maps long after Stow's time. So again in St Olave's parish along the river bank eastwards from London Bridge—"continual building on both sides, with lanes and alleys, up to Battle Bridge, to Horsedown, and towards Rotherhithe." In the Western Liberty, the lanes that had been laid out in Henry VIII.'s time, Shoe Lane, Fetter Lane and Chancery Lane, served as three main arteries to the densely populated area between Fleet Street and Holborn, but for the rest it was reached by a plexus or *rete mirabile* of alleys and courts, notorious even in the 19th century. In like manner Drury Lane and St Martin's Lane were the main arteries between High Holborn and the Strand. One piazza of Covent Garden was a new centre of regular streets, to which the haberdashers and other trades were beginning to remove from the City, for greater room, about 1662. The Seven Dials were a wonder when they were new, about 1694, and had the same intention of openness and regularity as in Wren's unused design for the City after the fire. The great speculative builder of the Restoration was Nicholas Barbone, son of Praise-God Barbones. He built over Red Lion Fields, much to the annoyance of the gentlemen of Gray's Inn[1], and his manner of building may be inferred from the following:

"He was the inventor of this new method of building by casting of ground into streets and small houses, and to augment their number with as little front as possible, and selling the ground to workmen by so much per foot front, and what he could not sell build himself. This has made groundrents high for the sake of mortgaging; and others, following his steps, have refined and improved upon it, and made a superfoetation of houses about London[2]."

In these mazes of alleys, courts, or "rents" the people were for the most part closely packed. Overcrowding had been the rule since the Elizabethan proclamation of 1580, and it seems to have become worse under the Stuarts. On February 24, 1623,

[1] Luttrell's *Diary* 10 June, 1684.
[2] Roger North's "Autobiography," in *Lives of the Norths*, new ed. 3 vols., 1890,

certain householders of Chancery Lane were indicted at the
Middlesex Sessions for subletting, "to the great danger of infectious disease, with plague and other diseases." In May, 1637,
one house was found to contain eleven married couples and
fifteen single persons; another house harboured eighteen lodgers.
In the most crowded parishes the houses had no sufficient
curtilage, standing as they did in alleys and courts. When we
begin to have some sanitary information long after, it appears
that their vaults, or privies, were indoors, at the foot of the
common stair[1]. In 1710, Swift's lodging in Bury Street, St
James's, for which he paid eight shillings a week ("plaguy
deep" he thought), had a "thousand stinks in it," so that he
left it after three months. The House of Commons appears to
have been ill reputed for smells, which were specially remembered
in connexion with the hot summer of the great fever-year 1685[2].

The newer parts of London were built over cesspools,
which were probably more dangerous than the visible nuisances
of the streets satirized by Swift and Gay. There were also
the "intramural" graveyards; of one of these, the Green Ground,
Portugal Street, it was said by Walker, as late as 1839; "The
effluvia from this ground are so offensive that persons living
in the back of Clement's Lane are compelled to keep their
windows closed." But that which helped most of all to make
a foul atmosphere in the houses of the working class, an
atmosphere in which the contagion of fever could thrive, was
the window-tax. It is hardly possible that those who devised
it can have foreseen how detrimental it would be to the public
health; it took nearly a century to realize the simple truth that
it was in effect a tax upon light and air.

[1] Willan, 1801: "The passage filled with putrid excremental or other abominable
effluvia from a vault at the bottom of the staircase." See also Clutterbuck, *Epid.
Fever at present prevailing.* Lond. 1819, p. 60. Ferriar, of Manchester, writing of
the class of houses most apt to harbour the contagion of typhus, says, "Of the new
buildings I have found those most apt to nurse it which are added in a slight manner
to the back part of a row, and exposed to the effluvia of the privies."
[2] C. Davenant to T. Coke, London, 14 Dec. 1700. *Cal. Coke MSS.*, II. 411, "I
heartily commiserate your sad condition to be in the country these bad weeks; but I
fancy you will find Derbyshire more pleasant even in winter than the House of
Commons will be in a summer season. For, though it be now sixteen years ago
[1685], I still bear in memory the evil smells descending from the small apartments
adjoining to the Speaker's Chamber, which came down into the House with irresistible
force when the weather is hot."

The Window-Tax.

Willan, writing of fever in London in 1799, mentions that
even the passages of tenement houses were "kept dark in order
to lessen the window-tax," and the air therefore kept foul[1].
Ferriar, writing of Manchester in the last years of the 18th
century, mentions, among other fever-dens, a large house in an
airy situation which had been built for a poor's-house, but
abandoned: having been let to poor families for a very trifling
rent, many of the windows and the principal entrance were
built up, and the fever then became universal in it[2]. The
Carlisle typhus described by Heysham for 1781 began in a
house near one of the gates, tenanted by five or six very poor
families; they had "blocked up every window to lessen the
burden of the window-tax[3]." John Howard's interest having
been excited in the question of gaol-fever, he noted the effects
of the window-tax not only in prisons but in other houses. The
magistrates of Kent appear to have paid the tax for the gaols
in that county from the county funds; but in most cases the
burden fell on the keepers of the gaols.

"The gaolers," says Howard, "have to pay it; this tempts them to stop
the windows and stifle their prisoners;" and he appends the following note:
"This is also the case in many work-houses and farm-houses, where the
poor and the labourers are lodged in rooms that have no light nor fresh
air; which may be a cause of our peasants not having the healthy ruddy
complexions one used to see so common twenty or thirty years ago. The
difference has often struck me in my various journeys[4]."

Such impressions are known to be often fallacious; but in
the history of the window-tax, which we shall now follow, it will
appear that there was a new law, with increased stringency, in
the years 1746–1748, corresponding to the "twenty or thirty
years ago" of Howard's recollection.

The window-tax was originally a device of the statesmen
of the Revolution "for making good the deficiency of the clipped
money." By the Act of 7 and 8 William and Mary, cap. 18,
taking effect from the 25th March, 1696, every inhabited house
owed duty of two shillings per annum, and, over and above such
duty on all inhabited houses, every dwelling-house with ten
windows owed four shillings per annum, and every house with

[1] *Report on the Diseases in London*, 1796–1800. Lond. 1801.
[2] John Ferriar, M.D., *Medical Histories and Reflections.* London 1810, II. 217.
[3] Heysham, *Jail Fever at Carlisle in 1781.* Lond. 1782, p. 33.
[4] John Howard, *State of the Prisons.*

twenty windows eight shillings. In 1710 houses with from twenty
to thirty windows were made to pay ten shillings, and those with
more than thirty windows twenty shillings. Various devices
were resorted to to check the evasions of bachelors, widows
and others. A farmer had to pay for his servants, recouping
himself from their wages. A house subdivided into tenements
was to count as one; which would have made the tax difficult
to gather except from the landlord. The machinery of collection was a board of commissioners, receivers-general and collectors.

But in the 20th of George II. (1746) the basis of the law
was changed. The tax was levied upon the several windows
of a house, so much per window, so that it fell more decisively
than before upon the tenants of tenement-houses, and not on
the landlords. The two-shillings house duty was continued;
but the window-tax became sixpence per annum for every
window of a house with ten, eleven, twelve, thirteen or fourteen
windows, or lights, ninepence for every window of a house with
fifteen, sixteen, seventeen, eighteen or nineteen windows, and
one shilling for every window of a house with twenty or more
windows. An exemption in the Act in favour of those receiving parochial relief was decided by the law officers of the
Crown not to apply to houses with ten or more windows or
lights, which would have included most tenement-houses; on
the other hand they ruled that hospitals, poor-houses, workhouses,
and infirmaries were not chargeable with the window duty. To
remove doubts and check evasions another Act was made in
21 George II. cap. 10. All skylights, and lights of staircases,
garrets, cellars and passages were to count for the purpose of
the tax; also certain outhouses, but not others, were to count
as part of the main dwelling whether they were contiguous or
not. The 11th paragraph of the Amendment Act shows how
the law had been working in the course of its first year: " No
window or light shall be deemed to be stopped up unless such
window or light shall be stopped up effectually with stone or
brick or plaister upon lath," etc.

This remained the law down to 1803, when a change was
made back to the original basis of rating houses as a whole,
according to the number of their windows, the rate being
considerably raised and fixed according to a schedule. The
tax for tenement houses was at the same time made recoverable

from the landlord. The window-tax thus became a form of the modern house-tax, rated upon windows instead of upon rental, and so lost a great part of its obnoxious character.

The law of 1747–48, which taxed each window separately, and was enforced by a galling and corrupt machinery of commissioners, receivers-general and collectors paid by results, could not fail to work injuriously; for light and air, two of the primary necessaries of life, were in effect taxed. Even rich men appear to have taken pleasure in circumventing the collectors[1]. But it was among the poor, and especially the inhabitants of tenement houses, that the effect was truly disastrous; a tax on the skylights of garrets and on the lights of cellars, staircases and passages, taught the people to dispense with them altogether. Towards the end of the 18th century the grievance became now and then the subject of a pamphlet or a sermon.

Gaol-Fever.

Besides these ordinary things favouring contagious epidemic fever both in town and country, there were two special sources of contagion, the gaols and the fleets and armies. I shall take first the state of the gaols, which has been already indicated in speaking of the window-tax. In the opinion of Lind, a great part of the fever, which was a constant trouble in ships of the navy, came direct from the gaols through the pressing of newly discharged convicts.

The state of the prisons in the first half of the 18th century was certainly not better than Howard found it to be a generation after; it was probably worse, for the administration of justice was more savage. About the beginning of the century, many petitions were made to Parliament by imprisoned debtors, complaining of their treatment, and a Bill was introduced in 1702. Sixty thousand were said to be in prison for debt[2]. On 25

[1] *Notes and Queries*, 4th ser. XII. 346. Jenkinson, who was a Minister under George II., was reputed to have set an example of stopping up windows in his mansion near Croydon:
You e'en shut out the light of day
To save a paltry shilling.
Others had boards painted to look like brickwork, which could be used to cover up windows at pleasure.
[2] Petition, undated, but placed in a collection in the British Museum among broadsides of the years 1696–1700. In 1725 the imprisoned debtors at Liverpool petitioned Parliament for relief, alleging that they were reduced to a starving condi-

February, 1729, the House of Commons appointed a committee "to inquire into the state of the gaols of this Kingdom"; but only two prisons were reported on, the Fleet and the Marshalsea, in London, the inquiries upon these being due to the energy of Oglethorpe, then at the beginning of his useful career. The committee found a disgraceful state of things :—wardens, tip-staffs and turnkeys making their offices so lucrative by extortion that the reversion of them was worth large sums, prisoners abused or neglected if they could not pay, some prisoners kept for years after their term was expired, the penniless crowded three in a bed, or forty in one small room, while some rooms stood empty to await the arrival of a prisoner with a well-filled purse. On the common side of the Fleet Prison, ninety-three prisoners were confined in three wards, having to find their own bedding, or pay a shilling a week, or else sleep on the floor. The "Lyons Den" and women's ward, which contained about eighteen, were very noisome and in very ill repair. Those who were well had to lie on the floor beside the sick. A Portuguese debtor had been kept two months in a damp stinking dungeon over the common sewer and adjoining to the sink and dunghill; he was taken elsewhere on payment of five guineas. In the Marshalsea there were 330 prisoners on the common side, crowded in small rooms.. George's ward, sixteen feet by fourteen and about eight feet high, had never less than thirty-two in it "all last year," and sometimes forty; there was no room for them all to lie down, about one-half of the number sleeping over the others in hammocks; they were locked in from 9 p.m. to 5 a.m. in summer (longer hours in winter), and as they were forced to ease nature within the room, the stench was noisome beyond expression, and it seemed surprising that it had not caused a contagion; several in the heat of summer perished for want of air. Meanwhile the room above was let to a tailor to work in, and no one allowed to lie in it. Unless the prisoners were relieved by their friends, they perished by famine. There was an allowance of pease from a casual donor who concealed his name, and 30 lbs. of beef three times a week from another charitable source. The starving person falls into a kind of hectic, lingers for a month or two and then dies, the right of his corpse to a coroner's inquest being often scandalously re-

tion, having only straw and water at the courtesy of the serjeant. *Commons' Journals,* xx. 375.

fused[1]. The prison scenes in Fielding's *Amelia* are obviously faithful and correct.

Oglethorpe's committee had done some good since they first met at the Marshalsea on 25th March, 1729, not above nine having died from that date to the 14th May; whereas before that a day seldom passed without a death, "and upon the advancing of the spring not less than eight or ten usually died every twenty-four hours." Two of the chief personages concerned were found by a unanimous vote of the House of Commons to have committed high crimes and misdemeanours; but when they were tried before a jury on a charge of felony they were found not guilty.

About a year after these reports to the Commons there was a tragic occurrence among the Judges and the Bar of the Western Circuit during the Lent Assizes of 1730. The Bridewell at Taunton was filled for the occasion of the Assizes with drafts of prisoners from other gaols in Somerset, among whom several from Ilchester were said to have been more than ordinarily noisome. Over a hundred prisoners were tried, of whom eight were sentenced to death (six executed), and seventeen to transportation. As the Assize Court continued its circuit through Devon and Dorset several of its members sickened of the gaol fever and died: Piggot, the high-sheriff, on the 11th April, Sir James Sheppard, serjeant-at-law, on 13th April at Honiton, the crier of the court and two of the Judge's servants at Exeter, the Judge himself, chief baron Pengelly, at Blandford, and serjeant-at-law Rous, on his return to London, whither he had posted from Exeter as soon as he felt ill[2]. It is said that the infection afterwards spread within the town of Taunton, where it arose, "and carried off some hundreds"; but the local histories make no mention of such an epidemic in 1730, and no authority is cited for it[3]. Something of the same kind is

---

[1] *Commons' Journals*, 20 March, 17$\frac{28}{29}$, 14 May, 1729, 24 March, 17$\frac{29}{30}$.
    "Mrs Mary Trapps was prisoner in the Marshalsea and was put to lie in the same bed with two other women, each of which paid 2s. 6d. per week chamber rent; she fell ill and languished for a considerable time; and the last three weeks grew so offensive that the others were hardly able to bear the room; they frequently complained to the turnkeys and officers, and desired to be removed; but all in vain. At last she smelt so strong that the turnkey himself could not bear to come into the room to hear the complaints of her bedfellows; and they were forced to lie with her on the boards, till she died."
[2] *Political State of Great Britain*, XXXIX. April, 1730, pp. 430-431, 448.
[3] *Gent. Magaz.*, XX. 235. This authority is twenty years after the event, the incident having been recalled in 1750, on the occasion of the Old Bailey catastrophe.

believed to have happened at a gaol delivery at Launceston in 1742, but the circumstances are vaguely related, and it does not appear that any prominent personage in the Assize Court died on the occasion[1].

The great instance of a Black Assize in the 18th century, comparable to those of Cambridge, Oxford and Exeter in the 16th[2], was that of the Old Bailey Sessions in London in April, 1750. It has been fully related by Sir Michael Foster, one of the justices of the King's Bench, who had himself been on the bench at the January sessions preceding, and was the intimate friend of Sir Thomas Abney, the presiding judge who lost his life from the contagion of the April sessions[3].

"At the Old Bailey sessions in April, 1750, one Mr Clarke was brought to his trial ; and it being a case of great expectation, the court and all the passages to it were extremely crowded ; the weather too was hotter than is usual at that time of the year[4]. Many people who were in court at this time were sensibly affected with a very noisome smell ; and it appeared soon afterwards, upon an enquiry ordered by the court of aldermen, that the whole prison of Newgate and all the passages leading thence into the court were in a very filthy condition, and had long been so. What made these circumstances to be at all attended to was, that within a week or ten days at most, after the session, many people who were present at Mr Clarke's trial were seized with a fever of the malignant kind ; and few who were seized recovered. The symptoms were much alike in all the patients, and in less than six weeks time the distemper entirely ceased. It was remarked by some, and I mention it because the same remark hath formerly been made on a like occasion [Oxford, 1577], that women were very little affected : I did not hear of more than one woman who took the fever in court, though doubtless many women were there.

"It ought to be remembered that at the time this disaster happened there was no sickness in the gaol more than is common in such places. This circumstance, which distinguisheth this from most of the cases of the like kind which we have heard of, suggesteth a very proper caution : not to presume too far upon the health of the gaol, barely because the gaol-fever is not among the prisoners. For without doubt, if the points of cleanliness and free air have been greatly neglected, the putrid effluvia which the prisoners bring with them in their clothes etc., especially where too many are brought into a crowded court together, may have fatal effects on people who are accustomed to breathe better air ; though the poor wretches, who are in some measure habituated to the fumes of a prison, may not always be sensible of any great inconvenience from them.

"The persons of chief note who were in court at this time and died of the fever were Sir Samuel Pennant, lord mayor for that year, Sir Thomas Abney, one of the justices of the Common Pleas, Charles Clarke, esquire,

[1] Huxham.
[2] See the former volume of this History, pp. 375-386.
[3] *A Report &c. and of other Crown Cases.* By Sir Michael Foster, Knt., some time one of the Judges of the Court of King's Bench.   2nd ed.   London, 1776, p. 74.
[4] The *Gentleman's Magazine* however says (1750, p. 235): "There being a very cold and piercing east wind to attack the sweating persons when they came out of court."

one of the barons of the exchequer, and Sir Daniel Lambert, one of the aldermen of London.   Of less note, a gentleman of the bar, two or three students, one of the under-sheriffs, an officer of Lord Chief Justice Lee, who attended his lordship in court at that time, several of the jury on the Middlesex side, and about forty other persons whom business or curiosity had brought thither."

The same thing was remarked here as at Exeter in 1586 that those who sat on the side of the Court nearest to the dock were most attacked by the infection[1].   When the cases of fever began to occur, after the usual incubation of "a week or ten days," there was much fear of the infection spreading, so that many families, it is said, retired into the country[2].   But Pringle wrote on 24 May, "However fatal it has been since the Sessions, it is highly probable that the calamity will be in a great measure confined to those who were present at the tryal[3];" and Justice Foster gives no hint of anyone having taken the fever who was not present in court.

The tragedy of gaol-fever at the Old Bailey in 1750 secured increased attention to the subject of scientific ventilation.   The great bar to fresh air indoors throughout the 18th century was the window-tax.   It bore particularly hard on prisoners, for the gaolers had to pay the window-tax out of their profits, and they naturally preferred to build up the windows.   Scientific ventilation of gaols was something of a mockery in these circumstances; but it is the business of science to find out cunning contrivances, and ingenious ventilators were devised for Newgate, the leading spirit in this work being the Rev. Dr Hales, rector of a parish near London, and an amateur in physiology at the meetings of the Royal Society.

A ventilating apparatus had been erected at Newgate about a year before the fatal sessions of 1650, but it does not seem to have answered.   It consisted of tubes from the various wards meeting in a great trunk which opened on the roof.   A committee of the Court of Aldermen in October 1750 resolved, after consulting Pringle and Hales, to add a windmill on the leads over the vent, and that was done about two years after. Pringle, who inspected the ventilator on 11 July, 1752, says that

---

[1] See Bancroft, *Essay on the Yellow Fever, with observations concerning febrile contagion etc.* Lond. 1811.

[2] *Gent. Magaz.* 1750, p. 274: "Many families are retired into the country, and near 12,000 houses empty"—an impossible number.

[3] Sir John Pringle, *Observations on the Nature and Cure of the Hospital and Jayl Fever.* Letter to Mead, May 24. London, 1750.

a considerable stream of air of a most offensive smell issued from the vent; and it appeared that no fewer than seven of the eleven carpenters who were working at the alterations on the old ventilator caught gaol-fever (of the petechial kind), which spread among the families of some of them[1]. Pringle and Hales were of opinion that the wards furnished with tubes were less foul than the others; and they claimed, on the evidence of the man who took care of the apparatus, that only one person had died in the gaol in two months, whereas, before the windmill was used, there died six or seven in a week[2]. But Oglethorpe had claimed an improvement of the same kind at the Marshalsea in 1729 merely from having the prisoners saved from hunger; and Lind, who was a most matter-of-fact person, did not think that the ingenious contrivances for ventilation had answered their end[3].

Howard's visitations of the prisons, which began in 1773 and were continued or repeated during several years following, brought to light many instances of epidemic sickness therein, which was nearly always of the nature of gaol-typhus. The following is a list compiled from his various reports, the two or three instances of smallpox infection being given elsewhere.

Wood Street Compter, London. About 100 in it, chiefly debtors. Eleven died in beginning of 1773; since then it has been visited by Dr Lettsom at the request of the aldermen.

Savoy, London. On 15 March, 1776, 119 prisoners. Many sick and dying. Between that date and next visit, 25 May, 1776, the gaol-fever has been caught by many.

Hertford. Inmates range from 20 to 30. In the interval of two visits, the gaol-fever prevailed and carried off seven or eight prisoners and two turnkeys. (The interval probably corresponded to the admission of an unusual number of debtors.)

Chelmsford. Number of inmates varies from 20 to 60, about one-half debtors. A close prison frequently infected with the gaol-distemper.

Dartford, County Bridewell. A small prison. About two years before visit of 1774 there was a bad fever, which affected the keeper and his family and every fresh prisoner. Two died of it.

Horsham, Bridewell. The keeper a widow: her husband dead of the gaol-fever.

[1] One of the cases was that of an apprentice: "Some of the journeymen working in Newgate had forced him to go down into the great trunk of the ventilator in order to bring up a wig which one of them had thrown into it. As the machine was then working, he had been almost suffocated with the stench before they could get him up." Pringle, "Ventilation of Newgate," *Phil. Trans.* 1753, p. 42.

[2] Thomas Stibbs to Sir John Pringle, Jan. 25, 1753. *Ibid.* p. 54.

[3] "Ventilators some years since when first introduced, it was thought, would prove an effectual remedy for and preservative against this infection in jails; great expectations were formed of their benefit, but several years' experience must now have fully shewn that ventilators will not remove infection from a jail." Lind, *Means of Preserving the Health of Seamen in the Royal Navy.* New ed. Lond. 1774, p. 29.

Petworth, Bridewell. Allowance per diem a penny loaf (7½ oz.). Th.
    Draper and Wm. Godfrey committed 6 Jan., 1776 : the former died on
    11 Jan., the other on 16th. Wm. Cox, committed 13 Jan., died 23rd.
    "None of these had the gaol-fever. I do not affirm that these men
    were famished to death ; it was extreme cold weather." After this the
    allowance of bread was doubled, thanks to the Duke of Richmond.
Southwark, the new gaol. Holds up to 90 debtors and felons. "In so
    close a prison I did not wonder to see, in March, 1776, several felons
    sick on the floors." No bedding, nor straw. The Act for preserving
    the health of prisoners is on a painted board.
Aylesbury. About 20 prisoners. First visit Nov., 1773, second Nov., 1774 :
    in the interval six or seven died of the gaol-distemper.
Bedford. About twenty years ago the gaol-fever was in this prison; some
    died there, and many in the town, among whom was Mr Daniel, the
    surgeon who attended the prisoners. The new surgeon changed the
    medicines from sudorifics to bark and cordials; and a sail-ventilator
    being put up the gaol has been free from the fever almost ever since.
    (This was the gaol which is often said to have started Howard on his
    inquiries when he was High Sheriff.)
Warwick. Holds up to fifty-seven. The late gaoler died in 1772 of the
    gaol-distemper, and so did some of his prisoners. No water then ;
    plenty now.
Southwell, Bridewell. A small prison. A few years ago seven died here of
    the gaol-fever within two years.
Worcester. Has a ventilator. Mr Hallward the surgeon caught the gaol-
    fever some years ago, and has ever since been fearful of going into the
    dungeon ; when any felon is sick, he orders him to be brought out.
Shrewsbury. Gaol-fever has prevailed here more than once of late years.
Monmouth. At first visit in 1774, they had the gaol-fever, of which died the
    gaoler, several of his prisoners, and some of their friends.
Usk (Monmouth) Bridewell. The keeper's wife said that many years ago
    the prison was crowded, and that herself, her father who was then
    keeper, and many others of the family had the gaol-fever, three of whom,
    and several of the prisoners, died of it.
Gloucester, the Castle. Many prisoners died here in 1773 ; and always
    except at Howard's last visit, he saw some sick in this gaol. A large
    dunghill near the stone steps. The prisoners miserable objects : Mr
    Raikes and others took pity on them.
Winchester. The former destructive dungeon was down eleven steps, and
    darker than the present. Mr Lipscomb said that more than twenty
    prisoners had died in it of the gaol-fever in one year, and that the
    surgeon before him had died of it.
Liverpool. Holds about sixty, offensive, crowded. Howard in March, 1774,
    told the keeper his prisoners were in danger of the gaol-fever. Between
    that date and Nov., 1775, twenty-eight had been ill of it at one time.
Chester, the Castle. Dungeon used to imprison military deserters. Two
    of them brought by a sergeant and two men to Worcester, of which
    party three died a few days after they came to their quarters. (For fever
    in this prison in 1716 see the text, p. 60.)
Cowbridge. The keeper said, on 19 August, 1774, that many had died of
    the gaol-fever, among them a man and a woman a year before, at which
    time himself and daughter were ill of it.
Cambridge, the Town Bridewell. In the spring of 1779, seventeen women
    were confined in the daytime, and some of them at night, in the
    workroom, which has no fireplace or sewer. This made it extremely
    offensive, and occasioned a fever or sickness among them, which so
    alarmed the Vice-Chancellor that he ordered all of them to be discharged.
    Two or three of them died within a few days.

Exeter, the County Bridewell. Between first visit in 1775 and next on 5 Feb., 1779, the surgeon and two or three prisoners have died of the gaol-fever. In 1755 a prisoner discharged from the gaol went home to Axminster, and infected his family, of whom two died, and many others in that town afterwards.

Exeter, the High Gaol for felons. Mr Bull, the surgeon, stated that he was by contract excused from attending in the dungeons any prisoners that should have the gaol-fever.

Winchester, Bridewell. Close and small. Receives many prisoners from other gaols at Quarter Sessions. It has been fatal to vast numbers. The misery of the prisoners induced the Duke of Chandos to send them for some years 30 lbs. of beef and 2 gallon loaves a week.

Devizes, Bridewell. Two or three years ago the gaol-fever carried off many. An infirmary added since then.

Marlborough. The rooms offensive. Saw one dying on the floor of the gaol-fever. One had died just before, and another soon after his discharge.

Launceston. Small, with offensive dungeons. No windows, chimneys, or drains. No water. Damp earthen floor. Those who serve there often catch the gaol-fever. At first visit, found the keeper, his assistant and all the prisoners but one sick of it (on 19 Feb., 1774, eleven felons in it). Heard that, a few years before, many prisoners had died of it, and the keeper and his wife in one night. A woman confined three years by the Ecclesiastical Court had three children born in the gaol.

Bodmin, Bridewell. Much out of repair. The night rooms are two garrets with small close-glazed skylight 17 in. × 12 in. A few years ago the gaol-fever was very fatal, not only in the prison but also in the town.

Taunton, Bridewell. Six years ago, when there was no infirmary provided, the gaol-fever spread over the whole prison, so that eight died out of nineteen prisoners.

Shepton Mallet. Men's night room close, with small window. So unhealthy some years ago that the keeper buried three or four in a week.

Thirsk. Prisoners had the gaol-fever not long ago.

Carlisle. During the gaol-fever which some years ago carried off many of the prisoners, Mr Farish, the chaplain, visited the sick every day.

I shall add some medical experiences of gaol-fever in London from the notes of Lettsom[1] :—

May, 1773. A person released from Newgate "in a malignant or jail-fever" was brought into a house in a court off Long Lane, Aldersgate Street; soon after which fourteen persons in the same confined court were attacked with a similar fever: one died before Lettsom was called in, one was sent to hospital, eleven attended by him all recovered, though with difficulty. Two deaths in Wood Street Compter: 1. Rowell, an industrious, sober workman, who had supported for many years a wife and three children; some of these having been lately sick, he fell behind with his rent, a little over three guineas; he offered all he had (more than enough) to the landlord, but the latter preferred to throw the man and his family into the Compter, where Rowell died of fever. 2. Russell, once a reputable tradesman on Ludgate Hill, fell into a debt of under three guineas, sent to the Compter with his wife and five children, took fever and died; attended in his sickness in a bare room by his eldest daughter, elegant and refined, aged seventeen; his son, aged fourteen, took the fever and recovered.

[1] J. C. Lettsom, M.D., *Medical Memoirs of the General Dispensary in London,* 1773-4. Lond. 1774.

There was one Black Assize at this period, at Dublin in April 1776. A criminal, brought into the Court of Sessions without cleansing, infected the court and alarmed the whole city. Among others who died of the contagion were Fielding Ould, High Sheriff, the counsellors Derby, Palmer, Spring and Ridge, Mr Caldwell, Messrs Bolton and Eriven, and several attorneys and others whose business it was to attend the court[1].

There were two notorious outbreaks of malignant fever among foreign prisoners of war, one in 1761[2] and another in 1780[3], the first among French and Spaniards at Winchester and Portchester, the second among Spaniards at Winchester.

Howard found so little typhus in the gaols in his later visits that it seemed as if banished for good. But it was heard of frequently about 1780–85—at Maidstone, at Aylesbury, at Worcester, costing the lives of some of the visiting physicians.

Circumstances of severe and mild Typhus.

The circumstances of the gaol distemper bring out one grand character of typhus which will have to be stated formally before we go farther. Ordinary domestic typhus was not a very fatal disease. Haygarth says that of 285 attacked by it in the poorer quarters of Chester in the autumn of 1774, only twenty-eight died. Ferriar, in Manchester, had sometimes an even more favourable experience than that: "The mortality of the epidemic was not great,...out of the first ninety patients whom I attended, only two died." This was before the House of Recovery was opened; so that the low mortality was of typhus in the homes of the people.

The fever was often an insidious languishing, without great heat, and marked most by tossing and wakefulness, which might pass into delirium; when it went through the members of a family or the inmates of a house, there would be some cases concerning which it was hard to say whether they were cases of typhus or not. Misery and starvation brought it on, and often it was itself but a degree of misery and starvation. "I have found," says Ferriar, "that for three or four days before the

---

[1] *Gent. Magaz.* 1776, April 22. p. 187.
[2] Lind, *Two Papers on Fevers and Infection.* Lond. 1763. pp. 90, 106. Many cases had buboes both in the groins and the armpits.
[3] Carmichael Smyth, *Description of the Jail Distemper among Spanish Prisoners at Winchester* in 1780. Lond. 1795.

appearance of typhus in a family consisting of several children, they had subsisted on little more than cold water." "It has been observed," says Langrish, "that those who have died of hunger and thirst, as at sieges and at sea, etc., have always died delirious and feverish." The fever was on the whole a distinct episode, but in many cases it had no marked crisis. "Those women who recovered," says Ferriar, "were commonly affected with hysterical symptoms after the fever disappeared;" and again : "Fevers often terminate in hysterical disorders, especially in women; men, too, are sometimes hysterically inclined upon recovering from typhus, for they experience a capricious disposition to laugh or cry, and a degree of the globus hystericus." These were probably the more case-hardened people, inured to their circumstances, their healthy appetite dulled by the practice of fasting or "clemming," or by opium, and their blood accustomed to be renovated by foul air. If the limit of subsistence be approached gradually, life may be sustained thereat without any sharp crisis of fever, or with only such an interlude of fever as differs but little from a habit of body unnamed in the nosology.

The worst kind of typhus, often attended with delirium, crying and raving, intolerable pains in the head, and livid spots on the skin, ending fatally perhaps in two or three days, or after a longer respite of stupor or waking insensibility, was commonly the typhus of those not accustomed to the minimum of wellbeing —the typhus of hardy felons newly thrown into gaol, of soldiers in a campaign crowded into a hospital after a season in the open air, of sailors on board ship mixing with newly pressed men having the prison atmosphere clinging to them, of judges, counsel, officials of the court and gentlemen of the grand jury brought into the same atmosphere with prisoners at a gaol-delivery, of the wife and children of a discharged prisoner returned to his home, of the gaol-keeper, gaol-chaplain, or gaol-doctor, of the religious and charitable who visited in poor localities even where no fever was known to be, and most of all of country people who crowded to the towns in search of work or of higher wages or of a more exciting life.

It was in these circumstances that the most fatal infections of typhus took place. Such extraordinary malignancy of typhus happened often when the type of sickness (if indeed there was definite disease at all) among the originally ailing failed to account for it; it was the great disparity of condition that accounted for it. There were, however, more special occasions when a higher degree of malignancy than ordinary was bred or cultivated among the classes at large who were habitually liable to typhus. But even the old pestilential spotted fever which used to precede, accompany, and follow the plague itself, was fatal to a comparatively small proportion of all who had it. Thus, towards the end of the great London plague of 1625, on 18th October, Sir John Coke writes to Lord Brooke: "In London now the tenth person dieth not of those that are sick, and generally the plague seems changed into an ague[1]." One in ten is probably too small a fatality for the old pestilential fever; but that is the usually accepted proportion of deaths to attacks in the typhus fever of later times. The rate of fatality is got, naturally, by striking an average. But in truth an aggregate of typhus cases, however homogeneous in conventional symptoms or type-characters, was not always really homogeneous. We have seen that ninety cases of typhus could occur in the slums of Manchester with only two deaths. On the other hand there were outbreaks of gaol-fever in which half or more of all that were attacked died; and I suspect that the average fatality in typhus of one in ten was often brought up by an admixture of cases of healthy and well-conditioned people who caught a much more malignant type of fever from their contact with those inured to misery. To strike an average is in many instances a convenience and a help to the apprehension of a truth; but for the average to be instructive, the members of the aggregate must be more or less comparable in their circumstances. It has been truly said that there is no common measure between Lazarus and Dives as regards their subjective views of things; it is not a little strange to find that they are just as incommensurable in their risk of dying from the infection of typhus fever. The rule seems to be that the degree of acuteness or violence of an attack of typhus was inversely as the habitual poor condition of the victim. In adducing evidence of the tragic nature of typhus infection conveyed across the gulf of misery to the other side, I shall endeavour to keep strictly to the scientific facts, leaving the moral, if there be a moral (and it is not always obvious), to point itself.

Let us take first the common case of country-bred people

[1] *Cal. Coke MSS.* Hist. MSS. Commiss. i. 218.

migrating to the towns. Any lodging in a crowded centre
of industry and trade would be high-rented compared with the
country cottage which they had left, and they would naturally
gravitate to the slums of the city.

"Great numbers of the labouring poor," says Ferriar of Manchester,
"who are tempted by the prospect of large wages to flock into the principal
manufacturing towns, become diseased by getting into dirty infected houses
on their arrival. Others waste their small stock of money without procuring
employment, and sink under the pressure of want and despair....The number
of such victims sacrificed to the present abuses is incredible." And again:

"It must be observed that persons newly arrived from the country are
most liable to suffer from these causes, and as they are often taken ill
within a few days after entering an infected house, there arises a double
injury to the town, from the loss of their labour, and the expense of supporting them in their illness. A great number of the home-patients of the
Infirmary are of this description. The horror of these houses cannot easily
be described; a lodger fresh from the country often lies down in a bed
filled with infection by its last tenant, or from which the corpse of a victim
to fever has only been removed a few hours before[1]."

Two instances from the same author will show the severe
type of the fever.

The tenant of a house in Manchester, who was herself ill of typhus along
with her three children, took in a lodger, a girl named Jane Jones, fresh
from the country. The lodger fell ill, but the fact was kept concealed from
the visiting physician until her screams discovered her: "She was found
delirious, with a black fur on the lips and teeth, her cheeks extremely
flushed, and her pulse low, creeping, and scarcely to be counted." Treatment was of no use; she "passed whole nights in shrieking," and in her
extremity, she was saved, as Ferriar believed, by affusions of cold water.
Another case, exactly parallel, proved fatal in three days:

"In 1792 I had two patients ill of typhus in an infected lodging-house.
I desired that they might be washed with cold water; and a healthy, ruddy
young woman of the neighbourhood undertook the office. Though apparently in perfect health before she went into the sick chamber, she
complained of the intolerable smell of the patients, and said she felt a
head-ache when she came down stairs. She sickened, and died of the fever
in three days[2]."

These are instances of country-bred people, plunging
abruptly into the fever-dens of cities and catching a typhus

---

[1] *Med. Hist. and Reflect.* ut infra.

[2] The following case, which happened five or six years ago, shows disparity of
conditions in a twofold aspect. A lady from a city in the north of Scotland travelled
direct to Switzerland to reside for a few weeks at one of the hotels in the High Alps.
Within an hour or two of the end of her journey she began to feel ill, and was
confined to her room from the time she entered the hotel. An English physician
diagnosed the effects of the sun; the German doctor of the place, from his reading
only, diagnosed typhus fever, which proved to be right, the patient dying with the
most pronounced signs of malignant typhus. An explanation of the mystery was soon
forthcoming. The lady had been a district visitor in an old and poor part of the
Scotch city; she had, in particular, visited in a certain tenement-house in a court,
from which half-a-dozen persons had been admitted to the Infirmary with typhus (an
unusual event) at the very time when she was ill of it on the Swiss mountain.

severe in the direct ratio of their ruddy, healthy condition. Another class of cases is that of persons carrying the atmosphere of a gaol into the company of healthy and otherwise favourably situated people. Howard gives a case: at Axminster a prisoner discharged from Exeter gaol in 1755 infected his family with the gaol-distemper, of which two of them died, and many others in that town. The best illustrations of the greater severity and fatality of typhus among the well-to-do come from Ireland, in times of famine, and will be found in another chapter. But it may be said here, so that this point in the natural history of typhus fever may not be suspected of exaggeration, that the enormously greater fatality of typhus (of course, in a smaller number of cases) among the richer classes in the Irish famines, who had exposed themselves in the work of administration, of justice, or of charity, rests upon the unimpeachable authority of such men as Graves, and upon the concurrent evidence of many.

Ship-Fever.

The prevalence of fevers in ships of war and transports from the Restoration onwards can be learned but imperfectly, and learned at all only with much trouble. Sir Gilbert Blane, who was not wanting in aptitude and had the archives of the Navy Office at his service, goes no farther back than 1779, from which date an account was kept of the causes of death in the naval hospitals. But the deaths on board ships of the fleet were not systematically recorded until 1811, when the Board of Admiralty instructed all commanders of ships of war to send to the Naval Office an annual account of all the deaths of men on board[1]. The sources of information for earlier periods are more casual.

The war with France, which dated from the accession of William III. and continued until the Peace of Ryswick in 1697, led to numerous conflicts with French and Spaniards in the West Indies, and to naval expeditions year after year. The loss of life from sickness in the British ships for a few years at the end of the century was such as can hardly be realized by us. Some part of it happened on the outward voyages, but by far the greater part of it was from the poison of yellow fever

---

[1] Blane, *Select Dissertations.* London, 1822, p. 1.

which had entered the ships in the anchorages of West Indian colonies. It was probably to that cause that the enormous mortality in the fleet under Sir Francis Wheeler was owing. After some ineffective operations against the French in the Windward Islands in the winter of 1693–4, he sailed for North America with the intention of attacking Quebec. This he failed to do, having sailed from Boston for home on the 3rd of August without entering the St Lawrence. The reason of the failure was probably the extraordinary fatality which Cotton Mather, of Boston, professes to have heard from the admiral himself, namely, that he lost by a malignant fever on the passage from Barbados to Boston 1300 sailors out of 2100, and 1800 soldiers out of 2400[1].

Another instance comes from Carlisle Bay, Barbados. The slave ship 'Hannibal' arrived there in November, 1694, during a disastrous epidemic of yellow fever. Phillips, the captain, whose journal of the voyage is published[2], had great difficulty in saving his crew from being pressed into the king's ships, which were short of men owing to the yellow fever. Captain Sherman, of the 'Tiger,' who convoyed the 'Hannibal' and other merchantmen back to England in April, 1695, told Phillips that he buried six hundred men out of his ship during the two years that he lay at Barbados, though his complement was but 220, "still pressing men out of the merchant ships that came in, to recruit his number in the room of those that died daily."

These and other similar experiences of yellow fever in the West Indies, which might be collected from the naval history, do not come properly into this chapter; and I pass from them to ship-fever proper, having indicated how much of the loss of life abroad was due to yellow fever.

Some light is thrown upon the state of health on board ships of war on the home station by Dr William Cockburn, physician to the fleet, afterwards the friend of Swift, who calls him "honest Dr Cockburn." He had a secret remedy for dysentery, which he succeeded in getting adopted by the Admiralty, greatly to his own emolument for many years after. Dining on

---

[1] Mather's *Magnalia*. 2 vols. Hartford, 1853, i. 226 "Life of Sir William Phipps." " Whereof there died, ere they could reach Boston, as I was told by Sir Francis Wheeler himself ['but a few months ago'], no less than 1300 sailors out of 21, and no less than 1800 soldiers out of 24." He had brought 1800 troops with him from England to Barbados in transports.

[2] Churchill's Collection, vi. 173.

board one of the ships at Portsmouth, in 1696, with Lord Berkeley of Stratton, he brought up the subject of his electuary, and arranged for a public trial of it next day on board the 'Sandwich.' An uncertain number, which looks to have been about seven in Cockburn's own account, but became seventy in the pamphlet which advertised the electuary after his death, were available for the trial and were speedily cured. Cockburn's three essays on the health of seamen[1] leave no doubt as to the extensive prevalence of scurvy and the causes thereof; while his references to " malignant fever," although they are, as usual, brought in to illustrate some doctrinal or theoretical point, give colour to the belief that ship-typhus may have been as common then as we know it to have been in the ships at Portsmouth and Plymouth, on the more direct testimony of Huxham in 1736, and of Lind twenty years later.

A naval surgeon of the time of William III. and Anne, was induced by his enthusiasm for blood-letting in fevers to record some of his experiences on board ship[2]. It was usually the lustiest, both of the young, strong and healthy people, and likewise of the elder sort, that died of fevers, the symptoms which proved so mortal having been delirium, phrenitis, coma or stupor, whether they occurred in the συνόχοι (of Sydenham) or in the συνεχεῖς (of the same author):

"I had observed in a ship of war whose complement was near 500, in a Mediterranean voyage in the year 1694, where we lost about 90 or 100 men, mostly by fevers, that those who died were commonly the young, but almost always the strongest, lustiest, handsomest persons, and that two or three escaped by means of such [natural] haemorrhagies, which were five or six pounds of blood"—the point being that the amount of blood drawn by phlebotomy should be in proportion to the robustness and body-weight of the patient.

In 1703 and 1704 he was surgeon to two of Her Majesty's ships "where a delirium, stupor and phrenitis" were found as symptoms of the fevers. In the summer of 1704, cruising in the latitudes of Portugal and Spain, the men brought on board from Lisbon unripe lemons with which they made great quantities of punch. This was the evident cause of a cholera morbus and dysentery: "after this we had a pretty many taken with the

---

[1] W. Cockburn, M.D. *An Account of the Nature, Causes, Symptoms and Cure of the Distempers that are incident to Seafaring People.* 3 Parts. London, 1696-97.

[2] J. White, M.D. *De recta Sanguinis Missione, or, New and Exact Observations of Fevers, in which Letting of Blood is shew'd to be the true and solid Basis of their Cure, &c.* London, 1712. His chief point, that the strongest and lustiest were most obnoxious to malignant fevers, had been urged by Cockburn in 1696.

synochus putris, and some with the *causus*" [malignant fever]. Most of these fevers went off by a crisis in sweating, "which was so large I had good reason to believe it judicatory." In several the fevers left on the 9th, 10th or 11th day, and in almost all by the 14th. "About the latter end of July, and in August, there were many taken with a delirium and stupor or coma, and some with the phrenitis in their fever." Among the symptoms was one which we find described for fevers on board ship on the West Coast of Africa at the same time— "soreness all over as if from blows with a cane," a symptom afterwards associated with dengue. "Sometimes the bones (as they term it) don't pain them much." In some cases there were petechial spots as well as a stupor. In the month of August "the fevers with a stupor and phrenitis" came on apace. The treatment was to take ten ounces of blood every day from the second to the eighth day of the fever, to give tartar emetic in five-grain doses at the outset, and to administer cathartic glysters in the second half of the fever. "Seeing the lustiest men now ran no more hazard of their lives than any other who were usually taken with this fever, nor indeed so much, in the beginning of September I resolved, after all the phlebotomy was done in these fevers, to try the cathartic sooner." Many of these who had accustomed themselves to the liberal use of spirituous liquors miscarried in the phrenitis.

White left the navy in 1704 and settled in practice at Lisbon, where he saw much fever. He had seen epidemics break out in British ships of war at anchor in the Tagus, crowded with men and prisoners. One case he mentions in a Lisbon woman, with continual synochus, stupor, and petechiae on the fifth day: "This was contagious, for she got it by going often to assist a gunner of a man-of-war, who came to her house with this distemper upon him : for many at the same time on board that ship were sick of that disease." Among the causes of fever on board ship he mentions the effluvia of the bilge-water.

Exposed to these emanations were "a multitude of people breathing and constantly perspiring in a close place, such as a ship's *allop* or lower deck next the hould, where is the entry to a certain vacant space near the ship's center, which leadeth to the bottom, for gathering all the water together which the ship draweth by leakage, and is called the well. Several times there is occasion for some people to go down to examine the quantity of the water, and in some ships to bore an augur hole to let in as much as will preserve a good air. I have often known two or three men killed at a time, as it is said; and the reason may be understood from what I said of the general effects of that fluid in ordinary fever [he is now writing on heat apoplexy], where there is not above two or three inches, but just as much as may make a surface, almost equal to the square of the well, of stagnant salt water which had been a long while in gathering; and the air over the whole *allop* extremely rarified, and here not at all ventilated[1]."

We owe it to the accident of the celebrated Dr Freind having accompanied Lord Peterborough's expedition to Spain in 1705 that some account has been preserved of the sickness among the troops ashore and afloat[2].

The expedition of some 8000 men being then in its second year, fever and dysentery were by far the most common diseases, so common that "we can hardly turn, whether at sea or in camp, without finding them as if our inseparable companions and as if domesticated among us." In the summer of the previous year there had been much fever both in the ships of the fleet and in the camp before Barcelona: "It was of the continual kind, though it usually remitted in the day time, and seemed to approach nearly to the stationary one which Sydenham has described in the years 1685 and 1686." He then gives symptoms, which were on the whole those of the hospital fever to be afterwards described from Pringle's medical account of the campaigns in 1743–48. Persons of a robust habit were affected more than others, and more severely, and carried off sooner. The others were generally taken away by a lingering death. "Some, when the fever seemed to have been wholly gone off lay four or five days without pain or sickness, though weak;

---

[1] Lind (*Two Papers on Fevers and Infection*, London, 1763, p. 113) gives an instance where the poisonous effluvia of the ship's well did not spread through the 'tween decks: "The following accident happened lately [written in 1761] in the Bay of Biscay. In a ship of 60 guns, by the carpenter's neglecting to turn the cock that freshens the bilge-water, which had not been pumped out for some time, a large scum, as is usual, or a thick tough film was collected a-top of it. The first man who went down to break this scum in order to pump out the bilge-water was immediately suffocated. The second suffered an instantaneous death in like manner. And three others, who successively attempted the same business, narrowly escaped with life: one of whom has never since perfectly recovered his health. Yet that ship was at all times, both before and after this accident, remarkably healthy." It was the contention of Renwick, a naval surgeon who wrote in 1794, that it was the stirring of the bilge-water in being discharged from the ship's well, or the adding of fresh water to the foul, that caused the offensive emanations. "Hence the first cause of febrile sickness in all ships recently commissioned." Renwick made so much of the foul bilge-water as a cause that he thought the fevers ought to be termed "bilge-fevers." *Letter to the Critical Reviewer*, p. 42.

[2] These particulars are not given in Freind's special work on Peterborough's campaign, which deals only with the military and political history, but in his *Nine Commentaries on Fever* (Engl. ed. by Dale, London, 1730), and in a Latin letter to Cockburn, dated Barcelona, 9 Sept. 1706, which was first printed in *Several Cases in Physic*. By Pierce Dod, M.D. London, 1746.

afterwards being suddenly seized with convulsions of the nerves they in a short time expired".—perhaps the phenomenon of relapse, which Lind recorded for ship-fever fifty years after and was seen among the troops landed from Corunna in 1809. In some few the parotids, or abscesses formed about the groin, carried off the disease.

He then gives the case of a lieutenant on board the 'Barfleur.' At first he was restless and delirious; on the 7th and 8th days he had *subsultus tendinum;* on the 8th day his tongue was sometimes fixed, and his eyes sparkled; on the 9th day, he was wholly deprived of his understanding; he pulled off the fringe of the bed and plucked the flocks ; when he had before faultered in his speech, he was sometimes seized with hiccough. But on the 10th day, after 12 oz. of blood had been drawn from the jugular vein, his delirium went off on a sudden, and he began to mend, making a perfect recovery.

Until the middle of the 18th century there are few other notices of ship-fever, but it is probable that Huxham's accounts of a very malignant typhus among the crews of ships of war at Plymouth in 1735 (as well as at Portsmouth according to report), and again in 1741, are to be taken as samples of what might have been recorded on many occasions[1].

Fever and Dysentery of Campaigns : War Typhus, 1742–63.

The war in Ireland after the accession of William III. produced two remarkable instances of war-sickness, which are fully given in another chapter. The campaigns of Marlborough against the armies of Louis XIV., from 1704 to the Treaty of Utrecht in 1713, appear to have found no historian from the medical side, nor does the duke refer to these matters in his dispatches or letters, beyond a remark in a letter to his wife from near Munich, 30 July, 1704, a fortnight before the battle

---

[1] Smollett joined the 'Cumberland' as surgeon's mate in 1740, before she sailed with the fleet sent out under Vernon and others to Carthagena. His account in *Roderick Random* of the sick-bay of the 'Thunder' as she lay at the Nore is doubtless veracious : " When I observed the situation of the patients, I was much less surprised that people should die on board, than that any sick person should recover. Here I saw about fifty miserable distempered wretches, suspended in rows, so huddled one upon another that not more than fourteen inches space was allowed for each with his bed and bedding ; and deprived of the light of the day, as well as of fresh air ; breathing nothing but a noisome atmosphere of the morbid steams exhaling from their own excrements and diseased bodies, devoured with vermin hatched in the filth that surrounded them, and destitute of every convenience necessary for people in that helpless condition." Chap. xxv. He wrote a separate account of the fatal Carthagena expedition in a compendium of voyages.

of Blenheim : " There having been no war in this country for above sixty years, these towns and villages are so clean that you would be pleased with them[1]."

The war of 1742–48, in which George II. joined Austria against France, produced the first good accounts of war typhus, on land and on board ship, in the writings of Pringle[2]. After the battle of Dettingen, 27 June, 1743, the men were exposed all night in the wet fields ; during the next eight days five hundred of them were attacked with dysentery, and in a few weeks near half the army were either ill of it or had recovered from it. The dysentery continued all July and part of August, while the army lay at Hanau. The village of Feckenheim, a league from the camp, was used as a hospital, some 1500 being quartered in it, most of them ill at first of dysentery. The latrines appear to have been ill designed and badly kept. " A malignant fever began among the men, from which few escaped: for however mild or bad soever the flux was for which the person was sent to hospital, this fever almost surely supervened. The petechial spots, blotches, parotids, frequent mortifications, and the great mortality, characterized a pestilential malignity: in this it was worse than the true plague....Of 14 mates employed about the hospital five died; and, excepting one or two, all the rest had been ill and in danger. The hospital lost nearly half of the patients; but the inhabitants of the village of Feckenheim, where the sick were, having first received the bloody flux, and afterwards the fever by contagion, were almost utterly destroyed[3]." The survivors from the sick troops in Feckenheim were removed to Neuwied, where they were relieved ; " but the rest, who were mixed with them, caught the infection." The mixed troops were sent still down the Rhine in bilanders, during which voyage " the fever became so virulent that above half the number died in the boats, and many of the remnant soon after their arrival." A parcel of tents sent in these bilanders to the Low Countries were given to a Ghent tradesman to refit; he employed twenty-three journeymen upon them, " but these unhappy men were quickly seized with

---

[1] Coxe's *Life of Marlborough*. Bohn's ed. I. 183.
[2] Grainger's essay, *Historia febris anomalae Bataviae annorum*, 1746, 1747, 1748, *etc.* Edin. 1753, is chiefly occupied with an anomalous "intermittent" or "remittent" fever with miliary eruption, and with dysentery.
[3] For a full discussion of the relation of dysentery to typhus, see Virchow, "Kriegstypus und Ruhr." *Virchow's Archiv*, Bd. LII. (1871), p. 1.

this fever, whereof seventeen died." They had no other communication with the infected but through the tents.

"These," says Pringle, "are instances of high malignity. The common course of the infection is slow, and only catching to those constantly confined to the bad air. Sometimes one will have this fever about him for several days before it confines him to his bed; others I have known complain for weeks of the same symptoms without any regular fever at all; and some, after leaving the infectious place, have afterwards fallen ill of it[1]."

After the battle of Fontenoy on 11 May, 1745, the army was in good health: "the smallpox was the only new disease; it came with the recruits from England, but did not spread; and indeed we have never known it of any consequence in the field."

On the Jacobite rebellion breaking out in Scotland later in the same year, some of the returning troops were ordered to disembark at Newcastle, Holy Island and Berwick. They had a long voyage, so that a kind of remitting fever which some of them had acquired in the autumn in the Low Countries was "by the crowds and the foul air of the hold soon converted into the jail distemper and became infectious." At Newcastle most of the nurses and medical attendants of the extemporized hospital were seized with it, of whom three apothecaries, four apprentices and two journeymen died. But the most remarkable experience was on Holy Island. Of ninety-seven men taken out of the ships there, ill of the gaol-fever, forty died, "and the people of the place receiving the infection, in a few weeks buried fifty, the sixth part of the inhabitants of that island." At Nairn and Inverness there was a singular experience in the spring of 1746. The ships which brought Houghton's brigade to Nairn carried also thirty-six deserters to be tried by court-martial at the headquarters at Inverness: these men had deserted to the French in Flanders, had been found on board of a captured French transport carrying men to aid the Pretender, and had been thrown into gaol in England till an opportunity arose of sending them to their trial. Three days after the landing at Nairn of the force with which these deserters sailed, six of the officers were seized with fever and many of the men,

---

[1] Sir John Pringle, *Obs. on the Nature and Cure of Hospital and Jayl Fever*, Lond. 1750 (Letter to Mead); and his *Obs. on Diseases of the Army*, Lond. 1752 (fullest account).

of whom eighty were left sick at Nairn; in the ten days that the regiment remained at Inverness it sent one hundred and twenty more to hospital, ill of the same fever, which became frequent also among the inhabitants of the town. "Though the virulence of the distemper diminished afterwards in their march to Fort Augustus and Fort William, yet the corps continued sickly for some time." From the middle of February, 1746, when the army crossed the Forth, to the end of the campaign, there were two thousand sick in hospital, including wounded, of which number near three hundred died, mostly of the contagious fever[1].

After the Peace of Aix-la-Chapelle in 1748, the English troops embarked at Willemstad for home; "but the wind being contrary, several of the ships lay above a month at anchor, and, after all, meeting with a tedious and stormy passage, during which the men kept mostly below deck, the air was corrupted and produced the jail or hospital fever." The ships that came to Ipswich were in the worst state, about four hundred men having been landed sick there, most of them ill of this contagious fever. The infection was at first as active and the mortality as great on shore as on board; but the virulence of the fever was at length subdued by dispersing the sick and convalescents as much as possible[2].

Monro gives a similar account of the camp sickness among the British troops during the campaigns in North Germany in 1760–63. In the autumn of 1760, before he joined the forces, there had been much malignant fever and dysentery: the camp at Warburg was near the battlefield (31 July, 1760), where many of the dead were scarce covered with earth; there were also many dead horses, and in a time of heavy rains, the camp, with the neighbouring villages and fields, was filled with the excrements of a numerous army. Not only the soldiers, but the inhabitants of the country, who were reduced to the greatest misery and want, were infected, and whole villages almost laid waste. When Monro joined at Paderborn in January, 1761, he found the hospitals overcrowded, and the malignancy of the fever thereby much increased, so that a great many died. "The 1st and 3rd regiments suffered most, owing to all the sick of each regiment being put into a particular hospital by themselves,

---

[1] Pringle, *Diseases of the Army*, pp. 40–45.
[2] *Ibid.* p. 68.

which kept up the infection, so that they lost one-third of those left ill of this fever, and many of the nurses and people who attended them were seized with it." He distributed the sick men of the Coldstreams among the houses in the town, and lost few in comparison with the 1st and 3rd regiments. The contagion, under this bold policy, did not spread.

Two points in the symptoms are noteworthy: first the occurrence of suppurating buboes of the groins and armpits in several; and, secondly, the frequency of round worms.

"In this fever it was common for patients to vomit worms, or to pass them by stool, or, what was more frequent, to have them come up into the throat or mouth, and sometimes into their nostrils, while they were asleep in bed, and to pull them out with their fingers. The same thing happened to most of the British soldiers brought to the hospitals for other feverish disorders as well as this."

He cannot explain the commonness of round worms in the sick, unless it was from the great quantity of crude vegetables and fruits eaten, and the bad water. Patients in convalescence often suffered from deafness, and from suppurating parotids. Some had frequent relapses into the fever, "which seemed to be owing to the irritation of these insects," namely the worms. Most of those who fell into profuse, kindly, warm sweats recovered, the sweats lasting from twelve to forty-eight hours, and carrying off the fever. He never saw any miliary eruptions, and only sometimes petechiae, or small spots, or marbling as in measles[1].

Ship-Fever in the Seven Years' War and American War.

Ship-fever would appear to have been at its worst after the middle of the 18th century. Dr James Lind joined Haslar Hospital in 1758, and brought to the naval medical service the same high qualities which Pringle and Monro brought to that of the army[2]. The smaller ships, such as the 'Saltash' sloop, the 'Richmond' frigate, and the 'Infernal' bomb were full of fever of the most malignant kind; of 120 men in the 'Saltash,' 80 were infected with a contagion much more virulent and dangerous than that in the guard-ships. The explanation was

[1] Donald Monro, M.D. *Diseases of British Military Hospitals in Germany, from Jan.* 1761 *to the Return of the Troops to England in* 1763. Lond. 1764. The same campaign called forth also Dr Richard Brocklesby's *Œconomical and Medical Observations from* 1758 *to* 1763 *on Military Hospitals and Camp Diseases etc.* London, 1764.
[2] *Essay on Preserving the Health of Seamen*, Lond. 1757; *Two papers etc.* u. s.

that the smaller ships were receiving vessels for the larger ships, and were manned from the gaols; drafts from them carried the infection to the guard-ships and to the ships fitting out for foreign service. Malignant fever also arose on the voyage home from America[1]. In September and October 1758, after the reduction of Louisburg, several of the ships arriving at Spithead were infected with a malignant fever; three hundred men were received from them at Haslar Hospital (some with scurvy), of whom twenty-eight died. The 'Edgar,' having been manned at the Nore from gaols, sailed for the Mediterranean, and lost sixty men from fever and scurvy. The 'Loestoffe,' having lain in the St Lawrence for eight months in perfect health, took on board six convalescent men from Point Levi Hospital before sailing for home; in forty-eight hours, fifty out of her two hundred men were seized with fevers and fluxes, and six died on the voyage home. The 'Dublin' on the homeward voyage from Quebec buried nineteen, and on her arrival reported ninety men sick of fever, fluxes and scurvy. The 'Neptune' was said to have lost one hundred and sixty men in a few months, and reported 136 sick. The 'Cambridge,' with 650 men in health, sent three of her crew to the 'Neptune' laid up, to prepare her for the dock; of these three, one on the fifth day became spotted and died, and another narrowly escaped with life. The 'Diana' developed fever during a rough passage home from America. The 'St George,' having sailed from Spithead in 1760, met with rough weather and had to return on account of sickness. On the other hand, Hawke's fleet of twenty ships of the line with fourteen thousand men, which defeated the French in November 1759, kept the Bay of Biscay for four months in the most perfect health.

From 1 July, 1758, to 1 July, 1760, there were 5743 admissions to Haslar Hospital, the chief diseases being as follows:

Fevers 2174
Scurvy 1146
Consumption 360
Rheumatism 350
Fluxes 245

Of the fevers some were of an intermittent type, but by far the most were continued ship-typhus. Relapses were common, even to the sixth or seventh time. The fever varied a good

---

[1] In 1755 a pestilential sickness raged in the North American fleet, the 'Torbay' and 'Munich' being obliged to land their sick at Halifax.

deal in malignity, but never produced buboes, livid blotches or mortifications, and seldom parotids. Twenty-four men received from January to March 1760 out of the 'Garland' had most of them petechial spots accompanied with other symptoms of malignity, and of these, five died or 20 per cent. But of 105 received during the same months from the 'Postilion' and 'Liverpool' only eight died, and those mostly of a flux. The infection had little tendency to spread among the attendants at Haslar. In the first six months only one nurse died; in 1759, two labourers and two nurses died, one of the nurses by infection, having concealed some infected shirts under her bed, the other by decay of nature. Of more than a hundred persons employed in various offices about the sick there died only those five in the course of eighteen months.

Although Lind's account of ship-fever in the British navy is bad enough, he has collected some far worse particulars of foreign ships. Febrile contagion destroyed two-thirds of the men in the Duc d'Anville's fleet at Chebucto (now Halifax), in 1746, the complete destruction of which was afterwards accomplished by the scurvy. It was ship-fever which ravaged the Marquis d'Antin's squadron in 1741, the Count de Roquesevel's in 1744, and the Toulon squadron in 1747. He takes the following from Poissonnier's *Traité de Maladies des Gens de Mer:* The fleet commanded by M. Dubois de la Mothe sailed in 1757 from Rochefort for Louisburg, Canada, having some men sickly. The ships touched at Brest, and sent 400 ashore sick. They sailed from Brest on 3 May, and arrived at Louisburg on 28 June. There was then sickness in only two ships, but in a short time it appeared in all the fleet. On 14 October the fleet sailed from Louisburg for home, embarking one thousand sick, and leaving four hundred supposed dying. In less than six days from sailing most of the thousand sick were dead. When the fleet arrived at Brest on 22 November there were few seamen well enough to navigate the ships ; 4000 men were ill, the holds and decks being crowded with the sick. The hospitals at Brest were already occupied, two ships from Quebec shortly before having sent a thousand men to them. Fifteen hospitals were soon filled, attended by five physicians and one hundred and fifty surgeons. Two hundred almoners and nurses fell victims. The infection passed to the lower class of the citizens, the havoc became general, and houses everywhere were filled with the dying and the dead. At length it got among the prisoners in the hulks. This dreadful infection began to abate in March, 1758, and ceased in April, having carried off in less than five months upwards of 10,000 people in the hospitals alone, besides a great number of the Brest townspeople. The stench was intolerable. No person could enter the hospitals without being immediately seized with headache; and every kind of indisposition quickly turned to fatal fever, as in the old plague times. The state of the bodies showed the degree of malignity that had been engendered: the lungs were engorged with blood, and looked gangrenous ; the intestines often contained a green offensive liquor, and sometimes worms. Lind's other instances are chiefly of the Dutch East Indiamen that anchored at Spithead with fever on board. In Nov., 1770, the 'Yselmonde' bound to Batavia, came to anchor at Spithead, and buried a number of men every day; two custom-house officers caught the fever and died. He gives two other instances of Dutch ships bound to

Batavia, which came in to Portsmouth with fever[1]. The Dutch were said to send annually 2000 soldiers to Batavia, and to lose three-fourths of them by the ship-fever before they arrived. In 1769 Lind saw ship-fever in the Russian fleet at Spithead.

Brownrigg, of Whitehaven, gives a good instance of the diffusion of typhus in a newly-commissioned ship of war, and thence to the civil population, which bears out Lind's favourite notion that the gaols and the press-gang had far-reaching effects. In the year 1757 a sloop of war had been hastily manned at the Nore to protect the shipping between the Irish and Cumberland ports. She reached Whitehaven in May, with fever on board. The men were landed and lodged in small houses. Brownrigg found about forty lying on the floor of three small rooms, very close together, many of them in a dying state; seven days after he was himself seized with fever, and had a narrow escape with life. The ship's surgeon died of it, his mate recovered with difficulty, two surgeons of the town died of it, and two more in Cockermouth. The contagion spread widely among the inhabitants of Whitehaven, Cockermouth and Workington[2].

Lind showed to Howard in one of the wards of Haslar Hospital a number of sailors ill of the gaol fever; it had been brought on board their ship by a man who had been discharged from a prison in London, and it spread so much that the ship had to be laid up[3].

With the outbreak of the American War we begin to hear of still more disastrous epidemics of fever in the English fleets. Some instances from Robertson's full collection must suffice[4]. The 'Nonsuch' left England in March, 1777, and fifty of her men were carried off by fever before December; in that month, the 'Nonsuch,' 'Raisonable' and 'Somerset' had each from 130

---

[1] The *Gentleman's Magazine* for December, 1772 (p. 589), records the following: "The bodies of two Dutchmen who were thrown overboard from a Dutch East Indiaman, where a malignant fever raged, were cast up near the Sally Port at Portsmouth; they were so offensive that it was with difficulty that anyone could be got to bury them."

[2] W. Brownrigg, M.D. *Considerations on preventing Pestilential Contagion.* London, 1771, p. 36.

[3] Lind writes in his book on the Health of Seamen, "The sources of infection to our armies and fleets are undoubtedly the jails: we can often trace the importers of it directly from them. It often proves fatal in impressing men on the hasty equipment of a fleet. The first English fleet sent last war to America lost by it alone two thousand men."

[4] R. Robertson, M.D. *Observations on Jail, Hospital or Ship Fever from the 4th April, 1776, to the 30th April, 1789, made in various parts of Europe and America and on the Intermediate Seas.* London, 1789. New edition.

to 150 men on the sick list, chiefly fever in the 'Somerset,' and scurvy in the other two.   In April, 1778, the 'Venus,' with a crew of 240, was at Rhode Island very sickly; the surgeon told Robertson that they had lost about fifty men of fever, which still continued to rage on board: they became sickly from being crowded with prisoners and cruising with them on board in bad weather.   The 'Somerset' had buried 90 men of the fever since she left England, 70 of them being of the best seamen.   On arriving at Spithead in October, 1779, Robertson found much fever in the Channel Fleet which had lately come in, especially in the 'Canada,' 'Intrepid, 'Shrewsbury,' London' and 'Namur,' three or four of which were put past service, so much were they disabled by sickness.   At Gibraltar Hospital from 12 January to 31 March, 1780, there were admitted 570 men from twenty-seven ships, of whom 57 died; of 110 sick from the 'Ajax,' 18 died; of 437 Spanish prisoners, 37 died.   Next year, in May, 1781, at Gibraltar, the 'Bellona' had buried 27 men since she left England, and had 108 on the sick list.   The 'Cumberland' had buried 15; of the 'Marlborough's' men, 40 had died at the hospital.   Robertson had to purchase at his own expense vegetable acids, fruit and vegetables for the sick.

Some statistics remain of the loss of men in the navy by sickness in the Seven Years' War (1756–62) and in the American War[1]. The House of Commons had ordered a return of the number of seamen and marines raised and lost in the former; but the return was too general to be of much use, the number "lost" having included all those men who had been sent to hospital and never returned to their ships, all those who had been discharged as unserviceable, and all deserters. The number raised was 184,899, and the number "lost" 133,708, besides 1512 killed. The Return by the Navy Board for the period of the American War was more specific, showing only the number of the dead and killed.

Seamen and Marines raised, dead or killed, during the American War,
29 *Sept.,* 1774, *to* 29 *Sept.,* 1780:

Year	Raised	Dead	Killed
1774	345	—	—
1775	4,735	—	—
1776	21,565	1679	105
1777	37,457	3247	40
1778	31,847	4801	254
1779	41,831	4726	551
1780	28,210	4092	293
	175,990	18,545	1243

[1] Given by Blane in a Postscript to his paper "On the Comparative Health of the British Navy, 1779–1814" in *Select Dissertations*, London, 1822, p. 62.

Fully a tenth part of the men raised were lost by sickness. Fever was the chief sickness, and as it happened rarely that more than one in ten cases of fever died, it will be easy to form an approximate estimate of the proportion of all the men raised for the ships that were on the sick list at one time or another with fever—nearly the whole, one might guess.

During the three last years of the period Haslar Hospital was constantly full of typhus fever. Admiral Keppel's fleet arrived at Spithead on 26 October, 1778, and soon began to be infected with contagious fever; before the end of December, 3600 men had been sent to Haslar, which could make up at a pinch 1800 beds. But the great epidemic at Portsmouth was the next year, 1779, when the very large Channel Fleet under Sir Charles Hardy came in. During the month of September, 2500 men were received into hospital, and more than 1000 ill of fevers remained on board for want of room in the hospitals. In the last four months of 1779, 6064 sick were sent to Haslar, which had 2443 patients on 1 January, 1780. There was an additional hospital at Foston, holding 200, as well as two hospital ships holding 600. The infection was virulent during the winter, when Portsmouth was crowded with ships; and in the first five months of 1780, when 3751 cases of fever were admitted during the decline of the epidemic, one in eight died. The following shows how much fever preponderated at Haslar Hospital in 1780. In 8143 admissions on the medical side, the chief forms of sickness were as follows[1]:

Continued Fevers	5539
Scurvy	1457
Rheumatism	327
Flux	240
Consumption	218
Smallpox	42

Blane gives the instance of the 'Intrepid,' one of the Channel Fleet under Hardy in 1779: "Almost the whole of her crew either died at sea or were sent to the hospital upon arriving at Portsmouth. This ship, after refitting, was pretty healthy for a little time; but probably from the operation of the old adhering infection, she became extremely sickly immediately after joining our fleet and sent 200 men to the hospital after arriving in the West Indies. Most of these were ill of dysentery[2]." During a voyage of three weeks of the 'Alcide' and 'Torbay' from the Windward Islands to New York in September, 1780, nearly a half of the men were unfit. In the 'Alcide' it was a fever that raged, in the 'Torbay' it was a dysentery[3].

---

[1] Blane, u. s. p. 47, from information supplied by Dr John Lind, of Haslar Hospital.

[2] *Diseases incident to Seamen*, p. 18.   [3] *Ibid.* p. 34.

These experiences of fever in the ships of the Royal navy continued to the end of the 18th century. In Trotter's time, as in Lind's, receiving ships were a source of contagion to others, one ship of the kind, the 'Cambridge' having diffused fever among many ships of the Channel Fleet by men drafted from her[1].

Ship typhus was also an incident of the voyages of the East India Company's ships, which nearly always carried troops. In the voyage of the 'Talbot,' 22 March—25 August, 1768, with 240 persons on board, "towards the end of July a fever of a very bad kind made its appearance, attended with delirium, low pulse, petechiae or livid vibices and hæmorrhages from the nose, of which one died and three or four escaped hard." The sick were isolated, and the infection did not spread. Such outbreaks of typhus were not uncommon at sea, although the loss of life from them was small beside that from the fevers of Madagascar, Sumatra, Batavia and Bengal. The ship typhus usually began on board among the soldiers. The most notable point is that relapses were common, as Lind also observed at Haslar Hospital ; some on board the 'Lascelles' in 1783 (150 attacks among 151 soldiers) had relapsed seven times. It does not appear, however, that the best class of merchantmen suffered greatly from fevers. Dr Clark, who compiled a report of the practice in fevers in the ships of the East India Company from 1770 to 1785, had reason to congratulate the Company on the general healthiness of their fleet :

"When ships set out at a proper season, when they are not too much crowded, when the weather is favourable, and no mismanagement appears, fewer lives are lost in these long voyages than in the most healthy country villages. And in perusing the medical journals I have the peculiar pleasure of finding that many ships have arrived in India without the loss of a single life by disease," e.g. the 'Valentine' in 1784, seven months out, with 300 souls, no deaths, and the 'Barrington' in 1789, no deaths outward bound[2].

[1] Trotter, *Medicina Nautica*, I. 61. His general abstracts of the health of the fleet in the first years of the French War, 1794–96, give many instances of ship-typhus.

[2] John Clark, M.D. *Observations on the Diseases which prevail in Long Voyages to Hot Countries, &c.* London, 1773. 2nd ed. 2 vols, 1792.

John Lorimer, M.D., published in *Med. Facts and Observations*, VI. 211, a " Return of the ships' companies and military on board the ships of the H. E. I. C. for the years 1792 and 1793."

	Outward voyages		Homeward voyages		In port
	Crew	Military	Crew	Invalids	
Number of men	2657	3919	2701	1075	—
Sick	1253	1751	1058	282	1533
Dead	28	50	51	27	96

On the other hand, these English reports give incidentally the most unfavourable accounts of the Dutch East Indian ships. Three Dutch ships, then in Praya Bay, St Jago (Cape de Verde Islands), had buried 70 to 80 men each, and had some hundreds of sick on board. Another report says: "Before we left Table Bay several Dutch ships arrived, some of which had buried 80 people in the voyage from Holland. None lost less than 40 men. I am informed that some of their ships last year buried 200 men"—the causes of the sickness being overcrowding, filth, and the slowness of the voyages. One experience of the very worst kind happened to an English expedition consisting of the 100th regiment, the 98th regiment, the second battalion of the 42nd, and four additional companies. They had formed part of the force for the reduction of the Cape of Good Hope, whence they re-embarked for Bombay. During the voyage from Saldanha Bay a contagious fever and scurvy broke out among the troops, who were crowded and badly clothed; dead men were thrown overboard by dozens, and the regiments were reduced to a third of their original numbers. Six officers of the 100th regiment died, and an equal if not greater proportion of those of the 98th and 42nd.

The other chief occasion of ship typhus was the emigration to the American and West Indian colonies from Britain and Ireland. The Irish emigration was especially active from the beginning of the 18th century, owing to rack-renting and other causes. Madden[1] professed to know that one-third of the Irish who went to the West Indies (perhaps he should have included Carolina) perished either on the voyage or by diseases caught in the first weeks after landing; and as we know that typhus attended the Irish emigration in the 19th century, we may infer that the same was the cause of mortality in the 18th.

The trouble from ship-fever in the navy was so great all through the 18th century that many ingenious shifts were tried to overcome it. Towards the end of the century, the favourite device was fumigation with the vapour of mineral acids; one such plan, for which the Admiralty paid a good sum, ended in the burning of several ships to the water's edge. An earlier plan was ventilation of the hold and 'tween decks ·by means of

---

[1] *Reflections and Resolutions for the Gentlemen of Ireland*, p. 28. Cited by Lecky.

Sutton's pipes[1], which found a strong advocate in the Rev. Stephen Hales, of the Royal Society[2].

Twice in the course of a paper to that learned body[3] he asserts that the noxious, putrid, close, confined, pestilential air of ships' holds and 'tween decks "has destroyed millions of mankind"; on the other hand, according to the testimony of a captain of the navy, Sutton's pipes had kept his ship free from fever. Lind caps this with the case of H.M.S. 'Sheerness,' bound to the East Indies. She was fitted with Sutton's pipes, the dietary being at the same time so arranged that the men had salt meat only once a week. After a very long passage of five months and some days she arrived at the Cape of Good Hope without having had one man sick. "As the use of Sutton's pipes had been then newly introduced into the king's ships, the captain was willing to ascribe part of such an uncommon healthfulness in so long a run to their beneficial effects; but it was soon discovered that, by the neglect of the carpenter, the cock of the pipes had been all this while kept shut[4]."

Ship-fever was at length got rid of by more homely and more radical means than scientific ingenuity. Lind had shown one root of the evil to lie in the pressing of men just out of gaol. Admiral Boscawen, by his unaided wits, discovered another means of checking it. He avoided the mixing of fresh hands with crews seasoned to their ships, unless when some evident utility or necessity of service made it proper; "and upon this principle he used to resist the solicitation of captains, when they requested to carry men from one ship to another when changing their command[5]." Towards the end of the 18th century many reforms were made in the naval service—in the dietary, in the allowance of soap, in keeping the bilges clean, in the use of iron and lead instead of timber; so that Blane dates from the year 1796 a new era in the health of the navy[6].

[1] Sutton, "Changing Air in Ships," *Phil. Trans.* XLII. 42; W. Watson, M.D. *ibid.* p. 62; H. Ellis, *ibid.* XLVII. 211.
[2] *Ibid.* XLIX. 332, "Ventilation of a Transport."
[3] *Ibid.* pp. 333, 339.
[4] Lind, *Essay on the Most Effectual Means of Preserving the Health of Seamen in the Royal Navy.* New Ed. London, 1774, p. 29.
[5] Blane, *Diseases incident to Seamen*, 1785, p. 243.
[6] *Id.* "On the Comparative Health of the British Navy from the year 1799 to the year 1814, with Proposals for its farther Improvement." *Select Dissertations*, 1822, p. 1.

The " Putrid Constitution " of Fevers in the middle third of the 18th Century.

Resuming the history of fevers among the people at large from the great typhus epidemic of 1741–42 to the end of the century, we find the conditions somewhat different in the earlier and later divisions of the period. The time of prosperity, when England exported large quantities of wheat in every year except two or three, is reckoned from 1715 to 1765 ; after the latter date England gradually ceased to be an exporting country, owing to various causes, including the increase of pasture farming and the growth of industrial populations in the northern counties. The year 1765 marks the beginning of what has been called the Industrial Revolution ; and it is also an important point of time in the history of the fevers of the country, for it is in the generation after that we obtain all the best information on what may be called industrial typhus, in the writings of a group of physicians who were at once philanthropic and exact. But there was an earlier period of fever, which is somewhat difficult to the historian. It is perhaps the last period in which Sydenham's language of " epidemic constitutions " seems to be appropriate, whether it be that the writers of the time were still under his influence, or because the prevalent maladies could not well be accounted for in any other way. The constitution in question was a " putrid " one. It coincided with the great outburst of putrid or gangrenous sore-throat, to be described elsewhere ; and it included an extensive prevalence of fevers which were also called putrid or nervous, and sometimes called miliary. Fevers of the same kind, and with the same miliary rash, are described by earlier writers, such as Huxham. Perhaps the most correct view of the matter is to consider this type of fever as corresponding roughly to the middle third of the century, and as having been interrupted by the typhus epidemic of 1741–42, during a time of special distress. Besides the great outburst of putrid or malignant sore-throat, there was also a disastrous murrain of cattle for several years ; and at Rouen there was a remarkable fever which some English writers of the time took to be the highest manifestation of the same " putrid " constitution that they discovered also in the English and Irish fevers.

The fever at Rouen which Le Cat specially described to the Royal Society was an outbreak from the end of November, 1753, to February, 1754. This outbreak was only one of a series; but as it attacked a great number of persons of distinction and made great havock among them, it attracted unusual notice and was regarded as something new, the rumour spreading over Europe that Rouen had been visited by plague. The same fever, however, had occurred there in previous years; and allied forms of sickness, of the same gangrenous character, including gangrenous sore-throat, could be traced back for twenty or thirty years. It will suffice to mention of these the malignant fever which appeared in 1748 and continued in 1749, 1750 and 1751. There was a fixed pain in the head, pain about the heart, a low fever with delirium, often miliary eruptions, continual faint sweating, drowsiness, scanty or suppressed urine, abdominal distension. After death the stomach was found "inflamed" at places, as well as the small intestine. In some cases there were ulcerations which almost penetrated the coats. The lungs were engorged with blood. In one case, of a young woman aged twenty, the mesentery was filled with obstructed glands and the intestines mortified in different places. In another, almost the whole mesentery was mortified and there was an anthrax or carbuncle at the upper fore part of the armpit. At the same time some cases of smallpox, with miliary eruption, also had ulcerations of the stomach, with inflammatory spots on other parts of it and of the intestine, the mesenteric glands being enlarged and hard. Some of the cases at the Hôtel Dieu in 1750 were traced to infection from bales of horsehair; but the type of the disease in those cases did not differ essentially from that of other cases. Some rapidly fatal cases in the winter of 1752–53 had suppurative inflammation about the heart. (In 1739 there had been deaths from continued fever at the Hôtel Dieu, after an illness of six or seven days, marked by frequent faintings, small abscesses being found after death in the substance of the heart near the auricles.) The fever among the upper classes in the winter of 1753–54 was marked, in its most mortal form, by lowness, continued fever, pain in the head, cough, sore-throat, nausea, dry black tongue, delirium, sweats, stupor, some oppression of the heart, spitting of blood, sometimes swelling of the belly, these symptoms being followed often by miliary eruption, and sometimes by a slight flux with blood. Many were affected with a dejection of spirits, and with a feeling of terror which made them tremble at the ordinary sound of the voice. The fever ran a full course of thirty or forty days (the miliary eruption coming about the 21st day), while death usually ensued about the 25th. The appearances after death were remarkable (many bodies were opened): "In some a part of the villous coat of the stomach and of the small guts was inflamed; and the rest of these organs were filled with an eruption of the miliary crystalline kind, except that it was larger; and there was likewise an obstruction in the glands of the mesentery. In others a strong inflammation had seized the whole stomach and a small portion of the oesophagus, but the intestines were free...In those cases where the delirium had continued long and violent, we found either ulceration on the stomach, or its villous coat separated, together with a great inflammation, and even some gangrenous spots, on the other coats of that organ." Some recovered by critical abscesses. Others who escaped death by the poison carried its terrible effects for many months; their limbs and joints were feeble, and they were troubled with vertigo, lassitude and fears[1].

Exactly covering the period of these fevers at Rouen, there were low putrid fevers in London, in Worcestershire, in Ireland, and among the English colonists in Barbados. It was certainly

[1] Le Cat, *Phil. Trans.* XLIX. 49.

not a mere fashion in medicine which produced the accounts of a similar fever, for these accounts came from places far apart and were independent of each other. Dr Fothergill, of Lombard Street, published in the *Gentleman's Magazine* every month for five years a short account of the weather and prevalent diseases of London, beginning with April, 1751, and ending with December, 1755. He had the weekly bills of mortality before him, and he makes various comments upon them ; but his accounts of prevalent diseases are from his own observation and by way of illustrating the bills. His first reference to a fever is under October, 1751 : "A slow continual fever, with acute pain in the forehead : not many attacked, few mortally." The year 1752 was remarkably free from fevers until November, when we read of a fatal fever which had rheumatic symptoms at first (as at Rouen in 1744), attacking the head later, with coma-vigil and a dark-coloured ichor on the tongue and lips. It continued into January and February, 1753, proving fatal to several. In the summer and autumn months there were fevers of the low, depressed kind, sometimes called "remittents," with copious sweats, or "slow, remitting, dangerous fever," or "slow, treacherous, remittent fever, too often fatal." The references to it are most numerous in the months from November, 1753, corresponding to Le Cat's Rouen narrative. It was slow and imperceptible in its approach, the sick often going about ill for a week before seeking advice ; it was attended with profuse sweats which never relieved, and was fatal to many. It continued more or less through the summer, and from August, 1754, it is again prominent. In September, it was the most alarming form of disease, and was then commonly vehement in its access, with lassitude, and pain in the head and back ; unrelieving sweats are again mentioned, with dry tongue, delirium, coma-vigil, and death about the 14th–15th day. Fothergill was at a loss to know whether he should order blood to be drawn, owing to the low depressed nature of the fever. In February, 1755, the fever is still "too much of the nature of those which prevailed in the preceding months to allow a repetition of bleeding." In April it is called the petechial and miliary fever, the miliary eruption being of a white sort with a very noisome scent ; the petechial spots turned livid, black and gangrenous ; few patients escaped who had been sweated at the beginning. The fever was truly malignant, the patient restless from the outset, the sweats weakening. Fothergill's last entries of it are important, under the months of May and June, 1755. In May, 1755, the fevers were "for the most part allied to that dangerous remittent which has for some years past more or less prevailed in different places of this kingdom." In June: "It does not appear that either in the hospitals or any part of the city a disease has broken out of so dangerous a nature as has been reported. The same kind of fever that has long continued in this city with some small variations in its type, still remains, but it is by no means more frequent than it has been in the preceding months, nor is it attended with more unfavourable symptoms."

It is impossible to say how general over England this fever may have been in the years 1751–57. Our fullest accounts come from Worcestershire; but the putrid fever is heard of more widely. Thus a short Latin piece in the *Gentleman's Magazine*, dated 14 April, 1755, is on the putrid fever lately epidemic, and not yet extinct, in some parts of the county of Somerset and adjoining places; its signs were contagiousness, pains of the head and loins, nausea and vomiting, diarrhoea, quick weak pulse, purple spots, delirium and coma[1]. Grainger, writing from Edinburgh in 1753, declares his motive for publishing an account of the anomalous fever of the Netherlands in 1746–48 to be that the same had lately been raging over almost the whole of Britain.

We have some particulars for Kidderminster, which can hardly have been exceptional for an industrial town, and according to the accounts were true also for villages and market towns near. Kidderminster was, in the year 1756, a town of about four thousand inhabitants, mostly hand-loom weavers of worsted and silk. There were no power-looms anywhere in England at that time; and the condition of the Kidderminster weavers' houses was doubtless what that of the Tiverton community had been fifteen years before. Many of the weavers, we are told, are lodged in small nasty houses, for the most part crowded with looms and other utensils[2]. Many of these houses were built on a low flat of the river Stour, whence rose putrid

---

[1] "Its cause seemed to be something contagious mixed with the contents of the stomach and intestines, especially the bile and alvine faeces, which absorbed thence contaminates the whole body and affects especially the cerebral functions." *Gent. Magaz.*, Article signed " S," 1755, p. 151.

[2] James Johnstone, M.D., senior, *Malignant Epidemic Fever of* 1756. London, 1758.

vapours after floods. Its situation had served to render the town specially unhealthy before, as in the epidemic of 1727–29[1].

The first notice by Dr Johnstone is of a low miliary fever from Midsummer 1752 to the end of the year. This was a comparatively mild affair, although it carried off several. But after Christmas it was succeeded by a fever which would then have been classed as of the putrid kind. The first great season was in 1753, it ceased in the fine years 1754–55, but came back in 1756 and 1757. It began with languor, lowness, flutterings, faintness, vague pains in the limbs, a low quick pulse, giddiness and slight sickness. Some had a propensity to loose stools and to profuse hurtful sweats; some bled at the nose, others coughed and spit blood; some had pain in the throat, and crimson-red tongue, the sweat and breath of the sick had a strong, offensive, putrid smell. In some of the worst cases livid petechiae, large livid blotches, and dark brown spots occurred over the trunk and limbs. The successful treatment was by mineral acids, bark, port wine, and vesication. "This malignant fever was very often (though not constantly) complicated with, and in general bore great analogy to the malignant sore-throat which at this time prevailed in many parts of England." The fever which prevailed during that remarkable year (1753) was very evidently contagious, for whole families were either all together or one after another seized with it. One of the most distinctive symptoms was a tendency to trembling of the whole body, as well as leaping of the tendons at the wrists. In some the tonsils were beset with aphthous sloughs, and towards the decline there would be aphthae of the mouth, but symptomatic only, and not the dominant lesion as in the ulcerous sore-throat. About the 15th day the fever was generally at its height. The miliary eruptions were critical to the few that had them; the flat livid petechiae appeared at all times of the disorder. Johnstone then compares the fever with that described by Le Cat at Rouen in the winter of the same year; and although he had been unable to satisfy his curiosity by opening any body dead of the fever, he felt sure that these dreadful symptoms arose from

---

[1] Nash, *Hist. of Worcestershire*, II. 39, found evidence in the Kidderminster registers that the fevers of 1727, 1728 and 1729 had "very much thinned the people, and terrified the inhabitants." Watson, "On the Medical Topography of Stourport," *Trans. Proc. Med. Assoc.*, II., had heard or read somewhere that fever was so bad in Kidderminster in the first part of the 18th century that farmers were afraid to come to market.

some affection of the stomach and small guts, at first erysipelatous, afterwards gangrenous, and at last truly sphacelous.

Johnstone's statement that the putrid fever in Worcestershire
in 1752–53 was often complicated with and bore great analogy
to the malignant sore-throat is borne out by Huxham's accounts
for Plymouth during the same season :

> "In all sorts of fevers," he writes, "there was a surprising disposition to
> eruptions of some kind or other [including miliary], to sweats, soreness
> of throat and aphthae." It is hardly possible to make out all his cases of
> "malignant anginose fever" to have been scarlet fever with sore-throat.
> Thus there occurred stench, swelling, and samious haemorrhages "commonly
> in those that died of malignant anginose fever above described. I have
> known the whole body swell vastly, even to the ends of the fingers and toes,
> with a cadaveric lividity, though almost quite cold, and an intolerable
> stench, even before the person was actually dead, blood issuing at the same
> time from the ears, nose, mouth and guts[1]."

The first years of this putrid or miliary fever were not
seasons of scarcity, there having been no failure of the crops since
1741 (unless in Ireland, in the province of Ulster mostly, in
1744); on the contrary, many of the seasons had been unusually
fine and abundant, the exports from England of wheat, barley,
malt and rye in the three years 1748, 1749 and 1750 amounting
to four million quarters. Prices were at the same time favourable
to the poorer classes[2]. But there had been a destructive murrain
for several years (30,000 cows are said to have died in Cheshire
in 1751), and the harvest of 1756 was a failure.

To the month of February, 1756, the season had been very
forward, but the early promise of spring was blighted by cold,
a wet summer and autumn ensued, the fruit crop was ruined,
and the corn harvest spoiled by long, heavy rains. A dearth,
bread-riots, &c. ensued[3]; but it is to be noted that the revival of
the dangerous malignant contagious fever began at Kidderminster
as early as April, becoming much worse after harvest. "Many
for weeks or months laboured under an uncommon depression
of spirits, felt their strength abate, with great lassitude, and very
often a great proneness to faint away." As the summer advanced
the fever became truly epidemic not only in Kidderminster but
in many other parts of the West and North-west of England.

---

[1] Huxham, *Dissertation on the Malignant Ulcerous Sore-Throat.* Lond. 1757,
p. 60.

[2] Tooke, *History of Prices.* Introduction.

[3] In Shrewsbury gaol, in 1756, thirty-seven colliers were confined for rioting
during the dearth. Four of them died in gaol, ten were condemned to death, of
whom two were executed. Phillips, *History of Shrewsbury*, 1779, p. 213.

It went through whole families, who succumbed either all together or one member after the other, and was carried from place to place by the attendants on the sick. "It prevailed chiefly in poor families, where numbers were lodged in mean houses, not always clean, but sordid and damp. It seemed to affect such poor families most where there was reason to think a sufficiency of the necessaries of life, on account of the dearth, had for some time been scantily supplied; yet the other poor persons, given to the intemperate use of malt liquors and ardent spirits, were observed to be very much liable to its influence. And not a few persons in easy circumstances of life were affected with this fever like others."

Frost in October checked it, and then measles of a malignant type had its turn among the children, the whooping-cough succeeding the measles. From November to Christmas the putrid fever, which chiefly affected persons from ten to fifty, and more women than men, returned with increased force. In fatal cases, the face was ghastly, sunken and livid (the facies Hippocratica), the patient sweated profusely, but seldom became cold till death was at hand. There was an abominable cadaverous stench in the breath, perspiration and stools. In these cases death took place from the 12th to the 14th day.

The intense and long frost of the opening months of 1757 nearly put a stop to the fever at Kidderminster.

"But in other neighbouring villages and market towns it has since the spring hitherto (Dec. 1757) been very frequent in places that were little affected with it last year. The families of the poorer sort of people universally are the most subject to it. And it is observable that the fever in some places first broke out in the parish workhouses, and from thence spread among the neighbouring people with great malignity. Wherever it has appeared it has given very apparent and fatal evidence of its infectious nature[1]."

Parliament was summoned to meet in December, 1756, on account of the dearth, which formed the topic of the Speech from the throne. The export of corn (which had reached a million quarters a year not long before) was prohibited, and the use of grain in distilling stopped for two months. The distress was more acute in 1757, and was enhanced by the greed of corn-dealers and millers, who used French bolting-mills to grind the mere husks of wheat, pease, rye and barley together into meal. Short, who practised at Sheffield, says that the fever in October and November, 1757, "was neither so rife nor fatal as in 1741[2]." It raged fiercely in several towns at a

[1] Johnstone, u. s. Short says: "a slow, malignant, putrid fever in some parts of Yorkshire, Cheshire, Worcestershire and the low parts of Leicestershire, which carried off very many." In October, 1757, it set in at Sheffield and raged all the winter.
[2] Short, *Increase and Decrease of Mankind in England, etc.* London, 1767, p. 109.

distance, " where it went by the name of the miliary fever," and was mostly among the poor, half-starved in the dearth of 1756–57. It is heard of again in the district of Cleveland in the winter of 1759–60, where it seems to have been mostly a disease of children complicated with sore-throat, and allied more to scarlet fever than to the putrid fever of adults[1]. But at Sunderland, near at hand, there was spotted fever at the same time, and in Newcastle there was dysentery.

The accounts of fever in Ireland in the same period as in England (see chapter II.) are not without value, as showing that the " putrid " or nervous type of fever, contrasting with the ordinary typhus of the country, had been remarked there also Rutty and Sims describe, during a certain period, the symptoms of the low, putrid fever, sometimes with miliary eruptions, identifying it both by name and in character with the fever then prevalent in England. The most significant thing in Rutty's annals is that there occurred in the midst of the low, putrid fever with miliary pustules in 1746, a more acute fever, ending after five or seven days in a critical sweat, and relapsing. The same fever, not very fatal, reappeared in 1748. Sims brings the history of the nervous or putrid or miliary fever in Ireland (Tyrone) continuously down to the year 1772, as elsewhere related. The remarkable phenomenon of tremors or shakings, which most witness to, was seen by him in perfection in the year 1771 :

The tremulousness of the wrists, he says, extended to all the body, "insomuch that I have seen the bed-curtains dancing for three or four days, to the no small terror of the superstitious attendants, who, on first perceiving it, thought some evil spirit shook the bed. This agitation was so constant a concomitant of the fever as to be almost a distinguishing symptom." These were not the shakings of an ague, for there might be no intermission for days[2].

Perhaps the most surprising testimony to the existence of an " epidemic constitution " of slow, continued nervous fever comes from the island of Barbados. Hillary, who had kept a record of the prevalent diseases at Ripon, continued the same when he settled in Barbados in 1751[3]. There can be no doubt as to

---

[1] Charles Bisset, *Essay on the Medical Constitution of Great Britain*, 1 Jan. 1758, to Midsummer, 1760. Together with a narrative of the Throat-Distemper and the Miliary Fever which were epidemical in the Duchy of Cleveland in 1760. London, 1762, pp. 265, 270, &c.

[2] James Sims, M.D., *Obs. on Epid. Disorders.* Lond. 1773, p. 181.

[3] W. Hillary, M.D., *Changes of the Air and Concomitant Epid. Disorders in Barbadoes.* 2nd ed., Lond. 1766.

the appearance of this fever in February 1753, its prevalence all over the island for eighteen months, and its disappearance in September 1754, when, as he writes, "It now totally disappeared and left the island, and, I think, has not been seen in it since" (1758). He gives the same account of it as the observers in England and Ireland, except that he does not describe miliary eruptions and describes jaundice in convalescent children. It was insidious in its onset (as in London), the patient often keeping afoot five or six days; the symptoms included pains in the head, vertigo, torpor, lassitude, vigil, delirium, faintings, partial sweats, involuntary evacuations, gulpings, tremors, twitchings, catchings, coma and convulsions. Recovery was marked by copious equable sweats and plentiful spitting. "This slow, nervous fever was certainly infectious, for I observed that many of those who visited, and most of them that attended the sick in their fever were infected by it, and got the disease, and especially those who constantly attended them and performed the necessary offices of the sick." It was last heard of in the remoter parts of the island.

Miliary Fever.

It will have been observed in the foregoing accounts of the predominant fevers of the years (roughly) from 1750 to 1760 that there was often a miliary eruption, but that it was far from constant. The constant things were the lowness, depression, ill-smelling sweats, tremors of the whole body or of the wrist-tendons, and other nervous or ataxic symptoms. But we hear more of a miliary eruption in connexion with that than with any other period of fevers in the history; and this was the time when a controversy arose as to whether there was in reality a distinctive kind of fever marked by miliary eruption. Some of the school of Boerhaave contended that the phenomenon of miliary vesicles was due solely to the heating and sweating treatment of the alexipharmac physicians. De Haën and others answered that miliary fever was a natural form, independent of the mode of treatment. The Boerhaavian contention may be admitted as good for such miliary fevers as were described under that name in 1710 by Sir David Hamilton[1]; nearly the

---

[1] *Tractatus duplex de Praxeos Regulis et de Febre Miliari*, Lond. 1710. Engl. transl. of the latter, Lond. 1737.

whole of his sixteen cases appear to have been made miliary by treatment, in so far as they became miliary at all. What this physician did was to foretell the approach of miliary symptoms in various maladies (about one-half of the cases being of lying-in women, and the rest various), and then to prescribe Gascoign's powder, Goa stone, Gutteta powder, Venice treacle or other diaphoretics, along with diluents and the application of blisters; the miliaria appeared about the breast, neck, and clefts of the fingers in due course (tenth to fourteenth day).

So far as his clinical cases are concerned, the late appearance of miliary vesicles, lasting a few days, is sufficiently explained by the powerful drenches administered; and it can hardly be doubted that much of what was called miliary·fever was of that factitious kind. But even in Hamilton's essay we find indications of a real miliary type of fever; thus he mentions a class of cases which look to be the same as those described by Johnstone, Rutty, Sims and others forty years after—cases with wakefulness, depression, tremblings of the tongue and hands, convulsive movements and delirium. He mentions also a complication of this with sore-throat in 1704, which destroyed many.

As to the association of miliary eruption with the low putrid fever so characteristic of the sixth decade of the 18th century, it is asserted by too many and in too various circumstances for any doubt as to its reality. There is nothing to show that the alexipharmac treatment was the one always used; and it is not certain that some in Ireland and elsewhere who had miliary eruption received any medical treatment at all. Again, miliary vesicles, not always with perspiration, were commonly found in the relapsing fever of Irish emigrants in London during the great famine of Ireland in 1846–47, by which time the powerful drenches of the alexipharmac treatment had been long disused[1]. The controversy as to the reality of miliary fever was one of the kind usual in medicine: certain physicians, of whom Hamilton in 1710 was an obvious instance, took up an untenable position; they were answered according to the weakness of their argument; and that has been held in later times to be an answer to all who alleged the existence of a type of fever marked by miliary eruptions. There can be no question as to a low, "putrid" kind of fever in which miliary eruptions were usual;

[1] Ormerod, *Clin. Obs. on Continued Fever*. London, 1848.

but offensive sweats were perhaps more usual, whence the name
of putrid in a literal sense, different from the theoretical sense of
Willis; more constant also were the starting of tendons, the
tremors and shakings, together with very varied hysteric
symptoms, from which the fevers received the name of nervous.
Dr John Fordyce in his 'History of a Miliary Fever' (1758)
really describes under that name the symptoms of the low,
nervous, putrid fever, often attended with miliary vesicles, which
had been the common type in England in the years immediately
preceding, and was a common type for some time after, although
less is heard of the miliary eruptions in the later history[1].

About the last quarter of the 18th century medical writers
were inclined to drop the names of nervous and putrid as
distinctive of certain fevers. Pringle, in his edition of 1775,
says he had been careful to avoid the terms nervous, bilious,
putrid and malignant, which conveyed either no clear idea or a
false one. Armstrong, another army physician, writing in 1773,
says: "Nervous, putrid, bilious, petechial or miliary, they are
all of the malignant family; and in this great town [London]
these are almost the only fevers that have for many years
prevailed, and do so still, to the great destruction of mankind.
For inflammatory fevers...have for many years been remarkably
rare[2]." Dr John Moore becomes sarcastic over the variety of
names given to continued fever, some such generic name as
Cullen's "typhus," then newly introduced, being what he desired[3].

Haygarth, writing of the Chester fevers in 1772, said that the
miliary fever had been "supposed" endemic there for more than
thirty years past, but he thought it probable that the eruption
had generally, or always, been fabricated "by close, warm rooms,
too many bed-cloaths, hot medicines and diet." He had seen
only one case in the epidemic that year, and he believed its
rarity at that time was due to the treatment by fresh air and by

[1] *Historia Febris Miliaris, et de Hemicrania Dissertatio.* Auctore Joanne Fordyce, M.D., Londini, 1758. Symptoms at p. 16. In an Appendix Dr Balguy makes the following curious division of the miliary vesicles: the white in malignant continued fever, the dull red in remittent fever, the "almost efflorescent" in intermittent. Fordyce makes them to appear as early as the third day, and to begin to disappear in four or six days in favourable cases.
[2] London, 1773, p. 9. See also Sir W. Fordyce's essay of the same year.
[3] John Moore, M.D., *Medical Sketches*, Lond. 1786. Part II. "On Fevers." Referring to the "putrid" fever in particular, he says that certain unbelievers, of whom he was probably one, "assert that mankind are tenacious of opinions, when once adopted, in proportion as they are extraordinary, disagreeable and incredible." Dr Moore is best known as the author of *Zeluco*.

"such regimen and medicines as are cooling and check putre-faction[1]." We shall see later that Percival, for Manchester, contents himself with saying that miliary fevers, which were formerly very frequent in that town and neighbourhood, now [1772] rarely occur[2]. In Scotland as late as 1782 the type was still nervous or low, and hardly ever inflammatory[3].

Mortalities in London from fever and all causes.

Year	Fever deaths	All deaths	Year	Fever deaths	All deaths
1741	7528	32169	1756	3579	20872
1742	5108	27483	1757	2564	21313
1743	3837	25700	1758	2471	17576
1744	2670	20606	1759	2314	19604
1745	2690	21296	1760	2136	19830
1746	4167	28157	1761	2475	21063
1747	4779	25494	1762	3742	26326
1748	3981	23069	1763	3414	26148
1749	4458	25516	1764	3942	23202
1750	4294	23727	1765	3921	23230
1751	3219	21028	1766	3738	23911
1752	2070	20485	1767	3765	22612
1753	2292	19276	1768	3596	23639
1754	2964	22696	1769	3430	21847
1755	3042	21917	1770	3214	22434

It is singular to observe that in the five successive years in this period with lowest fever-deaths and deaths from all causes, the years 1757–61 England was at war on the Continent. A similar low fever-mortality corresponded with the wars under Marlborough and Wellington.

The era of agricultural prosperity in England, which had its only considerable interruptions in the years 1727–29 and 1740–42, may be said to have met with a more serious check from the bad harvest of 1756. There was a recurrence of agrarian troubles in 1764–67, partly through actual scarcity caused by the extreme drought of 1764, partly through the pulling down of cottages and the discouragement of country villages, which Goldsmith has pathetically described in his poem of the time. Short says that the country in 1765 was in general very healthy but for children's diseases. "In some parts the putrid fever roamed about from place to place in the highest degree of putrefaction, so as several dead bodies were obliged to be buried the same day as they died." The price of provisions was excessive, meal riots broke out, and the export of corn was

[1] Haygarth, *Phil. Trans.* LXIV. 73. [2] Percival, *ibid.* LXIV. 59.
[3] Hutchinson, u. s.

stopped, Parliament having been summoned for the occasion in
November, 1766[1]. In 1769, at the time of the formation of
Chatham's ministry, the same train of incidents recurred,—bread-
riots, flour-mills wrecked, corn and bread seized by the populace
and sold at low prices, collisions with the military, the gaols full
of prisoners[2]. The long period of cheapness, having lasted half
a century, was coming to an end. Moralists and economists
had much to say as to the meaning of the national distress
which began to be felt in the sixties. Want of industry, want
of frugality, want of sobriety, want of principle, said one, had
brought trouble on the working class. "The tumults that have
lately arisen in many counties of England are no other than the
murmurs of the people, which have been heard for some years,
bursting forth at last into riot and confusion." The English, it
seems, had returned to their old medieval taste for the best food
they could get; they would not give up the finest bread,
although the Irish lived on potatoes, and the French on turnips
and cabbage: "The ploughman, the shepherd, the hedger and
ditcher, all eat as white bread as is commonly made in London,
which occasions a greater consumption of wheat." Women
must have tea and snuff, though children go naked and starved.
Another writes: "The poorest people will have the finest
or none." The enclosures had made a want of tillage. "What
must become of our poor, destitute of work for want of tillage?"
The country had for the most part been sickly, labourers scarce,
and the farmers not able to get their usual quantity threshed
out. The profligacy of the poor, profane swearing, etc., are
remarked upon[3].

In the last thirty years of the 18th century the accounts of

[1] *Annual Register*, 1766, p. 220. The King's Speech on 11 Nov. was chiefly
occupied with the dearth. The use of wheat for distilling was prohibited by an order
of Council of 16 Sept. 1766. *Gent. Magaz.* p. 399. To show the hardships of the
rural population at this time, Mr Gladstone, in a speech at Hawarden in 1891, read
the following words copied from a stone set up in the park of Hawarden to com-
memorate the rebuilding of a mill: "Trust in God for bread, and to the king for
protection and justice. This mill was built in the year 1767. Wheat was within this
year at 9s., and barley at 5s. 6d. a bushel. Luxury was at a great height, and charity
extensive, but the poor were starved, riotous, and hanged."
[2] Lecky, III. 115.
[3] *Gent. Magaz.*, series of letters by various hands in 1766. See also a long essay
in the *Annual Register* for 1767 (then edited by Edmund Burke), "On the Causes and
Consequences of the present High Price of Provisions," p. 165. The evidence of a
rise in the standard of living, in the matter of dress and luxuries as well as of food, is
equally clear from Scotland in the articles written by the parish ministers for the
'Statistical Account.'

fever in England became more detailed as to its circumstances, and more numerically precise. I shall accordingly bring together all that I can find relevant to fever in London, Liverpool, Newcastle and Chester, and thereafter in those towns, such as Manchester, Leeds, and others in the North, which were specially touched in their public health by the movement known as the Industrial Revolution.

Typhus Fever in London, 1770–1800.

In the London bills of mortality the item of fevers diminishes steadily during the latter part of the 18th century, the deaths from all causes diminish, the births come nearer to the number of the deaths, and in three years of the last decade they exceed them. This statistical result is doubtless roughly correct; but the bills were becoming more and more inadequate to the whole metropolitan area; and even for the original parishes which they included they have not the same value for fever in the later period as they had for plague at their beginning[1]. On the other hand, from about the year 1770 we begin to have more exact medical accounts of fever in London, which are not indeed numerically exhaustive, but good as samples of what was going on. Whatever improvement there was in the prevalence of typhus fever touched the richer classes. The Paving Act of 1766 is credited with having improved the health of the City, and there were many new streets and squares being built in the west end that were, of course, free from typhus. It is to these desirable residential quarters that the eulogies of Sir John Pringle[2], Dr John Moore[3] and others apply. The slums of London were as yet unimproved, and but little known to the physicians. Lettsom, who was one of the first of his class to visit among the poor in their homes, has much to say of typhus fever; but he is emphatic that it was nearly all an infection of the poor. "In the airy parts of this city," he writes in 1773, "and in large, open streets, fevers of a putrid tendency rarely

[1] For a judicious estimate of the value of the Parish Clerks' bills of mortality see the elaborate paper by Dr William Ogle, *Journ. Statist. Soc.* LV. (1892), 437.

[2] *Diseases of the Army.* New ed. 1775, pp. 334–5. Pringle admitted, however, that "in some of the lowest, moistest and closest parts of the town, and among the poorer people, spotted fevers and dysenteries are still to be seen, which are seldom heard of among those of better rank living in more airy situations."

[3] *Medical Sketches*, Lond. 1786, p. 464.

arise....In my practice I have attentively observed that at least forty-eight out of fifty of these fevers have existed in narrow courts and alleys." The same is remarked by Currie for Liverpool, by Clark for Newcastle, by Percival and Ferriar for Manchester, by Haygarth for Chester, and by Heysham for Carlisle.

The quarters of the rich had gradually become detached from those of the poor. I have shown this more especially for Chester, where the old walls made a clear division ; but it was general in the second half of the 18th century[1].

Medical practice lay mostly among the richer classes ; the physicians knew little of the state of health in the cellars and tenement-houses of large towns. Those physicians who did know how much typhus fever there was in these purlieus had to enter a caveat against the incredulity of the rest. Dr Currie of Liverpool, whose facts I shall give in their place, protested that he was not exaggerating; a protest the more necessary that a contemporary of his own, Mr Moss, a middle-class practitioner, who wrote a book specially on the medical aspects of Liverpool, declares that fever is "rare" in that city, while Currie was treating from his dispensary a steady average of three thousand cases of typhus every year. In the same years, in February, 1779, a physician to the army, Dr John Hunter, who had commenced practice in Mayfair, found on visiting in the homes of the poorer classes in the west of London cases of fever for which he had no other name than the gaol or hospital fever of his military experience ; it was so much a novelty to him, apart from campaigns or transport ships, that he gave an account of his discovery of domestic typhus to the College of Physicians[2]. At length he found so many cases steadily winter after winter that he had them sent to the infirmary of the Marylebone Work-house. The practitioners who knew most of the sicknesses of the poor were such as Robert Levett, Dr Samuel Johnson's

---

[1] Lecky, *History of England in the Eighteenth Century*, II. 636, generalizes the facts as follows: "The wealthy employer ceased to live among his people; the quarters of the rich and of the poor became more distant, and every great city soon presented those sharp divisions of classes and districts in which the political observer discovers one of the most dangerous symptoms of revolution."

[2] "This disease, as it appears in jails and hospitals, has been well described by Sir John Pringle; and other authors have given accounts of it on board of ships, especially crowded transports and prison-ships, but I do not find that its originating in the families of the poor in great cities during the winter has been taken notice of." *Med. Trans. Coll. Phys.* III. 345.

dependant, who lived with the doctor in the house in Gough Square. Levett had been a waiter in a Paris coffee-house frequented by the medical fraternity, and had acquired a taste for and perhaps some knowledge of the healing art. He made his modest living by the small fees or articles of food and drink which his poor patients gave him. He had only to issue from the back of Gough Square by the courts and alleys behind Fleet Street, and he would find in the region between Chancery Lane and Shoe Lane hundreds of families seldom visited by a physician or by a qualified surgeon-apothecary. The good Levett was only one of a class. There had always been such humble medical attendants of the poor in London. An Act of the third year of Henry VIII. was directed against them at the instance of the privileged practitioners; but the regular faculty is said to have proved in the sequel both greedy and incompetent, and after thirty years there came another Act, couched in terms that the bluff king himself might have indited (31–32 Henry VIII.), which asserts those qualities of the profession in so many words, and establishes the right of any subject of the king to practise minor surgery and the medicine of simples upon his or her neighbours. That Act is still part of the law of England, and under it Levett exercised a statutory right, perhaps without knowing it[1]. There were many other regions of courts and alleys all round the City on both sides of the water, which must have been medically served by such as Levett, if served at all. It was there that typhus was found and at length clinically described by competent physicians, among the earliest of whom was Lettsom.

The General Dispensary in Aldersgate Street having been started in 1770 with one physician, Lettsom was chosen additional physician in 1773, and threw himself into the work with great zeal[2]. In the first twelvemonth he saw many cases of fever, as in the following table:

---

[1] He has been immortalised by Johnson's verses:

> "Well tried through many a varying year
> See Levett to the grave descend,
> Officious, innocent, sincere,
> Of every friendless name the friend.
> In misery's darkest cavern known
> His ready help was ever nigh;" etc.

[2] John Coakley Lettsom, M.D., *Medical Memoirs of the General Dispensary in London, April* 1773 *to March* 1774. London, 1774.

Lettsom's practice in Fevers at the Aldersgate Dispensary.

Febris	April	May	June	July	Aug.	Sept.	Oct.	Nov.	Dec.	Jan.	Feb.	March	Total in 12 months	Died
				1773						1774				
hectica	2	2	4	13	4	2	3	4	9	12	18	13	86	3
inflammatoria	—	—	—	—	—	—	—	1	1	1	—	2	5	—
intermittens	3	1	7	1	1	1	1	—	2	1	2	2	22	—
nervosa	4	3	4	14	7	11	4	5	1	1	5	4	65	3
putrida	14	19	14	25	14	21	34	22	11	6	7	5	192	8
remittens	6	10	5	4	3	6	7	3	12	13	10	3	82	—
simplex vel diarium	—	2	1	6	2	5	4	5	—	—	—	4	29	—

The nervous, putrid and remittent fevers, belonging to the same group, make up the bulk of the fevers. The hectic fevers were almost all of children. The fatal cases of fever were fourteen, the fatal cases in all diseases for the year having been forty-four. What these putrid, nervous and remittent fevers were, will now appear from some of Lettsom's descriptions. Fevers with symptoms of putrescency were marked by nausea, bitter taste, and frequent vomiting, by laboured breathing and deep sighing, offensive breath, sweats offensive and sometimes tinged with blood, almost constant delirium, the tongue dry, the tongue, teeth and lips covered with black or brown tenacious foulness, thrush and ulceration in the mouth and throat, the urine with a dark sediment, the stools excessively nauseous and foetid, and blackish or bloody, the eyes horny or glassy, with the whites often tinged of a deep blood colour, spots on the skin like flea-bites, or larger haemorrhagic vibices, bleeding from the gums, nose or old ulcers, hiccup near death, often a cough through the fever. Lettsom's treatment consisted in good liquors, Peruvian bark, and above all fresh, or "cold" air: "When it is considered that putrid fevers originate in close unventilated places, the introduction of fresh air seems so natural a remedy that I have often admired its aid should have been so long neglected[1]." Accordingly he persuaded the poor people to open their windows, and dragged the sick out of doors as soon as it was safe to do so; the effects, he says, were wonderful. His fifty-one cases are most valuable illustrations of the perennial fever in the crowded parts of London:

[1] Nothing could be clearer than Dr John Arbuthnot's reasoning and advice on this matter half a century before.

Case 1 is of a man aged forty who had occasion to visit a miserable crowded workhouse in Spitalfields. He was instantly seized with such a nausea and debility as induced him to keep his room as soon as he got home. At the end of a week Lettsom found him in "the true jail-fever, or, what is the same, a true workhouse-fever." He had involuntary stools and leaping of the tendons, and took more wine in a week than he had done for many years.

Cases 2 to 12 were of several families in one house in a court in Long Lane, Aldersgate Street, who had been infected by a discharged prisoner from Newgate. Other cases follow, where the infection was caught from visiting the sick. In Case 17, Lettsom applied blisters "owing to the importunity of the friends," but without advantage. Case 30, on 26th October, 1773, was of a family of six persons near Christ Church, Lambeth, father, mother, boy of seventeen, child of two (slight attack) and two maids. Other localities were courts off Whitecross Street, Jewin Street, Little Moorfields, Chiswell Street, and St Martin's-le-Grand. Case 43 was of a woman, aged thirty, in Bunhill Row; she attended a relation who died of a putrid fever, and was herself attacked; her eyes were bloodshot, her skin marbled and interspersed with a general deep-coloured eruption, her cheeks and nose mortified. Cases 44–47 were of people in a "very helpless situation" in Gloucester Court, Whitecross Street.

The year 1773, to which these experiences in a small part of London relate, was one of high febrile mortality, according to the Bills. Two years after, Dr William Grant was moved to write an 'Essay on the Pestilential Fever of Sydenham, commonly called Gaol, Hospital, Ship and Camp Fever[1],' which, as he said in his preface, "I often see in this city: and though so common and fatal, appears not at present to be generally understood." It was, he says, "an indigenous plant, frequent in this city, being produced by close confinement; but it often passes unnoticed, because unknown." The deaths by "fever" in the London Bills were as follows until the end of the century:

Deaths from Fever and from all causes in London.

Year	Fever deaths	All deaths	Year	Fever deaths	All deaths
1771	2273	21780	1786	2981	20454
1772	3207	26053	1787	2887	19349
1773	3608	21656	1788	2769	19697
1774	2607	20884	1789	2380	20749
1775	2244	20514	1790	2185	18038
1776	1893	19048	1791	2013	18760
1777	2760	23334	1792	2236	20213
1778	2647	20399	1793	2426	21749
1779	2336	20420	1794	1935	19241
1780	2316	20517	1795	1947	21179
1781	2249	20719	1796	1547	19288
1782	2552	17918	1797	1526	17014
1783	2313	19029	1798	1754	18155
1784	1973	17828	1799	1784	18134
1785	2310	18919	1800	2712	23068

[1] London, 1775.

There were higher figures in the years immediately before 1771, the years to which the generalities of Fordyce and Armstrong relate.   There is a decline in the fever-mortality towards the end of the century; but it is just from the years 1799–1800 that we have an account by Willan of the prevalence and conditions of London typhus, than which nothing can well be imagined worse.   The intermediate glimpses we get of typhus in London in the writings of Dr Hunter, physician, and of Dr James Sims, show that the disease was perennial.

"In the month of February, 1779," says Hunter[1], "I met with two examples of fever in the lodgings of some poor people whom I visited that resembled in their symptoms the distemper which is called the jail or hospital fever.   It appeared singular that this disease should show itself after three months of cold weather.   Being therefore desirous of learning the circumstances upon which this depended I neglected no opportunity of attending to similar cases.   I soon found a sufficient number of them for the purpose of further information.   It appeared that the fever began in all in the same way and originated from the same causes.   A poor family, consisting of the husband, the wife, and one or more children, were lodged in a small apartment not exceeding twelve or fourteen feet in length, and as much in breadth.   The support of them depended on the industry and daily labour of the husband, who with difficulty could earn enough to purchase food necessary for their existence, without being able to provide sufficient clothing or fuel against the inclemencies of the season.   In order therefore to defend themselves against the cold of the winter, their small apartment was closely shut up, and the air excluded by every possible means.   They did not remain long in this situation before the air became so vitiated as to affect their health and produce a fever in some one of the miserable family. The fever was not violent at first, but generally crept on gradually…soon after the first a second was seized with the fever, and in a few days more the whole family perhaps were attacked, one after another, with the same distemper.   I have oftener than once seen four of a family ill at one time and sometimes all lying on the same bed.   The fever appeared sooner or later as the winter was more or less inclement, as the family was greater or smaller, as they were worse or better provided with clothes for their persons and beds, and with fuel, and as their apartment was more or less confined. The slow approach of the fever, the great loss of strength, the quickness of the pulse with little hardness or fulness, the tremors of the hands, and the petechiae or brown spots upon the skin, to which may be added the infectious nature of the distemper, left no doubt of its being the same with what is usually called the jail or hospital-fever."

Dr James Sims, who had seen much of Irish typhus in Tyrone in his earlier years, and had removed to London, wrote of typhus among the poor there in 1786, ten years before the more systematic and more circumstantial descriptions by Willan[1].

[1] *Med. Trans. of the Coll. Phys. Lond.* III. (1785), 345: "Observations on the Disease commonly called the Jail or Hospital Fever." By John Hunter, M.D., physician to the army.
[2] James Sims, M.D., "Scarlatina anginosa as it appeared in London in 1786," *Mem. Med. Soc. Lond.* I. 414.   Willan, who saw the same epidemic of scarlatinal sore-throat in London in 1786, believed that the angina was also "connected with a

This fever was exceedingly mortal, several medical men, he had reason to believe, falling sacrifices to it. Sims never saw the cases till the 7th or 8th day, when they were desipient, insensible, with pulse scarcely to be felt and not to be counted, all having petechiae. None had scarlet rash or sore-throat. They sank and died quietly; the strongest cordials did not produce the smallest effect, and blisters in many did not even raise the skin[1].

It is in the year 1796 that we begin to have the full and accurate records by Willan of the prevailing diseases of London month by month as he saw them at the Carey Street Dispensary, situated in the crowded quarter between Holborn and the Strand[2]. His first reference to typhus is as follows :

" In September, also, fevers usually appear which from their commencement exhibit symptoms of malignancy; being attended with a brown dry tongue, violent pain of the head, delirium, or coma, deep-seated pains of the limbs, petechial spots and haemorrhagy. These fevers become highly contagious, especially when they occur in close, confined situations, and in houses where little attention is paid to ventilation or cleanliness. The disease is extended by infection during the months of October and November, but its progress is generally stopped by the frosts of December."

Willan says little more of fever in London until September, 1798, when these contagious malignant fevers became more numerous, both in the city and adjacent villages, than had been known for many years before; also the fever was more fatal than usual, one in five or six dying, whereas one in seven was formerly a very unfavourable death-rate, and one in twenty not unknown. Haemorrhages, aphthae, diarrhoea, starting of the tendons, picking the bedclothes, violent delirium, ending in deafness, stupor, hiccough and involuntary evacuations, were the usual accompaniments of this fever. In the corresponding months of 1799 he recurs to the symptoms of this "malignant contagious fever," and depicts typhus as clearly as may be. In September, 1799, it was "attended with a dull pain of the head, great debility or sense of lassitude and pains referred to the bones, tremblings,

---

different species of contagion, namely, that of the typhus or malignant fever originating in the habitations of the poor, where no attention is paid to cleanliness and ventilation." *Cutaneous Diseases*, 1808, p. 333.

[1] The rumour of London fevers seems to have reached Barker, who kept an epidemiological record at Coleshill. Referring to the winter of 1788-89, he says: "At this time there were dreadful fevers in London, fatal to many, and a very infectious one in Coventry, of which many among the poor died, most of them being delirious, and many phrenetical."

[2] Robert Willan, M.D., *Reports on the Diseases of London, particularly during the years* 1796–97–98–99 *and* 1800. London, 1801.

restlessness with slight delirium, a querulous tone of voice, a small and frequent pulse, heat of the skin, thirst and a fur upon the tongue, first of a dirty white colour, but turning in the latter stage of the disease to a yellowish brown. In this form the fever continued thirteen days without any dangerous symptoms, and then suddenly disappeared, leaving the patient, for some time after, languid and dispirited. All the individuals of a family were successively affected with the same train of symptoms; many of them so slightly as not to be much confined to their beds." In October and November he describes the symptoms of the disease in a more dangerous form. By this fever, he was informed, some houses of the poor had been almost depopulated, the infection having extended to every inmate. "The rumour of a plague was totally devoid of foundation."

He then describes the state of the dwellings where such fevers occurred—the unwashed bed-linen, the numbers in one bed, the rooms encumbered with furniture or utensils of trade, the want of light and air in the cellars and garrets and in the passages thereto, the excremental effluvia from the vault at the bottom of the staircase. It cannot be wondered at, he concludes, that contagious diseases should be thereby formed, and attain their highest degree of virulence; and he estimates that "hundreds, perhaps thousands" of labourers in and near London, heads of families and in the prime of life, perished annually from such fevers. He denies that his account is exaggerated, and appeals for the truth of it to medical practitioners whose "situation or humanity has led them to be acquainted with" the localities[1].

Typhus in Liverpool, Newcastle and Chester in the last quarter of the 18th century.

Liverpool, in the last quarter of the 18th century, came next in size to London, having a population (in 1790) of 56,000 to the capital's estimated 800,000. According to a medical author,

[1] He names specially some streets of St Giles's parish, the courts and alleys adjoining Liquorpond Street, Hog-Island, Turnmill Street, Saffron Hill, Old Street, Whitecross Street, Golden Lane, the two Bricklanes, Rosemary Lane, Petticoat Lane, Lower East Smithfield, some parts of Upper Westminster, and several streets of Southwark, Rotherhithe, etc. "I recollect a house in Wood's Close, Clerkenwell, wherein the fomites of fever were thus preserved for a series of years; at length an accidental fire cleared away the nuisance. A house, notorious for dirt and infection, near Clare-market, afforded a farther proof of negligence: it was obstinately tenanted till the wall and floors, giving way in the night, crushed to death the miserable inhabitants."

whose experiences lay among the middle classes, it was everything that could be wished in the way of healthfulness and prosperity; but it had a dark side as well. About 7,000 of the people lived in cellars underground, and nearly 9,000 in back houses, in small confined courts with a narrow passage to the street. "Among the inhabitants of the cellars," says Currie[1], "and of these back houses, the typhus is constantly present; and the number of persons under this disease that apply for medical assistance to the charitable institutions, the public will be astonished to hear, exceeds three thousand annually...In sixteen years' practice I have found the contagious fever of Liverpool remarkably uniform among the poor. Seldom extending itself in any considerable degree among the other classes of the community, it has been supposed that Liverpool was little subject to fever; but this will be shewn from authentic documents to be a great and pernicious error." At the Dispensary in the year 1780 the cases of typhus averaged 160 per month, the numbers being as remarkably steady from month to month as from year to year. In the ten years from 1 January, 1787, to 31 December, 1796, 31,243 cases of fever were entered on the books of the Dispensary, an average of 3124 per annum[2].

Of 213,305 cases of all diseases at the Dispensary in seventeen years, 1780 to 1796, 48,367, nearly one-fourth, were labouring under typhus. Supposing that these were all the cases of typhus in Liverpool, and that 1 in 15 died, we should have some 150 deaths from typhus in a year. Supposing also that typhus was relatively as common at that time in London, it will follow that nearly all the deaths under "fever" in the bills of mortality might well have been from typhus fever; for London in its several densely populated out-parishes was the fever-quarter of Liverpool a dozen times over[3].

---

[1] *Medical Reports on the Effects of Water, Cold and Warm, as a Remedy in Fever and other Diseases.* 2nd ed., 1798. It need hardly be explained that Dr Currie was competent on fevers, his use of the clinical thermometer marking him as a man of precision. He is best known to the laity as the biographer of Robert Burns and the generous helper of the poet's widow and family.

[2] "If it be supposed," says Currie, "that some cases may be denominated typhus by mistake, let it be considered how many cases of this disease do not appear in the books of the Dispensary, though occurring among the poor, being attended by the surgeons and apothecaries of the Benefit Clubs to which they belong."

[3] Moss (*A Familiar Medical Survey of Liverpool,* 1784), who had not the same means of knowing the prevalence of typhus in Liverpool as Currie, declares that "there has been but one instance of a *truly* malignant fever happening in the town for many years; it was in the autumn of 1781, and appeared in Chorley Street, which is one of the narrowest and most populous streets in the town, and nine died of it in

The Newcastle Dispensary was opened in October, 1777, by
the exertions of Dr John Clark, who was in correspondence with
Lettsom in London [1]. Dr Clark had been in the East India Company's service, and had seen much of ship-fever and of the fevers
of the East. During a visit to his home in Roxburghshire in
the summer of 1770, between his voyages, he attended several
persons in continued fever. When he settled at Newcastle he saw
the worst kinds of contagious fever, in workhouses and " in the
sordid and crowded habitations of the indigent." Putrid fever,
or typhus, was by far the most common disease attended from
the new dispensary, although less than at Liverpool, the operations of the charity being on a much smaller scale. It was seldom
out of Newcastle a whole year; and in some years, as 1778,
1779, 1783, 1786 and 1787 it was unusually rife in particular
districts, often attacking whole families. Scarlet fever was
epidemic and very fatal in 1778 and 1779, while dysentery
attacked great numbers of the poor in the autumns of 1783 and
1785. The following Table shows the principal diseases attended
from the Dispensary during the first twenty-three months of its
working, 1 Oct. 1777, to 1 Sept. 1779:

Newcastle Dispensary 1777–79.

	Cases visited	Cured	Too far advanced	Dead
Putrid fever	391	357	9	16
Ulcerated sore-throat	146	125	11	9
Dysentery	72	55	5	4
Smallpox	45	29	5	6

From 1 Oct. 1777, to 1 Sept. 1789, the cases of typhus visited
were 1920, of which 121 were fatal. During the winter of 1790
and the spring and summer of 1791 it was prevalent amongst
the poor, and was frequently introduced into genteel families
and sometimes even into those of the first distinction. That
outbreak was supposed to have been generated in the Gateshead
poorhouse. For some time its ravages were confined chiefly to
the low, ill-aired, narrow street called Pipewell Gate. In Sep-

one week; it was only of short duration, and did not spread in any other part of the
town." He admits that the habitations of the poorer class were confined, being
chiefly in cellars; yet the diet of the *sober* and *industrious* is wholesome and sufficient,
the comfortable artizans being ship-carpenters, coopers, ropers and the like.
[1] John Clark, M.D., *Observations on the Diseases which prevail in Long Voyages,*
&c. 2nd ed., Lond. 1792; *Account of the Newcastle Dispensary from its Commencement in* 1777 *to March* 1789, Newcastle, 1789; and subsequent Annual Reports.

tember it made its appearance in Newcastle; at first the contagion was easily traced from Pipewell Gate, and afterwards from one house to another. In that outbreak, 188 poor persons were visited from the Newcastle Dispensary, the Gateshead poor having been attended by the parochial surgeon. Clark's ten cases recorded of the epidemic were all of people in good circumstances. The Dispensary Tables show cases of typhus every year down to 1850, the largest totals being in 1793 (374, 18 deaths), 1801 (435, 20 deaths), and 1819 (368, 14 deaths); and these, we may take it, were but a small fraction of all the cases in Newcastle.

Perhaps the most unexpected revelation of typhus is at Chester, from the time when Haygarth began to write upon its public health in 1772. Chester was then one of the most desirable places of residence in England. Boswell wrote to Johnson, " Chester pleases me more than any town I ever saw." The old city within the walls was occupied by a superior class of residents, including the cathedral clergy, county families, retired officers and Anglo-Indians, professional men, merchants and tradesmen. It had the best theatre out . of London. Squares, crescents and broad streets were replacing most of the old buildings. The six parishes that lay entirely within the walls had a population, in 1774, of 3502, and an annual average death-rate (in the ten years 1764 to 1773) of 1 in 58 or 17·2 per 1000, the central parish of St Peter having a rate of 1 in 62, and the cathedral parish 1 in 87. It passed as one of the healthiest cities in the kingdom, being far before Shrewsbury and Nottingham, to say nothing of the large towns where the burials exceeded the baptisms. But its moderate death-rate over all, 1 in 42 living, would have been much lower but for the four poor suburban parishes, with a population of 11,211 which had a death-rate of 1 in 35. Haygarth gives a deplorable account of them. The houses were small, close, crowded and dirty, ill supplied with water, undrained, and built on ground that received the sewage from within the walls. The people were ill-fed and they seldom changed or washed their clothes; when they went abroad they were noisome and offensive to the smell. Many of them worked on the large farms around Chester, others at shipbuilding and shipping (Chester had then a considerable foreign trade), others at the mills and markets, others at a nail-factory, while others were employed by the tradesmen within the walls. Fever seems to have been perennial among them, the deaths from typhus having been 23 in 1772, 33 in 1773 and 35 in 1774. "In these poor habitations," says Haygarth, "when one person is seized with a fever, others of the family are generally affected with the same fever in a greater or less degree." It became rifer than usual in August, 1773, and attacked 285, proving fatal to 28, or to one in ten. It had the common symptoms of malignant fevers produced by human effluvia, and particularly affected the head with pain, giddiness and delirium. It attacked in general the lowest, few of the middle rank, and none (or only one) of the highest rank[1].

Chester had no manufactures. Its population had grown rapidly of late, as that of Liverpool had grown, the poorer classes being the prolific part of the community; but it had no share in the industrial revolution, it did not employ its women and children in factories, and it was in some respects better than Leeds, Warrington, Manchester, or Carlisle. It is a good illustration of a town growing rapidly without manufactures, and of a community divided by the old walls into two quite distinct sections, a rich and a poor. Such had been the drift of things in England apart from the industrial revolution; but it is the latter which furnishes the best illustrations of a poor prolific populace, of a growing struggle, and of the attendant typhus fever.

Fever in the Northern Manufacturing Towns, 1770–1800.

The prosperity of the first two-thirds of the 18th century had been attended with a very small increase of population. From 1700 to 1750 the numbers in England are estimated to have grown no more than from about six millions to six millions and a half. The fecundity of many rural parishes was swallowed up by emigration to the American and West Indian colonies, by the army and navy, and by the great waste of life in London and some other towns. The increase was nearly all north of the Trent, while the old weaving towns of the south-west had actually declined. Gloucestershire, Somerset and Wilts were the most crowded counties in 1700. During the next fifty

---

[1] Haygarth, *Phil. Trans.* LXIV. 67; Hemingway, *History of Chester*, I. 344 *seq.*

years, the greatest increase was as in the following rough estimate [1]:

	1700	1750	Increase per cent.
Lancashire	166,200	297,400	78
West Riding of Yorks.	236,700	361,500	52
Warwickshire	96,600	140,000	45
Durham	95,500	135,000	41
Staffordshire	117,200	160,000	36
Gloucestershire	155,200	207,800	34

In the counties where population had increased most, much of the increase was still rural or semi-rural. Defoe describes how the land near Halifax was divided into lots of from two to six or seven acres, hardly a house out of speaking distance from another, at every house a tenter, and on almost every tenter a piece of cloth, or kersey or shalloon. Every clothier kept one horse at least, to carry his manufactures to the market, and nearly every one kept a cow, or two or more, for his family. The houses were full of lusty fellows, some at the dye-vat, some at the looms, others dressing the cloths, the women and children carding or spinning, being all employed from the youngest to the oldest: not a beggar to be seen, nor an idle person [2]. We have no accounts of the health of this population, except Nettleton's statistics of smallpox in and around Halifax in 1721 and 1722, given elsewhere, and the "epidemic constitutions" recorded by Wintringham at York during the same period, and by Hillary at Ripon.

Before the earliest of the inventions of spinning by machinery, the weavers were gathering to the towns of Yorkshire, Lancashire and other counties north of the Trent. The spinning-jenny of Hargreaves was wrecked by a Blackburn mob in 1768, and a mob wrecked the cotton-mill built by Arkwright at Chorley eleven years later. This was decidedly a time of movement from the country to the towns, a movement which preceded the spinning ingenuity of the sixties and may have been stimulated by the earlier use of the fly-shuttle in weaving.

[1] Arnold Toynbee, *Lectures on the Industrial Revolution of the 18th Century, etc.* London, 1884.

[2] Toynbee (u. s.) says of the time before the mills were built: "The manufacturing population still lived to a very great extent in the country. The artisan often had his small piece of land, which supplied him with wholesome food and healthy recreation. His wages and employments too were more regular. He was not subject to the uncertainties and knew nothing of the fearful sufferings which his descendants were to endure from commercial fluctuations, especially before the introduction of free trade."

Much of the country round Manchester, though it doubtless retained those farm-houses, hedgerows, and field paths which come into the idyllic opening of 'Mary Barton' more than half a century later, was "crowded with houses and inhabitants," as Percival says: so populous were the environs of Manchester that every house in the township had been found by a late survey to contain an average of six persons. The proportion of deaths was less than in 1757; but that was chiefly due to the accession of new settlers from the country, which raised the ratios of marriages and births[1]. Manchester had increased from a population of about 8000 in 1717 to one of 19,839 (inclusive of Salford) in 1757. When the inhabitants were next counted in 1773, they were found to be 22,481 in Manchester (5317 families in 3402 houses) and 4765 in Salford (1099 families in 866 houses). According to Percival, who gives these figures, the death-rate in 1773 was 1 in 28·4, the births exceeding the deaths by forty in a year. The poor, he says, were now better lodged, and some of the most dangerous malignant distempers were less violent and less mortal. Manchester, however, was still an unhealthy place compared with the country, especially to young children. Thus, the thirty-one townships in the parish of Manchester contained, exclusive of the city, 13,786 inhabitants (2525 families in 2371 houses), and of these only 1 in 56 died annually (compared with 1 in 28 in the city)—the births being to the deaths as 401 to 246 in the year 1772.

Again, the bleak upland parish of Darwen with a population in the year 1774 of 1850 souls mostly occupied in the cotton manufacture, had, during the seven years before, more than twice as many baptisms as burials (508 to 233), the birth-rate (1 in 25·5) being high and the death-rate (1 in 56) low.

Leeds had a population of some six or seven thousand at the time of the Civil Wars, and lost 1325 in nine months of the year 1645 from plague, all of them the poorer class. A generation or two later, in the time of Thoresby's 'Diary,' it was a centre of the cloth trade; and it appears to have grown steadily throughout the 18th century. In 1775 it had a population of 17,117. We hear from Lucas of an epidemic typhus in it previous to 1779[2]. Eighty persons had died of that fever in one year, and

[1] Percival, "Population of Manchester." *Phil. Trans.* LXIV. 54.
[2] James Lucas, "Remarks on Febrile Contagion." *London Medical Journal,* X. 260.

many who struggled through the disease died afterwards of lingering complaints. In two courts or yards (such as might have been the Lantern Yard which Silas Marner found pulled down when he revisited Leeds) forty persons were affected with the fever; some families had received ten shillings a week from the assessment for the poor. As early as 1779 Lucas proposed a house of reception for contagious fever, a proposal which was carried into effect in 1804, after a whole generation of typhus and at a time when there was little fever in Leeds or elsewhere, The infectious fevers, being chiefly confined to the poor, often prevailed, says this writer, for a length of time without exciting much alarm, or without their fatality being attended to; but, he adds about the year 1790, "should a few of the higher rank receive the infection, then the disease is described in most exaggerated terms."

Carlisle was a good instance of the increase of urban population and the breeding of typhus. In seventeen years, from 1763 to 1780, the inhabitants had increased from 4158 to 6229, many of the immigrants being Scots and Irish with their families. The chief industry was the making of calico, in which the women and children were employed as well as the men. When Dr Heysham surveyed the town and suburbs for his census of 1779, he had "opportunity of seeing many scenes of poverty and filth and nastiness[1]"; and in the bill of mortality for that year he confesses himself astonished that there should be so little fever.

The great outburst of typhus at Carlisle began in the end of March, 1781, with no very obvious special provocation[2]. Upwards of 600 had typhus to February 7th, 1782, at which date 12 or 15 were still suffering from it. The deaths were less than 1 in 10 of all attacked: viz. 2 in May, 4 in June, 8 in July, 8 in August, 7 in September, 9 in October, 8 in November, 6 in December, and 3 in January, 1782, a total of 55. Of this total of fatal cases, 3 were boys, 4 bachelors, and 15 husbands: 3 girls, 2 maids, 22 wives, and 6 widows. Two-thirds of all the deaths were of married people; Heysham saw no case in a child under three years. It affected about a tenth part of the inhabit-

---

[1] In Appendix to Hutchinson's *Cumberland*, 1794. Reprinted in Appendix to Joshua Milne's *Valuation of Annuities*, Lond. 1815.
[2] John Heysham, M.D., *Account of the Jail Fever, or Typhus Carcerum, as it appeared at Carlisle in* 1781. London, 1782.

ants of Carlisle (6299), and raged most among the lower class who lived in narrow, close, confined lanes and in small crowded apartments, of which there were a great many in Carlisle, generally going through all the inmates of a house where it had once begun. On seeking to trace the origin of the epidemic, he found that it began in the end of March, 1781, in a house in Richard-gate, which contained about half-a-dozen very poor families. Every window that could be spared was shut up, to save the window-tax. The surgeon who attended some of these poor wretches told Dr Heysham that the smell was so offensive that it was with difficulty he could stay in the house. One of the typhus patients in this house was a weaver, who, on his recovery, went to the large workshop where he worked, and there, it was supposed, gave the infection (in his clothes) to his fellow workmen, by whom new centres of infection were made in various other houses. In August, a young man just recovered from the fever went to his mother's in the small village of Rockliffe, four or five miles from Carlisle, to get back his strength in the country air; his mother soon took the fever and died, and a neighbour woman who came to her in her sickness likewise caught it and died. These were all the cases known in the village, and they show the enormously greater fatality of typhus in those not inured to its atmosphere and conditions.

The state of population and health at Warrington was peculiar, and is given fully in another chapter. There could be no more striking instance of the growth of what the foreign writers call the proletariat; an old market-town, with a small sail-cloth industry from Elizabethan times, it became a busy weaving town owing to the demand for sail-cloth during the war with the American colonies. The whole population of some 9000 men, women and children, were wage-earners; the women were all the while unusually prolific, and the sacrifice of infant life was enormous, especially by smallpox. We have no particular accounts of fevers; but in the bill of mortality for 1773, the year of a disastrous smallpox epidemic, there were 25 deaths from fever, of which 10 were of " worm fever," or the remittent of children[1].

By the year 1790, when Ferriar's accounts of fever in Manchester begin, the industrial revolution had been accomplished, mills were everywhere, and the characteristic hardships

[1] Aikin, *Phil. Trans.* LXIV. 473.

and maladies of a prolific working class in a time of slack trade were already much the same as we find them pictured with fidelity and pathos in the pages of Mrs Gaskell half a century after.

But, so as not to exaggerate the ill health of the working class in Manchester at the end of the 18th century, let us compare the births with the deaths according to the doubtless imperfect registers[1]:

Manchester, Births and Deaths, 1770–91.

Year	Births	Deaths	Year	Births	Deaths
1770	1050	988	1781	1591	1370
1771	1169	993	1782	1678	984
1772	1127	904	1783	1615	1496
1773	1168	923	1784	1958	1175
1774	1245	958	1785	1942	1734
1775	1359	835	1786	2319	1282
1776	1241	1220	1787	2256	1761
1777	1513	864	1788	2391	1637
1778	1449	975	1789	2487	1788
1779	1464	1288	1790	2756	1940
1780	1566	993	1791	2960	2286

The mean lodging-houses in the outskirts of the town, says Ferriar, in 1790[2], were the principal nurseries of febrile contagion: some of these were old houses with very small rooms, into each of which four or more people were crowded to eat, sleep, and frequently to work. They commonly bore marks of a long accumulation of filth, and some of them had been scarcely free from infection for many years past. As soon as one poor creature dies or is driven out of his cell he is replaced by another, generally from the country, who soon feels in his turn the consequences of breathing infected air. There was hardly any ventilation possible, many of these old houses being in dark narrow courts or blind alleys. In other parts of the town the lodging-houses were new, and not yet thoroughly dirty; but in these there was a long garret under the tiles, in which eight or ten people often lodged, the beds almost touching. Again, many lived in cellars, sleeping on the damp floor with few or no bedclothes; the cellars of Manchester, however, were better ventilated than those of Edinburgh, and

[1] John Aikin, M.D., *The Country from* 30 *to* 40 *miles round Manchester.* Lond. 1795, p. 584.
[2] John Ferriar, M.D., *Medical Histories and Reflections.* 4 vols., 1810–13, I. 172

freer from fever. These cellar-tenants were subject to the constant action of depressing passions of the mind. "I have seen patients," says Ferriar, "in agonies of despair on finding themselves overwhelmed with filth and abandoned by everyone who could do them any service, and after such emotions I have seldom found them recover." Addressing the Literary and Philosophical Society of Manchester previous to 1792, he pointed out in an *argumentum ad hominem* that "the situation of the poor at present is extremely dangerous, and often destructive to the middle and higher ranks of society[1]." And again, "the poor are indeed the first sufferers, but the mischief does not always rest with them. By secret avenues it reaches the most opulent, and severely revenges their neglect or insensibility to the wretchedness surrounding them[2]."

In an address to the Committee of Police in Manchester, he instances the following cases :

A family of the name of Turner in a dark cellar behind Jackson's Row : they have been almost constantly patients of the Infirmary for three years past on account of disorders owing to their miserable dwelling. There are other instances of the same kind in Bootle Street.

In Blakely Street, under No. 4, is a range of cellars let out to lodgers, which threatens to become a nursery of disease. They consist of four rooms communicating with each other, of which the two centre rooms are completely dark; the fourth is very ill-lighted and chiefly ventilated through the others. They contain four or five beds in each, and are already extraordinarily dirty.

In a nest of lodging-houses in Brook's entry near the bottom of Long-mill-gate, a very dangerous fever constantly subsists, and has subsisted for a considerable number of years. He had known nine patients confined in fevers at the same time in one of those houses and crammed into three small dirty rooms without the regular attendance of any friend or of a nurse. Four of these poor creatures died, absolutely from want of the common offices of humanity and from neglect in the administration of their medicines. Another set of lodging-houses constantly infected is known by the name of the Five Houses, in Newton Street[3].

The fever in Manchester was not always malignant typhus : sometimes it had the symptoms and low rate of mortality that suggest relapsing fever. Thus, in the winter epidemic of 1789–90, very prevalent in Manchester and Salford, out of Ferriar's first ninety patients only two died ; in some the skin had a remarkable, pungent heat, in others there were profuse watery sweats ; women were commonly affected with hysterical symptoms during convalescence, which was often tedious[4]. A certain

---

[1] Ferriar, I. 261. [2] *Ibid.* I. 234. [3] *Ibid.* II. 213–20.
[4] *Ibid.* I. 153–6; and II. 57.

number of these cases would run into "a formed typhus," with petechiae and all the other signs of malignity; and in some seasons, as in the distressful year 1794, typhus was the usual form. Two fatal cases in children, examined after death, had peritonitis; "in the one no marks of the disease were discernible within the cavity of the [intestinal] tube;" in the other, the patient was covered with petechiae[1]. These cases of localized inflammation in typhus he compares with Pringle's cases of spotted fever complicated with abscess of the brain.

The years 1792 and 1793 passed, says Ferriar, without any extraordinary increase of fever patients, although the noxious influences were always present. But in the summer and autumn of 1794 "the usual epidemic fever" became very prevalent among the poor in some quarters of the town, particularly after a bilious colic had raged among all ranks of people. This was a time when work was slack; many workmen enlisted and left their families. In November and December 1794, as many as 156 sent applications to the Infirmary in a week to be visited in fever at their homes.

This was a memorable time of scarcity and distress all over the country, the beginning of a twenty-years' period of so-called " war-prices," when farmers' profits were so large that they could afford to double or treble their rents to the landlords. The history of epidemics comes at this point into close contact with the economic history, which I shall touch on in the sequel, after giving a few more particulars of typhus in England and Scotland generally, previous to the outbreak of the war with France in 1793.

Typhus in England and Scotland generally, in the end of the 18th century.

The introduction of machinery and the building of mills brought typhus fever to places much less crowded than Leeds, or Manchester, or Carlisle.

Dr David Campbell of Lancaster saw much of typhus in that town, and in mill villages near it, in the years 1782, 1783, and 1784. In Lancaster town he saw about 500 cases, of which 168 were in men, with 20 deaths, 236 in women, with 11 deaths,

---

[1] Ferriar, I. 166–8.

and 94 in children under fourteen, with 3 deaths. At Backbarrow cotton mill, twenty miles from Lancaster, there were 180 cases, of which 38 were in men, with 5 deaths, 11 in women, with 2 deaths, and 131 in children under fourteen, with no deaths[1] At this mill there was an extremely offensive smell in the rooms, which came from the privy; the doors of the latter, "for indispensable reasons in the economy of these works, where so many children are employed, always communicate with the workrooms." Every care had been taken to keep the air sweet, but without effect. The offensive smell was in all the cotton mills from the same cause; and in the Radcliffe mill belonging to Mr Peel, the typhus was ascribed to that source, the nuisance having been at length got rid of. Both at Backbarrow and Radcliffe the houses of the workpeople were new, airy and comfortable. In the same years typhus raged with uncommon severity at Ulverston and in various parts of Lancashire, where cotton-mills had been set up[2].

The typhus of Liverpool and Newcastle was reproduced in Whitehaven and Cockermouth on a scale proportionate to their size. Whitehaven, the port of the Cumberland coal-field, was the Newcastle of the west coast, and had a large trade with Ireland. Many of the labourers lived in cellars. Brownrigg's experiences of typhus fever in it went back to near the middle of the 18th century. The Whitehaven Dispensary was opened in 1783, the occasion for it being thus explained:—

"Previous to the establishment of dispensaries Whitehaven and Cockermouth were infested by nervous and putrid fever. Many of their respectable inhabitants became its victims; and among the lower class of people it prevailed with deplorable malignancy. The present period happily exhibits a different picture. Notwithstanding our connection with the metropolis of Ireland, and other commercial places, contagion rarely appears; or, when accidentally introduced, is readily suppressed[3]."

The following is the abstract of "contagious fever cases" from the records of the Whitehaven Dispensary from 30 June, 1783, to 9 June, 1800[4]:

---

[1] This is perhaps the first numerical evidence of the slight fatality of typhus in children. A more elaborate proof of the same was given long after by Geary for Limerick. An early age-table for Whitehaven is given under Smallpox, *infra.*

[2] David Campbell, M.D., *Observations on the Typhus or Low Contagious Fever.* Lancaster, 1785.

[3] Joshua Dixon, M.D., *Annual Reports of the Whitehaven Dispensary*, 1795 *to* 1805. Details for 1773-4 in his note in *Memoirs of Lettsom*, III. 353.

[4] Dixon, *Literary Life of Dr Brownrigg*, pp. 238-9.

Year	Cured	Dead	Total		Year	Cured	Dead	Total
1783	75	1	76		1792	17	2	19
1784	401	9	410		1793	7	3	10
1785	350	20	370		1794	13	1	14
1786	91	6	97		1795	28	2	30
1787	21	1	22		1796	48	1	49
1788	53	7	60		1797	35	2	37
1789	103	2	105		1798	12	1	13
1790	288	21	309		1799	11	1	12
1791	74	6	79		Total	1627	85	1712

The year 1790 is indicated as an unhealthy one, by the excess of burials over christenings, also at Macclesfield, where there were 316 christenings to 380 burials, the proportion being usually the other way[1].

Dr John Alderson of Hull wrote in 1788 an essay on the contagion of fever, in which there are no authentic details for Hull: "The calamity itself is the constant complaint of every neighbourhood, and almost every newspaper presents us with an example of the direful consequences of infection"—the reference being to gaols more particularly[2]. Whatever was the reason, there was undoubtedly a great deal of typhus in England in the eighties of the eighteenth century. Oxfordshire, Gloucestershire, Worcestershire, Wiltshire and Buckinghamshire experienced much typhus from 1782 to 1785, although we have few particulars. "The remembrance of its ravages at Gloucester, Worcester and Marlborough," says Dr Wall of Oxford, "is still fresh in every mind, where its virulence proved so peculiarly fatal to the medical world." At Aylesbury, Dr Kennedy survived an attack of the "contagious fever," to write an account (1785) of the epidemic, which he traced to the gaol (the date, be it observed, is subsequent to Howard's visitations)[3]. At Maidstone, also, in 1785, the gaol fever was the subject of a special account[4].

At Worcester in 1783 the younger Dr Johnstone caught typhus while visiting the gaol, which was thereafter rebuilt at great expense. A prisoner took it to Droitwich where 14 died[5].

Dr Wall gives clinical details of fifteen cases of typhus treated by him in private practice at Oxford in 1785; one of his patients was an apothecary whose business had exposed him very much to the influence of contagion, as he was much

[1] Aikin, *Country round Manchester*. Lond. 1795, p. 616.
[2] *Nature and Origin of the Contagion of Fevers*. Hull, 1788.
[3] *Account of a Contagious Fever at Aylesbury*. Aylesbury, 1785.
[4] Thomas Day, *Some Considerations...on the Contagion in Maidstone Jail*, 1785.
[5] See Barnes, in *Mem. Lit. Soc. Phil. Manchester*, II. 85. Dr Samuel Parr wrote his epitaph in the Cathedral. Also Johnstone sen. to Lettsom, *Memoirs*, III. 241.

employed amongst the poor in the suburbs of the town and neighbouring villages and in the House of Industry[1]." In the year 1783–85, much of the epidemic fever was of the nature of ague, as described in another chapter. It is not always easy to separate it from typhus; but there is no doubt that both were prevalent together. Thus in the parish of Painswick, Gloucestershire, in the spring of 1785 there occurred both "a contagious fever" and an "epidemic ague," the latter having left a good many persons dropsical and cachectic[2]. This had been part of an epidemical fever which had raged for some time in the county of Gloucestershire, and is said to have lately carried off a great number of poor. At Norton, within five miles of Gloucester, there lived in two adjoining tenements two families: in one a man and his wife and three children, in the other a man and his wife, of whom only one remained alive on the 1st of March, 1785[3].

The extraordinary failure of the harvest in Scotland in 1782 produced much distress, and with it fever, in the winter following. The Glasgow and Edinburgh municipalities imported grain for the public benefit. Various traces of the scarcity and fever appear in the Statistical Account written a few years after. Thus, in Holywood parish, Dumfriesshire, some fevers were wont to appear in February and March among people of low circumstances living in a narrow valley; and the unusual mortality in the dear year 1782 was owing to an infectious fever in the same cottages. In the regular bills of mortality of Torthorwald parish, Dumfriesshire, the deaths from "fever" fall in the dear years, 1782–3, 1785, &c. In Dunscore parish, in the same county, the burials of 1782 rose to the most unusual figure of 30 (the baptisms being 17), "owing to a malignant fever[4]."

[1] Martin Wall, M.D., *Clin. Obs. on the Use of Opium in Low Fevers and in the Synochus.* Oxford, 1786.

[2] J. C. Jenner, in *Lond. Med. Journal*, VII. 163.

[3] *Gent. Magaz.* 1785, I. 231, March 1.

[4] This is the period and the district to which Robert Burns refers, under date of 21 June, 1783, in a letter to his cousin, James Burness, of Montrose: "I shall only trouble you with a few particulars relative to the wretched state of this country. Our markets are exceedingly high, oatmeal 17*d*. and 18*d*. per boll, and not to be got even at that price. We have, indeed, been pretty well supplied with quantities of white peas from England and elsewhere; but that resource is likely to fail us, and what will become of us then, particularly the very poorest sort, heaven only knows." The lately flourishing silk and carpet weaving had declined during the American War, and the seasons had been adverse to farmers. The lines in Burns' poem, "Death and Dr Hornbook":
'This while ye hae been mony a gate
       At mony a house.'
'Ay, Ay,' quoth he, and shook his head.—
are explained by a note, "An epidemical fever was then raging in the country."

But Scotland was now past the danger of actual famine from even a total failure of the harvest. Some farmers were ruined, and many more were unable to pay the year's rent; but the very poorest were enabled to find food, one source being "the importation of white pease from America." From Delting, in Shetland, one of the poorest parishes, the report is: "There is reason to believe that none died from mere want; but there is no doubt that many, from the unwholesome food, contracted diseases that brought them to their graves."

The following relating to the parishes of Keithhall and Kinkell, Aberdeenshire, in the scarcity following the lost harvest of 1782, is a curiously detailed glimpse of the time:

"Several families who would not allow their poverty to be known lived on two diets of meal a day. One family wanted food from Friday night till Sunday at dinner. On the last Friday of December, 1782, the country people could get no meal in Aberdeen, as the citizens were afraid of a famine; and a poor man, in this district, could find none in the country the day after. But the distress of this family being discovered, they were supplied. Next day the [Kirk] session bought at a sale a considerable quantity of bere, which was made into meal. This served the poor people until the importation at Aberdeen became regular, and every man of humanity rejoiced that the danger of famine was removed[1]."

We hear most of fevers in the Highland parishes, with their subdivisions of holdings and an excess of population. Thus of Gairloch, Ross-shire, it is said: "Fevers are frequent, sometimes they are of a favourable kind, at other times they continue long and carry off great numbers"—the poor in this parish, upon the Kirk Session roll, numbering 84 in the year 1792, and the aggregate money paid to the whole number averaging £6. 7s. in a year, whereas the fertile parish of Ellon, Aberdeenshire, with 40 on the poor's roll, paid them £43 per annum.

Again, of the fishing village of Eyemouth, it is said: "The only complaints that prove mortal in this place are different kinds of fevers and consumptions; and these are mostly confined to the poorest class of people, and ascribed to their scanty diet." And of another fishing parish, in Banffshire, Fordyce, including Portsoy, it is said: "The most prevalent distemper is a fever, and that for the most part not universal, but confined to particular districts. It is sometimes thought to arise from infection and communication with other parts of the country; at other times from local situations and circumstances of the people's houses and habits of living in particular districts[2]."

[1] Account by Rev. Geo. Skene Keith, *Statist. Act.* II. 544.   [2] Also Banff, *ibid.* XX. 347.

The beginning of the great French war was the occasion of a considerable increase of fever; although no records make it appear so fatal a time as the years 1783–86. The commercial distress and want of work which began in the autumn of 1792, were intensified by the bad harvests of 1794 and 1795, which followed two harvests also deficient. This was the period of distress and of epidemic fever to which Wordsworth referred in the passage in the first book of the 'Excursion,' where he is relating the story of Margaret's ruined cottage[1].

There is little medical writing upon the epidemic fever of 1794–95 ; and, in the very district of Wordsworth's story, the records of the Whitehaven Dispensary bear no traces of a great concourse of patients. There is reason to think that the fever, if slow and weakening, was seldom fatal, that it was *typhus mitior*, and that it was sometimes, perhaps often, relapsing. One glimpse we get of it in the family of the afterwards celebrated Dr Edward Jenner of Berkeley, in the winter of 1794–95. He thus writes to a friend about the visitation of "grim-visaged typhus:"

"You shall hear the history of our calamities. First fell Henry's [his nephew and assistant] wife and sister. From the early use of bark, they both appeared to recover; but the former, after going about her ordinary business for some days, had a dreadful relapse which nearly destroyed her. It was during my attendance on this case that the venomed arrow wounded me...Like Mrs Jenner's fever, at an early period there was a clear inter-

1   " Not twenty years ago, but you I think
            Can scarcely bear it now in mind, there came
            Two blighting seasons, when the fields were left
            With half a harvest. It pleased heaven to add
            A worse affliction in the plague of war, &c."
Trotter, *Medicina Nautica*, I. 182, 1797, gives these real cases :—"During the short time that I attended the dispensary at Newcastle, just at the beginning of the [French] war, I was sent for to a poor man in a miserable and low part of the town called Sandgate. He was ill with what is called a spotted fever." Six children were standing round his bed, the oldest not more than nine. They had been ill first, then his wife, who was recovered and had gone out to pawn the last article they had to buy meal for the children. The man worked on the quay at 1*s.* 2*d.* per diem. Again, "When I practised as a surgeon and apothecary at the end of the late [American] war in a small town in Northumberland, with an extensive country business, some similar scenes came under my view. Two servants of two opulent farmers applied to me for relief. The first had seven children, who took the fever one by one till the whole became sick. His wages were 1*s.* per diem. His master, a rich man, thought himself charitable by allowing them to pull turnips from his field for food. The other servant was a shepherd; but his herding, as the saying is, was a poor one. The first and second of six children were able to work a little, till they got a fever in a severe winter, and down they fell, one after another, the father and mother at last." They wanted to sell the cow; but some charitable ladies raised a small subscription, by which means the comforts of wine and diet came within their reach; their master, for his part, sent them the carcase of a sheep, which had been found dead in a furrow, with a request that the skin should be returned.

mission for four days...On the eighth day after the first seizure it again set in, in good earnest, and continued one-and-twenty days...Dr Parry was with me from Bath five times, Dr Hicks and Dr Ludlow as many, and my friend George was never absent from my bedside...But, to return to that mansion of melancholy, Henry's. His infant girl has now the fever; a servant maid in the house is dying with it; and to complete this tragical narrative, about five days ago fell poor Henry himself. His symptoms at present are such as one might expect: violent pain in the head, vertigo, debility, transient shiverings....His pulse this evening is sunk from 125 to 100. The stench from the poor girl is so great as to fill the house with putrid vapour; and I shall remove him this morning by means of a sedan-chair to a cottage near my own house[1]."

This is a tolerably clear picture of a short-period fever with relapses, or of relapsing fever strictly so-called; the stench, also, of one patient is characteristic. Barker, of Coleshill or Birmingham, has much to say under the same year 1794, of a slow, tedious fever, marked by " sluggish action and comatose symptoms," and much subject to relapses ; but he does not give the duration of the first or subsequent paroxysms, as Jenner does, or the usual length of the clear intervals, his most definite case being of a young woman who died in twenty-four hours from a relapse which came on about three weeks after the fever had left her[2].

It was the access of fever in 1794–5, and the alarm that it caused among the richer classes, that led to the opening of the Manchester House of Recovery in 1796. In certain streets in the neighbourhood chosen for the hospital, Portland Street, Silver Street and others in the same block, the cases of contagious fever for nearly three years before the hospital was opened are given by Ferriar as follows:

Sept. 1793 to Sept. 1794, cases of fever, 400
Sept. 1794 to Sept. 1795, „ „ „ 389
Sept. 1795 to May 1796, „ „ „ 267

The cases began to be sent to the hospital on the 27th May, 1796, and an attempt was made to extinguish contagion in the houses, by white-washing, disinfecting and the like; so that in the same group of streets there were only 25 cases of fever from 13 July, 1794 to 13 March, 1797. Meanwhile the admissions to the hospital were few until the dearth of 1799–1802. One of the manufacturing towns which is known to have shared in the epidemic fever of 1794–96 was Ashton-under-Lyne, where upwards of three hundred cases (with few deaths)

---

[1] Jenner to Shrapnell, Baron's *Life of Jenner*, I. 106-7.
[2] John Barker, *Épidemicks*, pp. 201-6.

occurred in less than three months at the end of 1795. This epidemic must have been somewhat special to Ashton, for it produced much alarm in neighbouring places and caused Ashton to be avoided from fear of infection.

Shortly after 1796, Ferriar made an inquiry into an epidemic of fever at a village within a mile of Manchester; the houses were many of them new, built for the convenience of a large cotton mill; but even the new houses were offensive, with cellars occupied by lodgers, and almost every house overcrowded. This was the first fever in the village, and it was traced to a family who had come from Manchester with infected clothes. Stockport about the same time erected a House of Recovery, having "the same general causes of fever which render the disease so common in Manchester"; and Ferriar adds: "I believe there is not a town in the kingdom containing four thousand inhabitants which would not be greatly benefited by similar establishments."

The bad harvest of 1794 raised the price of wheat to 55*s.* 7*d.* on 1 January, 1795, and the prospect of another short harvest to 77*s.* 2*d.* on 1 July. A famine being threatened, the Government caused neutral ships bound to French ports with corn to be seized, and brought into English ports, the owners receiving an ample profit. Agents were also sent to the Baltic to buy corn. By these means the price of wheat, which had risen in August to 108*s.* 4*d.*, fell in October to 76*s.* 9*d.* Parliament met on the 29th October, and various measures were taken[1]. In the spring

---

[1] The dearth of 1794–95 called forth one notable piece, the 'Thoughts and Details on Scarcity,' drawn up by Mr Burke, from his experience in Buckinghamshire, originally for the use of Mr Pitt, in November, 1795. Burke takes an optimist line, and preaches the economic doctrine of *laissez faire:* "After all," he asks, "have we not reason to be thankful to the Giver of all good? In our history, and when 'the labourer of England is said to have been once happy,' we find constantly, after certain intervals, a period of real famine; by which a melancholy havock was made among the human race. The price of provisions fluctuated dreadfully, demonstrating a deficiency very different from the worst failures of the present moment. Never, since I have known England, have I known more than a comparative scarcity. The price of wheat, taking a number of years together, has had no very considerable fluctuation, nor has it risen exceedingly within this twelvemonth. Even now, I do not know of one man, woman, or child, that has perished from famine; fewer, if any, I believe, than in years of plenty, when such a thing may happen by accident. This is owing to a care and superintendence of the poor, far greater than any I remember...Not only very few (I have observed that I know of none though I live in a place [Beaconsfield] as poor as most) have actually died of want, but we have seen no traces of those dreadful exterminating epidemicks, which, in consequence of scanty and unwholesome food, in former times not unfrequently wasted whole nations. Let us be saved from too much wisdom of our own, and we shall do tolerably well." The last sentence is his favourite principle of "a wise and salutary neglect" on the part of Government.

of 1796, the climax of distress was reached, wheat being at 100s. per quarter. The harvest of 1796 was abundant and wheat fell to 57s. 3d. The harvests of 1797 and 1798 were not equally good, but they were not altogether bad, and the price of wheat kept about 50s. for nearly three years, which were years of comparative comfort between the dearth of 1794–96 and the dearth of 1799–1802.

Fevers in the Dearth of 1799–1802.

Although Willan chooses the end of the year 1799 to enlarge upon the London fever, he does not connect it with the dearth that was already beginning to be felt (soup kitchens having been opened in various parts of London). The price of wheat, which had been steadily about 50s. in 1797 and 1798, rose in May, 1799 to 61s. 8d., after a hard winter which had probably injured the autumn-sown corn. The harvest turned out ill, and the price of wheat rose in December, 1799, to 94s. 2d. Bounties were offered on imported foreign grain, but in June, 1800, the price was 134s. 5d., falling in August to 96s. 2d. on the crops promising well. The latter end of harvest proved wet, much of the grain being lost, so that the price per quarter of wheat rose to 133s. in December. There was much suffering, and some rioting. Parliament met on the 11th November, 1800, on account of the dearth, the opinions of the members being much divided as to the causes of the high prices. In March, 1801, wheat was at 156s. 2d. per quarter, beef from 10d. to 10½d. per pound, mutton 11d. to 12d. per pound. It is to this year, when the quartern loaf was at one-and-eightpence, that a comparison by Arthur Young belongs, showing the great change in the purchasing power of wages[1]. By the end of summer, 1801,

---

[1] A labourer at Bury St Edmunds, receiving a weekly wage of five shillings, was able to buy therewith at the old prices :

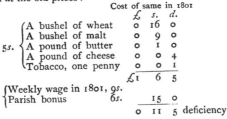

		Cost of same in 1801		
		£	s.	d.
	A bushel of wheat	0	16	0
	A bushel of malt	0	9	0
5s.	A pound of butter	0	1	0
	A pound of cheese	0	0	4
	Tobacco, one penny	0	0	1
		£1	6	5
	Weekly wage in 1801, 9s.			
	Parish bonus 6s.		15	0
		0	11	5 deficiency

wheat rose to 180*s.*, and the quartern loaf was for four weeks
at 1*s.* 10½*d.*

Whatever statistics were then kept of fever-cases, show a
decided rise in the years 1800 and 1801 :

Year	Manchester House of Recovery (fever-cases)	Glasgow Royal Infirmary (fever-cases)	Newcastle Dispensary (fever-cases)	London Bills of Mortality (fever-deaths)
1796	371	43	201	1547
1797	339	83	65	1526
1798	398	45	67	1754
1799	364	128	—	1784
1800	747	104	—	2712
1801	1070	63	425	2908
1802	601	104	—	2201
1803	256	85	352	2326
1804	184	97	255	1702
1805	268	99	74	1307

The London Fever Hospital was not opened until February,
1802, a small house in Gray's Inn Lane containing sixteen beds.
It came at the end of the epidemic, and was in small request
during the next fifteen years. The same epidemic at Leeds
was the occasion of opening a House of Recovery there in 1804,
twenty-five years after Lucas had first called for it. The state
of affairs in Leeds, which at length moved the richer classes
to that step, is thus described by Whitaker[1]:

"In the years 1801 and 1802 an alarming epidemic fever spread in Leeds
and the neighbourhood. The contagion extended so rapidly and proved so
fatal that some hundreds were affected at the same time, and two medical
gentlemen, with several nurses, fell victims to the disease...In 1802 whole
streets were infected house by house; in one court, of crowded population,
typhus raged for four months successively."

One of the Leeds physicians, Dr Thorp, seized the occasion
to urge the need of a fever hospital, in a pamphlet written
in 1802, in which he said:

"In a visit made a few days ago to those abodes of misery, I saw in one
particular district upwards of twenty-five families ill in contagious fever. In
some houses two, in others six or seven [families] were confined, many
of whom appeared to be in extreme danger." The superintendent of the
sick poor stated to Dr Thorp "that sixty families in epidemic fever are
under his care at this time. New applications are making daily. In some
families three, in others six or seven, are in the disease. Forty persons in
fever have applied to him for medical aid within the present week[2]."

[1] *Loidis and Elmete*, 1816, p. 85.
[2] Thorp, Tract of 1802, cited by Hunter, *Ed. Med. Surg. Journ.* April, 1819,
p. 239.

The wonder is that, with the enormous prices of food, things were not worse. At the time when provisions were dearest, work was slack in several industries. A commercial report of 1 April, 1801, speaks of the trade of Birmingham as very distressed, a large proportion of the men being out of work; the ribbon trade of Coventry was deplorable, and the woollen trade of Yorkshire still worse. Evidence of epidemic typhus in various parts of England came out in connexion with the reports on influenza in 1803. Holywell, in Flintshire, with a large cotton-making industry, had not been free from a bad kind of typhus for two years previous to the influenza of 1803[1]. In Bristol there was a good deal of fever in 1802–3, which found its way, through domestic servants, into good houses in Clifton, "and proved fatal in some instances[2]." It is probable that these are only samples, the writings on epidemics being singularly defective at this period. The following, dated 10th April, 1802, by a surgeon at Earlsoham, near Framlingham, Suffolk, gives us a glimpse of malignant contagious fever in a farm-house:

"The most prevailing epidemics for the last twelve months have been typhus maligna and mitior, scarlatina anginosa, measles, and mumps. Many of the former have proved alarmingly fatal in several of our villages, whilst those of the second class of typhoid fevers have put on the appearance of the low nervous kind attended with great prostration of strength, depression of spirits, loss of appetite, etc., which frequently continue many weeks before a compleat recovery ensues." Five cases, of "the most malignant kind of typhus," occurred in a farmer's family: one of the sons, aged eighteen, died in a few days with delirium, and black sordes of the mouth, tongue and throat; then the father, two daughters, and another son, took the infection but all escaped with their lives. Of four persons who nursed them, one caught the fever, and died. Four persons in a neighbouring family, who visited them, took infection, of whom two died[3].

There was perhaps nothing very unusual in such instances of country fevers at the beginning of the century. The incident is exactly in the manner of one that figures prominently in a story of Scottish life and customs at the same period, which long passed current as a faithful picture and as enforcing a much-needed moral[4].

---

[1] Currie, *Med. Phys. Journ.* X. 213.   [2] Beddoes.
[3] Goodwin, *Med. Phys. Journ.* IX. 509. Cf. Gervis, *Med. Chir. Trans.* II. 236.
[4] Elizabeth Hamilton, *The Cottagers of Glenburnie*, Edin. 1808: "The only precaution which the good people, who came to see him [the farmer] appeared now to think necessary, was carefully to shut the door, which usually stood open...The prejudice against fresh air appeared to be universal...The doctor did not think it probable that he would live above three days; but said, the only chance he had was in removing him from that close box in which he was shut up, and admitting as much air as possible into the apartment...While the farmer yet hovered on the brink of death, his wife and Robert, his second son, were both taken ill...Peter MacGlashan

Comparative immunity from Fevers during the War and high prices of 1803–15.

From 1803 to 1816 there was comparatively little fever in this country. This was notably the case in London, but it was also true of all the larger towns where fever-hospitals had been established, and it was as true of Ireland as of England. This was, indeed, a time of great prosperity, which reached to all classes, the permanent rise of wages having more than balanced the increased cost of the necessaries of life. The following prices of wheat will show that a dear loaf did not necessarily mean distress while the war-expenditure lasted:

Prices of wheat (from Tooke).

		s.	d.			s.	d.			s.	d.
1802		57	1	1810	June	113	5	1817	Sept.	77	7
1803		52	3		Dec.	94	7	1818	Dec.	78	10
1804	Lady Day	49	6	1811	June	86	11	1819	Aug.	75	
	Dec.	86	2		Nov.	101	6	1820		72	
1805	Aug.	98	4	1812	Aug.	155		1821	July	51	
	Dec.	74	5		Nov.	113	6		Dec.	50	
1806		73	5	1813	Aug.	112		1822		42	
1807	Nov.	66			Dec.	73	6	1823	Feb.	40	8
1808	May	73	6	1814	July	66	5		June	62	5
	Dec.	92		1815	Dec.	53	7		Oct.	46	5
1809	March	95		1816	May	74			Dec.	50	8
	July	86	6		Dec.	103		1824		65	
	Dec.	102	6	1817	June	111	6				

The only years in the period from 1803 to 1816 in which there was some slight increase of fever were about 1811–12. There was undoubtedly some distress in the manufacturing districts at that time, owing to the much talked-of Orders in Council, which had the effect of closing American markets to British manufactures[1].

had taken to his bed on going home and was now dangerously ill of the fever...All the village indeed offered their services; and Mrs Mason, though she blamed the thoughtless custom of crowding into a sick room, could not but admire the kindness and good nature with which all the neighbours seemed to participate in the distress of this afflicted family."

[1] Charlotte Brontë's story of *Shirley* falls in this period and turns upon the industrial crisis in Yorkshire; but it is on the whole a happy idyllic picture. Harriet Martineau wrote in *Household Words*, vol. I. 1850, Nos. 9–12, a story entitled "The Sickness and Health of the People of Bleaburn," a Yorkshire village supposed to have been Osmotherly. It is, in substance, an account of a terrible epidemic of fever in the year 1811, the story opening with the news of the victory of Albuera and the rejoicings thereon. It appears to have been constructed very closely from the real events of the plague of 1665–66 in the village of Eyam, in the North Peak of Derbyshire, and had probably a very slender foundation in any facts of fever in Yorkshire or elsewhere in the year 1811. "Ten or eleven corpses," says the novelist, "were actually lying unburied, infecting half-a-dozen cottages from this cause." Cf. infra, Leyburn, p. 167.

The small amount of fever in London between the year 1803 and the beginning of the epidemic of 1817–19 rests on the testimony of Bateman[1], who in 1804 took up Willan's task of keeping a systematic record of the cases at the Carey Street Dispensary. He has only two special entries relating to typhus: one in the autumn of 1811, when some cases occurred in the uncleanly parts of Clerkenwell and St Luke's ("but I have not learned that it has existed in any other districts of London"); the other in October and November 1813, when there was more typhus among the Irish in some of the filthy courts of Saffron Hill, near Hatton Garden, than for several years past, the infection having spread rapidly and fatally in several houses. The best evidence of this lull in typhus in London is the almost empty state of the new fever-hospital:

Year	Admissions		Year	Admissions
1802	164		1810	52
1803	176		1811	43
1804	80		1812	61
1805	66		1813	85
1806	93		1814	59
1807	63		1815	80
1808	69		1816	118
1809	29		1817	760

Until it was removed to Pancras Road, in September, 1816, the London fever-hospital had only sixteen beds. But Bateman says that no one was refused admission, and that for several years the house was frequently empty three or four weeks together. Also at the Dispensary, in Carey Street, he had an opportunity during the period 1804–1816,

"Of observing the entire freedom from fevers enjoyed by the inhabitants of the numerous crowded courts and alleys within the extensive district comprehended in our visits from that charity." And again, writing in the winter of 1814–15, Bateman says: "To those who recollect the numerous cases of typhoid fevers [this term did not then mean enteric] which called for the relief of dispensaries twelve or fourteen years ago, and the contagion of which was often with great difficulty eradicated from the apartments where it raged, and even seized the same individuals again and again when they escaped its fatal influences, the great freedom from these fevers which now exists, even in the most close and filthy alleys in London, is the ground of some surprise." And once more, in the summer of 1816, just as the new epidemic period was about to begin, he says: "The extraordinary disappearance of contagious fever from every part of this crowded metropolis during the long period comprehended by these Reports [since 1804], cannot fail to have attracted the attention of the reader."

[1] T. Bateman, M.D., *Reports on the Diseases of London...from* 1804 *to* 1816. Lond. 1819.

Bateman concluded, not without reason, that this immunity of London from fever was due to the high degree of well-being among the poorer classes in times of plenty; and although he made out that the poor of Dublin, Cork and some Scotch towns did not profit by times of plenty so much as those in London, yet his reason for the abeyance of fever from 1804 to 1816 applied to England, Ireland and Scotland at large, and was doubtless the true reason.

The following figures from Manchester[1], Leeds[2] and Glasgow[3] hospitals, as well as the Irish statistics elsewhere given, are closely parallel with those of London:

Manchester House of Recovery.

Year	Cases	Deaths	Year	Cases	Deaths
1796–7	371	40	1807–8	208	15
1797–8	339	16	1808–9	260	21
1798–9	398	27	1809–10	278	30
1799–1800	364	41	1810–11	172	15
1800–1	747	63	1811–12	140	18
1801–2	1070	84	1812–13	126	13
1802–3	601	53	1813–14	226	17
1803–4	256	33	1814–15	379	29
1804–5	184	34	1815–16	185	14
1805–6	268	29	1816–17	172	6
1806–7	311	33			

Leeds House of Recovery.

Year	Cases	Deaths	Year	Cases	Deaths
1804 (2 mo.)	10	0	1812	80	12
1805	66	6	1813	137	11
1806	75	2	1814	79	4
1807	35	1	1815	146	15
1808	80	3	1816	121	13
1809	93	8	1817	178	8
1810	75	14	1818 (10 mo.)	254	20
1811	92	4			

Glasgow Royal Infirmary (Fever Wards).

Year	Cases	Year	Cases
1795	18	1807	25
1796	43	1808	27
1797	83	1809	76
1798	45	1810	82
1799	128	1811	45
1800	104	1812	16
1801	63	1813	35
1802	104	1814	90
1803	85	1815	230
1804	97	1816	399
1805	99	1817	714
1806	75	1818	1371

[1] Parl. Committee's Report on Contag. Fev. 1818, p. 33. Table by P. M. Roget.
[2] Adam Hunter, *Ed. Med. Surg. Journ.*, April, 1819.
[3] Cleland, *Glasgow and Clydesdale Statist. Soc. Transactions*, Pt. I. Nov. 2, 1836.

Even such fever as there was in Britain from 1804 to 1817 was not all certainly typhus. The high death-rates at the Manchester fever-hospital in 1804 and 1805 (1 death in 7·5 cases and 1 death in 5·25 cases) may mean a certain proportion of enteric cases in those years. "From 1804 to 1805," says Ferriar, "many cases were admitted of a most lingering and dangerous kind....Many deaths took place from sudden changes in the state of the fever, contrary to the usual course of the disease, and only imputable to the peculiar character of the epidemic. Similar cases occurred at that time in private practice." Next year, 1806, there was an epidemic among the troops at Deal, described under the name of "remittent fever," which Murchison claims to have been enteric[1]. In September, 1808, says Bateman, several were admitted into the London House of Recovery, with malignant symptoms; "and some severe and even fatal instances occurred in individuals in respectable rank in life." He still uses the name of typhus; but he is aware that the cases of continued fever, especially in the summer and autumn of 1810, had often symptoms pointing to a bowel-fever rather than to a head-fever[2].

The years 1807 and 1808 appear to have been the most generally unwholesome during this period of comparative immunity from fever; they were marked by the occurrence of dysenteries, agues, and infantile remittents, as well as of fevers of the "typhus" kind. The chief account comes from Nottingham[3]. The cases of "typhus" there were very tedious, but not violent, nor attended with any unfavourable symptoms, only one case having petechiae, and all having diarrhoea. The following

---

[1] Sutton, *Account of a Remittent Fever among the Troops in this Climate.* Canterbury, 1806.

[2] In the first three months of 1811 a singular fever occurred among working people in part of a suburb of Paisley, one practitioner having 32 cases in 13 families. It was marked by rigors at the onset, pain in the back, headache, dry skin, loaded very red tongue, quick fluttering pulse, watchfulness, delirium-like fatuity, abdominal pain in many, foetid stools, great prostration, gradual recovery after fifteen or sixteen days without manifest crisis, and relapses in some. In this fever Murchison discovers enteric or typhoid. Its limitation to a part of one of the suburbs of Paisley is, of course, in the manner of enteric fever; on the other hand, only one of those 32 cases died, which is a rate of fatality perhaps not unparalleled in typhoid but much more often matched in typhus or relapsing fever of young and old together; while the length of the fever, fifteen or sixteen days or sometimes more, is too great for the abortive kind of enteric and too little for enteric fever completing both its first and second stages. James Muir, *Edin. Med. and Surg. Journ.* VIII. 134. Murchison, *Continued Fevers,* p. 428.

[3] James Clarke, M.D., "Medical Report for Nottingham from March 1807 to March 1808," *Edin. Med. and Surg. Journ.* IV. 422. His account of the unwholesome state of the weavers' houses is as bad as any of those already given.

table of admissions for various kinds of fever (as classified by Cullen) at the Nottingham General Hospital, 25 March, 1807, to 25 March, 1808, shows the preponderance of "synochus" and next to it, of infantile remittent :

Admitted to the Nottingham General Hospital, 1807.

Intermittent fever	7
Synocha	10
Typhus	27
Febris nervosa	26
Synochus	155
Febris infantum remittens	88
Dysentery	5

The state of war in the Peninsula was favourable to epidemic or spreading diseases, and there is a good deal to show that such diseases did exist among the British troops[1]. But there is only one good instance of England getting a taste of that experience of war-typhus which the Continent had to endure for many years. This was on the return of the remnant of the army after the defeat at Corunna on 16 January, 1809. The troops were crowded pell-mell on board transports, which had a very rough passage home. Dysentery broke out among them, and was the most urgent malady when they landed at Plymouth in a state of filth and rags. Typhus fever followed, but in the first three weeks at Plymouth, to the 18th of February, it was not of a malignant type, only 8 dying of it in the Old Cumberland Square Hospital; in the next three weeks, 28 died of it there. Up to the 27th of March, 1809, the sick at Plymouth from the Corunna army numbered 2432, of whom 241 died. Of 4 medical officers, 3 took the contagion, of 29 orderlies, 25 took it. The fever was in some cases followed by a relapse, which was more often fatal than the original attack[2]. This was a typical instance of typhus bred from dysentery or other incidents of campaigning, a contagion more dangerous to others than to those who had engendered it. "Within a few yards of the spot where I now write," says Dr James Johnson, of Spring Gardens, London, "the greater part of a family fell sacrifices to the effects of fomites that lurked in a blanket purchased from one of these soldiers after their return from Corunna[3]." In

---

[1] McGrigor, "Med. Hist. of British Armies in Peninsula," *Med. Chir. Trans.* VI. 381.

[2] Richard Hooper, "Account of the Sick landed from Corunna," *Edin. Med. and Surg. Journ.* V. (1809), p. 398. See also Sir James McGrigor, *ibid.* VI. 19.

[3] James Johnson, *Influence of Tropical Climates*, p. 20.

August, 1813, an Irish regiment passing through Leyburn, a small market-town of the West Riding of Yorkshire, in an airy situation, was obliged to leave behind a soldier ill of typhus, who died of the fever after a few days. The infection appeared soon after in the cottages adjoining, and remained in that end of the town for several months, choosing the clean and respectable houses. In a farmer's family, a son, aged twenty-nine, died of it, while another son and two daughters had a narrow escape. The disease appeared also in the village of Wensby, a mile distant, and in other villages. Few lives were lost[1].

These were, perhaps, not altogether solitary instances in Britain of typhus spread abroad by the movements of troops during the great French war. Let us multiply such instances by hundreds, and we shall vaguely realize the meaning of the statement that the period of the Napoleonic wars, and more particularly the period from the renewal of the war in 1803 until its close in 1815, was one of the worst times of epidemic typhus in the history of modern Europe. It was precisely in those years that England, Scotland and Ireland enjoyed a most remarkable degree of freedom from contagious fever.

The Distress and Epidemic Fever (Relapsing) following the Peace of 1815 and the fall of wages.

The long period of comparative immunity from typhus near the beginning of the 19th century was first broken, both in Great Britain and in Ireland, by the very severe winter of 1814–15; but it was not until the great depression of trade following the peace of 1815 (which made a difference of forty millions sterling a year in the public expenditure) and the bad harvest of 1816 that typhus fever and relapsing fever became truly epidemic, chiefly in Ireland but also in Scotland and England. The lesson of the history is unmistakable: with all the inducements to typhus from neglect of sanitation in the midst of rapidly increasing numbers, there was surprisingly little of the disease so long as trade was brisk and the means of subsistence abundant. The reckoning came in the thirty years following the Peace.

[1] J. Terry, in *Ed. Med. and Surg. Journ.*, Jan. 1820, p. 247.

In London, says Bateman[1], the epidemic began in the autumn of 1816, before the influence of scarcity was acutely felt, in the courts about Saffron Hill, the same locality in which he mentioned fever in the winter of 1813-14 among the poor Irish. But this means little more than that the Irish, whether in Ireland or out of it, are the first to feel the effects of scarcity in producing fever. At the very same time that it began among them in Saffron Hill, it began among some young people at a silk factory in Spitalfields. In March, 1817, there was a good deal more of it in Saffron Hill, as well as among the silk-weavers in Essex Street, Whitechapel, in Old Street, in Clerkenwell, and in Shadwell workhouse. Many poor-houses, and especially those of Whitechapel, St Luke's, St Sepulchre's and St George's, Southwark, were getting crowded in 1817 with half-starved persons, among whom fever was rife in the summer and autumn. There was also much of it in the homes of working people in the eastern, north-eastern and Southwark parishes, with more occasional infected households in Shoe Lane, Clare Market, Somers Town and St Giles's in the Fields ("in the filthy streets between Dyot Street and the end of Oxford Street")[1]. The hospitals and dispensaries were fully occupied with fever, and the new House of Recovery in Pancras Road, with accommodation for seventy patients, was soon full. At the Guardian Asylum for young women, more than half of the forty inmates were seized with the fever in one week. The cases were on the whole milder than in ordinary years; of 678 admitted to the House of Recovery in 1817, fifty died or 1 in 13·5. In two-thirds of these patients the fever lasted two weeks or to the beginning of the third week; of the remaining third, a few lost the fever on the 7th, 8th or 9th day, a larger number on the 12th to the 14th day, while a considerable number kept it to the end of the third week or beginning of the fourth. Of the whole 678, only 75 had a free perspiration, and in only 19 of these was the perspiration critical so as to end the fever abruptly. The fever relapsed in 54 of the 678, a proportion of relapsing cases which seemed to Bateman to be "remarkably great[2]." In most

---

[1] Bateman, *Account of the Contagious Fever of this Country.* Lond. 1818.
[2] The following from the "Observations on Prevailing Diseases," Oct.—Nov., 1818 (perhaps by Dr Copland), in the *London Medical Repository*, X. 525, shows that the relapses in the earlier part of this epidemic had been commonly remarked in London: "Fevers are still prevalent...Relapses have been noticed as of frequent occurrence in the instances of the late epidemic. To what are these to be attributed?

the symptoms continued without break throughout the illness. Besides other febrile symptoms, there were pains in the limbs and back, aching of the bones, and soreness of the flesh, as if the patients had been beaten. There was a certain proportion of severe complicated cases of typhus. Bateman held that the differences in type depended on the differences of constitution, giving the following reason for and illustration of his opinion :

"Thus, in the instance of a man and his wife who were brought to the House of Recovery together, the former was affected with the mildest symptoms of fever, which scarcely confined him to bed, and terminated in a speedy convalescence; while his wife was lying in a state of stupor, covered with *petechiae* and *vibices*; in a word, exhibiting the most formidable symptoms of the worst form of typhus. Yet these extreme degrees of the disease manifestly originated from the same cause; and it would be equally unphilosophical to account them different kinds of fever and give them distinct generic appellations as in the case of the benign and confluent smallpox, which are generated in like manner from one contagion." Besides this woman, only eight others had petechiae.

The House of Commons Committee were unable to find out with numerical precision how much more prevalent the fever was in 1817–18 than in the years preceding[1]. To their surprise they found that in six of the general hospitals of London, which admitted cases of fever, "no register is kept in the hospital to distinguish the different varieties of disease." The apothecary of St Luke's Workhouse told them that he attended, on an average of common years, about 150 cases of fever; in the last year [1817] the number rose to 600; and they were assured by several besides Bateman, that the great decrease of the deaths from "fever" in the London bills of mortality during a space of fourteen years at the beginning of the century (1803–17), was not a mere apparent decrease, from the growing inadequacy of the bills, but was a real decrease.

The epidemic which began in 1817 continued in London throughout the years 1818 and 1819, chiefly in the densely populated poorer quarters of the town. Two instances of the London slums of the time came to light before the House

Are we to ascribe them to the influence of the atmosphere, to anything in the nature of the disorders themselves, or to the vigorous plans of treatment which are adopted for their removal? These relapses are more common in hospital than in private practice...It has recently become the fashion to consider the state of recovery from fever as one which will do better without than with the interposition of the cinchona bark. Has the prevalence of this negative practice anything to do with the admitted fact of frequent relapse?"
[1] *Report of the Select Committee of the House of Commons on Contagious Fever*, Parl. Papers, 1818.

of Commons Committee on Mendicity and Vagrancy in 1815–16: firstly, Calmel's Buildings, a small court near Portman Square, consisting of twenty-four houses, in which lived seven hundred Irish in distress and profligacy, neglected by the parish and shunned by everyone from dread of contagion; and, secondly, George Yard, Whitechapel, consisting of forty houses, in which lived two thousand persons in a similar state of wretchedness. The dwellings of the poorer classes in London at this period, before the alleys and courts began to disappear, were described thus generally by Dr Clutterbuck[1]:

"The houses the poor occupy are often large, and every room has its family, from the cellar to the garret. Thirty or forty individuals are thus often collected under the same roof; the different apartments must be approached by a common stair, which is rarely washed or cleansed; there are often no windows or openings of any kind backwards; and the *privies* are not unfrequently within the walls, and emit a loathsome stench that is diffused over the whole house. The houses are generally situated in long and narrow alleys, with lofty buildings on each side; or in a small and confined court, which has but a single opening, and that perhaps a low gateway: such a court is in fact little other than a well. These places are at the same time the receptacles of all kinds of filth, which is only removed by the scavenger at distant and uncertain intervals, and always so imperfectly as to leave the place highly offensive and disgusting."

In England, generally, this epidemic of 1817–19 is somewhat casually reported. One writes from Witney, Oxfordshire, "on the prevailing epidemic," which began there in July, 1818, among poor persons, in crowded, filthy and ill-ventilated situations. At first it was like the ordinary contagious fever of this country, "a disease familiar to common observation"; but afterwards it showed choleraic and pneumonic complications. Sometimes the parotid and submaxillary glands were inflamed; petechiae were absent[2]. The type of fever at Ipswich in the spring of 1817 was contagious (e.g. six cases in one family) and sthenic, or of strong reaction, admitting of bloodletting, according to the teaching which Armstrong, Clutterbuck and others had been reviving for fevers[3]. Those instances, one from Oxfordshire the other from Suffolk, must stand for many. Hancock says that the fever of 1817–19 "visited almost every town and village of the United Kingdom[4]." Prichard says that

---

[1] *On the Epidemic Fever at present prevailing.* Lond. 1819, p. 40.
[2] J. B. Sheppard, "Remarks on the prevailing Epidemic." *Edin. Med. Surg. Journ.*, July 1819, p. 346. Also for Taplow, Roberts, *Lond. Med. Repos.* XIV. 186.
[3] W. Hamilton, M.D., *Med. and Phys. Journ.*, June 1817, p. 451.
[4] *Laws and Phenomena of Pestilence*, Lond. 1821, p. 39. Christison says: "All great towns, with the exception it is said of Birmingham."

it began in Ireland, "where the distress was most urgent, and afterwards prevailed through most parts of Britain," some of the more opulent also being involved in the calamity. As to its prevalence in the manufacturing towns of Yorkshire we have ample testimony. The Leeds House of Recovery, which had not been fully occupied at any time since its opening in 1804, received 178 cases in 1817, and 254 in the first ten months of 1818. Of the latter, 66 came from low lodging-houses, of whom upwards of 50 were strangers. Of 50 admitted in January, 1818, 20 came from four or five lodging-houses in March Lane, and from another locality equally bad—Boot and Shoe Yard ; while the rest of the 50 in that month came from houses and streets in the same vicinity. March Lane was one of the worst seats of the great Leeds plague in 1645. By the month of April, 1820, the epidemic had decreased a good deal in Leeds, the cases becoming at the same time more anomalous[1].

The following is one of the Rochdale cases :

June 2, 1818, Alice Eccles, a delicate young woman living in a crowded and filthy court from which fever had not been absent for nearly a year, was bled to ten ounces, purged, and recovered. On September 20th the same woman returned, desiring to be bled again. She was labouring under her former complaint; "since her last illness she had been repeatedly exposed to contagion, or rather, she had been living in an atmosphere thoroughly saturated with infectious effluvia, the house in which she resided, and generally the room in which she slept, having had one or more cases of fever in them," and the windows kept closed[2].

At Halifax in the summer of 1818, typhus (or relapsing fever) had increased so much that fever-wards were added to the Dispensary. It had been alarmingly fatal in a high-lying village near Settle. It was prevalent in Ripon, Huddersfield and Wakefield ; and had been brought from Leeds to Atley. A Bradford physician visited 27 cases of fever in one day at a neighbouring village. Throughout Yorkshire, it was confined to the lower orders, and was not very fatal[3]. At Carlisle it began about July, 1817, and became somewhat frequent in the winter and spring following; of 457 cases treated from the Dispensary 46 died, or 1 in 10[4]. At Newcastle, a mild typhus (typhus mitior) broke out in the autumn of 1816, not in the poorer quarters, but mostly among the domestics of good

[1] Adam Hunter, *Edin. Med. Surg. Journ.*, Apr. 1819, p. 234, and Apr. 1820.
[2] Wood, "Cases of Typhus." *Edin. Med. Surg. Journ.*, April, 1819.
[3] Adam Hunter, u. s.
[4] T. Barnes, *Edin. Med. Surg. Journ.*, April, 1819.

houses in elevated situations. There was much privation at Newcastle, as elsewhere, at this time, among the poor. Murchison takes this fever of the autumn of 1816 at Newcastle to have been enteric or typhoid; but it is described as a simple continued fever, with vertigo, headache, and bloodshot eyes, lasting from five or six days to four or five weeks, ending usually without a marked crisis, and causing few deaths[1]. The epidemic continued in Newcastle for three years, the admissions to the Fever Hospital from 4 Sept. 1818, to 4 March, 1819, having been 160, with 12 deaths. Dr McWhirter wrote, in April, 1819, that he saw on his rounds as dispensary physician "too many of the obvious causes of fever," including the filth and wretchedness of the poor inhabitants: "one rather wonders that so many escape it than that some are its victims[2]."

Thus far there has been little besides Bateman's essay to indicate the nature or type of the fever in England. In Ireland it was to a large extent relapsing fever, and, as we shall see, it was so also in Scotland. Bateman found less than a tenth part of the cases at the London Fever Hospital to have relapses, which was an unusually large proportion, in his experience. Elsewhere in England the tendency to relapse was either wanting or the relapses were described or accounted for in other ways; to understand this it has to be kept in mind that the epidemic was the occasion of a great revival of blood-letting, a practice which had fallen into disuse in fevers since the last half of the 18th century, and was something of a novelty in 1817. The fever of that year was undoubtedly abrupt in its onset, strong, "inflammatory," with full bounding pulse, beating carotids, hot and dry skin, intense headache, suffused eyes, and the like symptoms, which seemed to call for depletion. The common practice was to bleed *ad deliquium*, which meant to ten, or fourteen, or twenty ounces, at the outset of the fever. There was hardly one of the writers upon the epidemic, unless it were Bateman, an advocate of the cordial and supporting regimen, who did not consider the stages or duration of the fever as artificially determined by the blood-letting, and not as belonging to the natural history.

In order to show how much the treatment by blood-letting dominated the view of the fever itself, of its type, its stages,

---

[1] H. Edmonston, *ibid.* xiv. (1818), p. 71.
[2] T. McWhirter, *ibid.* April, 1819, p. 317.

or duration, I shall take the Bristol essay of Prichard, who adopted phlebotomy, as he says, at first tentatively and with some fear and trembling, but at length practised it vigorously, having found it to answer well[1]. The epidemic of fever in Bristol began about June, 1817, and lasted fully two years. The first cases brought to St Peter's Hospital, which was the general workhouse of the city, were of wretched vagrants found ill by the wayside or abandoned in hovels. About the same time forty-two felons in the Bristol Newgate, "one of the most loathsome dungeons in Britain, perhaps I might say in Europe," were infected, of whom only one died, and he of a relapse. From June, 1817, to the end of 1819, there were 591 cases in the poor's house, 647 in the General Infirmary, and 975 treated from the Dispensary, making 2213 cases, of which a record was kept. But there were also many cases in private practice among the domestics, children, and others in good houses, such as those on Redcliff Hill. The cases in the poor's house were classified by Prichard as follows:

	1817	1818	1819
Simple Fever	22	45	40
with cephalic symptoms	24	27	25
„ pneumonic symptoms	7	10	16
„ gastric symptoms	3	11	5
„ enteric symptoms	3	4	5
„ hepatic symptoms	5	3	3
exhausted and moribund	1	6	4
not characterised	30	44	2
	95	150	105
Of these there died	20	16	11

The "genuine form," or ground-type, according to Prichard, was "simple fever," of which the cases with cephalic symptoms were merely the more protracted or more serious. "The pneumonic, hepatic, gastric, enteric and rheumatic forms may be regarded as varieties"—the gastric and hepatic being cases mostly in summer with jaundice, the enteric in autumn and winter with diarrhoea and dysentery. Nearly all these patients were bled within four or five days from the commencement of the disease: "in a very large proportion of the cases the fever was immediately cut short"; when it did not end thus abruptly,

[1] J. C. Prichard, M.D., *History of the Epidemic Fever which prevailed in Bristol,* 1817–19. Lond. 1820.

its symptoms declined gradually, and the attack was over within eight or ten days. After the blooding "sleep very frequently followed, and a partial or sometimes a complete remission of the symptoms." Only one case of relapse is mentioned, No. 118, of the year 1818, and that was a relapse in a very prolonged case: the patient was admitted on 6 October, had a relapse on 18 November, and was discharged on 23 December. Prichard has not one word in his text to suggest relapsing fever; the bulk of his cases were simple continued fever, with or without cephalic or other local symptoms, ending in four, six, eight or ten days, while some were cases of *typhus gravior*. The fever was undoubtedly contagious: it spread through whole families, and in St Peter's Hospital itself it attacked seventy of the ordinary pauper inmates, including a good many lunatics.

The Epidemic of 1817–19 in Scotland: Relapsing Fever.

Let us now turn to the epidemic in Scotland, where the relapsing type was as marked as in Ireland, if not more so. The destitution in the Scots towns in the autumn of 1816, and following years, was fully as great as anywhere in the kingdom, although the peasantry of Scotland were not famine-stricken, as those of Ireland were. The state of the poorer classes in Edinburgh was graphically set forth in an essay by Dr Yule, in 1818[1], and in an article in *Blackwood's Magazine* the year after. Vigorous efforts to relieve the distress were made by the richer classes, and a special fever-hospital was opened at Queensbery House, the admissions to which, together with the fever-cases at the Royal Infirmary, were as follows:[2]

Year	Admitted	Died	Ratio of deaths
1817	511	33	1 in $15\frac{18}{33}$
•1818	1572	75	1 in 21
1819	1027	30	1 in 34
(to 1 Dec.)			

Of this epidemic several accounts were published at the time, including one by Welsh, superintendent of the fever hospital, which is dominated, like the Bristol account of Prichard, by the idea that blood-letting cut short the fever[3]. Christison,

[1] *Obs. on the Cure and Prevention of the Contagious Fever now in Edinburgh.* Edin. 1818.
[2] *Edin. Med. Surg. Journ.* XVI. 146.
[3] Benj. Welsh, *Efficacy of Bloodletting in the Epidemic Fever of Edinburgh.* Edin. 1819.

who had experience of the relapsing form in his own person[1], describes also two other forms mixed with the cases of relapsing fever: a mild typhus, the *typhus mitior* (*typhus gravior* being exceedingly rare in that epidemic), and a form which began like the inflammatory relapsing *synocha*, and gradually after a week put on the characters of mild typhus.

The admissions for fever to the Glasgow Infirmary, which was then the only charity that received fever cases, had been at a somewhat low level since the last epidemic in 1799–1801. They began to rise again with the distress of 1816 :—

Admissions for Fever, Glasgow Infirmary.

Year	Cases	Year	Cases
1814	90	1819	630
1815	230	1820	289
1816	399	1821	234
1817	714	1822	229
1818	1371	1823	269

At the height of the epidemic in 1818 an additional fever hospital was opened at Spring Gardens, to which 1929 cases were admitted in that and the following year. Great efforts were made in Glasgow to "stamp out" the contagion by disinfectants and removal to hospital[2]; but the course of the epidemic seemed to follow the economic conditions more than anything else.

The outbreak at Aberdeen was later than in the south of Scotland, having begun in August, 1818. The infection was said to have been brought to the city by a woman who found a lodging in Sinclair's Close. A group of houses in the close, covering an area of seventy by fifty feet and containing one

[1] *Life of Sir Robert Christison*, Edin. 1885, I. 142 :—"I had been scarcely three weeks at my post in the fever hospital when I was attacked suddenly—so suddenly, that in half-an-hour I was utterly helpless from prostration. I had nearly six days of the primary attack, then a week of comfort, repose and feebleness, and next the secondary attack, or relapse, for three days more. My pulse rose to 160, and continued hard and incompressible even at that rate. My temperature under the tongue was 107° &c." He was bled to 30 oz. and next day to 20 oz. more. Before the end of the epidemic, in August, 1819, he had another attack of relapsing fever, for which he was bled to 24 oz. and a third, after exposure to chill, the same autumn, which last was a simple five-days' fever without relapse, also treated by the abstraction of 24 oz. of blood. In 1832 he had two attacks of the same *synocha* without relapses, and throughout the rest of his life many more: e.g. 16 June, 1861, "I have had something like the relapsing fever of my youth"—a five-days' fever with a relapse on the 18th day; and again, on 19 March, 1868, "Incomprehensible return of mine ancient enemy." These experiences coloured Christison's view of relapsing fever, the so-called relapses being, in his opinion, comparable to the returning paroxysms of ague.
[2] Cleland.

hundred and three inmates, became the first centre of the fever. The scenes described are like those of the Irish epidemics : in one room, a man, his wife, and five children were lying ill on the floor; in another, a man, his wife and six children; in a third, a young girl, whose mother had just died of fever, was left with three infant brothers or sisters. More than three-fourths of the denizens of the close were " confined to bed in fever, and all the others crawling about during the intervals of their relapses." The value of all the furniture and clothing belonging to 103 persons could little exceed £5. There was a horrible stench both within and without the houses (relapsing fever being remarkable for its odour). Yet this close was usually as healthy as any other part of the town. A House of Recovery, with sixty beds, was opened in the Gallowgate, and thirty beds were given up to fever-cases in the Infirmary of the city. Besides those ninety hospital cases at the date of 17 December, 1818, it was estimated that were three hundred more. Begging had been put down, so that the contagion had not spread to the richer classes. Despite these removals to hospital, the epidemic became more general about the New Year, 1819, and of a worse type; two physicians died of it, and some others had a narrow escape. At the outset, the fever had been of the relapsing kind—"subject to relapses for a third and fourth time, more especially when they return too early to their usual labour[1]." At a later period the epidemic seems to have become ordinary typhus, as it did also in Ireland and elsewhere; and it was called typhus in the essay upon it by Dr George Kerr[2].

The extent of this epidemic of 1818–19 over Scotland generally is not known; but the following notice of it in a country parish of Forfarshire was probably a sample of more that might have been given.

Early in the summer of 1818 an epidemic of continued fever appeared in a manufacturing village seven miles from Lintrathen; it attacked at first young and plethoric subjects, and ran through whole families. In August it reached Lintrathen parish, in which one practitioner had forty cases, with no deaths. The fever was of an inflammatory nature; the bulk of the cases fell in October, and were nearly all of young women. They were bled to syncope, which then meant usually to 32 ounces. There was a prejudice

[1] Report signed A. Brebner, provost, printed in Harty, *Historic Sketch of the Contagious Fever in Ireland*, 1817–19. Dublin, 1820, Appendix, p. 110.
[2] *Memoir concerning the Typhus Fever in Aberdeen*, 1818–19. By George Kerr, Aberdeen, 1820.

against blooding among the old people, who said "they had had many fevers, and in their time no such thing was ever allowed." But, according to the doctor, this withholding of the lancet had the effect of protracting their illnesses : "they toasted sick for six weeks, and were often confined to bed for months[1]."

The epidemic of 1817–19 brought into prominence two questions, the one theoretical, the other practical. The theoretical question (not debated at the time) was touching the place or affinities of relapsing fever in the nosology. Christison maintained that it was the inflammatory fever, or *synocha* of Cullen, showing a peculiar tendency to relapse. The fever of the same epidemic period in England was also undoubtedly a fever of strong or inflammatory reaction, corresponding to Cullen's definition of *synocha*, but it relapsed much less frequently than in Ireland and Scotland in the same years. Even in Ireland and Scotland there were always many cases of "relapsing fever" which did not relapse. The law of its relapses was reduced to great simplicity by a physician learned in fevers, Dr John O'Brien, in the Dublin epidemic of 1827. The bulk of that epidemic was a fever of short periods—three, five, seven or nine days, most of the attacks ending on the fifth or seventh night of the fever. The attack being ended in a free perspiration, there might or might not happen, after an interval, a relapse, and again a relapse after that, or even a third. The five-days' fever was more liable to relapse than the seven-days' fever, the seven-days' fever more liable than the nine-days' fever, the fevers of the longest periods not liable at all. In other words, the sooner the patient "got the cool," by a night's sweating, the more liable he was to have one or more relapses[2].

The logical position of relapsing fever was completed by Dr Seaton Reid, of Belfast, when he proposed, in his account of the epidemic in 1846–7, to call it Relapsing Synocha[3]. Other fevers have shown a tendency to relapse in certain circumstances. Three fevers which have many points in common, the sweating sickness, dengue and influenza, are all subject to relapses. It was doubtless of the sweating sickness that Sir Thomas More was thinking when he wrote : " Considering there is, as physicians say, and as we also find, double the peril in the relapse that

---

[1] William Gourlay, " History of the Epidemic Fever as it appeared in a Country Parish in the North of Scotland." *Edin. Med. and Surg. Journ.*, July, 1819, p. 329, dated 20 Nov. 1818.
[2] *Trans. K. and Q. Col. Phys. Ireland*, V. 527.   [3] *Dub. Q. J. Med. Sc.* VIII. 297.

12

was in the first sickness." Plague, also, might relapse, or recur in an individual once, twice, three times, or oftener in the same epidemic season. Enteric is an instance of a long-period fever which has at times a tendency to relapses[1]. None of these, however, can dispute the claim of relapsing synocha to be relapsing fever *par excellence.* For whatever reason, the short-period fever of times .of distress and dearth or famine has shown a peculiar tendency to relapse, and has shown that tendency more in the 19th century than in the 18th, and more among the Irish and Scotch poor than among the English.

The practical question that came to the front in the epidemic fever of 1817–19 was that of isolation hospitals for the sick. It was thus stated by Dr Millar, of Glasgow, in a letter of advice to the authorities of Aberdeen :

"It is only by a universal, or nearly universal sweep of the sick into Fever Hospitals, joined to a universal or nearly universal purification of their dwellings, that anything is to be hoped for in the way of suppressing our epidemic. So far as this grand object is concerned, all the rest is folly : it is worse than folly[2]."

This was the well-meant but somewhat fanatical application of a trite and commonplace notion. It was well understood by reflective persons at that time, who were quite sound on the contagiousness of fever, that the whole question of segregating the poor in fever hospitals was beset with difficulties, not merely of expense but also of expediency. A Select Committee of the House of Commons sat upon it in 1818, and published their report, with the minutes of evidence, on the 20th May. So much had been said in Parliament by Peel and others, and said so truly, of the spreading of fever all over Ireland by whole families turned adrift in beggary, that the Select Committee were full of ideas of contagion, and of the great opportunity of suppressing fever by destroying its germs or seeds. But they had soon occasion to learn that a fever may be potentially contagious, yet not contagious in all circumstances, and that segregation in fever hospitals had a rival in dispersion through general hospitals. Half-a-dozen London physicians of position, answering respectively for Guy's, St Thomas's, the London, St Bartholomew's, St George's, the Westminster and the

---

[1] A succession of thirty-one cases of relapsing typhoid at Charing Cross Hospital in 1877–78 were made the subject of an able essay by J. Pearson Irvine, M.D., *Relapse of Typhoid Fever*, London, 1880.

[2] Cited in Aberdeen Report, 17 Dec. 1818, in Harty, App. p. 110.

Middlesex Hospitals, declared that they mixed their cases of contagious fever in the ordinary wards among the other patients; and when asked by the astonished Committee whether the fever did not spread, they answered one after another with singular unanimity, "Never," which under cross-examination, became in one or two instances, "hardly ever," as, for example, in the evidence for St Thomas's Hospital, where a sister and a nurse had caught fever and died. The point of this London evidence was that the great safeguard against febrile contagion was free dilution with air, and that the great provocation of a contagious principle was to "concentrate" the cases of fever[1]. The Bristol experience in the same epidemic, although it did not come before the Select Committee, was wholly in agreement with medical opinion in London. The fever-cases there were received either into St Peter's Hospital, which was the city poor-house, or into the General Infirmary. The former was an old irregular building, badly ventilated, in which the contagion spread freely to the ordinary inmates and became very virulent. Contrasting with the apartments of the old poor's house, the wards of the Bristol General Infirmary were spacious, lofty, well-ventilated :

"Here the patients labouring under fever were dispersed among invalids of almost every other description; so that, whatever effluvia emanated from infected bodies became immediately diluted in the mass of air free from such pollution. Here, accordingly, no instance occurred of the propagation of fever. None of the nurses were attacked, nor were patients lying in the adjacent beds in any instance infected, though cases of the worst description, some of them exhibiting all the symptoms of typhus gravior, were placed promiscuously among the other patients, scarcely two feet of space intervening between the beds[2]."

The same practice was kept up in the Edinburgh Infirmary until 1858 or longer; Christison, who gives a diagram of an ordinary ward with four fever-beds in it, declared in 1850 that there had been no spread of fever for fifteen years before, except on one occasion, when the rules of the house were neglected[3]. The bold policy of dispersing fever-patients among the healthy was begun by Pringle and Donald Monro during the campaigns of 1742–48 and 1761–63 in the Netherlands and North Germany. They found that concentration raised the contagion to high degrees of virulence and that dispersion

---

[1] *Report of Select Committee*, u. s. p. 6, and minutes of evidence.
[2] Prichard, pp. 74, 88.
[3] Christison, *Month. J. Med. Sc.* x. ; Bennett, *Princip. and Pract. of Med.* 944–5.

weakened it to the point of non-existence, Monro's success at Paderborn in 1761 having been of the most signal kind[1].

The Select Committee of 1818 were more influenced by what they were told of the good effects of the earliest Houses of Recovery, at Waterford, Manchester and other places in the end of the last century. For several years after their opening they were little needed, the epidemic which gave the immediate impulse to their establishment having subsided in due time both in the towns provided with Houses of Recovery and in the innumerable places where no such provision had been made. The recommendations of the Committee do not appear to have been carried out; for the London Fever Hospital, in Pancras Road, which had been enlarged to seventy beds when the epidemic began in 1817, remained the only special fever hospital in London until the establishment of the hospitals of the Metropolitan Asylums Board in 1870[2].

The confusion of commerce, depression of trade and lack of employment which followed the Peace of Paris, and gave occasion to the British and Irish epidemic fevers of 1817–19, gradually righted themselves. The price of wheat, which would have been still higher after the four-months drought of 1818, but for large imports, gradually fell, and was about 50s. in 1821, and 40s. in the winter of 1822–23. After that, it rose somewhat again, and the third decade of the century, in the middle of which occurred the great speculative crash of 1825, was on the whole a hard time for the working classes. The history of fever has few illustrations between the epidemic of 1817–19 and that of 1826–27, excepting the great famine-fever of Connemara and other parts of the West of Ireland

---

[1] See above, p. 110–11.

[2] A complementary measure, namely, notification of contagious sickness to the authorities, was put in practice at Leeds in 1804 on the opening of the House of Recovery there. The Leeds House of Recovery, with fifty beds, was opened on 1 November, 1804, the epidemic of fever being then about over. One of its officers was an inspector, whose duty was "to detect the first appearance of infection, to cause the removal of the patient to the House of Recovery, and to superintend the fumigating and whitewashing of the apartment from which he is removed. So great is the solicitude of the physicians to promote early removal that rewards are offered to such as shall first give information of an infectious fever in their neighbourhoods." It was claimed that this had been a great success, Leeds having been for twelve years previous to the epidemic of 1817 nearly exempted from two of the most infectious and fatal diseases, namely, typhus and scarlet fever. (It happened, however, that the whole of England, Scotland and even Ireland were exempted to the same remarkable, and of course gratifying degree.) Whitaker, *Loidis and Elmete*, 1816, p. 85.

in 1822, elsewhere described, which coincided with a somewhat prosperous time in England and called forth a princely charity[1].

The Relapsing Fever of 1827-28.

The epidemic of relapsing fever which was at a height in Dublin in 1826, did not culminate in Edinburgh, Glasgow. and other towns of Scotland until 1828. It was a somewhat close repetition of the epidemic of 1817-19, except that it was chiefly an affair of the towns, owing to depression of trade and want of work following the great crash of commercial credit in 1825-26. In Glasgow, the admissions for fever to the Royal Infirmary began to rise in 1825[2]:

Glasgow: Admissions for Fever.

Year		Year	
1824	523	1828	1511*
1825	897	1829	865
1826	926	1830	729
1827	1084*		

* Some of these were treated at the extra fever-hospital in Spring Gardens.

At Edinburgh the cases of fever treated in hospital were fewer in ordinary years than at Glasgow, but they rose to a higher point in the epidemic years[3]:

Edinburgh: Admissions for Fever.

Year		Year	
1824	177	1828	2013
1825	341	1829	771
1826 (nine months)	456	1830	346
1827	1875		

[1] A strange epidemic of the early summer of 1824 in a semi-charitable girls' school at Cowan Bridge, between Leeds and Kendal, which is the subject of a moving chapter in 'Jane Eyre,' was inquired into by Mrs Gaskell, the biographer of Charlotte Brontë. Forty girls were attacked with fever. A woman who was sent to nurse the sick, saw when she entered the school-room from twelve to fifteen girls lying about, some resting their heads on the table, others on the ground; all heavy-eyed and flushed, indifferent and weary, with pains in every limb, the atmosphere of the room having a peculiar odour. The symptoms, so far as known, and the circumstances of the school, point more to relapsing fever than to typhus, which is the name given to it by Charlotte Brontë. None died of the fever (it is otherwise in the tale), but one girl died at home of its after-effects. Dr Batty, of Kirby, who was called in, did not consider the type of fever to be alarming or dangerous. The dietary of the school had undoubtedly been most meagre for growing girls, and its discipline severe. The house was old and unsuited for the purposes of a boarding-school.
[2] Cowan, *Journ. Statist. Soc.* III. (1840) p. 271; *Glas. Med. Journ.* III. 437.
[3] From the table by Christison, *Edin. Med. Journ.*, Jan. 1858, p. 581.

Christison gives the following account of the epidemic in Edinburgh in 1827–28 :

"Like that of 1817–19, it arose in Edinburgh during a protracted period of want of work and low wages among the labouring classes and tradespeople; it prevailed only among the working classes and unemployed poor— in the Fountainbridge and West Port districts, the Grassmarket 'closes,' the Cowgate and the narrow 'wynds' descending on either side of the long sloping back of the High Street and Canongate." The fever had the same three types as in 1817–19—many cases of inflammatory, or relapsing, or synocha, a few of low fever (typhus), and some between the two—militant or inflammatory for a week, then becoming low, and running the continuous course of typhus..."The inflammatory fever presented the same extreme violence of reaction as in the former epidemic—the same tendency to abrupt cessation, with profuse sweating—the same liability to return abruptly a few days afterwards—and the same disposition to depart finally in a few days more, and again abruptly with free perspiration. The cases of typhus were more frequently severe than in 1818–19. Icteric synocha occurred also oftener, although far from frequently[1]."

The epidemic of relapsing fever in 1826–28, which made a great impression in the towns of Ireland and Scotland, has left few traces in specially English records. But it is clear that there was some increase of fever about the same time in London; and it becomes a matter of interest, as well as of no little difficulty, to ascertain the type or types of the same. It was just after this quasi-epidemic in London that Dr Burne published his essay on fevers, the preface bearing the date of 28th February, 1828[2]. The materials of this essay came from Guy's Hospital, and they were both clinical and anatomical. The author seeks to find a common name for all varieties of continued fever, the name that he chooses being " Adynamic Fever." " By far the greater number of cases," he says, " are of the first or second degree only of severity, and not dangerous." These were cases of " simple continued fever," or fever of short duration, with flushed face, suffused eyes and other signs of the " inflammatory " type, or of synocha. Although Burne does not give the exact proportion of cases with relapse, as Bateman had done for the London epidemic of 1817–18, yet he makes it clear that relapses did occur, and he discusses the phenomenon in a manner which makes his testimony interesting : " Convalescents are more liable to a relapse after the adynamic fever than after any other disease; and this may be accounted for by the very enfeebled and exhausted state in which the powers

[1] *Life of Christison,* " Autobiography."
[2] John Burne, M.D., *Pract. Treatise on the Typhus or Adynamic Fever.* London, 1828.

of the system are left." His relapses were obviously a return of the original fever, beginning again suddenly in the midst of convalescence with flushing of the face, headache, dry tongue, and scanty urine, and with a great access of febrile heat in the night, a disturbance of the system which generally continued for several days, while in some it went off sooner with a diarrhoea. He assigned three principal causes for the relapse —overloading the enfeebled but craving stomach, walking out in the open air too soon, and giving way to emotion[1].

The references to relapse apply almost certainly to fevers of the shorter periods (synocha or "inflammatory" fever), and not to those cases of enteric fever which did undoubtedly occur in the practice of Guy's Hospital in the same seasons.

Typhoid or Enteric Fever in London, 1826.

The identification of enteric fever and relapsing fever respectively, or the separation of each from typhus, became actual in Britain at one and the same time. I have already said all that seems necessary as to the earlier appearances of relapsing fever on the stage of epidemiological history. This will be the fitting point in the chronology, the third decade of the 19th century, to bring in the question of enteric or typhoid fever. As to its identification, or recognition as a distinct species, that was not really completed, to the satisfaction of everyone, until the elaborate analysis of the symptoms respectively of typhus and enteric fevers by Sir William Jenner in 1849–51[2]. But, for ten years before that, the co-existence with maculated typhus of a different long-period fever, having abdominal symptoms and abdominal lesion, had been recognised,

---

[1] To show the effect of emotion in causing a relapse, he gives an instance, almost the only concrete illustration in all his book: An Irishwoman, Ann McCarthy, aged 26, was admitted to Guy's Hospital on 20 June, 1827, with "adynamic fever of the second degree," having been already ill for two weeks: the course of her fever was favourable and she was "soon convalescent." While still in the ward mending her strength, she lent her bonnet to another female patient to go out with; finding that her kindness had been abused by the woman forgetting to return the bonnet, she became exceedingly angry, relapsed into the fever on the 10th of July, was wildly delirious for several days, and died on the 19th of July. At this time it was the practice at Guy's to examine the bodies after death; but permission was refused in the case in question, so that Burne was unable to say "whether the bowels were affected." The case, therefore, may have been one of relapsing enteric fever. A similar ambiguity is discussed by Hughes Bennett in his *Principles and Practice of Physic* (p. 923), and decided in favour of relapsing fever proper, or relapsing synocha.

[2] Sir William Jenner, M.D., *Lectures and Essays on Fevers and Diphtheria*, 1849 to 1879. London, 1893.

and the characteristic ulceration or sloughing of the lymph-follicles of the ileum, with sphacelation of the mesenteric lymph-glands, had been clearly described by several London physicians and depicted in coloured plates, in the years 1826 and 1827, during an unusual prevalence of such cases in London. The authentic history of enteric fever in Britain really begins with these writings by physicians of St George's and Guy's Hospitals. But, as it is improbable that the type of fever was absolutely new in the years 1825 and 1826, it may be asked whether the enteric type cannot be discovered in the old accounts of British fevers, and if so, whether we may assume in the past as much enteric fever relatively to spotted typhus, relapsing fever, or simple continued fever, as in the period after 1850.

Having adverted to this point from time to time in the preceding history as it arose, for example in connexion with Willis's fever of 1661, Strother's fever of 1727–29, the Rouen fever of 1750, and other instances both in children (remittent or convulsive or comatose fever of children) and in adults, I shall not recapitulate farther back than the beginning of the 19th century.

There was a certain amount of post-mortem observation in the 18th century, especially in camp sicknesses, by Pringle and others; but there is no trace of intestinal ulceration among their fatal fevers. It was found, however, in the epidemic of 1806 among the troops at Deal, and it is probable that Ferriar's cases at Manchester about 1804, and Bateman's cases of continued fever in London from 1804 to 1816, were in some part enteric, although the anatomical test is wanting. That was a period when there was singularly little of the old London fever in the houses of the poorer class. Then came the remarkable "constitution" of relapsing or simple continued fever, from about 1816 to 1828, the relapsing character of which was far more obvious in Ireland and Scotland, than in London, Bristol, or elsewhere in England, but was not altogether unobserved in London, whether in 1817–19 or in 1827–28. The relapsing type disappeared after that for fifteen or twenty years, and was replaced by typhus more maculated than had been seen for many years. But, before the relapsing or simple continued fever disappeared for a time, enteric fever was seen in London in company with it.

The chief season of enteric fever in London was the autumn of 1826, following a long period of great drought and heat. The remarkable weather of that season was the same in England, Ireland and Scotland, and is thus described for the last by Christison :

"The spring and summer seasons of that year were remarkable for the extraordinary drought and heat which prevailed for many continuous months. No such seasons could be recollected by anybody, and assuredly there has been nothing similar in this country since....The fine weather set in with the beginning of March, and continued, with scarcely a check, well into the autumn....The drought prevailed and the heat increased till the middle of June, when a thunderstorm with heavy rain cooled the air for a day or two. But the heat then became greater than ever, and there was continuous sunshine and no rain till after the middle of July, when again there was thunder and rain, after which sun, heat and drought ruled the season once more." The shade temperature at Edinburgh was 84° Fahr., at 3 p.m. on three successive days of July[1]. The two summers preceding had also been exceptional, that of 1824 having been hot and moist, that of 1825 hot and dry, with dysentery in Dublin.

In August, 1826, Dr Cornwallis Hewett, of St George's Hospital, published ten fatal cases of enteric fever, four of which had occurred in his own practice, six in the practice of his colleagues[2]. The first was admitted on 23 April, 1825, the latest on 3 July, 1826. While his paper was under hand, he had read in the *Medico-chirurgical Review* for July, 1826, some extracts from Bretonneau's paper on " Dothiénentérite" (enteric fever), and he pronounced the London cases to be the same as those recently observed at Tours. Several other cases occurred at St George's Hospital in the autumn of 1826, three of them reported by Dr Chambers[3]. At the very same time, there was a run of enteric cases at Guy's Hospital. Dr Bright says: " Fever occurred with considerable frequency among the patients who presented themselves for admission into Guy's Hospital, during the months of October, November and December, 1826. On the whole, the disease was not severe." The more comprehensive account of these cases was given by Burne, early in 1828, from which it appears that the bulk of them were fevers of the shorter period, that there were relapsing cases among them, and that some were cases of enteric fever, verified by post-mortem

[1] Christison, *Life*, u. s. I. 341.
[2] " Cases showing the frequency of the occurrence of Follicular Ulceration in the Mucous Membrane of the Intestine during the progress of Idiopathic Fever, with Dissections, and Observations on its Pathology." *Lond. Med. and Physical Journ.*, Aug. 1826, p. 97.
[3] *Ibid.* p. 351.

examination[1].   It was the enteric cases that attracted the notice of Dr Bright, who says nothing of the relapsing cases, or of cases of simple continued fever.   The fact that the intestinal mucous membrane may become diseased during fever was, he says, "long known in particular cases, but never suspected to be so general till brought into view by the French physicians, and which has lately been illustrated in this country with great beauty [this does not mean in plates] by the pens of my able and assiduous friends Dr Chambers and Dr Hewett." He gives ten fatal cases, with coloured plates of the intestinal or mesenteric lesion in some of them, the earliest coloured plate having been made from a case admitted on 13 October, 1825, and the most typical plate of the sloughing Peyer's follicles from a case admitted on 25 November, 1826.   He gives also eleven cases of recovery, to show the benefit of treating the diarrhoea by calomel[2].   Nearly all the cases occurred in the end of the year, either of 1825 or 1826; and Burne confirms this when he says that the cases with enteric lesion were found at Guy's Hospital only in autumn.   Some two years after, in 1830, Drs Tweedie and Southwood Smith, physicians to the London Fever Hospital, described cases of fever with ulcerated intestine and sphacelated mesenteric glands.   After that, the interest shifted to typhus, which reappeared in London of an unusually maculated type; so that the years 1826–30 make a somewhat distinct period in which the new fever, with enteric lesion, was an engrossing medical topic.   It is tolerably certain that it was the unusual seasons of 1825 and 1826 which brought enteric fever into prominence; while, as soon as it became frequent, it could hardly have escaped the systematic apparatus of clinical case-taking and post-mortem examination, with preservation and drawing of specimens, for which Guy's Hospital was already noted under the influence of Bright and his colleagues, and in which the staff of St George's Hospital would appear to have been not less competent.   Although Dr Hewett, in 1826, identified his cases with the *dothiénentérite* of Bretonneau, yet neither he nor Dr Bright took the abdominal ulcerations or sloughs as distinctive of a new kind of fever.   They regarded them rather as a new complication of "idiopathic" typhus fever, a "complication" which appealed to them more on the side

[1] Burne, u. s.
[2] Richard Bright, M.D., *Reports of Medical Cases.*   Part I., 1827.

of treatment than of systematic nosology; hence the writings of both physicians are occupied mainly with the benefit of calomel in relieving the congestion of the bowels and in checking the diarrhoea.

It is undoubted that cases of enteric fever in 1826–27 were relatively more numerous in London than in Dublin and Edinburgh, where the epidemic fever was almost wholly of the relapsing type. In Edinburgh, at least, the comparative infrequency of enteric fever for years after it had been recognized in Paris, Tours and other French cities, and had been found in London as a common autumnal type, can be proved beyond cavil. Writing long after of the first epidemic of relapsing fever in Edinburgh, Christison said :

"Of enteric typhus (typhoid fever) we saw nothing then [1817–20], nor for many years afterwards. If it might have been overlooked during life, it could not have been missed after death. For our dissections were many, and, to meet the bias of the day for finding a local anatomical cause for all fevers [the doctrine of Broussais], every important organ in the body was habitually looked to. Nevertheless we were constantly met with the want of morbid appearances anywhere, unless slight signs of vascular congestion in various membranous textures be considered such[1]."

These vascular congestions were, indeed, scanned closely for traces of ulceration, after Bright's plates of 1828, and any little irregularity on the surface of a congested Peyer's patch was liberally construed in that sense, as in Craigie's reports subsequently. But in the Edinburgh epidemic of 1827–29, the anatomical signs of enteric fever were wanting until the end of it. Writing in 1827, Alison said that he had dissected 26 cases dead of the epidemic fever, without finding intestinal ulceration in one of them. Christison, however, says that a very few cases of enteric fever were dissected in Edinburgh in 1829[2].

In Dublin, also, the anatomical mark of enteric fever was missed in 1826–27, in the few dissections that were made during the epidemic[3]. An opinion in a widely different sense was given on that point by Stokes twelve years after the event, to which I refer in a note[4].

---

[1] *Life of Sir Robert Christison*, I. 144. Also in *Trans. Soc. Sc. Assn.* 1863, p. 104.
[2] *Edin. Med. Journ.*, Jan. 1858, p. 588. Cf. *infra*, under Dysentery, 1828.
[3] Reid, *Trans. K. and Q. Coll. of Phys. in Ireland*, v. ; O'Brien, *ibid.*
[4] Writing in 1839, Dr Stokes, of Dublin, made the following remarkable assertion (*Dub. Journ. Med. and Chem. Sc.* xv. p. 3, note) : "In the epidemic of 1826 and 1827 we observed the follicular ulceration (dothienenteritis of the French) in the greater number of cases." As the epidemic of 1826–27 was almost wholly one of relapsing

Return of Spotted Typhus after 1831 : " Change of Type." Distress of the Working Class.

A fever with relapses, and a fever with sloughing of the follicles and lymph glands of the intestine, were not the only novelties in the first thirty or forty years of the 19th century. Relapsing fever and enteric or typhoid fever were each clearly separated, at a later date, from typhus fever. But what was the "typhus fever" from which they were at length separated ? It was a fever which came prominently into notice after the "constitution" of 1826–29 was ended—a fever with a mottled, measly, or rubeoloid rash, and with various other spots, on account of which it was described by Dr Roupell in 1831, in a lecture before the College of Physicians of London, as a "new fever[1]." It was a new fever only in the sense in which each new febrile "constitution," whether it were an influenza, an epidemic ague, or a malignant typhus, was apt to be called popularly "the new fever," in the 16th and 17th centuries. There were, of course, erudite men at the College of Physicians in 1831 who knew that a fever with a mottled rash, with vibices and petechiae, and with all other symptoms of typhus gravior, had often occurred in England, Scotland and Ireland in former times. The "spotted fever" was perhaps the most familiar name of typhus in the 17th century. The mottled rash, like that of measles, was described for the fever of Cork by Rogers in the beginning of the 18th century, and for various other English and Irish epidemics by Huxham, O'Connell, Rutty and others. But undoubtedly the maculated typhus was somewhat new to the generation who saw it about 1830 and following years, the continued fevers which had prevailed in England, Scotland and

fever, the statement is at least puzzling. It was made twelve years after the epidemic, at a time when the discrepancies between British and French observers, as to the occurrence of ulceration of the ileum in continued fever, were much discussed. Dr Lombard, of Geneva, having visited Glasgow, Dublin and other places, and confirmed the fact that the characteristic lesion of enteric fever was at that time only occasional, went on to say that Irish typhus was a species of disease by itself, a *morbus miseriae.* Whereupon the editor of the ' Dublin Journal of Medical Science' (XII. 503, in a review of Cowan's Glasgow Statistics) gave the following truly Irish reply : " Had Dr Lombard made more inquiries, he would have found that Ireland is not so sunk in misery and debasement but that she can produce occasionally a fever which, in abdominal ulcerations, can compete with the sporadic diseases of her wealthier and more enlightened neighbours." It may have been in the same patriotic spirit that Stokes declared " the greater number of cases " in the epidemic of 1826 and 1827 to have had follicular ulceration.

[1] G. L. Roupell, M.D., *Some Account of a Fever prevalent in* 1831. Lond. 1837.

Ireland since 1816 having been for the most part the simple continued, or synocha, with or without the relapsing character, and to some extent enteric fever[1].

It was from 1830 to 1834 that a change in the reigning type of fever began to be remarked in London, Dublin, Edinburgh and Glasgow, the new type becoming more and more evident as fevers became more prevalent in the 'thirties' and 'forties.' Typhus at length became so much a spotted fever that the question arose whether it should not be classed among the exanthemata. In 1840, Dr Charles West, having observed "the alteration in character which fever has undergone within the last few years," went over the history (but more the foreign than the English) with a view "to illustrate the question whether typhus ought not to be classed among the exanthematous fevers[2]:" of course he found many old descriptions of a mottled rash or other spots, but saw no reason to make spotted typhus one of the exanthemata. Dr Kilgour, of Aberdeen, who treated more than a thousand cases in his fever-ward at the infirmary there from 1838 to 1840, wrote in 1841, "I am perfectly satisfied that this fever, call it by what name we will, is truly an exanthematous fever[3]." Previous to 1835, the spots of fever-cases in the Glasgow Infirmary had hardly been remarked; but after that date all cases were classed either as spotted or not, the spotted cases being three-fourths of the whole. Besides being spotted, the fever of the new constitution was insidious in its approach and low in its reaction, very unlike the sthenic, militant, inflammatory synocha of the generation before. The blood-letting which had been all but universally used in the fever from 1816 to 1828, and had seemed to answer well, was continued for a time in the fever of the 'thirties.' But it was soon found to be injurious: the patients in the new fever were apt to faint when only a few ounces of blood (four or six) had been drawn, whereas in the other fever (whether relapsing or

---

[1] In addition to what has been said on this point already, for particular epidemics, I shall give a statement for ordinary years by Dr Carrick, of Bristol, in his 'Medical Topography' of that city: *Trans. Prov. Med. Assocn.* II. (1834), p. 176. "Continued fever is common enough, but nine-tenths of the cases are of a simple character, terminating for the most part within seven days, and unaccompanied with anything more serious than slight catarrhal or rheumatic disorder. Typhus gravior is rare—much more so than might be expected."

[2] Charles West, M.D., "Historical Notices designed to illustrate the question whether Typhus ought to be classed among the Exanthematous Fevers." *Edin. Med. and Surg. Journ.* 1840, April, p. 279.

[3] Alexander Kilgour, M.D., *ibid.* Oct. 1841, p. 381.

simple continued) they had often lost thirty ounces before
deliquium was reached. It was found, on the other hand,
that fever-cases in the 'thirties' needed wine and other cordial
regimen.   There was nothing new in these revolutions, whether
of the fevers themselves, or of the opinions as to their treatment.
Sydenham's method of taking his cue for treatment from the
"constitution" of the season, which was the method of Hippocrates, appeared to be once more the best suited to the circumstances.

It is not easy to make out what were the circumstances of
the time that led to the supersession of simple continued fever
(or relapsing fever in Ireland and Scotland), by spotted fever or
typhus gravior in all parts of the kingdom.   Sydenham would
have looked, among other things, to the weather and the character of seasons ; but from 1830 onwards there was no season
so notable as the dry and hot summer of 1826, although the end
of the year 1836 was remarkably wet.   The period of typhus
gravior was a time of much sickness of other kinds—the Asiatic
cholera of 1831–32, the influenza of 1831, 1833, and 1836–37,
and the general unhealthiness of the year 1837.   This was also
the decade when the "condition-of-England question" was a
common topic, a time of strikes and of much distress among the
working classes, as shown in the reports of the Poor Law
Commission.

In Glasgow there was a considerable prevalence of fevers
year after year from the relapsing-fever epidemic of 1827–29,
according to the following table of admissions for fever to the
Royal Infirmary and the special fever-hospitals[1] :

Admissions for Fever, Glasgow.

Year	Fever cases	Year	Fever cases
1827	1084	1833	1288
1828	1511	1834	2003
1829	865	1835	1359
1830	729	1836	3125
1831	1657	1837	5387 [3]
1832	1589) [2] 1148)	1838	2047
		1839	1529

The worst year of the series for fever was 1837, and the
worst month of that year was May, when the fever-deaths were

[1] Cowan, "Vital Statistics of Glasgow," *Journ. Statist. Soc.* III.
[2] Cases at Mile-End Fever Hospital.
[3] Including 906 male fever-patients at Albion Street temporary hospital.

1 in 3·22 of the mortality from all causes. That great access of fever in Glasgow followed immediately upon the great strike of the cotton-spinners, on 8th April, 1837, by which eight thousand persons, mostly women, were thrown out of work[1]. The death-rate in Glasgow was in those years as high as anywhere in the kingdom, and was higher in the nine years from 1831 than in the nine years preceding. The population of Glasgow, says Cowan, had increased on the industrial side, out of proportion to its middle and wealthiest class[2]; and to that he would attribute the higher death-rates in the second period (right-hand side), of the following table :

Glasgow Death-rates.

	1822—1830			1831—1839	
Year	Death-rate over all. One in	Death-rate under five. One in	Year	Death-rate over all. One in	Death-rate under five. One in
1822	44·4	101	1831	33·8	79
1823	36·4	78	1832	21·67	63
1824	37·0	81	1833	35·7	77
1825	36·3	81	1834	36·3	81
1826	40·6	105	1835	32·6	67
1827	37·0	84	1836	28·9	62
1828	33·0	79	1837	24·6	65
1829	37·9	100	1838	37·9	83
1830	41·5	97	1839	36·1	72

The high death-rates in some of the years in the second column were owing to special causes—Asiatic cholera in 1832, smallpox of children in 1835 and 1836, and to influenza, as well as to typhus, in 1831, 1833 and 1837. As to the fever which prevailed from 1831 to 1836, as it was not relapsing in type, so it was not associated with scarcity.

"The increase of fever in Glasgow," says Cowan, "during the seven years prior to 1837, had taken place, not in years of famine or distress, but during a period of unexampled prosperity, when every individual able and willing to work was secure of steady and remunerating employment. From the close of 1836, one of those periodical depressions in trade, arising from the state of our monetary system, had visited this city, and deprived a large proportion of the population of the means of subsistence[3]."

It was then that the cases of typhus trebled in number.

[1] *Blackwood's Magazine*, March, 1838, p. 289.

[2] In 1819 the Irish in Glasgow had been estimated at 1 in 9·67 : in 1831 the Irish part of the population had risen to 1 in 5·69. Dr Cowan, however, said of them : "From ample opportunities of observation, they appear to me to exhibit much less of that squalid misery and habitual addiction to the use of ardent spirits than the Scotch of the same grade."

[3] Robert Cowan, M.D., "Statistics of Fever in Glasgow for 1837." *Lancet*, April 10, 1839.

The epidemic of fever reached its height in Dundee about the same time as in Glasgow, and in both towns sooner than anywhere else in Scotland or England. One reason of this was the labour-troubles culminating in strikes. In the twelve-month from 15 June, 1836, to 12 June, 1837, more than three-fourths of all the admissions to the Dundee Infirmary on the medical side were for fever (700 cases). After the wet autumn of 1836 there were a good many cases of dysentery, of which 22 were treated in the infirmary, with two deaths[1].

At Edinburgh, as at Glasgow, there had been an unusual amount of fever in 1831 and 1832, and a steady prevalence of it thereafter. The epidemic of 1836–39 was for the most part typhus of the winter seasons, declining each spring and disappearing each summer, except in the summer of 1836, when many cases came in June, July and August from airy parts of the town[2]. The climax of the epidemic was in 1838, a year later than in Glasgow and Dundee, according to the admissions to the fever-wards of the infirmary[3]:

Admissions for Fever, Edinburgh Infirmary.

Year	Cases		Year	Cases
1831	758		1836	652
1832	1394		1837	1224
1833	878		1838	2244
1834	690		1839	1235
1835	826		1840	782

At Aberdeen the epidemic appears to have been later even than at Edinburgh, if the following admissions to one of the two fever-wards (Dr Kilgour's) may be taken as a fair measure of it[4]:

Admissions for Fever, Aberdeen.

Year	Cases	Deaths
1838 (March to December)	189	26
1839	286	29
1840	534	53

In all these large towns of Scotland, the fever was purely typhus. The various observers all describe the fever as of the spotted kind, the proportion of cases with spots varying somewhat.

[1] James Arrott, M.D., *Edin. Med. and Surg. Journ.*, Jan. 1839, p. 121.
[2] Craigie *ibid.* April, 1837.
[3] Christison, *Monthly Journ. Med. Sc.* x. 1850, p. 262.		[4] Kilgour, u. s.

Thus, at Glasgow Infirmary, from 1835 to 1839, there were 4202 cases with eruption, 1270 without eruption, and 143 doubtful. And, that the cases without eruption were not cases of enteric or typhoid, is probable from the record kept of the fatalities in Dr Anderson's fever-wards[1]:

In 1885 cases with eruption,   275 deaths, or 14·58 per cent.
„   324 cases without eruption,   11 deaths, or 3·33 per cent.
„   143 cases doubtful,   7 deaths, or 4·89 per cent.

At Aberdeen, Kilgour counted 59 cases spotted in a total of 189 in 1838, 96 in a total of 286 in 1839, and 278 in a total of 534 in 1840, all the cases, whether spotted or not, being of the same fever, which he considered an exanthematous malady as a whole. Of 169 cases tabulated by Craigie at Edinburgh, from 28 June, 1836, to 12 February, 1837, there were 79 with an eruption, which was usually the mottled or rubeoloid rash.

The fatalities were relatively more in Edinburgh than in Dundee, comparing two periods which were not the same. Of 700 cases at Dundee, from June, 1836, to June, 1837, only 50 died, or 1 in 14, notwithstanding a good many complications from chest complaints and bowel complaints[2]. At Edinburgh during fifteen months of 1838–39, there died 276 in 2037 cases, or 1 in 7·3 ; of those cases, 1075 were in females, with 116 deaths, or 1 in 9, and 962 males, with 160 deaths, or 1 in 6[3]. The most common age for the fever at Dundee was from twenty to forty years (416 out of 700 cases, with 26 deaths, or 1 in 16), while the most fatal age, as usual, was from forty to sixty years, at which one person died of three attacked. At Aberdeen, in the last year of the epidemic, the years of life from ten to twenty had more cases (233 in a total of 657) than any other decade of life. The average stay of a patient in the Aberdeen fever-wards was 18·67 days. The great preponderance of deaths in adolescents or adults was clearly shown in the Glasgow fever-statistics, 1835–39.

Deaths from typhus fever	Under ten years	Over ten years	Fever-deaths per cent. of deaths from all causes
4788	752	4036	11·57

The corresponding epidemic of typhus in England had the fortune to be recorded in great part under the new system of Registration, which came into force on the 1st of July, 1837. At the beginning of registration of the causes of death, and until a good many years after, no distinction was made in the published tables between typhus fever and enteric fever. But we happen to know that the epidemic of 1837–38 was in London

---

[1] Cowan, *Journ. Statist. Soc.* III. 1841.
[2] Arrott, u. s.   [3] Craigie, u. s.

almost wholly typhus, just as it was in the large towns of Scotland. Of sixty cases in 1837–38, of which notes were kept by West, under Latham at St Bartholomew's Hospital, none that died and were examined post-mortem had ulcerations, although some had congestion, of Peyer's patches, the cases being all reckoned typhus exanthematicus[1]. Sir Thomas Watson, who was then physician to the Middlesex Hospital, says of the ulceration of Peyer's patches in continued fever:

"Since attention has been drawn to the subject, the patches of glands, and the whole tract of mucous membrane, from the stomach to the rectum, have been diligently explored, and the result seems to be that, at certain times and places (in other words, in certain epidemics), the ulceration of the inner surface of the intestine is far less common than at others. It was comparatively rare in an epidemic of which I witnessed some part in Edinburgh [1827–29]. Then I came to London; and for several years I never saw a body opened after death by continued fever without finding ulcers of the bowels. More recently, however, and especially during the present epidemic (1838), I have looked for them carefully, in many cases that have proved fatal in the Middlesex Hospital, and have discovered neither ulceration nor any other apparent change in the follicles of the intestines." And elsewhere he confirms the purely typhus character of the epidemic of 1838: "Our wards at the Middlesex are full of it, and scarcely a case presents itself without these spots. We speak of it familiarly as the *spotted* fever; or, from the resemblance which the rash bears to that of measles, as the *rubeoloid* fever[2]."

From which it would appear that not even the ordinary average number of endemic cases of enteric fever, such as might have been expected at a hospital in the west end of London, were forthcoming in the epidemic of 1837–38, so purely was the type of fever typhus.

The deaths from this epidemic in London, from the 1st of July, 1837, to the 31st of December, 1838, were as follows[3]:

1837		1838			
3rd Quarter	4th Quarter	1st Quarter	2nd Quarter	3rd Quarter	4th Quarter
826	1107	1285	1176	829	788

—a total of 6011 deaths from fever, nearly all typhus, in eighteen months. The worst London parishes were Whitechapel and St Pancras, in which latter the fever-hospital was situated. The high mortality from fever, which had begun before the 1st of July, 1837, continued into the year 1839, when the deaths in London (probably including some enteric) were 1819.

---

[1] *Edin. Med. and Surg. Journ.* July, 1838.
[2] *Principles and Practice of Physic*, 3rd ed. 1848, II. 742, 732.
[3] *First Report of the Registrar-General*, London, 1839.

Over all England and Wales, including London, the last six months of 1837 produced 9047 deaths from "typhus," and the twelve months of 1838, 18,775 deaths, the winter of 1837–38 having been the most fatal period. After London, the large towns most affected by the epidemic in the latter half of 1837 were as follows :

	Deaths from typhus in six months			Deaths from typhus in six months
Liverpool	524		Dudley	54
Manchester and Salford	274		Abergavenny	53
			Wolverhampton	45
Birmingham	75		Newcastle	44
Bolton	75		Wigan	43
Sunderland	72		Chorley	41
Leeds	71		Swansea	36
Sheffield	68		Halifax	33
Bradford	65		Macclesfield	33
Stockport	63		Norwich	27

In each of the next two years the number of deaths from typhus in the four largest towns was as follows :

	Typhus deaths in 1838	Typhus deaths in 1839
Manchester and Salford	627	416
Liverpool	573	358
Leeds	245	150
Birmingham	123	141

From nearly all the registration districts of England and Wales, deaths from fever were returned in 1837–39, so that the contagion must have been very widely spread in town and country[1]. In London the epidemic declined greatly in 1839, but in many parts of England the deaths registered as "typhus" were hardly less numerous than in 1838, and in some country divisions they were more, as if the contagion had taken longer to reach the villages[2]. One village epidemic in North Devon in the latter half of the year 1839 had been observed by Dr W. Budd, afterwards of Bristol:

[1] The district registrars had hardly organised their work in the first two or three years of registration. Some gave much more complete returns than others. There was a reluctance to register births, and the marriages were not all registered. But the totals of deaths came out very nearly as the actuaries had expected.

[2] The Third Report of the Registrar-General gives the mortality in all parts of England from typhus in 1839 (as well as from scarlatina) in an elaborate table of the registration districts and sub-districts.

The first case in the village (North Tawton, 1100 to 1200 inhabitants) was of a young woman in a poor and crowded cottage, who sickened on 11 July, 1839; her mother, brother, and sister sickened in succession, her father and a young infant escaping the infection. In another cottage, four out of six were ill of fever, in another, three persons had it, and so on, the whole number of cases treated by Dr Budd in the village until the beginning of November being about eighty. It was carried from North Tawton to neighbouring hamlets : thus, a sawyer who lodged next door to the first infected cottage sickened of the fever and, on 2 August, returned to his home in the hamlet of Morchard. As he lay there, he was visited by a friend, who assisted to raise him in bed : "While thus employed, the friend was quite overpowered by the smell from the sick man's body," and on the tenth day thereafter sickened of fever, which spread to two of his children and to a brother who came from a distance to see him. Another sawyer who lodged with the former left North Tawton ill a week after him (9 August) for his home, also at Morchard, where he died after a period not stated; ten days after his death his two children took the fever, his widow escaping it. In a third instance, a widow L—— left North Tawton on 21 August to visit her brother, a farmer in the hamlet of Chaffcombe, seven miles distant. Two days after her arrival she fell ill of fever and recovered slowly. In the same farmhouse the mistress caught it a month or two later and died on 4 November; the farmer himself took to bed with the fever on the day his wife died, and came safe through the attack. Three weeks after, an apprentice on the farm sickened, then a lad (the fifth in order) in the end of December, then the farmer's sister, then another apprentice, then a serving-man, then a maidservant, and lastly the daughter of the widow L—— from North Tawton, who had been the first case in the house months before. This farmhouse at Chaffcombe sent off two distinct offshoots of contagion. The lad, who was fifth in the above series, was sent home ill to his mother's cottage, between Bow and North Tawton, in the end of December. His mother sickened on 24 January, 1840, and died on 2 February. Next door to her lived a married daughter, whose whole household were attacked. Another married daughter, who came from a distance to visit the sick, took the infection on her return home, and so started a new focus. From the same farm at Chaffcombe, the maid, who was ninth in order in the above series, was sent home to her father's cottage in the hamlet of Loosebeare, four miles away; her father caught the fever from her, and a farmer K——, who lived across the road, having visited this man several times in his illness, took the fever next, other cases following under farmer K's. roof, and thereafter throughout the whole hamlet of Loosebeare[1].

---

[1] W. Budd, M.D., *Lancet*, 27 Dec. 1856, and 2 July, 1859. Dr Budd, who had been studying in Paris and seeing much typhoid fever, but little or no typhus, in the service of Louis at La Pitié hospital, took the whole of these cases for enteric or typhoid, and insisted, in his later life, on the ground of his North Tawton experiences in 1839, that typhoid fever spread by contagion. He published numerous papers on this theme (*Lancet*, 27 Dec. 1856, another series in the same journal from 2 July to Nov. 1859, *Brit. Med. Journ.* Nov.-Dec. 1861, and, finally, a volume of reprints with additions, *Typhoid Fever, its Nature, Mode of Spreading and Prevention*, London, 1873). But he published no clinical cases nor post-mortem notes, to make good his 1839 diagnosis, on which the whole matter turned, contenting himself with an assurance that he knew typhoid well from studying it under Louis (who, at that time, believed that the typhus of armies, gaols, &c. and of the British writers, was the same as the fever which he, and others after him, named typhoid). He also made the following six statements, as if he were making affidavit : (1) that the great majority of the cases had early diarrhoea, (2) that three had profuse intestinal haemorrhage, (3) that more or less of tympanitis was almost universal in the epidemic, (4) that in nearly every case he found the rose-coloured lenticular spots, (5) that one case, which was the only one examined post-mortem, had the characteristic ulceration of the intestine,

This was doubtless the way the epidemic spread in all the country districts of England, the unwholesome state of labourers' cottages, as revealed in the reports of the Poor Law Commission, favouring it. In the chapter on the fevers of Ireland we shall find that the contagion of typhus and relapsing fever was dispersed in the same way, but to a much greater extent, owing to the amount of vagrancy.

In the manufacturing towns of the North of England the fever continued at a somewhat steady epidemic level for several years. The pathetic scenes of typhus among the poor of Manchester in Mrs Gaskell's famous tale of *Mary Barton* belong to the early part of the year 1839; but they might have been drawn from almost any months of the two or three years following, according to the passage cited below from the same work[1].

and (6) that one fatal case had the symptoms of perforation of the gut. This summary manner, asking in effect to be taken on trust, is not usually accepted from innovators, none of the great discoverers having resorted to it. Hitherto, however, no one has thought proper to question Budd's diagnosis of the epidemic fever in his North Tawton practice, nor even to remark upon his strange error of treating the epidemic of 1838–39 all over Britain as purely one of typhoid (*Lancet,* 27 Dec. 1856). But everyone knew that typhoid fever did not spread in the way that he described (doubtless correctly for the above cases). After the publication of his book in 1873 an attempt was made by an influential layman in the *Times* (9 Nov. 1874) to popularize Budd's fallacies or paradoxes on the contagiousness of typhoid. "How," it was asked, after a summary of the North Tawton epidemic in 1839, "could a disease whose characters are so severely demonstrable, have ever been imagined to be non-contagious? How could such a doctrine be followed, as it has been, to the destruction of human life?"

[1] "For three years past trade had been getting worse and worse, and the price of provisions higher and higher. This disparity between the amount of the earnings of the working classes and the price of their food occasioned, in more cases than could well be imagined, disease and death. Whole families went through a gradual starvation. They only wanted a Dante to record their sufferings. And yet even his words would fall short of the awful truth; they could only present an outline of the tremendous facts of the destitution that surrounded thousands upon thousands in the terrible years 1839, 1840, and 1841. Even philanthropists who had studied the subject were forced to own themselves perplexed in their endeavour to ascertain the real causes of the misery; the whole matter was of so complicated a nature that it became next to impossible to understand it thoroughly....The most deplorable and enduring evil that arose out of the period of commercial depression to which I refer, was this feeling of alienation between the different classes of society. It is so impossible to describe, or even faintly to picture, the state of distress which prevailed in the town [Manchester] at that time, that I will not attempt it; and yet I think again that surely, in a Christian land, it was not known even so feebly as words could tell it, or the more happy and fortunate would have thronged with their sympathy and their aid. In many instances the sufferers wept first, and then they cursed. Their vindictive feelings exhibited themselves in rabid politics. And when I hear, as I have heard, of the sufferings and privations of the poor, of provision shops, where ha'porths of tea, sugar, butter, and even flour, were sold to accommodate the indigent—of parents sitting in their clothes by the fireside during the whole night for seven weeks together, in order that their only bed and bedding might be reserved for the use of their large family—of others sleeping upon the cold hearthstone for weeks in succession, without adequate means of providing themselves with food or fuel—and this in the depth of winter—of others being compelled to fast for days together, uncheered by any hope of better fortune, living, moreover, or rather starving, in a crowded garret, or damp

In 1839 the Lancashire deaths from typhus were 1343; in Wales, Monmouth and Herefordshire they were 1548. There is, indeed, little improvement in the statistical returns as late as 1842. The deaths from "typhus" were as follows in all England and Wales:

1838	1839	1840	1841	1842
18,775	15,666	17,177	14,846	16,201

The deaths from the epidemic maladies of infants and children during the same five years were also very high.

	1838	1839	1840	1841	1842
Smallpox	16,268	9,131	10,434	6,368	2,715
Measles	6,514	10,937	9,326	6,894	8,742
Hooping cough	9,107	8,165	6,132	8,099	8,091
Scarlatina	5,802	10,325	19,816	14,161	12,807
Croup	4,463	4,192	4,336	4,177	4,457
Diarrhoea	2,482	2,562	3,469	3,240	5,241

The epidemic of smallpox corresponded closely to the epidemic of fever, the former being fatal chiefly to infants and young children, the latter fatal chiefly to adults. Before the smallpox epidemic had subsided scarlet fever became unusually mortal, especially in 1840, and kept its higher level of deaths for a generation after. The epidemic of fever, although it affected the mortality of the young comparatively little, was indirectly a reason why many of them died of other diseases; for the prostration of the parents, the impoverishment, and all the other troubles associated with an epidemic of typhus, led to inevitable sufferings among the young, which weakened their power of resistance.

The registration returns were not tabulated (except for London) from the end of 1842 to the beginning of 1847, but there is reason to think that the epidemic fever was not active in the interval. It is undoubted that the enormous construction of railroads in England during those years gave employment and wages to multitudes, and ended the distress the sooner. This effect of railroad-making in England was so obvious that Lord George Bentinck desired to relieve the distress in Ireland in 1846–47 by the same means.

Enteric Fever mixed with the prevailing Typhus, 1831–42.

While there is complete agreement among the hospital physicians of the great towns that the fever of 1837–39 was maculated typhus, to the total exclusion of cases with ulceration

cellar, and gradually sinking under the pressure of want and despair into a premature grave; and when this has been confirmed by the evidence of their careworn looks, their excited feelings, and their desolate homes—can I wonder that many of them, in such times of misery and destitution, spoke and acted with ferocious precipitation?" Mrs Gaskell, *Mary Barton.*

of the bowel, as in the experience of Watson at the Middlesex Hospital and of West (under Latham) at St Bartholomew's, yet some allowance should be made, in interpreting the figures of fever mortality in those years throughout England and Wales, for admixture of enteric fever. Budd's statement that the only case which was dissected in the epidemic at North Tawton, Devonshire, in 1839, had the bowel-lesion of enteric fever, if it is to count in the absence of the usual details (place, date, objective description), would mean that at least one case there was not of the prevailing type of contagious epidemic typhus. The coincidence of some such cases is made the more probable by the evidence from Anstruther, Fifeshire, reported by John Goodsir, afterwards Professor of Anatomy at Edinburgh, who was assisting his father in practice there from 1835 to 1839. During that period, which was the time of the typhus epidemic in the larger towns of Scotland, he attended about one hundred cases of fever annually in Anstruther and the neighbourhood; the fever was usually mild, only some sixteen of the cases having proved fatal; of those sixteen he examined ten after death, finding "ulceration" of the Peyer's patches in all, and perforation of the intestine in four of them. These facts he gave orally to Dr John Reid, pathologist to the Edinburgh Infirmary, whose experience of the morbid anatomy of fever was altogether different. Goodsir, having kept the specimens, made them the subject of a paper some years after (1842), in which he described very minutely the stages and degrees of congestion, ulceration, sloughing and perforation in the lymph-follicles of the intestine in fever, placing congestions at one end of the scale and sloughing at the other, as the French pathologists then did[1]. Reid examined, at the Edinburgh Infirmary from October, 1838, to June, 1839, forty-one bodies dead of fever, to see whether the intestinal lesion, which Goodsir had told him of, occurred in them. The distinctness of the Peyer's patches varied a good deal (differences which are known to be in part congenital and in part to depend on age), and in only two instances were they elevated and seemingly "ulcerated."

---

[1] John Goodsir, "On a Diseased Condition of the Intestinal Glands," *Lond. and Edin. Monthly Journ. of Med. Science*, April, 1842. He does not enter on the question "as to whether the subject of the present paper constitutes a distinct species of disease, or be merely a form of the ordinary continued fever"; but he appears to recognize that a certain district may have a form of fever special to it, as Reid had probably told him.

One of these was the case of an Irishman, from Sligo, aged 25, who had been so constipated that he was purged with colocynth, etc.: "at the lower part of thè ileum, the elliptical patches were irregular on the surface, and presented several superficial and ill-defined depressions (ulcerations)." The other was the case of a girl, aged 15, who had not suffered from diarrhoea, but had the intestinal patches elevated and superficially "ulcerated[1]." Neither of these cases would probably be reckoned typhoid or enteric fever at the present time on the anatomical evidence only. The early French observers, Chomel, Louis, Andral and others, included in a scale all the appearances of the Peyer's patches in fever that they thought morbid, from mere prominence of the lymphatic tissue and distinctness of the follicular pits, up to extensive sloughing and ulceration of the same, as if they were all the signs of one and the same fever in its various stages of development. But simple prominence or congestion of Peyer's patches may occur in typhus fever, or in relapsing fever; nor would a slight erosion, or "superficial ulceration" raise in all cases a suspicion of enteric fever.

The observations of Home, Reid's predecessor as pathologist to the Edinburgh Infirmary, from 1833 to 1837, were however conclusive that true enteric fever had occurred now and again during the steady prevalence of typhus fever from year to year. In that space he made 101 post-mortem examinations in fever-cases; in 29 the Peyer's patches were distinct, in 7 of those 29 there was "a greater or less degree of ulceration," and in 2 of those 7 there was perforation[2]. Murchison examined the post-mortem register of the Edinburgh Infirmary for the years 1833 to 1838, and found only fifteen cases of fever with ulceration of the bowel. But in the eight months from 1 November, 1846, to June, 1847, there were nineteen dissections with the characteristic lesion of typhoid, the season having been remarkable everywhere for that disease.

In the following series of years the fatal cases of fever in the Edinburgh Infirmary with ulceration were few[3]:

Year	Enteric deaths		Year	Enteric deaths
1854	5		1858	1
1855	2		1859	2
1856	1		1860	1
1857	8		1861	6

It was thought remarkable that the form of continued fever which was most usually found in the great continental cities, in Paris, Berlin, Prague and Vienna, namely that with ulceration of the lymph-follicles of the intestine, should be but occasionally mixed with the old typhus in England, Ireland and Scotland

---

[1] John Reid, M.D., "Analysis and Details of Forty-seven Inspections after Death," *Edin. Med. and Surg. Journ.*, Oct. 1839, p. 456.

[2] Reid, u. s., from Home's records.

[3] Murchison, *Continued Fevers*, 2nd ed. 1873, p. 444.

in the very same years. But there was nothing to discredit the British observations, anatomical and clinical; and in 1836 Dr Lombard, of Geneva, having visited various cities in England, Scotland and Ireland bore witness to the matter of fact, strange as it was to him. Writing to Graves, of Dublin, on 16 June, 1836, he said : "Before I leave Ireland, allow me to express to you my great astonishment at what I have seen in this country respecting your continued fever;" and in a second letter, of 18 July, after his return to Geneva, he added, that in Liverpool, ulceration of the ileum in continued fever was "occasional," that in Manchester he had been told it occurred "by no means always," that in Birmingham the cases of fever were not many, but "always" with intestinal ulceration, and that in London "not a fourth part" of the cases of fever had the latter condition, and these mostly in autumn[1]. This was before the great epidemic of typhus had begun in the English towns. To the same non-epidemic period (1834) belongs the statement of Carrick, for Bristol, that fever was often observed to be infrequent or altogether absent in the most crowded· and dirty parts of the city at times when there were a good many cases "in institutions and dwellings where cleanliness and free air are most carefully attended to," and that ulceration of the bowel was the most common post-mortem appearance[2].

The comparative rarity of enteric fever in the chief towns of Scotland and Ireland continued for a good many years longer, indeed until after the differences between typhus and typhoid were perceived and admitted by all. Even at the London Fever Hospital, during twenty-four years (1848–71) after Sir William Jenner's diagnostic points were strictly looked to in its wards, much the greater part of the admissions were of typhus; in only two periods, 1850–55 and 1858–61, during both of which there was comparatively little fever of any kind in London, did the admissions for enteric fever slightly exceed those for typhus; on an annual average of the twenty-four years ending 1871, the cases of the former were only about a fifth part of the

---

[1] Lombard, in *Dublin Journal of Med. Sc.* X. (1836), p. 17. He bore witness, also, to the rarity of the bowel-lesion in the Glasgow fevers. This was confirmed by Dr Perry, of that city, *Ibid.* X. 381. See also Julius Staberoh, M.D., "Researches on the Occurrence of Typhus in the Manufacturing Cities of Great Britain," *Ibid.* XIII. 426.

[2] *Trans. Prov. Med. Assoc.* II. (1834), p. 176.

whole. The cases of enteric fever increased decidedly after 1865. Murchison thought that the increase might be accounted for in part by the enlargement of the Fever Hospital, and by the unusually high temperature of certain years, the summers and autumns of 1865, 1866, 1868 and 1870 having been remarkable for their great heat and prolonged drought; but, he adds, "it is not a little remarkable that this increased prevalence of enteric fever in the metropolis has been contemporaneous with the completion of the main drainage scheme[1]."

Still more recently, the relative proportions of typhus and enteric fever have been reversed, so that there have been years with little or no typhus but with a good deal of enteric fever. There are some persons, unacquainted with the history, who cannot imagine that it was ever otherwise than now, who think of the former times of medicine, not as differing in social, economic, and various other respects from their own, but only as being less clever at diagnosis. There are others who realize clearly enough the historical matter of fact, but find it necessary to explain the almost contemporaneous decline of typhus and rise of typhoid by some hypothesis of the latter being "evolved" out of the former. This evolutional doctrine makes the mistake of ascribing to the species of disease the same comparative fixity of characters that belongs to the species of animals and plants. Beside the latter, the species of disease are the creatures of a day. In the nosological field, the origin of species is not analogous to the evolution of a new species of animal or plant out of an old, as in the hypothesis of Darwin, for the reason that every species of disease is evolved directly and, as it were, *pro re nata*, out of a few simple conditions of human life, variously mixed but always there to give occasion to one infective malady or another, which may have a shorter existence, like sweating sickness, or a longer, like plague. Edinburgh experiences offer a ready criticism of the evolutional doctrine. Typhus declined, and typhoid rose; but it was in the old tenement houses of the Canongate, Cowgate, Grassmarket, and High Street that typhus declined, and it was mostly in the new streets across the valley, or in the New Town of Edinburgh, that enteric fever arose, having sometimes no more mysterious an origin than the results of defective or cheap plumber-work,

[1] *Continued Fevers*, 2nd ed. 1873, p. 443.

for example, the leakage of a soil-pipe fermenting, a foot deep, beneath the basement floor. But it was not until a good many years after that these new experiences became common; and meanwhile Edinburgh and other towns in Scotland saw much of typhus and relapsing fever.

Relapsing Fever in Scotland, 1842–44.

The epidemic of 1836–39 had been typhus of a specially maculated kind. The period or "constitution" of synocha, rising twice to epidemics of relapsing fever, had lasted from near the beginning of the century until 1828 or 1829. Then came the new constitution of low, depressed, spotted fever, which would not stand blood-letting. But in 1842–44 relapsing fever reappeared in Scotland. This reappearance was a blow to two doctrines of the time—first that Ireland was the original breeding-place of all such fevers, and secondly, that a return of the "constitution" of relapsing fever would warrant a return to the practice of blood-letting, which had fallen into disuse during the epidemic of typhus. The epidemic of 1842–44 was at first purely a Scots affair, with some extension to England, but none to Ireland. As to blood-letting, once it had been given over in fevers it was not readily taken up again, notwithstanding the theory that relapsing fever belonged to those sthenic or inflammatory types of sickness in which the lancet was still thought admissible. Moreover, Christison, who remembered the relapsing synocha of 1817–19 and of 1827–28, said of the third epidemic: "The synocha of 1843–44, though so prevalent, by no means presented the same strong phlogistic or sthenic character as in the earlier epidemics of 1817–20 and 1826–29. The pulse was neither so frequent nor so strong; the heat was not so pungent; the glow of the integuments was less lively and less general[1]."

I take conveniently from Murchison the following succinct account of the Scots relapsing fever of 1842–44[2]:

" The next epidemic of fever in 1843 differed from those that preceded it, inasmuch as it did not originate in or implicate Ireland, but was mainly confined to Scotland. There was no increase of fever in the Irish hospitals

[1] Christison, " On the Changes which have taken place in the Constitution of Fevers and Inflammations in Edinburgh during the last forty years." Paper read at Med. Chir. Soc. Edin. 4 March, 1857. *Edin. Med. Journ.* Jan. 1858, p. 577.
[2] *Continued Fevers*, under the head of " Typhus," p. 47.

during this year, whereas the number of admissions into the Glasgow Infirmary rose from 1,194 to 3,467; in the Edinburgh Infirmary from 842 to 2,080; and in the Aberdeen Infirmary from 282 to 1,280. These numbers, too, are far from representing the true extent of the epidemic, for thousands of sick were sent from the hospital doors. The fever was almost exclusively relapsing fever; typhus was comparatively rare. The first cases were observed on the east coast of Fife, in 1841–2 (by H. Goodsir), and not in the crowded localities of large towns. In Dundee, where the proportion of typhus cases was comparatively great, the fever appeared early in the summer of 1842, and raged to a considerable extent during the whole of the autumn, before it showed itself elsewhere. In Glasgow the first cases occurred in September, 1842; but the fever was not generally prevalent until December, from which month the cases rapidly increased until October, 1843, when the epidemic began to decline. The number of cases in Glasgow was estimated at 33,000, or 11½ per cent. of the entire population. In Edinburgh relapsing fever was first observed in February, 1843. It rapidly spread until October, after which it gradually abated, until, by the following April, it had well nigh disappeared. In the month of October, 1843, the number of fever cases admitted into the Edinburgh Infirmary amounted to 638, and during several months, from thirty to fifty cases were daily refused admission. The total number of cases in Edinburgh was calculated by Alison at 9,000. In Aberdeen the epidemic commenced about the same time, and followed the same course as in Edinburgh. At Leith, curiously enough, it did not appear until September, 1843; it then spread rapidly for two months, after which it declined, and by the end of February, 1844, it had almost ceased; but during this brief period it attacked 1,800 persons, or one in every fourteen of the population. The disease was general over Scotland, and was not restricted to the large towns; it prevailed in Greenock, Paisley, Musselburgh, Tranent, Penicuick, Haddington, Dunbar, the Isle of Skye, etc. Although the epidemic was mostly confined to Scotland, the same fever was observed in some of the large towns of England. The number of admissions into the London Fever Hospital rose from 252 in the preceding year to 1,385 in 1843: and the annual report for 1843 makes it evident that a large proportion of these cases were relapsing fever. The rate of mortality of the epidemic was small, not exceeding from two-and-a-half to four per cent. Although this was the same fever as prevailed in 1817–19, even local bleeding was rarely resorted to, and many of the cases were thought to demand stimulants. All accounts agree in stating that the epidemic supervened upon a period of great distress among the Scottish poor, and that it was restricted throughout to the poorest and most wretched of the population."

This epidemic, which was the subject of an altogether unusual amount of writing in Edinburgh[1], partly on the supposition that relapsing fever was a "new disease," proved once for all that one had not to go to Ireland for the engendering or making of a famine-fever. The demonstration came just in time; for the epidemic was hardly over in Scotland, when the series of great potato-famines in Ireland began in 1845, soon to be followed by the disastrous epidemics of dysentery, relapsing

[1] See especially John Rose Cormack, M.D., *Natural History, Pathology and Treatment of the Epidemic Fever at present prevailing in Edinburgh and other towns.* Lond. 1843; and the papers by Wardell, *Lond. Med. Gaz.* N. S. II—V.

fever and typhus from 1846 to 1848. Indeed, so near was the Scots epidemic to the Irish, that in the North of Ireland the first of the relapsing fever, in 1846, was called "the Scotch Fever," on the supposition that it had reached them from its recent focus in the West of Scotland[1]. The Irish and original part of the great epidemic of 1846–48 has been fully described in another chapter; much of the mortality was due to dysentery, and the most prevalent fever was relapsing fever, with a very low rate of fatality among the poorer classes. But in Ireland itself there was also much typhus, very mortal to the richer classes who came in contact with the starving multitudes.

The "Irish Fever" of 1847 in England and Scotland.

The contagion that reached England and Scotland from the scene of famine in Ireland was more apt to produce typhus than relapsing fever. That the Irish contagion was the principal source of the great epidemics in England and Scotland in 1847–48, seems to be proved by every fact in their progress, direction and other circumstances. But it is not so clear that England and Scotland would not have had an unusual amount of typhus in the same years even if the Irish had been kept out by an ideally strict quarantine. What touched Ireland most, touched Scotland and England in a measure. The seasons were bad in all parts of the kingdom; many were out of work in the manufacturing towns; but as soon as the price of provisions fell in 1848, the epidemic in England came to a sudden end.

The epidemic of fever in England in 1847 was almost wholly typhus; in Scotland, it was to some extent relapsing fever, but there also it was mainly typhus. It was more severe, while it lasted, than the epidemic of 1837 and following years; but it was of shorter duration, ceasing almost abruptly in 1848. The rise of the epidemic of 1847 in London is shown by the following quarterly returns of the deaths from fever:

1st Quarter	2nd Quarter	3rd Quarter	4th Quarter
442	568	895	1279

In the last quarter of 1846, the deaths from fever in London

[1] Dr Betty, of Lowtherstown, Fermanagh, *Dubl. Quart. Journ. Med. Sc.* VII. 125.

had been 619.   In all England, the last quarter of 1846 was also
most unhealthy, its deaths from all causes being 53,055 (only
43,850 in the first quarter of the year).   The summer of 1846 had
been remarkable for heat and drought, and the end of the year
was, according to precedent, an unwholesome time.   It was just
the season for enteric fever, as in the still more memorable
circumstances of 1826.   There is evidence from various parts
of England and Scotland that much of the fever of the end of
1846 was enteric; and it was doubtless the unusual prevalence
of that disease, and of other maladies that are favoured, like it,
by extreme fluctuations of the ground-water, that explains the
very high mortality of the last quarter of 1846[1].   But it is
equally certain that it was typhus which raised the fever deaths
in London in the last quarter of 1847 to 1,279, and the deaths
from all causes in all England to the enormous total of 57,925.
In the whole of the year 1847, typhus alone claimed 30,320
deaths in England and Wales, the total in 1848 falling to 21,406.
Lancashire and Cheshire had the largest share of this epidemic,
and Liverpool the largest share in Lancashire.   In that Registration Division (the North-western) the deaths from typhus in
1847 were 9,076, and in 1848 they were 3,380.   Next in order
(excluding London and suburbs) came the West Midland Division, and next to that Yorkshire.   At Liverpool, and in other
places of the north-west of England, the fever was very clearly
connected with the enormous Irish immigration, and was in
great part among the Irish.   There were floating lazarettos on
the Mersey, filled with fever and dysentery, workhouses over-
flowing, and sheds hastily built to hold each 300 patients.   The
following returns from the several sub-divisions of Liverpool
for the months of July, August and September, 1847, show the
proportions of dysentery and fever, as well as the mortality from

[1] Murchison says that the enteric fever of the end of 1846 was prevalent at many
places in England where the epidemic of typhus never made its appearance, and that
in Edinburgh (according to an unpublished essay by Waters) most of the enteric cases
not only occurred prior to the outbreak of the epidemic of Irish fever, but came from
localities in the neighbouring country and from the best houses of the New Town—
not from the crowded courts of the Old Town, to which the later epidemic of typhus
and relapsing fever was restricted.   Murchison, u. s. p. 49.   The following papers
relate to the autumnal typhoid of 1846 in England : Sibson, "Fever at Nottingham
and neighbourhood in Summer and Autumn of 1846," *Med. Gaz.* XXXIX.; Taylor,
" Fever at Old and New Lenton in 1846," *Med. Times*, XV. 159 and *Med. Gaz.*
XXXVIII. 127; Turner, "Fever at Minchinhampton in Autumn 1846," *Med. Gaz.*
XLII. 157; Brenchley, "Fever in Berkshire in 1846," *Med. Gaz.* XXXVIII. 1082; Bree,
" Epidemic Fever at Great Finborough in Autumn of 1846," *Prov. Med. and Surg.
Journ.* 1847, p. 676.

diarrhoea, which last was mostly an affair of the infants and young children[1]:

Liverpool deaths, July—Sept. 1847.

	Fever	Dysentery	Diarrhoea
St Martin's	291	82	174
Dale Street	250	20	111
St Thomas	(301 deaths on the floating lazarettos)		
Mount Pleasant	324	18	73
Islington	105	37	78
Great Howard Street	(the fever extending to the upper classes)		

In his report for the quarter before (April, May and June, 1847) the registrar of the Great Howard Street sub-district says: "Eight Roman Catholic priests, and one clergyman of the Church of England, have fallen victims to their indefatigable attentions to the poor of their church[2]."

In Manchester there were causes of fever independently of the Irish contagion. The registrar of the Deangate sub-district writes in the third quarter of 1847: "In the calamitous season just passed, manufactures have been almost at a stand-still; food has been unattainable by the poor, for employment they had none; Famine made her dwelling in their homes &c." The hardships of the children caused an immense mortality from summer diarrhoea. The same registrar gives an account of the epidemic fever in his report for the second quarter of 1847, from which it appears that, although nearly all the hospital cases were distinctly maculated, and the fever was undoubtedly typhus in all other respects and in its conditions, yet tympanitis, with abdominal tenderness and diarrhoea, were specially noted[3].

Besides Liverpool and Manchester, many other towns in Lancashire had the "Irish fever" in them; also Birmingham, Dudley, Wolverhampton, Shrewsbury, Leeds, Hull, York and Sunderland. Except in London, the fever mortality was not unusual in the southern half of England[4].

---

[1] In the *Report of the Registrar-General for the year* 1847.

[2] This was the occasion which furnished Father Newman with a famous argument for the *bona fides* of his co-religionists: "The Irish fever cut off between Liverpool and Leeds thirty priests and more, young men in the flower of their days, old men who seemed entitled to some quiet time after their long toil. There was a bishop cut off in the North; but what had a man of his ecclesiastical rank to do with the drudgery and danger of sick calls, except that Christian faith and charity constrained him?" John Henry Newman, D.D., *History of My Religious Opinions*, London, 1865, p. 272.

[3] Leigh, in *Report Reg.-Gen. for* 1847, x. p. xx.

[4] H. M. Hughes, "On the Continued Fever at present existing in the southern districts of the metropolis," *Lond. Med. Gaz.* Nov. 1847; Laycock, "Unusual

In Scotland the epidemic was a mixture of relapsing fever and typhus. The following were the proportions of each admitted to the Glasgow Royal Infirmary:

Year	Relapsing Fever	Typhus
1846	777	500
1847	2,333	2,399
1848	513	980
1849	168	342

In the Barony Fever Hospital, Glasgow, open from 5 August 1847 to July 1848, the relapsing cases were double the typhus cases at the opening of the hospital, at the end of 1847 they were nearly equal, and from February 1848 the typhus cases were double the relapsing. In Edinburgh, where the epidemic was less severe, the same relations were observed—relapsing fever most at the beginning, typhus fever (much more fatal) most at the end[1]. Some relapsing fever occurred also in London, among destitute Irish, which was often attended by a miliary eruption (Ormerod).

Subsequent Epidemics of Typhus and Relapsing Fevers.

By midsummer, 1848, there was a most marked improvement in the public health, corresponding with the great fall in the prices of food, under the influence of free trade, and with a good harvest and the commencement of an era of steady employment for workers. The improvement is strikingly shown in the following comparison of the deaths from all causes in

prevalence of Fever at York," *Lond. Med. Gaz.* Nov. 1847; Bottomley, "Notes on the Famine Fever at Croydon in 1847," *Prov. Med. and Surg. Journ.* 1847; Ormerod, *Clinical Observations on Continued Fever at Bartholomew's Hospital,* Lond. 1848; Art. in *Brit. and For. Med. Chir. Rev.* 1848, I. 285; Duncan, *Journ. Pub. Health,* I. 200 (Liverpool); Paxton, *Prov. Med. Journ.* 1847, pp. 533, 596 (Rugby).

[1] The following papers relate to the epidemic in Scotland in 1847: Orr, "Historical and Statistical Sketch of the progress of Epidemic Fever in Glasgow during 1847," *Edin. Med. and Surg. Journ.* LXIX.; Stark, "On the Mortality of Edinburgh and Leith for 1847," *Ibid.* and LXXI.; R. Paterson, "Account of the Epidemic Fever of 1847–8" in Edinburgh, *Ibid.* LXX.; W. Robertson, "Notes on the Epidemic Fever of 1847–8," *Month. Journ. of Med. Sc.* IX. 368; J. C. Steele, "View of the Sickness and Mortality in the Glasgow Royal Infirmary during 1847," *Edin. Med. and Surg. Journ.* LXX.; J. C. Steele, "Statistics of the Glasgow Infirmary for 1848," *Ibid.* LXXII. 241; J. Paterson, "Statistics of the Barony Parish Fever Hospital of Glasgow in 1847–8," *Ibid.* LXX. 357.

Lancashire and Cheshire in the third quarter of each of the years 1846, 1847 and 1848:

	1846	1847	1848
Deaths in the 3rd Quarter	15,221	17,080	11,720

Since the epidemic of 1847, which was not unfairly called "the Irish fever," there has been no such extensive and fatal outbreak of typhus or relapsing fever in England, Scotland or Ireland. The fever deaths rose somewhat in Ireland and in Glasgow in 1851–53, the type of disease being relapsing and typhus. In London there was a considerable increase of typhus in 1856, at the end of the Crimean War. From 1861 to 1867 there was a considerable epidemic of the same fever in England and Scotland (not much of it in Ireland until 1864), the chief centres in England having been the Lancashire towns, Preston, Manchester, Accrington, Chorley, Salford and Blackburn, and the occasion of it the "cotton famine" of the American Civil War[1]. Greenock was the chief seat of typhus in 1863–64 in Scotland; indeed, in the whole kingdom, its death-rate from that cause was approached by that of Liverpool only. Fevers had been very mortal there in the epidemic of 1847 (it is said 353 deaths); in the next fever-period they rose as follows[2]:

1860	1861	1862	1863	1864
19	57	63	98	274

This epidemic was more easily dealt with than those of the same kind before it. Very large sums were subscribed by the wealthy, of which, indeed, a considerable balance remained undistributed. Rawlinson, as engineer, and Villiers, as Minister, devised extensive relief works, in the form of main drainage for the distressed Lancashire towns, the whole cost being defrayed eventually by the municipalities themselves. The following table, from Murchison, shows the admissions for typhus to the fever hospitals of various towns, subsequently to the great epidemic of 1847–48. The first rise in London was in 1856; the next rise, which was somewhat prolonged, coincided with the epidemic in Lancashire.

---

[1] Buchanan, *Report Med. Officer Privy Council, for* 1864, and *Trans. Epid. Soc.* 1865, II. 17; Hamilton, *Lancet*, II. 1867, p. 608 (Liverpool); Martyn, *Brit. Med. Journ.* July, 1863; Davies, *Med. Times and Gaz.* II. 1867, p. 427 (Bristol); Thompson, *St George's Hosp. Reports*, I. (1866), p. 47 (London); Allbutt, *ibid.* p. 61 (Leeds).

[2] Buchanan, *Report Med. Off. Privy Council for* 1865, p. 210.

Hospital Cases of Typhus, 1849—71.

Year	London Fever Hosp.	Edin. Royal Infirm.	Glasgow Royal Infirm.	Glasgow Fever Hosp.	Dundee Royal Infirm.	Aberdeen Royal Infirm.	Cork Fever Hosp.
1849	155	—	342	—	—	—	—
1850	130	—	382	—	—	—	—
1851	68	—	919	—	—	—	—
1852	204	—	1293	—	—	—	—
1853	408	—	1551	—	—	—	—
1854	337	—	760	—	—	—	—
1855	342	—	385	—	—	—	—
1856	1062	—	385	—	—	—	—
1857	274	—	314	—	—	—	—
1858	15	—	175	—	17	—	—
1859	48	—	175	—	128	—	—
1860	25	—	229	—	67	—	—
1861	86	—	509	—	129	—	116
1862	1827	14	780	—	54	—	272
1863	1309	74	1286	—	236	379 (4 mos.)	692
1864	2493	212	2150	—	264	811	1021
1865	1950	447	2334	1154	891	422	791
1866	1760	847	1055	384	706	167	247
1867	1396	303	761	795	225	68	124
1868	1964	280	620	1023	502	78	245
1869	1259	259	1430	2023	402	170	136
1870	631	287	947	702	232	61	165
1871	411	101	418	511	257	3	397

During the unusual prevalence of fever in Scotland, 1863–65, it was made clear by the diagnosis in hospitals, that the excess was caused by typhus, and not by enteric.

Of 440 cases of fever treated in the Royal Infirmary of Edinburgh, in 1864, 212 were cases of pure typhus, 140 were enteric fevers, while 88 were simple continued fever and febricula. In the Royal Infirmary of Glasgow in 1864, of 2,190 cases of fever, 2,150 were reported to be cases of typhus fever, while only 40 were cases of enteric fever. In the Aberdeen Royal Infirmary not a case of enteric fever was observed: of 396 cases in the year 1863, 387 were pure typhus, and 9 febricula; and in 1864, of 926 cases, 897 were pure typhus and 29 febricula. In the Royal Infirmary of Dundee, of 355 cases of fever treated in 1864, 318 were typhus, 16 enteric fever, and 21 febricula. It was only at Perth, and there not exclusively in hospital practice, that an excess of typhoid fever was observed; from 1st August, 1863, to 30th April, 1864 (months which included the special typhoid season), there were 101 cases of gastro-enteric or typhoid fever, 46 cases of typhus, 19 of relapsing fever, and 59 of simple continued fever[1].

The last considerable prevalence of contagious fever in England and Scotland was in 1869 and 1870. It was relapsing fever, mixed with some typhus, and it was restricted almost to

---

[1] James Stark, M.D., "Remarks on the Epidemic Fever of Scotland during 1863–64–65" etc., *Trans. Epidem. Soc.* N. S. II. 312. See also Russell, *Glasg. Med. Journ.* July, 1864, and R. Beveridge (for Aberdeen), *Lancet*, I. 1868, p. 630.

a few large towns, including London, Liverpool, Manchester, Leeds, Bradford, Glasgow, and Edinburgh[1]. It was first seen in London in 1868 among Polish Jews. It was heard of as late as 1872 at Newcastle. It was observed during this epidemic in Liverpool, Bradford and Edinburgh that the subjects of the relapsing fever were not suffering from want[2]. The same observation has been made in some foreign countries. Still, on the great scale and in a broad view, relapsing fever has been *typhus famelicus* or famine-fever, occurring in association with other maladies due to want, and especially in the circumstances which have been discussed fully in the chapter on fevers in Ireland.

Relative prevalence of Typhus and Enteric Fevers since 1869.

It was not until the year 1869, or about the time when typhus fever ceased to be epidemic or common, that the deaths from typhus fever, simple continued fever and enteric fever began to be tabulated separately in the Registrar-General's reports. The following tables show for England and Wales and for London a steady decline of the deaths from typhus and simple continued fever since the end of the epidemic period 1869–71, which was the last epidemic of typhus and relapsing fever in this country hitherto. The deaths from enteric fever, it will be seen, remained somewhat steady (in a growing population) for about ten years after the separation, and then began to decline.

---

[1] Weber, *Lancet*, I. 1869, pp. 221, 255; Murchison, *ibid*. II. 1869, pp. 503, 647; Gee (Liverpool), *Brit. Med. Journ*. II. 1870, p. 246; Robinson (Leeds), *Lancet*, I. 1871, p. 644; Muirhead (Edinburgh), *Edin. Med. Journ*. July, 1870, p. 1; Rabagliati (Bradford), *ibid*. Dec. 1873; Tennant (Glasgow), *Glasgow Med. Journ*. May, 1871, p. 354; Armstrong (Newcastle), *Lancet*, I. 1873, p. 48.

[2] Muirhead (l. c.) says: "In no single instance which came under my observation could starvation be said to be the immediate cause of the disease. Not one of those individuals could be said to be emaciated....On strict and repeated inquiry, not one of them would confess to having been in destitute circumstances." During the winter of 1870–71 I attended from the Edinburgh New Dispensary several relapsing-fever patients at their homes, and can clearly remember having been surprised at the condition of decency and comfort in which I found them. The appearance of comfort was certainly due in part to the district visitors, who were numerous and active during the epidemic.

Continued-fever Deaths in England and Wales, 1869–91

Year	Typhus	Simple or Ill-defined	Enteric
1869	4281	5310	8659
1870	3297	5254	8731
1871	2754	4248	8461
1872	1864	3352	8741
1873	1638	3081	8793
1874	1762	3089	8861
1875	1499	2599	8913
1876	1192	1974	7550
1877	1104	1923	6879
1878	906	1776	7652
1879	533	1472	5860
1880	530	1490	6710
1881	552	1159	5529
1882	940	1016	6036
1883	877	963	6068
1884	328	768	6380
1885	318	662	4765
1886	245	505	5061
1887	211	502	5165
1888	168	436	4848
1889	140	413	4971
1890	160	361	6146
1891	148	325	5075

Continued-fever Deaths in London, 1869–91.

Year	Typhus	Simple or Ill-defined	Enteric
1869	716	615	1069
1870	472	570	976
1871	384	436	871
1872	174	322	867
1873	277	325	968
1874	312	337	879
1875	128	272	817
1876	159	202	769
1877	157	194	901
1878	151	197	1033
1879	71	160	849
1880	74	134	702
1881	92	134	971
1882	53	95	975
1883	55	102	963
1884	32	75	925
1885	28	78	597
1886	13	73	618
1887	19	44	612
1888	9	35	694
1889	16	42	538
1890	10	35	604
1891	11	44	557

Such being the proportions of typhus and enteric fever since 1869, when the separation was made, it remains to ask what share each of them may have had in the total of "typhus," or of continued fever generally, in the years before the two forms were distinguished in the annual registration reports. Of course, they were distinguished by many of the profession long before that; so that there are means of forming a judgment. At the London Fever Hospital, enteric fever and typhus were distinguished after 1849. If the admissions of each kind of fever to that hospital be assumed to have been proportionate to the prevalence of each in London from year to year, we should get in the following table a means of estimating which of the two forms of continued fever furnished most of the deaths in all London, as given in the first column :

Year	Deaths in London from both fevers	Admissions to London Fever Hospital	
		Typhus	Typhoid
1838	4078	—	—
1839	1819	—	—
1840	1262	—	—
1841	1151	—	—
1842	1184	—	—
1843	2094	—	—
1844	1721	—	—
1845	1324	—	—
1846	1838	—	—
1847	3297	—	—
1848	3685	—	—
1849	2564	155	138
1850	2032	130	137
1851	2374	68	234
1852	2183	204	140
1853	2617	408	212
1854	2816	337	228
1855	2410	342	217
1856	2717	1062	149
1857	2195	274	214
1858	1919	15	180
1859	1840	48	176
1860	1476	25	95
1861	1848	86	161
1862	3673	1827	220
1863	2871	1309	174
1864	3782	2493	253
1865	3217	1950	523
1866	2688	1760	582
1867	2184	1396	380
1868	2468	1964	459

From this it will appear that every great annual rise in the London deaths from "fever," since the last great typhus epidemic of 1847–48, has corresponded to a greatly increased admission, not of enteric cases, but of typhus cases into the London Fever Hospital. On the other hand, enteric fever has been at a somewhat steady or endemic level for a good many years. Even at that level it would have had a small share of the whole fever-mortality in the old London; in modern London, especially in its residential quarters, its rate has probably been higher than in former times; while in recent years, owing to the absolute decline of typhus, it has been by far the most common continued fever. If the conditions were the same in London as in Edinburgh, it was the very creation of residential streets and new quarters of the town that called forth typhoid fever; while the more the town was remodelled, the more were the *fomites* of typhus destroyed. Thus it seems probable that the same progress in well-being among all classes, which has gradually brought typhus down almost to extinction (or apparently so for the present), has been attended with an increase of typhoid, an increase which has happily fallen within the last few years from its highest point.

The disappearance, during the last twenty years, of typhus and relapsing fevers from the observation of all but a few medical practitioners in England, Scotland and Ireland, is one of the most certain and most striking facts in our epidemiology. Most of the recent English cases have occurred in Lancashire, especially in Liverpool, and in Sunderland, Gateshead, Newcastle and other shipping places of the north. In the decennial period 1871–80 the death-rate from typhus, per 1000 living, was 0·58 in Liverpool and 0·33 in Sunderland, rates which were about the same as those from enteric fevers. The rates in 1881–83 were also high in the same group of towns. As to other industrial centres, including the coal-districts of Cumberland, Wales and Scotland, it is probable that a good deal of typhus passes under the name of "typhoid," the change in medical fashion having outrun somewhat the real change in the relative prevalence of each fever[1]. In Scotland the disease is still heard of from time to time in Glasgow, Edinburgh, Leith, Dundee, Aberdeen, Inverness and Thurso. In London the recent immunity from it is remarkable, but intelligible. First, the populace is better housed: we have got rid of the window-tax,

[1] Spear, "Typhus Fever in various parts of England, 1886-87." *Rep. Med. Off. Loc. Gov. Bd.* N. S. XVI. p. 169.

rebuilt the houses in regular streets opening upon wide thoroughfares, pulled down most of the back-to-back houses, dispersed the working population over square miles of suburbs easily accessible from the heart of the town by tramways and railways, perfected the sewerage and the water-supply. These great structural changes are so far an earnest that typhus cannot come back in the old way. Secondly, food has been for a long time cheap and wages good. During the remarkable lull in typhus from 1803 to 1816, Bateman pointed out that the unwholesome state of the dwellings of the working class remained the same as before, but that money was flowing freely among all classes (thanks to the special war-expenditure). Under free trade, the same abundance of the necessaries of life has been secured in another way. Typhus, it need hardly be said, is an indigenous or autochthonous infection ; the conditions of its engendering are never very far off. In a small and remote island off the coast of Skye, which I happened to know in its pleasing aspects from having landed upon it during a summer vacation, typhus fever was reported by the newspapers a few months after to have broken out in the hamlet of twenty or thirty families, the winter storms having prevented the fishers from leaving their cottages or any stranger from approaching the island. In a sparsely populated parish of the east coast of Scotland, two cases of genuine typhus (one of them fatal), and two only, have occurred, to medical knowledge, within the last ten years, each in a very poor cottage in a different part of the parish and in a different season. So long as our cheap supplies of food, fuel and clothing are uninterrupted, there is small chance of typhus or relapsing fever. But the population of England being now twice as great as the home-grown corn can feed, a return of those fevers on the great scale is not out of the question in the event of the foreign food-supply being interfered with, or the necessaries of life becoming permanently dearer from any other cause.

The following Table of the fever-deaths in Scotland since the beginning of Registration does not distinguish enteric from typhus, relapsing and simple continued during the first ten years of the period ; but it is probable, from all that is known non-statistically or by hospital figures only, as to the history of enteric fever in Scotland, that it made the smaller part of the generic total of fever-deaths so long as typhus and relapsing fevers were common.

*Scotland—Deaths from the Continued Fevers since the
beginning of Registration.*

Year		
1855	2419	
1856	2363	
1857	3087	
1858	2790	
1859	2436	Inclusive of typhus, relapsing, enteric
1860	2344	and other continued fevers.
1861	2579	
1862	3021	
1863	3441	
1864	4804 [1]	

	Typhus	Enteric	Relapsing	Simple continued	Infantile Remittent	Cerebro-Spinal
1865	3272	1048	62	839	164	—
1866	2172	1404	34	249	159	—
1867	1745	1378	40	105	119	—
1868	1561	1404	45	100	132	—
1869	2059	1335	29	121	157	—
1870	1460	1207	205	151	141	—
1871	1129	1234	411	108	124	—
1872	795	1223	115	103	118	—
1873	628	1495	31	192	117	—
1874	726	1455	27	104	80	—
1875	615	1625	17	98	85	—
1876	471	1448	18	65	88	—
1877	265	1427	5	164	—	—
1878	263	1477	2	147	—	—
1879	210	1013	5	133	—	—
1880	170	1338	4	155	—	—
1881	229	1004	0	115	—	—
1882	180	1204	2	90	—	—
1883	152	998	1	71	—	7
1884	138	1050	2	63	—	9
1885	111	889	1	58	—	8
1886	80	755	2	62	—	10
1887	126	835	7	65	—	4
1888	102	665	6	58	—	6
1889	69	795	1	45	—	2
1890	77	777	—	30	—	3
1891	107	799	4	23	—	6

Circumstances of Enteric Fever.

The circumstances of typhus and relapsing fevers need no
general stating after what has been said of particular epidemics
in England and Scotland, or remains to be said, for the most
distinctive instances of all, in the chapter on fevers in Ireland.
There has been so little typhus in the country at large since the

[1] 2303 of these fever deaths in 1864 occurred in the eight principal towns of
Scotland, classified as follows : typhus, 1450, relapsing fever, 371, gastric, enteric, or
typhoid, 382.

disease began to be registered apart in the mortality returns, in 1869, that hardly anything can be inferred except the fact of its disappearance. It is significant, however, that Sunderland, one of the two great towns which have kept typhus longest and in largest measure (Liverpool being the other) is distinguished for the overcrowding of its dwelling-houses (7·24 persons to a house in the Census of 1881, 7·00 in the Census of 1891).

But the circumstances of enteric fever are not only not so obvious as those of typhus in the historical way; they are also more complex and disputable. One fact in the natura history of enteric fever has been made clear in the chronology, namely, its greater frequency after a severe drought. It was in the autumn of 1826, after the driest and hottest summer of the century, that cases of fever with ulceration of the bowel were first described and figured in London. It was in the autumn of 1846, after the next very dry and hot summer, that cases of the same fever again became unusually common in many parts of England and Scotland. The same sequence has been remarked on more recent occasions and in various countries. It is explained by taking into account some other facts in the natural history of enteric fever. In nearly all countries in our latitudes, autumn is its principal season, and autumn is the season when the level of the water in the soil, or in the wells, is lowest. Virchow states the law of enteric fever in the following simple and concrete way: "We [in Berlin] have a certain number of cases of typhoid at all times. The number increases when the sub-soil water falls, and decreases when it rises. Every year, at the time of the lowest level of the sub-soil water, we have a small epidemic." A sharp rise above the mean level of the year, from the first week of September to the end of October, has been well shown for London from the admissions to the hospitals of the Metropolitan Asylums Board, 1875–1884. The curve has an equally sharp descent, passing below the mean line of the year in the second week of December[1]. There are indications that it is the partial filling of the pores of the sub-soil with water, after they have long been occupied with air only, that makes the virus of typhoid active, or, in other

---

[1] G. B. Longstaff, M.D., *Trans. Epid. Soc.* 1884–5, p. 72, reprinted in his *Studies in Statistics*, Lond. 1891, p. 402. The seasonal curve for the typhoid admissions to the London Fever Hospital over a longer period is nearly the same, as well as that of the registered deaths by typhoid in all London, 1869–84.

words, that the rains of late summer and autumn are the occasion of the seasonal increase of the infection.

Yet it is not the changes in the ground-water by themselves, just as it is not rainfall and temperature by themselves, that make enteric fever to prevail. The soil in which those vicissitudes of drought and saturation are potent for evil must be one that is befouled with animal organic matters, more especially with excremental matters. For that and other reasons (such as the geological formation), enteric fever shows, in its more steady or endemic prevalence from year to year or from decade to decade, certain marked preferences of locality. Since 1869, when the deaths from it began to be registered apart, it has been much more common, per head of the population, in the quick-growing manufacturing and mining towns than in any other parts of England and Wales, the districts with highest enteric death-rates being the mining region of the East Coast from the mouth of the Tees to somewhat north of the Tyne, the mining region of Glamorgan, certain manufacturing towns of Lancashire and the West Riding of Yorkshire, and some districts in the valley of the Trent in Staffordshire and Nottinghamshire. The following Table shows, by comparison with all England and Wales and with London, the excessive death-rates from enteric fever in the registration divisions which head the list:

Highest mortalities from Enteric Fever in Registration Divisions of England and Wales[1].

	Decennium 1871—80			Decennium 1881—90
	Annual death-rate, all causes per 1000 living	Annual death-rate, Enteric, per 1000 living	Enteric Deaths in 10 years	Deaths, Enteric, in 10 years
England and Wales	21·27	0·32	78421	53509
London	22·37	0·24	8536	7497
Durham co.	23·77	0·56	4525	2590
South Wales	21·09	0·45	3715	2550
W. Riding, Yorks.	23·24	0·45	9166	5170
N. Riding, Yorks.	19·68	0·44	1259	896
Nottinghamshire	21·23	0·43	1707	1263
Lancashire	25·17	0·39	12388	9874

[1] The following large registration districts besides those in the Table, had enteric-fever death rates of ·5 and upwards per 1000 persons living, in the ten years 1871–80; in nearly all of them there has been a marked decline in the ten years 1881–90:—

Durham Mining Districts.

Stockton incl. part of Middlesborough (4¾ years)	26·64	1·09	561	—
Stockton (5¼ years)	22·49	0·62	208 (5¼ years)	258
Guisborough, incl. part of Middlesborough (4¾ years)	24·80	1·17	251	—
Guisborough (5¼ years)	20·45	0·38	71	106
Middlesborough[1] (5¼ years)	19·93	0·63	272 (5¼ years)	460
Auckland	24·52	0·71	541	318

South Wales Mining Districts.

Pontypridd[2]	23·16	0·71	515	541
Merthyr Tydvil	24·23	0·62	639	249
Swansea	22·38	0·63	505	387
Llanelly	20·93	0·83	330	165

In the second decennium of the Table, 1881–90, the total deaths from enteric fever (the death-rates are still unpublished) are much below those of 1871–80. All the counties of England and Wales have shared in that notable decline, including Durham and Glamorgan. But these two great districts of the coal and iron mining are, by the latest returns, still keeping the lead; and it is probable that we shall find in them, or in particular towns within them, the conditions that have been most favourable to enteric fever in the earlier decennia of this century and are still favourable to it. First it is to be observed that one of the most noted of the old typhoid centres in Glamorgan, namely Merthyr Tydvil, has ceased to be in that class; its enormous rate of growth has been checked (to 18·9 per cent. from 1881 to 1891) and it has at the same time become a more uniform and better-ordered municipality.

Durham, Hartlepool, Easington, Houghton-le-Spring, Darlington, Gateshead (county Durham); Morpeth (Northumberland); Aysgarth, Todmorden, Dewsbury, Pontefract, Barnsley, Rotherham (Yorkshire); Dudley, Leigh, Ormskirk (Lancashire); Crickhowell (Wales); Worksop, Radford (Nottingham); Shrewsbury; Peterborough; Portsea Island (Hants). Of the London districts, Hackney had the highest enteric fever, 0·46 per 1000 in a general death-rate of 20·78. The high rate of a decennium is not unfrequently brought up by one great explosion. In many of the Lancashire, Yorkshire and Midland towns, with rates about ·4 per 1000 persons, the rate has been somewhat steady from year to year. In the decennium 1871–80, many special outbreaks, some of them in villages, were reported on by the inspectors of the Medical Department, and traced for the most part to water-supplies tainted by the percolation of excrement.

[1] The Registration District of Middlesborough was carved out of Stockton and Guisborough in 1875.

[2] Registration District containing a population of 72,707 on a mean between the census of 1871 and that of 1881. In 1891 the population was 146,812.

On the other hand, on the same river Taff, and in the tributary valley of the Rhondda, there is an immense population of miners, among whom the enteric fever death-rate will probably be found to have been higher in 1881–90 than in any other registration district. The most populous part of the district is the town of Ystradyfodwg, which had 44,046 inhabitants in 1881 and 68,720 in 1891, an increase of over fifty per cent., the highest urban rate of increase in the country. On the mean of the last three years, 1891–93, its enteric fever death-rate has been ·62 per 1000. There are several populous towns or townships in the mining districts of the north-east which have in like manner kept their high rate of typhoid mortality—Auckland, Easington, Bellington (Morpeth) and Middlesborough. It is held by many that enteric fever has been most characteristically a product of the modern system of closet-pipes and sewers. It is, of course, the defects of the system that are, in this hypothesis, to blame, including its partial adoption, the transition-state from the older system, the tardy extension to new streets, as well as cheap and faulty construction. All those things, together with the inherent difficulty of connecting with a main sewerage the irregular squattings of a mining community, are probably to be found in highest degree in those districts of Durham and South Wales that are most subject to enteric fever. While enteric fever is in some places steady or endemic from year to year, in others its force is felt mostly in great and sudden explosions.

One such happened in the city and district of Bangor in the summer of 1882. The registration district had only 95 deaths from enteric fever in the ten years 1871–80, but in the single year 1882 it had 87 deaths registered under that name. Of 548 attacks (with 42 deaths) which were known from 22 May to 12 September, 407 fell in August and the first twelve days of September[1]. In the following year and throughout the rest of the decennium the district had its usual low average of enteric-fever deaths. One thing relevant to the explosion was probably the excessive rainfall of June and July (9·5 inches, as compared with 4·8 inches about London).

Another explosion, probably unique in the history of enteric fever, took place at Worthing, on the Sussex coast, in the summer of 1893. The enteric death-rate of the town had been much below the average of England and Wales from 1871 to 1880, the rate being 0·15 per 1000 and the whole deaths in ten years 36. During the next ten years, 1881–90, the whole enteric deaths were 43 in the entire registration district (population in 1891,

---

[1] F. W. Barry, M.D., in *Rep. Med. Off. Loc. Gov. Board for* 1882, p. 72. The contention of the inspector was that the water-supply had been tainted by enteric-fever evacuations from a case which began on 22 May in a cottage some half-mile distant from the reservoir but in communication with it through ditches and brooks. The area of the water-supply did not correspond with the area of the fever.

32,394). In 1891 the typhoid deaths were two, in 1892 they were six. In 1893 a severe outbreak of typhoid took place within the municipal borough (population 16,606): In the first quarter of the year Worthing was one of the places mentioned for typhoid, having had 5 deaths; in April there were no deaths, in May 25, in June 19, in July 61, in August 64, in September 11, and in the last quarter of the year 8, making 193 deaths in the year. The highest weekly number of cases notified was 253 in the second week of July. The enormously wide dispersion of the poison, in a town little subject to enteric fever, caused suspicion to fall on the water-supply, the more reasonably that the district of West Worthing, which had a separate water-supply, was said not to have suffered from the outbreak. A new water-supply was at once undertaken. A relief fund of £7000 was raised for the sufferers.

The towns of Middlesborough, Stockton and Darlington, in the lower valley of the Tees, were together the scene of two remarkable explosions of enteric fever, the first from 7 September to 18 October, 1890, the second from 28 December, 1890, to 7 February, 1891. The phenomenal nature of these outbreaks in the autumn and winter of 1890–91 will appear from the following table of deaths by enteric fever :

	Darlington	Stockton	Middlesborough
Ten years 1881–90	104	258	460
1890	21	66	130
1891	17	59	93

In the first of the two explosions the three towns were almost equally attacked per head of their populations; in the second explosion, in mid-winter, Darlington had relatively only half as many cases as each of the other two, which had about the same number of cases as in the former six-weeks' period. In both periods, of six weeks each, the three towns had together 1334 cases of typhoid, while the country districts near them had a mere sprinkling. A flooded state of the Tees appeared to be a relevant antecedent to each of the explosions. The Tees is a broad shallow river flowing rapidly, subject to frequent inundations, tortuous in its lower course, forming at its mouth, where Middlesborough stands, a wide estuary bordered by low flat grounds. The rainfall at Middlesborough was 6·3 inches in August, of which 2·2 inches fell on the 12th of the month, the river being high in flood thereafter. There were again high floods in November, chiefly caused by the melting of snow in the upper basin (5 inches fell at Barnard Castle in November, 3·1 inches at Middlesborough, while the December fall was 1·2 inches at the former and 1·4 inches at the latter). To apply correctly the ground-water doctrine of enteric fever to these explosions, other particulars would have to be known, more especially the extent of the previous dryness of the subsoil (the rainfall at Middlesborough was 9·3 inches in the first half of 1890, 15·6 in the second half, and below average for the whole year). But the flooded state of the Tees valley in August and November must have changed abruptly the state of the ground-ferments within the areas of the respective towns and so afforded, according to the general law, the conditions for an abrupt increase of enteric fever in these its endemic or perennial soils[1].

[1] The report for the Medical Department by F. W. Barry, M.D. (*Enteric Fever in the Tees Valley*, 1890–91, Parl. papers, Nov. 1893), is an elaborate argument to prove that the flooded state of the Tees was indeed the relevant antecedent, not as indexing the rise of the ground-water in the respective towns, but as dislodging and sweeping down the slops, sewage and dry refuse of the market town of Barnard Castle, in upper Teesdale, whereby the water taken in from the Tees two miles above Darlington to the tanks, filters and reservoirs of the Darlington Corporation, and of the Stockton and Middlesborough Water Board, was tainted in some unusual degree—a hypothesis the more remarkable that the refuse, such as it was, had been suspended or dissolved in an unusual volume of water, that little refuse could have collected between the

While the more or less steady or endemic prevalence of
typhoid fever is due to the formation and reproduction in the
soil of an infective principle (probably of faecal origin) which
affects more or less sporadically the individuals living thereon,
after the manner of a miasma rising from the ground, there have
been some hardly disputable instances of the infection being
conveyed to many at once from a single source in the drinking
water and by the medium of milk[1]. But such instances, suggestive though they be and easy of apprehension by the laity, must
not be understood as giving the rule for the bulk of enteric
fever. In like manner, the escape or reflux of excremental
gases from pipes or sewers, or the leakage into basements or
foundations from faulty plumber-work, are causes, real no doubt,
but of limited application, which do not conflict with, as they do
not supersede, the more comprehensive and cognate explanation
of enteric fever as an infection having its habitat in the soil and
an incidence upon individuals after the manner of other miasmatic infections. Sex has little or nothing to do with the
incidence of the infective virus. As to age, enteric fever rarely
befalls infants, and, in the general belief of practitioners, is a less
frequent cause of death among children than among adolescents
and adults.

In the following Table from the Registrar-General's Decennial Review,
1871–80, enteric fever is not separated from other continued fevers. It is
probable that a considerable ratio of the deaths from 0 to 5 years are due to
febrile disorders other than enteric.

*Annual Mortality per million living at all ages and at eleven groups of
ages, males and females, from fever (including Typhus, Enteric Fever
and Different Forms of Continued Fever) 1871–80.*

	All ages	0—	5—	10—	15—	20—	25—	35—	45—	55—	65—	75+
Both sexes	484	651	518	439	543	509	411	379	402	458	553	498
Males	494	644	483	390	513	579	436	395	437	503	629	593
Females	477	658	550	487	573	445	387	362	369	418	488	425

first floods and the second, and that no cases of enteric fever were known in the upper
valley of the Tees. This judicial deliverance has not been accepted by the authorities
of Darlington, Stockton and Middlesborough, nor by the Royal Commission on Water
Supply, before whom it was laid.

[1] Besides the epidemic at Worthing in 1893, which is still *sub judice*, the best
known instance of typhoid following a certain water-supply is the explosion at
Redhill and Caterham in Jan.—Feb. 1879, *Rep. Med. Off. Loc. Gov. Board, for* 1879,
Parl. papers, 1880, p. 78. The first instance alleged of the distribution by milk was
the Islington explosion in July—August 1870 (Ballard, *Med. Times and Gaz.* 1870,
II. 611). It was soon followed by the Marylebone explosion in the summer of 1873
(*Rep. Med. Off. L. G. B.*, N.S. II. 193); but such instances have become less common,
while instances of scarlatina and diphtheria following a milk-supply have become
more common.

The cases notified under the Act in 1891 and 1892 have been found to average five or six for every death registered in the corresponding districts, the rate of fatality ranging widely. It is matter of familiar knowledge that many of the attacks and fatalities occur among the richer classes. New comers to an endemic seat of the disease are most apt to take it (this has been elaborately shown for Munich, and holds good for the British troops in India). There are undoubtedly constitutional proclivities to it among individuals, which may run strongly in families. As in other miasmatic infective diseases, such as yellow fever, Asiatic cholera, and (formerly) plague, there seem to be occasions in the varying states of body and mind, as well as in the external circumstances, when the infection of enteric fever is specially apt to find a lodgement and to become effective. The old plague-books gave lists of the things that were apt to invite venom or to stir venom (see former volume pp. 212, 674); and it is probable that some of these hold good also for the incidence of enteric fever.

CHAPTER II.

FEVER AND DYSENTERY IN IRELAND.

THE history of the public health in Ireland has been so remarkable that it may be useful to take a continuous view of it in a chapter apart, so far as concerns flux, or dysentery, and typhus with relapsing fever.

Ireland is a country which would have given Hume, had he thought of it, the best of all his illustrations of the difficult problem handled in the essay "Of National Characters"—how far the habits, customs, temperaments and, he might have added, morbid infections have been determined by climate, and how far by laws and government, by revolutions in public affairs, or by the situation of the nation with regard to its neighbours. Not only is there something special and peculiar in the actual epidemiology of Ireland, but its political and social history has been apt to borrow the phrases of medicine in a figure. "First the physicians are to take care," says Burke, "that they do nothing to irritate this epidemical distemper. It is a foolish thing to have the better of the patient in a dispute. The complaint, or its cause, ought to be removed, and wise and lenient arts ought to precede the measures of vigour[1]." And this singular use of the imagery of disease in Irish history might be illustrated from many other passages of the same orator and essayist, just as it may be seen any day in the columns of newspapers in our own time. Giraldus Cambrensis began it, within a few years of the first English conquest of Irish territory by Henry II. Writing of that singular effect upon the English settlers by contact with the native Irish, whereby they

[1] *Second Letter to Sir Hercules Langrishe*, May, 1795.

became, in the words of another medieval author, *ipsis Hibernis hiberniores*, he resorts to the medical figure of "contagion" as the best way to account for it. So again, to overleap six centuries, Bishop Berkeley in his query "whether idleness be the mother or daughter of spleen[1]," is trying upon the Irish both Hume's problem of national character and the use of the medical figure. And, to take a modern instance, Lord Beaconsfield used the same figure of the old humoral pathology, and gave his adhesion to a theory of national characters adverse to the sense of Hume, when he ascribed the habits and manners of the Irish, and the course of their national history, to their propinquity to a "melancholy" ocean.

As far back as we can go in the history, two diseases are conspicuous—the flux or "the country disease," and the sharp fever or "Irish ague." When Henry II. invaded Ireland in 1172, his army suffered from flux, which the contemporary chronicler, Radulphus de Diceto, dean of St Paul's, set down to the unwonted eating of fresh meat (*recentium esus carnium*), the drinking of water, and the want of bread[2]. Less than a generation after, Giraldus of Wales wrote his "Topography of Ireland," wherein he remarks that hardly any stranger, on his first coming to the country, escapes the flux by reason of the juicy food (*ob humida nutrimenta*)[3]. At that time Ireland was almost wholly a pastoral country, and a pastoral country it has remained to a far greater extent than England or Scotland. It is to this comparative want of tillage, an almost absolute want when Giraldus was there, that we shall probably have to look in the last resort for an explanation of the two national maladies that here concern us—the "country disease" and the "Irish ague." The same dietetic reason that the dean of St Paul's gave in 1172 for the prevalence of flux in the army of Henry II., the want of bread and the eating of fresh meat, can be assigned for the country disease long after, and, in some periods, on the explicit testimony of observers. As to the Irish ague, or typhus fever, Giraldus mentions it in the medieval period; and Higden, copying him exactly, says: "The inhabitants of Ireland are vexed by no kind of fever except the

---

[1] Berkeley's *Querist*, Q. 362.
[2] Radulphus de Diceto, *Imag. Histor.* Eng. Hist. Soc. ed. I. 350.
[3] "Topogr. Hiberniae" in *Opera*, Rolls ed. v. 67. This and the preceding reference had escaped the notice of Dr John O'Brien, in the historical introduction to his *Observations on the Acute and Chronic Dysentery of Ireland*. Dublin, 1822.

acute, and that seldom "—the word *acuta* being the original of
" the ague," or, as in another translation of the passage, " the
sharp axes[1]." In this pastoral country, according to Giraldus,
there was little sickness and little need of physicians ; but there
is hardly an instance of military operations by the English
unattended with sickness among the troops, and famine with
sickness among the native Irish.

The generalities of Fynes Moryson, a traveller of the time
of James I., who included Ireland among the many countries
that he visited and described, throw light upon the dietetic
peculiarities of the Irish. Having little agriculture, and at
that time no general cultivation of the potato (although they
adopted it much sooner than the English and Scots), they
lived, says Moryson, mostly on milk (as Giraldus Cambrensis
also records in the twelfth century), and upon the flesh of
unfed calves, which they cooked and ate in a barbarous fashion.
" The country disease " is also noted. The experience in Ireland
from time immemorial, that a bellyful was a windfall, must have
been the origin of a habit observed by Moryson :

> " I have known some of these Irish footemen serving in England to lay
> meate aside for many meales to devoure it all at one time." And again :
> " The wilde Irish in time of greatest peace impute covetousnesse and base
> birth to him that hath any corne after Christmas, as if it were a point of
> nobility to consume all within these festivall dayes." The Irish slovenliness
> or filthiness in their food, raiment and lodging was apt, he says, " to infect"
> the English who came to reside in their country[2].

About a generation after we come to the earliest medical
account of the sicknesses of Ireland, by Gerard Boate, compiled
during the Cromwellian occupation[3]. The following occurs
under the head of The Looseness :

---

[1] *Polychronicon*, Rolls ed. I. 332–3.
[2] " Many of the English-Irish have by little and little been infected with the Irish
filthinesse, and that in the very cities, excepting Dublin and some of the better sort in
Waterford, where the English continually lodging in their houses, they more retain
the English diet." And again : " In like sort the degenerated citizens are somewhat
infected with the Irish filthinesse, as well in lowsie beds, foule sheetes, and all linnen,
as in many other particulars...Touching the meere or wild Irish, it may truely be said
of them, which was of old spoken of the Germans, namely, that they wander slovenly
and naked, and lodge in the same house (if it may be called a house) with their
beasts." Fynes Moryson, *Itinerary*, Pt. IV. p. 180.
[3] *Ireland's Natural History*, *&c*. Written by Gerard Boate, late Doctor of
Physick to the State in Ireland. And now published by Samuel Hartlib, Esquire.
Lond. 1652. The author died at Dublin, shortly after his arrival there, on $\frac{9}{19}$ January

$16\frac{50}{49}$. His information would seem to have come in part from his brother Arnold
Boate, resident in Ireland.

The English have given it the name of the Country Disease. The subjects of it are often troubled a great while, but take no great harm. It is easily cured by good medicines : " But they that let the looseness take its course do commonly after some days get the bleeding with it ;......and last it useth to turn to the bloody flux, the which in some persons having lasted a great while, leaveth them of itself; but in far the greatest number is very dangerous, and killeth the most part of the sick, except they be carefully assisted with good remedies."

The other reigning disease is the " Irish Ague," a continued fever of the nature of typhus :

"As Ireland is subject to most diseases in common with other countries, so there are some whereunto it is peculiarly obnoxious, being at all times so rife there that they may justly be reputed for Ireland *endemii morbi*, or reigning diseases, as indeed they are generally reputed for such. Of this number is a certain sort of malignant feavers, vulgarly in Ireland called Irish agues, because that at all times they are so common in Ireland, as well among the inhabitants and the natives, as among those who are newly come thither from other countries. This feaver, commonly accompanied with a great pain in the head and in all the bones, great weakness, drought, loss of all manner of appetite, and want of sleep, and for the most part idleness or raving, and restlessness or tossings, but no very great nor constant heat, is hard to be cured." If blood-letting be avoided and cordial remedies given, "very few persons do lose their lives, except when some extraordinary and pestilent malignity cometh to it, as it befalleth in some years." Those who recover "are forced to keep their beds a long time in extreme weakness, being a great while before they can recover their perfect health and strength."

The occasion of Boate's writing was the subjugation of Ireland by Cromwell, in the course of which we hear from time to time of sickness. The greatest of the calamities was the utter destruction of the prosperity of Galway by the frightful plague of 1649–50, and by the suppression of the Catholics, who had brought the port of Connaught to be a place of foreign commerce[1].

Cromwell's troops in 1649 incurred dysentery through the hardships of campaigning. On 17 September, 1649, the Lord General writes from Dublin to Mr Speaker Lenthall after the storming of Tredah or Drogheda : " We keep the field much ; our tents sheltering us from the wet and cold. But yet the country-sickness overtakes many : and therefore we desire recruits, and some fresh regiments of foot, may be sent us." And on 25 October, " Colonel Horton is dead of the country-disease[2]."

[1] Hardiman, *History of Galway*, p. 126 *seq.* The plague from July 1649 to Lady Day 1650 is said to have swept away 3700 of the inhabitants, including 210 of the most respectable burgesses and freemen, with their families. The capitulation on 5 April, 1652, was followed by famine throughout the country, and by a revival of plague for two years, "during which upwards of one-third of the population of the province was swept away."

[2] *Cromwell's Letters and Speeches*, II. 55, 77.

Another general reference to the "country disease" of Ireland, by Borlase, is very nearly the same as Boate's. It is introduced early in the history, on the occasion of the death in 1591 of Walter, Earl of Essex, earl marshal of Ireland :

"The dysentery, or flux, so fatal to this worthy person, is commonly termed the country disease; and well it may, for it reigns nowhere so epidemically as in Ireland; tainting strangers as well as natives. But whether it proceeds from the peculiar disposition of the air, errour in diet, the laxity and waterishness of the meat, or some occult cause, no venomous creature living there to suck that which may be thought (in other countries) well distributed amongst reptilious animals, I shall not determine, though each of these circumstances may well conduce to its strength and vigour. Certain it is that regular diet preserves most from the violence, and many from the infection of this disease; yet as that which is thought very soveraign—I must say that the stronger cordial liquors (viz. brandy, usquebeh, treacle and Mithridate waters) are very proper, or the electuaries themselves, and the like[1]."

From the Restoration to the Revolution little is known of epidemics in Ireland. It is probable that Dublin and the other considerable towns fared much the same as English towns. A Dublin physician writing to Robert Boyle on 27 February, 1682, speaks of a petechial fever, marked by leaping of the tendons, which had been fatal to very many in that city for these twelve or fourteen months[2]. With the Revolution the troubles of the country begin again, and enter on their peculiarly modern phase. For our history, two characteristic incidents come at the very beginning of the new period of disorder among the Irish— the sicknesses of the siege of Londonderry and the unparalleled havoc of disease among the troops of Schomberg in the camp of Dundalk. In both, the old "country disease," which had affected Cromwell's troops, was the primary malady, occurring, of course, in circumstances special enough to have bred it anywhere; in both, the dysentery was attended or followed by typhus fever, the old "Irish ague;" and although the epidemics of Londonderry and Dundalk in 1689 are properly examples of war sickness, yet the circumstances of each may help to realize the connexion between dysentery and typhus in the ordinary history of the Irish.

[1] Edmund Borlase, *History of the Reduction of Ireland to the Crown of England.* 1675, p. 172.
[2] Boyle's *Works*, fol. Lond. 1744, V. 92.

Dysentery and Fever at Londonderry and Dundalk, 1689.

The siege of Londonderry[1] by the Catholic Irish army of James II. began in April and ended on 28 July, having lasted 105 days. On 19 April the garrison numbered 7020 men, and the total of men, women and children in the town was estimated at 30,000, a number which included refugees from the neighbouring country and would have been more but for many Protestants at the beginning of the siege leaving the city and taking "protection" at the hands of the besiegers. On 21 May, a collection was made for the poor, who began to be in want. Sickness is heard of on 5 June, when several that were sick were killed in their beds by the enemy's bombs. The dread of the bombs in the houses caused the people to lie about the walls or in places remote from the houses all night, so that many of them, especially the women and children, caught cold, which along with the want of rest and failing food, threw them into fluxes and fevers. The pinch of hunger began to be felt before the middle of June, about which time and for six weeks after the fluxes and fevers were rife. A great mortality spread through the garrison as well as the inhabitants ; fifteen captains and lieutenants died in one day, and it was estimated that ten thousand died during the siege, "besides those who died soon after." The want, the dysentery, the fever and the vast numbers of dead every day must have produced a horrible state of things; when, on 2 July, five hundred useless persons were put outside the walls, to disperse as they best could, the besiegers are said to have recognized them when they met them " by the smell."

---

[1] The war-pestilence at Londonderry in 1689 is the third recorded epidemic of the kind there, not including what may have happened in the capture of the town by the Catholics in O'Neill's rebellion, when Derry was destroyed, to be rebuilt in 1613 by the London Companies with a new charter under the name of Londonderry. The first historical occasion of sickness was in 1566. The troops of Elizabeth were landed on Loch Foyle in October and built their huts on the site of the old monastery. In the course of the winter the greater part of a force of 1100 men perished by dysentery and the infection which it breeds (see former volume, p. 372). On 12 Dec. 1642, a year after the outbreak of the Rebellion of Confederate Catholics, a petition of the agents of the distressed city of Londonderry to the Commons represented that there were 6059 persons in the city, whereof 5123 were women and children, or sick, aged or impotent ; only 2000 were inhabitants of the city, the rest having fled there for safety. Spotted fever had broken out. (*Hist. MSS. Comis.* v. "MSS. of the House of Lords.")

About the middle of June large quantities of provisions were found in cellars and places of concealment under ground; after that the garrison had always bread, although the allowance was small. An ingenious man discovered how to make pancakes of starch and tallow, of which articles there was no lack; the pancakes not only proved nutritious, but are said to have been an infallible cure of the flux, or preservative from it. At length, on 28 July some of the victuallers and ships of war which had been in Lough Foyle since the 15th of June, sailed up to the head of the Lough on the evening flood tide, finding little resistance from the enemy's batteries and none from "what was left of" the tide-tossed boom of logs across the mouth of the river. Provisions poured in, and the siege was raised; but it is clear that the infection continued for some time after, having been found among such of the released garrison as repaired to Schomberg's camp at Dundalk.

The Catholic army is said (by the Protestants) to have lost 8000 or 9000 before the walls of Londonderry, "most by the sword, the rest of fever and flux, and the French pox, which was very remarkable on the bodies of several of the dead officers and soldiers[1]."

Not far off, at Dundalk, there began, a few weeks after, an extraordinary outbreak of war-sickness, which, unlike the pestilence in Londonderry, was altogether inglorious in its circumstances. In many respects it resembled the disaster to Cromwell's troops at the first occupying of Jamaica in 1655–56[2]; but it was worse than that, and it is probably unexampled in the military annals of Britain[3].

Supplies had been voted in Parliament for quelling the Catholic rebellion in Ireland, and an expedition was got together under the illustrious Marshal, Duke of Schomberg. The force consisted of some ten thousand foot, most of them raw levies from the English peasantry, with one regiment of seasoned

[1] With the exception of the last quoted piece of information, the most minute particulars of the siege of Londonderry are in an essay by an army chaplain, John Mackenzie, *A Narrative of the Siege of Londonderry*, London, 1690, which was written to correct and augment *A True Account of the Siege of Londonderry* by the Rev. Mr George Walker, rector of Donoghmoore in the county of Tyrone, and late Governor of Derry. London, 1689.
[2] See former volume, pp. 634–43.
[3] Minute particulars of it are given in *An Impartial History of the Wars in Ireland* [1689–1692]. By George Story, Chaplain to Sir Thomas Gower's Regiment. London, 1693. Part I.

Dutch troops ("the blue Dutch"), and cavalry. While the bulk of the force was undisciplined, their clothes, food, tents and other munitions of war were bad or insufficient through the fraud of contractors. The expedition embarked at Hoylake on the Dee and landed on the 15th of August, 1689, nearly three weeks after the relief of Londonderry, at Bangor, on the south side of Belfast Lough. Schomberg took Carrickfergus, and began to advance on Dublin; but finding the towns burned and the country turned into a desert, he threw himself into an entrenched camp around the head of Dundalk Bay, nearly a mile from the town of Dundalk. His camp was on a low moist bottom at the foot of the hills. The Irish Catholic army took up a position among the hills "on high sound ground," not more than two miles distant from the English lines, and, being in superior force, in due time they offered battle, which was declined. Schomberg, who had been joined by the Enniskillen regiments of dragoons and by men from Londonderry, had under him some 2000 horse and not less than 12,000 foot at the time when James II. offered battle. The undisciplined state of his English troops and the suspected treachery of a body of French Protestants were among the causes that held Schomberg back; but he had to reckon also with sickness almost from the moment of sitting down at Dundalk. At a muster on 25 September, several of the regiments were grown thin "by reason of the distemper then beginning to seize our men." The distemper was dysentery and fever. The two maladies were mixed up, as they usually are in war and famines, the flux commonly preceding the fever, and perhaps affording the virulent matters in the soil and in the air upon which the epidemic prevalence of the fever depends. It was easy to account for the dysentery among the troops at Dundalk; but as to the fever, there was an ambiguity at the outset which Story is careful to note: "And yet I cannot but think that the feaver was partly brought to our camp by some of those people that came from Derry; for it was observable that after some of them were come amongst us, it was presently spread over the whole army, yet I did not find many of themselves died of it." Where the cause of death is specially named, it is fever, as in the cases of Sir Thomas Gower, Colonel Wharton and other officers on the 28th and 29th October. The fever was a most malignant form of typhus, marked by the worst of all symptoms, gangrene of the extremities, so that the toes or a whole foot would fall off when the surgeon was applying a dressing[1].

It seems probable that most of the enormous mortality was caused by infection, and not by dysentery due to primary exciting causes.

The primary exciting causes were obvious, but seemingly irremovable. Schomberg had a great military reputation, but he was now over eighty, and it does not appear that he made himself personally felt in the camp, although he issued incessantly orders to inspect and report. As the mortality proceeded apace during the six or eight weeks of inactivity, murmurings arose against the commander. He was unfortunate in his choice of a camping ground, and in an unusually cold and wet season. The newly raised English troops seem to have been lacking equally in intelligence and in moral qualities. Their foul language and debauchery were the occasion of a special proclamation; their laziness and inability to make themselves comfortable called forth numerous orders, but all to no purpose. The regiment of Dutch troops were so well hutted that not above eleven of them died in the whole campaign; but the English would not be troubled to gather fern or anything else to keep themselves dry and clean withal: "many of them, when they were dead, were incredibly lousy."

The camping ground not only received the drainage of the hills, but, strange to say, the rain would be falling there all day while the camp of the enemy, only a few miles farther inland, would not be getting a drop. On 1 October the tents on the low ground were moved a little higher up. On the same date there were distributed among the regiments casks of brandy—Macaulay says it was of bad quality—which appears to have been the trusted remedy against camp sickness, as in the Jamaica expedition of 1655. There were twenty-seven victuallers or other ships riding in Dundalk Bay; but the stores were bad, and the regimental surgeons had come unprovided with drugs that might have been useful in flux or fever. While the weather continued cold and wet, there was also a scarcity of firing and forage. On 14 October all the regimental surgeons were ordered to meet at ten in the morning to consult with

[1] Gangrene of the extremities was one of the symptoms of the "plague of Athens" as described by Thucydides. There is no need to invoke ergotism for an explanation of it, as some have done.

Dr Lawrence how to check the sickness[1]. Several officers having died on the 16th and 17th, the camp was shifted on the 20th to new ground, the huts being left full of the sick. Gower's regiment had sixty-seven men unable to march, besides a good many dead before or sent away sick. Story, the chaplain, went every day from the new camp to visit the sick of his regiment in the huts, and always at his going found some dead. He found the survivors in a state of brutal callousness, utterly indifferent to each other, but objecting to part with their dead comrades as they wanted the bodies to sit or lie on, or to keep off the cold wind. The ships at anchor had now received as many sick as they could hold, and the deaths on board soon became as many as on shore. On 25–27 October, the camp was again shifted, but the sickness continued apace. At length on 3 November, the Catholic army having dispersed to winter quarters, the sick were ordered to be removed to Carlingford and Newry. " The poor men were brought down from all places towards the Bridge End, and several of them died by the way. The rest were put upon waggons, which was the most lamentable sight in the world, for all the rodes from Dundalk to Newry and Carlingford were next day full of nothing but dead men, who, even as the waggons joulted, some of them died and were thrown off as fast." Some sixteen or seventeen hundred had been left dead at Dundalk. The ships were ordered to sail for Belfast with the first wind, and the camp was broken up. There was snow on the hills and rain in the valleys ; on the march to Newry, men fell out of the ranks and died at the road side. When the ships weighed anchor from Dundalk and Carlingford, they had 1970 sick men on board, but not more than 1100 of these came ashore in Belfast Lough, the rest having died at sea in coming round the coast of County Down. Such was the violence of the infection on board that several ships had all the men in them dead and nobody to look after them whilst they lay in the bay at Carrickfergus. An infective principle, once engendered in circumstances

---

[1] At that time there was little systematic knowledge of military hygiene. Nearly two generations after, the experiences of Pringle, Donald Monro and Brocklesby in the campaigns of 1743–48 and 1758–63 in Germany and the Netherlands, yielded many valuable hints, some of which Virchow made use of in compiling his "Rules of Health for the Army in the Field," in the Franco-Prussian War of 1870–71. See his *Gesammelte Abhandlungen aus dem Gebiete der öffentlichen Medicin und Seuchenlehre.* 2 Bde. Berlin, 1879, II. 193.

of aggravation such as these, is not soon extinguished.   Belfast
was the winter quarters, and in the great hospital there from
1 November, 1689, to 1 May, 1690, there died 3762, "as appears
by the tallies given in by the men that buried them."   These
numbers together make fully six thousand deaths, which agrees
with the general statement that Schomberg lost one half of the
men whom he had embarked at Hoylake in August.   The Irish
Catholic army began to sicken in their camp in the hills above
Dundalk Bay just before they broke up, and they are said to
have lost heavily by sickness in their winter quarters.

The war ended with the Treaty of Limerick, in 1691.   The
Seven Ill Years followed,—ill years to Scotland, in a measure
to England, and almost certainly to Ireland also ; but it does
not appear that the end of the 17th century was a time of
special sickness and famine to the Irish, and it may be inferred
from the fact of Scots migrating to Ireland during the ill years
that the distress was not so sharp there.   The epidemiology of
Ireland is, indeed, a blank until we come to the writings of
Dr Rogers, of Cork, in some respects the best epidemiologist
of his time, which cover the period from 1708 to 1734.   His
account of the dysentery and typhus of the chief city of Munster
in the beginning of the 18th century will show that the old
dietetic errors of the Irish, noted in medieval times, had hardly
changed in the course of centuries.

A generation of Fevers in Cork.

Rogers is clear that typhus fever was never extinct, while
the three several times when it "made its appearance amongst us
in a very signal manner," are the same as its seasons in England,
namely 1708–10, 1718–21 and 1728–30[1].   His experience relates
only to the city of Cork, and, so far as his clinical histories go,
only to the well-to-do classes therein ; and although those
seasons were years of scarcity and distress all over Ireland, yet
Rogers does not seem to associate insufficient food with the
fever, and never mentions scarcity.   The fevers were in the
winter, for the most part, and were usually accompanied by
epidemic smallpox of a bad type, which in 1708 "swept away
multitudes."   Nothing is said of dysentery for the earliest of the

[1] Joseph Rogers, M.D. *Essay on Epidemic Diseases.* Dublin, 1734.

three fever-periods; but for 1718 and following years we read that "dysentery of a very malignant sort, frequently producing mortification in the bowels," prevailed during the same space; and that the winters of the third fever-period, namely, those of 1728, 1729 and 1730 were "infamous for bloody fluxes of the worst kind." It is clear that the fever spread to the richer classes in Cork, for his five clinical histories are all from those classes. The following is his general account of the symptoms:

The patient is suddenly seized with slight horrors or rather chilliness, to which succeed a glowing warmth, a weight and fixed pain in the head, just over the eyebrows; soreness all over his flesh, as if bruised, the limbs heavy, the heart oppressed, the breathing laboured, the pulse not much altered, but in some slower; the urine mostly crude, pale and limpid, at first, or even throughout, the tongue moist and not very white at first, afterwards drier, but rarely black. An universal petechial effloresence not unlike the measles paints the whole surface of the body, limbs, and sometimes the very face; in some few appear interspersed eruptions exactly like the *pustulae miliares*, filled with a limpid serum. The earlier these petechiae appear, the fresher in colour, and the longer they continue out, the better (p. 5). The fixed pain in the head increasing, ends commonly in a coma or stupor, or in a delirium with some. Some few have had haemorrhage at the nose, a severe cough, and sore throat. In some he had observed a great tendency to sweats, even from the beginning: these are colliquative and symptomatic, not to be encouraged. In but few there have appeared purple and livid spots, as in haemorrhagic smallpox: some as large as a vetch, others not bigger than a middling pin's head, thick set all over the breast, back and sometimes the limbs, the pulse in these cases being much below normal. The extremities cold from the 6th or 7th day, delirium constant, tongue dry and black, urine limpid and crude, oppression greater, and difficulty of breathing more. It is a slow nervous fever (p. 18).

Rogers believed that mere atmospheric changes could not be the cause of these epidemics: "they may favour, encourage and propagate such diseases when once begun; but for the productive cause of them we must have recourse to such morbid effluvia as above described [particles of all kinds detached from the animal, vegetable and mineral kingdoms]; or resolve all into the θεῖον τί so often appealed to by Hippocrates[1]."

But, as regards Cork itself, special interest attaches to the following "four concurring causes:"

"1st, the great quantities of filth, ordure and animal offals that crowd our streets, and particularly the close confined alleys and lanes, at the very season that our endemial epidemics rage amongst us.

---

[1] In further illustration of the power of morbid effluvia, he says: "We see how small a portion of a putrid animal juice, taken into the blood by inoculation, like a most active *leaven* sets all in a ferment; and in a very short time brings the whole juices of a sound body into an equal state of corruption with itself,"—instancing war-typhus, plague from cadaveric corruption (according to Paré), the Oxford gaol fever, and "a later instance at Taunton not more than five or six years ago."

2nd, the great number of slaughter-houses, both in the north and south suburbs, especially on the north ridge of hills, where are vast pits for containing the putrefying blood and ordure, which discharge by the declivities of those hills, upon great rains, their fetid contents into the river.

3rd, the unwholesome, foul, I had almost said corrupted water that great numbers of the inhabitants are necessitated to use during the dry months of the summer.

4th, the vast quantities of animal offals used by the meaner sort, during the slaughtering seasons: which occasion still more mischief by the quick andsudden transition from a diet of another kind."

In farther explanation of the fourth concurring cause, he says that in no part of the earth is a greater quantity of flesh meat consumed than in Cork by all sorts of people during the slaughtering season—one of the chief industries of the place being the export of barrelled beef for the navy and mercantile marine. The meat, he says, is plentiful and cheap, and tempts the poorer sort "to riot in this luxurious diet," the sudden change from a meagre diet, with the want of bread and of fermented liquors, being injurious to them[1].

Famine and Fevers in Ireland in 1718 and 1728.

Thus far Rogers, for the city of Cork in the three epidemic periods, 1708–10, 1718–21, and 1728–30, two of which, if not all three, were periods of dysentery as well as of typhus. But it was usual in Ireland for the country districts and small towns to suffer equally with the cities. The circumstances of the Irish peasantry in the very severe winter of 1708–9 are not particularly known ; if there was famine with famine-fever, it was not such as to have become historical. But for the next fever-period, 1718–20, we have some particulars. Bishop Nicholson, of Derry, writes: "Never did I behold even in Picardy, Westphalia or Scotland, such dismal marks of hunger and want as appeared

---

[1] Dr Rogan of Strabane, in his *Condition of the Middle and Lower Classes in the North of Ireland*, 1819, was of a different opinion (p. 90) : " No police regulations exist in Strabane to prevent the slaughtering of cattle in any part of the town. The butchers, therefore, most of whom live in the narrow streets near the shambles, have their slaughter-houses immediately behind their dwellings. The garbage is thrown into a large pit, which is generally cleaned but once in the year, at the season when the manure is required for planting potatoes, and at this time an offensive smell pervades the whole town, and is perceptible for a considerable distance around. The families exposed constantly to the effluvia arising from these heaps of putrid offal might have been expected to suffer severely from fever ; but on the contrary, they were found to be much less liable to it than others in the same rank of life. This was no doubt owing to their living chiefly on animal food, and thus escaping the debility induced by deficient nourishment, which certainly had the chief share in creating a predisposition to the disease."

in the countenances of most of the poor creatures I met with on the road." One of the bishop's carriage horses having been accidentally killed, it was at once surrounded by fifty or sixty famished cottagers struggling desperately to obtain a morsel of flesh for themselves and their children[1].

This was a time when the population was increasing, but agriculture, so far from increasing in proportion to the number of mouths to feed, was positively declining, unless it were the culture of the potato. In a pamphlet of about 1724, on promoting agriculture and employing the poor, the complaint is of beef and mutton everywhere, and an insufficiency of corn. "Such a want of policy," says one, "is there, in Dublin especially, on the most important affair of bread, without a plenty of which the poor must starve." Another, a Protestant, has the following threat for the clergymen of the Established Church: "I'll immediately stock one part of my land with bullocks, and the other with potatoes—so farewell tithes[2]!" From this it is to be inferred that potatoes were not made tithable until a later period, pasture being exempted to the last. For whatever reason, grazing, and not corn-growing, was then more general in Ireland than in the generations immediately preceding, much land having gone out of tillage. The culture of the potato was driven out of the fertile lowlands to the hill-sides, so as to leave the ground clear for ranges of pasture. Rack-renting was the rule, doubtless owing to the same reason as afterwards, the competition for farms. While the Protestants emigrated in thousands, the Catholics multiplied at home in beggary. A pamphleteer of 1727 says: "Where the plough has no work, one family can do the business of fifty, and you may send away the other forty-nine." Thus we find the pasturing of cattle preferred to agriculture long after the barbaric or uncivilized period had passed, preferred indeed by English landlords or farmers[3].

There were three bad harvests in succession, 1726, 1727 and 1728, culminating in a famine in the latter year. Boulter, archbishop of Armagh, who then ruled Ireland, was able to buy oats or oatmeal in the south and west so as to sell it below

[1] Bp. Nicholson to Archbp. of Canterbury, cited by Lecky (II. 216) from *Brit. Mus. Add. MS.* 6116.
[2] Cited by O'Rourke, *History of the Great Irish Famine of* 1847. Dublin, 1875, from pamphlet in the Halliday Collection of the Royal Irish Academy.
[3] See Boulter's *Letters to the English Ministers.*

the market price to the starving Protestants of Ulster, an interference with the distribution of food which led to serious rioting in Cork, Limerick, Clonmel and Waterford in the first months of 1728[1]. No full accounts of the epidemic fever of that famine remain. Rutty, of Dublin, says it was "mild and deceitful in its first attack, attended with a depressed pulse, and frequently with petechiae[2];" while, according to Rogers and O'Connell[3], the epidemic fever of Munster was the same. Of the famine itself we have a glimpse or two. Primate Boulter writes to the Duke of Newcastle on 7 March, 1727:

> "Last year the dearness of corn was such that thousands of families quitted their habitations to seek bread elsewhere, and many hundreds perished; this year the poor had consumed their potatoes, which is their winter subsistence, near two months sooner than ordinary, and are already, through the dearness of corn, in that want that in some places they begin already to quit their habitations[4]."

Quitting their habitations to beg was a regular thing at a later time of the year. It was in the course of these bad years, in 1729, that Swift wrote his 'Modest Proposal for preventing the Children of Poor People in Ireland from being a Burden to their Parents or Country.' The scheme to use the tender babes as delicate morsels of food for the rich, was a somewhat extreme flight of irony, not so finished as in Swift's other satires, but the circumstances out of which the proposal grew were more real than usual.

> "It is a melancholy object," says the Dean of St Patrick's, "to those who walk through this great town, or travel in the country, when they see the streets, the roads and cabin doors crowded with beggars of the female sex followed by three, four, or six children, all in rags, and importuning every passenger for an alms." Having ventilated his project for the children, he proceeds to show that "their elders are every day dying and rotting by cold and famine, filth and vermin, as fast as can be reasonably expected."

All the while there was a considerable export of corn from Ireland. In the beginning of 1730, two ships laden with barley were stopped at Drogheda by a fierce mob and were compelled to unload[5].

The interval between those years of epidemic typhus in

---

[1] Wakefield's *Ireland*, ii. 6, cited by Barker and Cheyne.
[2] John Rutty, M.D. *Chronological History of the Weather and Seasons and prevailing Diseases in Dublin during Forty Years.* London, 1770.
[3] Maurice O'Connell, M.D. *Morborum acutorum et chronicorum Observationes.* Dublin, 1746.
[4] Boulter's *Letters.* Oxford, 1769, I. 226.
[5] Lecky, ii. 217.

Ireland and the next, 1740–41, was filled, we may be sure, with at least an average amount of the endemial fever. Rutty specially mentions it in Dublin in the autumn and winter of 1734–35: "We had the low fever, called nervous (and sometimes petechial from the spots that frequently attended, although probably not essential)." He then adds: "It is no new thing with us for this low kind of fever to prevail in the winter season;" and gives figures from the Dublin Bills of Mortality for forty years. He mentions the petechial fever as being frequent next in January and February, 1736, corresponding to a bad time of it in Huxham's Plymouth annals. In 1738 and 1739 the type of the Dublin fever was relapsing, in part at least, the same type having been seen at Edinburgh shortly before.

The economics of Ireland, at this time, gave occasion to Berkeley's *Querist*, a series of weekly essays written in 1737 and 1738, and collected in 1740, on the eve of the next great famine and mortality[1]. A few of the bishop's sarcasms, in the form of queries, will serve to show how anomalous was the economic condition of the country, and how easily a crisis of famine and pestilence could arise.

"169. Whether it is possible the country should be well improved while our beef is exported, and our labourers live upon potatoes?

"173. Whether the quantities of beef, butter, wool and leather, exported from this island, can be reckoned the superfluities of a country, where there are so many natives naked and famished?

"174. Whether it would not be wise so to order our trade as to export manufactures rather than provisions, and of those such as employ most hands?

"466. Whether our exports do not consist of such necessaries as other countries cannot well be without?

"353. Whether hearty food and warm clothing would not enable and encourage the lower sort to labour?

"354. Whether in such a soil as ours, if there was industry, there would be want?

"418. Whether it be not a new spectacle under the sun, to behold in such a climate and such a soil, and under such a gentle government, so many roads untrodden, fields untilled, houses desolate, and hands unemployed?

"514. Whether the wisdom of the State should not wrestle with this hereditary disposition of our Tartars, and with a high hand introduce agriculture?

"534. Why we do not make tiles of our own, for flooring and roofing, rather than bring them from Holland?

"539. Whether it be not wonderful that with such pastures, and so many black cattle, we do not find ourselves in cheese?"

[1] Berkeley's *Works.* Ed. Fraser, Oxford, 1871, III. 369.

In several of his queries (381, 383) Bishop Berkeley is driving at the expediency of domestic slavery. It was two hundred years since the same expedient had been tried by Protector Somerset in England, during the intolerable state of vaga-bondage which followed the rage for pasture farming under the first Tudors. In Scotland, it was hardly more than a generation since the institution of domestic slavery had commended itself to Fletcher of Saltoun, as the only expedient that could free that country from the vagabondage of a tenth, or more, of the population. England had surmounted the difficulty long ago, Scotland got over it easily and speedily when she was admitted to the English and colonial markets for her linen manufacture by the Treaty of Union[1]. But in Ireland in the year 1740, and until long after, disabilities of all kinds, not only economic, but political and religious, were fastened upon the weaker nation by the stronger, the unfortunate cause of their long continuance having been the costly inheritance of loyalty to James II. and the Mass.

The Famine and Fever of 1740–41.

At the time when the bishop of Cloyne was issuing his economic queries from week to week (not much to the satis-faction of Primate Boulter), things were making up for the greatest crisis of famine and pestilence that Ireland experienced in the 18th century. There had been relapsing fever among the poor in Dublin in the autumn of 1738, and it appeared among them again in the summer and autumn of 1739. Rutty's account of it is as follows:

"It was attended with an intense pain in the head. It terminated some-times in four, for the most part in five or six days, sometimes in nine, and commonly in a critical sweat. It was far from being mortal. I was assured of seventy of the poorer sort at the same time in this fever, abandoned to the use of whey and God's good providence, who all recovered. The crisis, however, was very imperfect, for they were subject to relapses, even some-times to the third time, nor did their urine come to a complete separation."

In October 1739, there appeared some dysenteries in Dublin. The winter of 1739 set in severely with cold and wet in November, and about Christmas there began a frost of many

---

[1] Lord John Russell used these historical parallels from England and Scotland in his great speech in the House of Commons, during the debate on Ireland, 25th January, 1847.

weeks' duration which was more intense than anyone remembered. It is said to have made the ground like iron to the depth of nine inches; the ice on all the rivers stopped the corn mills, trees and shrubs were destroyed, and even the wool fell out of the sheep's backs. In January 1740 the destitution was such that subscription-lists were opened in Dublin, Cork, Limerick, Waterford, Clonmel, Wexford and other places. Bishop Berkeley distributed every Monday morning twenty pounds sterling among the poor of Cloyne (near Cork) besides what they got from his kitchen. One morning he came down without powder on his wig, and all the domestics of the episcopal palace followed suit[1]. The distress became more acute as the spring advanced. The potato crop of 1739 had been ruined, not by disease as in 1845–46, but by the long and intense frost. It was usual at that time to leave the tubers in the ridges through most of the winter, with the earth heaped up around them. The frost of December found them with only that slight covering, and rotted them: "a dirissimo hoc et diuturno gelu penitus putrescebant," says Dr O'Connell. Besides putrid potatoes, the people ate the flesh of cattle which had died from the rigours of the season. Owing to the want of sound seed-potatoes, the crop of 1740 was almost a blank. The summer was excessively dry and hot. In Dublin, the price of provisions had doubled or trebled, and some of the poor had died of actual starvation. In July dysenteries became common, and extended to the richer classes in the capital. Smallpox was rife at the same time, and peculiarly fatal in Cork. Dysentery continued in Dublin throughout the autumn and winter of 1740 (the latter being again frosty), and became the prevailing malady elsewhere.

On 8 February, 1741, Berkeley writes that the bloody flux had appeared lately in the town of Cloyne, having made great progress before that date in other parts of the country. A week after he writes (15 Feb.), "Our weather is grown fine and warm: but the bloody flux has increased in this neighbourhood, and raged most violently in other parts of this and the adjacent counties[2]." This prevalence of dysentery, and not of fever, as the reigning malady of the winter of 1740–41 in Munster is

---

[1] Fraser, "Life and Letters of Berkeley," in *Works*, IV. 262.
[2] Berkeley to Prior, Feb. 8 and 15, 174$\frac{0}{1}$.

confirmed by Dr Maurice O'Connell, who says that the typhus of the previous summer gave place to it. Dysentery in the winter and spring, preceding the fever of summer, was also the experience in the famine of 1817. Berkeley treated the subjects of dysentery, not with tar water, but with a spoonful of powdered resin dissolved in oil by heat and mixed in a clyster of broth[1].

As the year 1741 proceeded, with great drought in April and May, typhus fever (which had appeared the autumn before) and dysentery were both widely epidemic, so that it is impossible to say which form of disease caused most deaths. In Dublin during the month of March, 1741, the deaths from dysentery reached a maximum of twenty-one in a week, "though it was less mortal than in the country, to which the better care taken of the poor and of their food undoubtedly contributed." Bishop Berkeley writes on the 19th of May:

"The distresses of the sick and poor are endless. The havoc of mankind in the counties of Cork, Limerick and some adjacent places, hath been incredible. The nation probably will not recover this loss in a century. The other day I heard one from county Limerick say that whole villages were entirely depeopled. About two months since I heard Sir Richard Cox say that five hundred were dead in the parish where he lives, though in a country I believe not very populous. It were to be wished that people of condition were at their seats in the country during these calamitous times, which might provide relief and employment for the poor[2]."

It was said that there were twenty-five cases of fever in the bishop's own household, which were cured by the panacea, tar-water, drunk copiously—a large glass, milk-warm, every hour in bed, the same method being practised by several of his poor neighbours with equal success[3]. In a "Letter from a country gentleman in the Province of Munster to his Grace the Lord Primate[4]" it is said:

"By a moderate computation, very near one-third of the poor cottiers of Munster have perished by fevers, fluxes and downright want...The charity of the landlords and farmers is almost quite exhausted. Multitudes have perished, and are daily perishing, under hedges and ditches, some by fevers, some by fluxes, and some through downright cruel want in the utmost agonies of despair. I have seen the labourer endeavouring to work at his spade, but fainting for want of food," etc.

[1] He published the receipt in a Dublin journal.
[2] Berkeley to Thomas Prior, in "Life and Letters," u. s., p. 265. Some attempts at relief-works had been made the year before, two of which are still to be seen in the obelisks on Killiney Hill near Dublin and on a hill near Maynooth ("Lady Conolly's Folly." O'Rourke, u. s.).
[3] Rutty, p. 93.
[4] (Dublin, 1741).

The loss of life must have been great also in Connaught. A letter of 8 July, 1741, from Galway, says: "The fever so rages here that the physicians say it is more like a plague than a fever, and refuse to visit patients for any fee whatever[1]." The Galway Assizes were held at Tuam[2], the races also being transferred to the same neighbourhood, not without their usual evening accompaniments of balls and plays.

Of this famine and sickness it might have been said, in the stock medieval phrase, that the living were hardly able to bury the dead[3].

As in later Irish famines, there appear to have been, in 1740–41, three main types of sickness—dysentery, relapsing fever and typhus fever. In Dublin, as we know from the direct testimony of Rutty, there was relapsing fever in 1739, before the distress had well begun, and again in the summer of 1741, when the worst was over. So much is said of dysentery that we may well set down to it, and to its attendant dropsy, a great part of the deaths, as in the famine of 1846–47. But it is probable that true typhus fever, sometimes of a malignant type, as at Galway, was the chief infection in 1741, which was the year of its great prevalence in England. It was characterized by a mild and deceitful onset, like a cold. Spots were not invariable or essential; they were mostly of a dusky red, sometimes purple, and sometimes intermixed with miliary pustules. O'Connell mentions, for Munster, bleeding from the nose, a mottled rash as in measles, and pains like those of lumbago. One of the worst features of the Irish epidemic of 1740–41 was the prevalence of fever in the gaols. At Tralee above a hundred were tried, most of them for stealing the means of subsistence; the gaol was so full that there was no room to lie down, and fifty prisoners died

---

[1] Cited by O'Rourke. Short, a contemporary, also says that the fever in Galway was like a plague.

[2] Dutton, *Statistical Survey of the County of Galway.* Dublin, 1824, p. 313: "1741. A fever raged this year that occasioned the judges to hold the assizes in Tuam. Numbers of the merchants of Galway died this year, and multitudes of poor people, caused partly by fever and by the scarcity, as wheat was 28s. per cwt."

[3] The author of *The Groans of Ireland* (Dublin, 1741) says: "On my return to this country I found it the most miserable scene of distress that I ever read of in history: want and misery in every face; the rich unable to relieve the poor; the road spread with dead and dying bodies; mankind of the colour of the docks and nettles which they fed on; two or three, sometimes more, on a car going to the grave for want of bearers to carry them, and many buried only in the fields and ditches where they perished." Skelton, a Protestant clergyman, says: "Whole parishes in some places were almost desolate; the dead have been eaten in the fields by dogs, for want of people to bury them." Skelton's *Works,* Vol. v. Cited by Lecky.

in six weeks. Limerick gaol had dysentery and fever among its inmates, and the judge who held the Munster Circuit died of fever on his return to Dublin[1].

Rutty says that the fever fell most upon strong middle-aged men, less upon women, and least of all upon children. The number of orphans was so great after the famine that Boulter, the Anglican primate, seized the opportunity to start the afterwards notorious Charter Schools for the education of the rising generation according to the Protestant creed. In all the subsequent Irish famines it was the enormous swarms of people begging at a distance from their own parishes that spread the infection of fever; and there seems to have been as much of beggary in 1741, when Ireland was underpeopled with two millions, as in 1817–18, when it was overpeopled with six millions. A few years after the famine, Berkeley wrote in 1749:

"In every road the ragged ensigns of poverty are displayed; you often meet caravans of poor, whole families in a drove, without clothes to cover, or bread to feed them, both which might be easily procured by moderate labour. They are encouraged in their vagabond life by the miserable hospitality they meet with in every cottage, whose inhabitants expect the same kind reception in their turn when they become beggars themselves."

The estimates of the Irish mortality in 1741 varied greatly, as they have done in the Irish famines of more recent times. One guessed a third of the cottiers of Munster, another said one-fifth; and it is known that, whereas in Kerry the hearth-money was paid in 1733 by 14,346, it was paid in 1744 by only 9372[2]. The largest estimates are 200,000 deaths or even 400,000 deaths in all Ireland in a population of less than two millions. But Dr Maurice O'Connell, who practised in Cork, and saw in Munster the mortality at its worst, estimated the deaths in all Ireland, in the two years 1740 and 1741, from fevers, fluxes and absolute want, at 80,000. Those who saw the famine, fever and dysentery of 1817–18 in a population increased by three times were inclined to doubt whether even the smallest estimate of 80,000 for 1740–41 was not too large; but it is clear that the famished and fever-stricken in the 18th century were in many places allowed to perish owing to the

---

[1] Report by Dr Phipps to Baron Wainwright, 10 March, 1741. Cited by F. C. Webb, *Trans. Epidem. Soc.* 1857, p. 67.

[2] Smith's *Kerry*, p. 77. He adds that many were excused the hearth-tax on account of their poverty, by certificate of the magistrates; so that the decrease in 1744 may mean a greater proportion excused the tax, as well as a depopulation.

indifference of the ruling class or the exhaustion of their means, so that a much higher rate of fatality may be assumed for that epidemic than for the first of the 19th century Irish famines.

The distress came to an end before the winter of 1741, when food was so cheap in Dublin that a shilling bought twenty-one pounds of bread. The subsequent prevalence of typhus fever and dysentery in Ireland, whether epidemic or endemic, is very imperfectly known to the end of the century. It may be inferred that there was in that period no epidemic so great as that of 1740–41 ; but it is clear from the records kept by Rutty in Dublin down to 1764, and by Sims in Tyrone to 1772, that the indigenous fevers and fluxes of the country were never long absent, being more common in some years than in others[1].

The year 1744 was remarkable for a destructive throat distemper among children, described elsewhere, and the year 1745 for smallpox dispersed by swarms of beggars. In 1746 and 1748, the Dublin fever was relapsing in part, "terminating," says Rutty, "the fifth, sixth, seventh or eighth day with a critical sweat. A relapse commonly attended, which however was commonly carried off by a second critical sweat." In 1748, though the season was sickly, the diseases were not mortal, several of the fevers being "happily terminated by a sweat the fifth or sixth day." But there were also fevers of the low kind, sometimes with petechiae, sometimes with miliary pustules, though not essentially with either. In the autumn of 1754 Rutty begins to adopt the language of the time concerning a "putrid" constitution, identifying the fever with the dangerous remittents which Fothergill was then writing about in London ; "it is probable that ours was akin to them and owing to the same general causes." In February, 1755, the fevers were fatal to many, raising the deaths to double the usual number; they attacked all ages, were of the low, depressed kind, and commonly attended with miliary pustules. He again identifies them with the low, putrid fever in London. From that time on to 1758, Rutty has frequent references to the same fever, under

---

[1] How near the verge of want the people were is brought out by an experience in Galway county in 1745 : a great fall of snow smothered vast numbers of cattle and sheep, which caused a great many farmers to surrender their lands. Wheat rose from six to eighteen shillings the hundredweight, while, after the distress, the best land in Connaught could be rented for five shillings an acre. Dutton's *Galway*, p. 313.

the names of low, putrid, petechial and miliary. It was at its worst in 1757, and was marked by the remarkable tremors described by Johnstone at Kidderminster, as well as by miliary eruptions and by a gangrenous tendency at the spots where blisters had been applied. In November, 1757, it was fatal to not a few of the young and strong in Dublin, " and we received accounts of a like malignity attending this fever in the country[1]." It was still prevalent in the North and West of Ireland in the spring of 1758. He describes also an unusual amount of fever in the end of 1762. Sims, of Tyrone, an epidemiologist in the same manner as Rutty, does not begin his full annals until 1765; but he sums up the years from 1751 to 1760 as unhealthy by agues in spring, dysenteries and cholera morbus in autumn, and " low, putrid or nervous fevers throughout the year[2]." He adds :

"To the unhealthiness of these years the bad state and dearth of provisions might not a little contribute; the poor, being incapable to procure sufficient sustenance, were often obliged to be contented with things at which nature almost revolted ; and even the wealthy could not by all their art and power render wholesome those fruits of the earth which had been damaged by an untoward season."

Much of the distress, however, was owing to the continual spread of pasture-farming, which made the labour of villagers unnecessary[3].

The nearest approach to a great Irish epidemic in the second half of the 18th century was in 1771, as described by Sims, the type of fever being clearly the same low, putrid or nervous fever, with offensive sweats and muscular tremors, that was commonly observed in England also in the middle third of the 18th century. Early in the summer of 1771 a fever began to appear which, as autumn advanced, raged with the greatest violence; nor was it overcome by a severe winter. It claimed the prerogative of the plague, almost all others vanishing from before its presence. It began twelve months sooner in the

---

[1] For Kinsale, Cork and Bandon, see Marjoribanks, *Med. Press and Circ.* 1867, II. 8.

[2] James Sims, M.D. *Observations on Epidemic Disorders, with Remarks on Nervous and Malignant Fevers.* London, 1773, p. 10. The preface is dated from London, whither Sims had removed from Tyrone. He rose to eminence in the London profession.

[3] *A Letter to a Member of the Irish Parliament relative to the present State of Ireland.* By Philo-Irene. London, 20 May, 1755. The turning of hundreds of acres into one dairy-farm had caused the depopulation which Goldsmith described in the *Deserted Village* : " By this unhappy policy several villages have been deserted at different times by the inhabitants, and numbers of them set a-begging," p. 6.

eastern parts of the kingdom, pursuing a regular course from East to West. Some symptoms suggest cerebro-spinal fever.

The symptoms were languor, precordial oppression, want of appetite, slight nausea, pains in the head, back and loins, a thin bluish film on the tongue, turbid urine, eyes lifeless and dejected. After the fourth day, constant watchfulness, the eyes wild, melancholy, sometimes with bloody water in them, constant involuntary sighing, the tendons of the wrists tremulous, the pulse quick and weak, most profuse sweats, small dun petechiae principally at the bend of the arm and about the neck. At the height of the fever, on the ninth or tenth day, the tremulousness of the wrists spread to all the members, "insomuch that I have seen the bed-curtains dancing for three or four days to the no small terror of the superstitious attendants, who on first perceiving it, thought some evil spirits shook the bed. This agitation was so constant a concomitant of the fever as to be almost a distinguishing symptom." The patients lay grinding their teeth; when awake, they would often convulsively bite off the edges of the vessel in which drink was given them. They knew no one, their delirium being incessant, low, muttering, their fingers picking the bed covering. The face was pale and sunk, the eyes hollow, the tongue and lips black and parched. Profuse clammy sweats flowed from them; the urine was as if mixed with blood: the stools were involuntary. Petechiae almost black came out, having an outer circle with an inner dark speck; sometimes there were the larger vibices. Bleedings at the nose were frequent. Those who were put to bed and sweated almost all died. Death took place about the 13th day.

Curiously enough this disease showed itself even among the middle ranks of the people, especially those who lived an irregular life, used flesh diet and drank much. Among the poorer sort, who used vegetable food, the fever was more protracted and less malignant, but in the winter and spring it made much greater havoc among them. "Bleeding, that first and grand auxiliary of the physician in treating inflammatory disorders, seemed here to lose much of its influence." It was, indeed, the long prevalence of this low or nervous type of fever in Britain and Ireland in the middle of the 18th century that drove blood-letting in fevers out of fashion until the return of a more inflammatory type (often relapsing fever) in the epidemic of 1817. In 1770, while such fevers more or less nervous, putrid, miliary, were beginning to be prevalent among the adults, there was a good deal of "worm fever" among children. They suffered from heat, thirst, quick, full pulse, vomiting, coma, and sometimes slight convulsions, universal soreness to the touch, and a troublesome phlegmy cough. When not comatose they were peevish. The fever was remitting, the cheeks being highly flushed at its acme, pale in its remission. It lasted several days, but seldom over a week, nor was it often fatal. In children under five or six years, it could hardly be distinguished from

hydrocephalus internus[1]. The same association of the worm
fever or remittent fever of children with the putrid or nervous
fever of adults had been noticed at Edinburgh in 1735. Neither
the fever of the adults nor that of the children will be found, on
close scrutiny, to have had much in common with our modern
enteric fever.

The Epidemic Fevers of 1799–1801.

Sims left Tyrone to practise as a physician in London, and
with his departure what seems to have been the only contemporary record of epidemics in Ireland ceased. The last
quarter of the 18th century in Ireland had probably as much
epidemic fever as in England; but it is not until the years
1797–1801 that we again hear of fever and dysentery, on the
testimony of the records of the Army Medical Board, of the
Dublin House of Industry, and of the Waterford Fever
Hospital. At the end of the year 1796 the health of the
regiments in Ireland was everywhere good; but in December of
that year, and in January 1797, the poor in the towns began to
suffer more than usual from fever, and in the course of the year
1797 fever appeared in several cantonments of troops—at
Armagh as early as February or March, at Limerick, at
Waterford and in Dublin[2]. The summer and autumn were
unusually wet, so that the peasantry of the southern and
western counties were unable to lay in their usual supply of turf
for fuel. In the course of the winter 1797–98 a considerable
increase of fever and dysentery was remarked among them, and
these two maladies appeared in various regiments in the early
months of 1798. This was the year of the rebellion in the
south-east of Ireland, pending the efforts for the union with
England. The British troops were much engaged with the
insurgents throughout the summer, and got rid in great part of
the maladies of their quarters while they were campaigning.
But in the end of the year fever began to spread, both among
the inhabitants and among the troops. It was nothing new for
English and Scots regiments to suffer from fever or dysentery
during the greater part of their first year in Ireland; but the

---

[1] Sims, u. s. pp. 164–5.
[2] F. Barker and J. Cheyne, *Account of the Fever lately epidemical in Ireland.*
2 vols. London, 1821. This work relates mainly to the epidemic of 1817–19, but
there is a short retrospect, the valuable part of which is for the years 1797–1802.

epidemics in the end of 1798 were more than ordinary. The Buckinghamshire Militia quartered in the Palatine Square of the Royal barracks, Dublin, lost by "malignant contagious fever" 13 men in October, 13 in November, and 15 in December. From November to January, the Warwick regiment suffered greatly in the same barrack. The Herefordshire regiment, 833 strong, lost 47 men at Fermoy, mostly from fever contracted in bad barracks; the Coldstream Guards at Limerick, the 92nd regiment at Athlone, and the Northamptonshire Fencibles at Carrick-on-Shannon, also lost men by fever. In July, 1799, not a single regiment in Ireland was sickly; but a wet and very cold autumn made a bad harvest, aggravating the distresses of the poor and causing much sickness, which the troops shared. The county of Wexford, the principal scene of the rebellion, suffered most, and next to it the adjacent county of Waterford. The fever-hospital of the latter town, the earliest in Ireland[1], was projected in 1799; the statement made in the report of a plan for the new charity, that fifteen hundred dependent persons suffered from contagious fever every year there, showed that the need for it was nothing new, although hardly a tenth part of the number sought admission to the hospital when it was at work. Next year, 1800, the managers of the newly-opened hospital gave some particulars of the causes of fever in Waterford—want of food, causing weakness of body and depression of mind, but above all the excessive pawning of clothes and bedding, whereby they suffered from cold and slept for warmth several in a bed. In the winter and spring of 1799–1800 the poor of Waterford had epidemic among them fever and dysentery, as well as smallpox. In Donagh-a-gow's Lane nine persons died of dysentery between October 1799 and March 1800. The harvest of 1800 was again a failure, from cold and wet, bread and potatoes being dear and of bad quality. In the autumn and winter the distress, with the attendant fever and dysentery, became worse. At that time in Dublin all fever cases among the poor were received into the House of Industry (the Cork Street and Hardwick Hospitals were soon after built for fever-cases), at which the deaths for four years were as follows:

---

[1] The history of the Limerick and Belfast fever-hospitals is carried back to a few years before the founding of the Waterford hospital; but the latter was the first that was formally organised as a fever-hospital.

Year	Died in the Dublin House of Industry
1799	627
1800	1315
1801	1352
1802	384

The enormous rise of the deaths in 1800 and 1801 shows how severe the epidemic of fever must have been. Compared with the epidemic of 1817–18, it has few records, perhaps because the political changes of the union engrossed all attention. But the significant fact remains that the deaths in the Dublin House of Industry in 1800 and 1801 were nearly as many as in all the special fever-hospitals of Dublin during the two years, 1 Sept. 1817 to 1 Sept. 1819. At Cork, in 1800, there were 4000 cases of fever treated from the Dispensary; at Limerick the state of matters is said to have been as bad as in the great famine of 1817–18; and there is some reason to think that the same might have been said of other places. All the relief in 1800–1801 came from private sources, the example of Dublin in opening soup-kitchens having been followed by other towns. The troops shared in the reigning diseases, especially at Belfast and Dublin; in the latter city, the spotted fever was severe both among the military and all ranks of the civil population in August, 1801. The harvest of 1801 was abundant, and the fever quickly declined. It had been often of the relapsing type[1]. Dysentery appeared in the end of September, and became severe in many places in October and November, being attributed to the rains after a long tract of dry, hot weather. Ophthalmias and scarlatinal malignant sore-throats were common at the same time.

The Growth of Population in Ireland.

When the history of the great famine and epidemic sicknesses of 1817–18 was written, it was found that this calamity had fallen upon a population that had grown imperceptibly until it had reached the enormous figure of over six millions, the census of 1821 showing the inhabitants of Ireland to be 6,801,827. The increase from an estimated one

---

[1] "The fever in 1800 and 1801 very generally terminated on the fifth or seventh day by perspiration; the disease was then very liable to recur. The poor were the chief sufferers by it; and it was much more fatal amongst the middling and upper classes in proportion to the number attacked." Barker and Cheyne, *op. cit.* p. 20.

million and thirty-four thousand in 1695 was, according to Malthus, probably without parallel in Europe. According to Petty, the inhabitants in 1672 numbered about one million one hundred thousand, living in two hundred thousand houses, of which 160,000 were "wretched, nasty cabins without chimney, window or door-shut, and wholly unfit for making merchantable butter, cheese, or the manufacture of woollen, linen or leather." In 1695, the war on behalf of James II. having intervened, the population as estimated by South was 1,034,000. When the people were next counted in 1731, by a not incorrect method in the hands of the magistracy and Protestant clergy, they were found to have almost doubled, the total being 2,010,221. This increase, the exactness of which depends naturally upon the accuracy of Petty's and South's 17th century estimates, had been made notwithstanding the famines and epidemics of 1718 and 1728, and an excessive emigration, mostly of Protestants, to the West Indian and American colonies, which was itself attended by a great loss of life through disease. For the rest of the 18th century, the estimates of population are based upon the number of houses that paid the hearth-tax. In the following figures six persons are reckoned to each taxed hearth:

Year	Persons
1754	2,372,634
1767	2,544,276
1777	2,690,556
1785	2,845,932

The hearth-money was not altogether a safe basis of reckoning, for the reason that many were excused it on account of their poverty by certificate from the magistrates, and that hamlets in the hills, perhaps those which held their lands in rungale or joint-lease, often compounded with the collectors for a fixed sum ; so that cabins might multiply and no more hearth-tax be paid[1]. It is probable that a considerable increase had taken place which was not represented in the books of the tax-collectors; for in 1788, only three years from the last date given, the number of hearths suddenly leapt up to the round figure of 650,000 (from 474,322), giving a population of 3,900,000, at the rate of six persons to a cabin or house. But it is undoubted that a new impulse was given to population in the last twenty years of the 18th century, firstly by the bounties on

[1] Smith's *Kerry*. Dublin, 1756, p. 77.

Irish corn exported, dating from 1780, which caused much grazing land to be brought under the plough, and secondly by the gradual removal, after 1791, of various penalties and disabilities which had rested on the Roman Catholics since the reign of Anne, affecting their tenure of land, and serving in various ways to repress the multiplication of families. Accordingly we find the hearths rated in 1791 at the number of 701,102, equal to a population of 4,206,612. The estimates or enumerations from 1788, to the census of 1831, show an increase as follows :

Year	Persons	Year	Persons
1788	3,900,000	1812	5,937,856
1791	4,206,612	1821	6,801,827
1805	5,395,456	1831	7,784,539

The secret of this enormous increase was the habit that the Irish peasantry had begun to learn early in the 17th century of living upon potatoes. From that dietetic peculiarity, it is well known, much of the economic and political history of Ireland depends. At the time when it was losing its tribal organization (rather late in the day, although not so late as in the Highlands of Scotland), the country was in a fair way to pass from the pastoral state to the agricultural and industrial. It is conceivable that, if Ireland had peacefully become an agricultural country, wheaten bread would have become the staple food of the people, as in England in early times and again in later times; or that the standard might have been oatmeal in the northern province, as in Scotland: in which case one may be sure that the population would not have increased as it did. "Since the culture of the potatoes was known," says a topographer of Kerry in 1756, "which was not before the beginning of the last century, the herdsmen find out small dry spots to plant a sufficient quantity of those roots in for their sustenance, whereby considerable tracts of these mountains are grazed and inhabited, which could not be done if the herdsmen had only corn to subsist on[1]." Twenty years later Arthur Young found an enormous extension of potato culture, the pigs being fed on the surplus crop[2]. The motive, on the part of the landlord or the farmer, was to have the peat bogs on the hill-sides reclaimed by the spade; the surface of peat having

[1] Smith's *Kerry*, p. 88.
[2] *A Tour in Ireland...in* 1776-78. London, 1780.

been removed, a poor subsoil was exposed, which might be made something of after it had grown several crops of potatoes, but hardly in any other way. Another motive was political; namely, the multiplication by landlords of forty-shilling freeholder dependent votes among the Catholics as soon as they became free to exercise the franchise[1].

Malthus relied so much upon statistics, that he found the case of Ireland, notable though it was, little suited to his method, and dismissed it in a few sentences. But he indicated correctly the grand cause of over-population :

"I shall only observe, therefore, that the extended use of potatoes has allowed of a very rapid increase of population during the last century (18th). But the cheapness of this nourishing root, and the small piece of ground which, under this kind of cultivation, will in average years produce the food for a family, joined to the ignorance and depressed state of the people, which have prompted them to follow their inclinations with no other prospect than an immediate bare subsistence, have encouraged marriage to such a degree that the population is pushed much beyond the industry and present resources of the country; and the consequence naturally is, that the lower classes of people are in the most impoverished and miserable state."

In another section he showed that the cheapness of the staple food of Ireland tended to keep down the rate of wages :

"The Irish labourer paid in potatoes has earned perhaps the means of subsistence for double the number of persons that could be supported by an English labourer paid in wheat...The great quantity of food which land will bear when planted with potatoes, and the consequent cheapness of the labour supported by them, tends rather to raise than to lower the rents of land, and as far as rent goes, to keep up the price of the materials of manufacture and all other sorts of raw produce except potatoes. The indolence and want of skill which usually accompany such a state of things tend further to render all wrought commodities comparatively dear...The value of the food which the Irish labourer earns above what he and his family consume will go but a very little way in the purchase of clothing, lodging and other conveniences...In Ireland the money price of labour is not much more than the half of what it is in England."

Lastly, in a passage quoted in the sequel, he showed how disastrous a failure of the crop must needs be when the staple was potatoes; the people then had nothing between them and starvation but the garbage of the fields[2].

What the growth of population could come to on these terms was carefully shown for the district of Strabane, on the borders of Tyrone and Donegal, by Dr Francis Rogan, a writer

[1] The forty-shillings freeholder of Ireland was a life-renter whose farm was worth forty shillings annual rent more than the rent reserved in his lease.
[2] Malthus, *Essay on the Principle of Population.* Bk. II. chap. 10, Bk. III. chap. 8, and Bk. IV. chap. 11.

on the famine and epidemic fever of 1817–18[1].   Strabane stood at the meeting of the rivers Mourne and Fin to form the Foyle ; and in the three valleys the land was fertile.   All round was an amphitheatre of hills, in the glens of which and among the peat bogs on their sides was an immense population.   The farms were small, from ten to thirty acres, a farm of fifty acres being reckoned a large holding.   The tendency had been to minute subdivisions of the land, the sons dividing a farm among them on the death of the father :

"The Munterloney mountains," says Rogan, "lie to the south and east of the Strabane Dispensary district.   They extend nearly twenty miles, and contain in the numerous glens by which they are intersected so great a population that, except in the most favourable years, the produce of their farms is unequal to their support.   In seasons of dearth they procure a considerable part of their food from the more cultivated districts around them ; and this, as well as the payment of their rents, is accomplished by the sale of butter, black cattle, and sheep, and by the manufacture of linen cloth and yarn, which they carry on to a considerable extent."

These small farmers dwelt in thatched cottages of three or four rooms, in which they brought up large families[2].   Besides the farmers, there were the cottiers, who lived in cabins of the poorest construction, sometimes built against the sides of a peat-cutting in the bog.   The following table shows the proportion of cottiers to small farmers on certain manors of the Marquis of Abercorn, near Strabane, at the date of the famine in 1817–18 (Rogan, p. 96) :

[1] Francis Rogan, M.D., *Observations on the Condition of the Middle and Lower Classes in the North of Ireland, as it tends to promote the diffusion of Contagious Fever; with the History and Treatment of the late Epidemic Disorders.* London, 1819.
[2] William Carleton, the *vates sacer* of the Irish peasantry, was born, in 1798, in one of those Tyrone thatched cottages, in the parish of Clogher.   His father had changed his holding three times before William, the youngest child, was fourteen years old; the last of the four was a farm of sixteen or eighteen acres in the north of Clogher parish, and "nearer the mountains."   Carleton says that he "lived among the people as one of themselves" until he was twenty-two, which would have been until the year 1820; so that he probably saw the famine and fever of 1817–18 among that very Tyrone peasantry whom Dr Rogan brings before us from the medical side. The scenes of famine and fever in the 'Black Prophet' are those "which he himself witnessed in 1817, 1822, and other subsequent years," having been recalled by him in the form of a tale which was published in 1846, at the beginning of the Great Famine of that and the following year.   His early recollections of famine and fever come into other tales, such as the 'Clarionet,' the 'Poor Scholar' and 'Tubber Derg,' in which last is related the almost inevitable reduction to poverty and at length to beggary of a most upright and industrious farmer owing to the fall of prices, without fall of rents, after the Peace of 1815.   Carleton's work has always the quality of fidelity, and he may be credited when he says that the scenes of famine and fever are not exaggerated.

Manors	Number of Families	
	Farmers	Cottiers
Derrygoon	368	335
Donelong	243	322
Magevelin and		
Lismulmughray	319	668
Strabane	302	415
Cloughognal	328	279

The cottiers rented their cabins and potato gardens from the farmers, paying their rent, on terms not advantageous to themselves, by labour on the farm. For a time about the beginning of the century the practice by farmers of taking land on speculation to sublet to cottiers was so common that a class of "middlemen" arose. One pamphleteer during the distress of 1822 speaks of the class. of middlemen as an advantage to the cottiers, and regrets that they should have been personally so disreputable as to have become extinct. It is not easy to understand how they served the interests of the cottiers: for the latter were answerable to the landlord for the middleman's rent, and were themselves over-rented and underpaid for their labour. The system of middlemen did not in matter of fact answer; they hoped to make a profit from the tenants under them, and neglected to work on their own farms; it appears that they were a drunken class, and that they were at length swallowed up in bankruptcy. After the first quarter of the century the cottiers and the landlords (with the agents and the tithe proctors) stood face to face; but at the date of the famine of 1817 there was subletting going on, of which Rogan gives an instructive instance in his district of Ulster[1].

Under this system of subdividing farms and subletting potato gardens with cabins to cottiers, the following enormous populations had sprung up in four parishes within the

---

[1] Rogan, u. s. p. 95: "A farmer within my knowledge, who holds fifteen acres of arable land, with nearly an equal quantity of cut-out bog, for which he pays £28 per annum, has erected six cabins for labourers. They are built with mud, instead of lime, and are thatched, so that they cannot each have cost more than three or four pounds. For some time he received from three of his tenants six guineas per annum, and from the others two guineas each, the latter only holding a cottage and a small garden [the former three having also grazing for a milch cow, half a rood of land for flax, and half an acre for oats, with privileges of cutting turf and planting as many potatoes as they could each provide manure for]; but they have been all so reduced in circumstances by the late scarcity as to be now unable to keep a cow, and for the two last years have rented their cabins and potato gardens alone. All the straw raised on the farm would scarcely suffice to keep the houses water-fast if applied solely to this purpose." One of the first things that the Marquis of Abercorn did in the epidemic of 1817 was to call upon the subletting farmers on his manors to repair the roofs of their cottiers' cabins.

Dispensary district of Strabane and in four manors of the Marquis of Abercorn adjoining them, but not included in the Dispensary District :

Town of Strabane	3896
Parish of Camus	2384
„ „ Leck	5092
„ „ Urney	4886
Manor of Magevelin and Lismulmughray	5548
Manor of Donelong	3126
„ „ Derrygoon	2568
„ „ Part of Strabane	2796

In the language of the end of the 19th century, this would have been called a "congested district" of Ireland; but all Ireland was then congested to within a million and a half of the utmost limit, so that the famine, which we shall now proceed to follow in this part of Ulster, has to be imagined as equally severe in Connaught, in Munster, and even in parts of Leinster.

The Famine and Fevers of 1817–18.

The winter of 1815–16 had been unusually prolonged, so that the sowing and planting of 1816 were late. They were hardly over when a rainy summer began, which led to a ruined harvest. The oats never filled, and were given as green fodder to the cattle; in wheat-growing districts, the grain sprouted in the sheaf; the potatoes were a poor yield and watery; such of them as came to the starch-manufacturers were found to contain much less starch than usual. The peat bogs were so wet that the usual quantity of turf for fuel was not secured[1]. This failure of the harvest came at a critical time. The Peace of Paris in 1815 had depressed prices and wages and thrown commerce into confusion. During the booming period of war-prices, from 1803 to 1815, farms and small holdings had doubled or even trebled in rent, and had withal yielded a handsome profit to the farmers and steady work to the labourers. When the extraordinary war expenditure stopped, this factitious prosperity came to a sudden end. The sons of Irish cottiers were not wanted for the war, and the daughters were no longer

---

[1] Carleton, in one of his tales, has given a vivid picture of the lurid or gloomy appearance of the country in the late autumn of 1816, as if it foreboded the distress of the following spring.

profitable as flax-spinners to the small farmers. Weavers could hardly earn more than threepence a day, and labourers who could find employment at all had to be content with fourpence or sixpence, without their food. A stone of small watery potatoes cost tenpence; but the value of cattle fell to one-third, and butter brought little. By Christmas the produce of the peasants' harvest of 1816 was mostly consumed. "Many hundred families holding small farms in the mountains of Tyrone," says Rogan, "had been obliged to abandon their dwellings in the spring of 1817 and betake themselves to begging, as the only resource left to preserve their lives[1]." At Galway, in January, a mob gathered to stop the sailing of a vessel laden with oatmeal. At Ballyshannon the peasants took to the shore to gather cockles, mussels, limpets and the remains of fish. In some parts the seed potatoes were taken up and consumed. The people wandered about in search of nettles, wild mustard, cabbage-stalks and the like garbage, to stay their stomachs. It was painful, says Carleton, to see a number of people collected at one of the larger dairy farms waiting for the cattle to be blooded (according to custom), so that they might take home some of the blood to eat mixed with a little oatmeal. The want of fuel caused the pot to be set aside, windows and crevices to be stopped, washing of clothes and persons to cease, and the inmates of a cabin to huddle together for warmth. This was far from being the normal state of the cottages or even of the cabins, but cold and hunger made their inmates apathetic. Admitted later to the hospitals for fever, they were found bronzed with dirt, their hair full of vermin, their ragged clothes so foul and rotten that it was more economical to destroy them and replace them than to clean them.

Some months passed before this state of things produced fever. The first effect of the bad food through the winter, such as watery potatoes eaten half-cooked for want of fuel, had been dysentery, which became common in February, and was aggravated by the cold in and out of doors. It was confined

[1] Probably their cattle had been impounded for rent and tithe. The author of the pamphlet *Lachrymae Hiberniae* (Dublin, 1822), a resident on the western coast, says (p. 8), with reference to the seizures for rent and tithe: "Oh what scenes of misery were exhibited in Ireland in this way during the years 1817, '18 and '19; by that time the people were left without cattle; after this their potatoes and corn were seized and sold, and in some cases their household furniture, even to their blankets." The hardness of landlords in general is alleged by Dr Rogan, with an exception in favour of the Marquis of Abercorn in his own district.

C. II. 17

to the very poorest, and was not contagious, attacking perhaps one or two only in a large family. Comparatively few of those who were attacked by it in the country places came to the Strabane Dispensary; but the dropsy which often attended or followed it brought in a larger number. The following table of cases at the Dispensary shows clearly enough that dysentery and dropsy preceded the fever, which became at length the chief epidemic malady[1]:

Cases at Strabane Dispensary.

1817	Dropsy	Dysentery	Typhus
June	23	2	10
July	107	31	60
August	40	22	206
September	9	23	287

At a few of the larger towns in each of the provinces typhus had risen in the autumn of 1816 somewhat above the ordinary low level which characterized the years from 1803 to 1816 in Ireland as well as in Britain. At that time there was steadily from year to year a certain amount of typhus in the poorest parts of the towns and here or there among the cabins of the cottiers. Statistically this may be shown by the table of regular admissions to the fever hospitals of some of the chief towns from the date of their opening.

Admissions to Irish Fever Hospitals, 1799–1818.

Year	Dublin, Cork St. Hospital	Dublin House of Industry	Cork Fever Hospitals	Waterford Fever Hospital	Limerick Fever Hospital	Kilkenny Fever Hospital
1799	—	—	—	146	—	—
1800	—.	—	—.	409	—	--
1801	—	—	—	875	—.	—
1802	—.	—	—-	419	446	.—.
1803	—	—	254	188	86	73
1804	415	82	190	223	95	80
1805	1024	709	200	297	90	69
1806	1264	1276	441	165	86	56
1807	1100	1289	191	166	84	81
1808	1071	1473	232	157	100	96
1809	1051	1176	278	222	109	116
1810	1774	1474	432	410	120	135
1811	1471	1316	646	331	196	153
1812	2265	2006	617	323	146	156
1813	2627	1870	550	252	227	183
1814	2392	2398	845	175	221	236
1815	3780	2451	717	403	394	249
1816	2763	1669	1026	307	659	162
1817	3682	2860	4866	390	2586	1100
1818	7608	17894	10408	2729	4829	1924

[1] There was dysentery also in the autumn of 1818. Cheyne, *Dubl. Hosp. Rep.* III. 1.

In 1812 the first step was taken towards the adoption of the Poor Law, namely the division of the country into Dispensary Districts, which remained the units of charitable relief until 1839, when the old English system of a poor-rate and parochial Unions was applied to Ireland. During that intermediate period much was left to the medical profession, which contained many well-educated and humane men, to the priests and clergy, and to charitable persons among the laity. There was fever in many places where there were no fever hospitals. A physician at Tralee reported that the back lanes of the town, crowded with cabins, were seldom free from typhus. Rogan gives two instances from the Strabane district in the summer and winter of 1815, at a time when the district was remarkably healthy. A beggar boy was given a night's lodging by a cottier at Artigarvan, three miles from Strabane. Next morning he was too ill to leave; he lay three weeks in typhus, and gave the disease to twenty-seven persons in the eight cabins which formed the hamlet. A few months after, about a mile from Strabane, a mother fell into typhus and was visited many times by her two married daughters and by others of her children at service in the neighbourhood. Nineteen cases were traced to this focus; "but the actual number attacked was probably more than three times this, as the disease, when once introduced into the town, spread so widely among the lower orders as to create general alarm, and led to the establishment of the small fever ward attached to the Dispensary." It was in April, 1816, that this was done, two rooms, each with four beds, having been provided at Strabane for fever cases; but at no time until the summer of 1817 were they all occupied at once.

The epidemic really began there in May, 1817, in a large house which had been occupied during the winter by a number of families from the mountains; they had brought no furniture with them, nor bedding except their blankets, and lay so close together as to cover the floors. Each room was rented at a shilling a week, the tenant of a room making up his rent by taking in beggars at a penny a night. The floors and stairs were covered with the gathered filth of a whole winter; the straw bedding, never renewed, was thrown into a corner during the day to be spread again at night. Every crevice was stopped to keep out the cold; the rain came in through the roof, the floors were damp, and the cellars of the house full of stagnant water turned putrid. Meanwhile more than a fourth part of the families resident in Strabane, to the number of 1026 persons, were being fed from a soup-house opened early in the spring of 1817, while there were others equally destitute but too proud to ask relief. The rumour of this charity soon brought crowds of people from the surrounding country, with gaunt cheeks, says Carleton, hollow eyes, tottering gait and a look of "painful abstraction" from the unsatisfied craving for food. In the crowd round the soup-shop, the timid girl, the modest mother, the decent farmer scrambled "with as much turbulent solicitation and outcry as if they had been trained, since their very infancy, to all the forms of impudent cant and imposture." These soup-shops were opened in all the Irish towns. At Strabane some of the richer class lent money to procure supplies, for sale at cost price, of oatmeal, rice and rye-flour, the last being in much request in the form of loaves of black bread.

The fever, having begun among the houseful of vagrants above mentioned, made slow progress until June, when it spread through the town, and in the autumn became a serious epidemic. Meantime the soup-kitchen was closed, the supplies having ceased, and the country people returned to their cabins carrying the infection of typhus everywhere with them. By the middle of October, 1817, the epidemic was general in the country round Strabane.

The following table shows the rise and decline of the epidemic of typhus in the town itself.

Cases of Fever attended from Strabane Dispensary[1].

	1817	1818		1817	1818
Jan.	9	83	July	60	106
Feb.	13	46	Aug.	206	90
March	6	60	Sept.	287	57
April	13	48	Oct.	233	49
May	3	39	Nov.	193	40
June	10	71	Dec.	140	38

The exact particulars from the Dispensary district of Strabane show clearly how famine in Ireland is related to fever. The epidemic of typhus was an indirect result of the famine, and was due most of all to the vagrancy which a famine was bound to produce in Ireland, in the absence of a Poor Law. In the

[1] Rogan, p. 31.

spring of 1817, said a gentleman near Tralee, "the whole country appeared to be in motion." "It was lamentable," said Peel, in the Commons debate, on 22 April, 1818, "at least it was affecting, that this contagion should have arisen from the open character and feelings of hospitality for which the Irish character was so peculiarly remarkable." They gathered also at funerals, and, as Graves said of a later epidemic, they were "scrupulous in the performance of wakes." The concourse of people at the daily distributions of soup was another cause of spreading infection, many of them having come out of infected houses[1]. Of such houses, the lodging-houses of the towns, we have several particular instances. At Strabane, there were four such, which sent ninety-six patients to the fever hospital in eighteen months. At Dublin, a house in Cathedral-lane sent fifty cases to the fever hospitals in a twelvemonth; the house No. 4, Patrick's close sent thirty cases in eight months; No. 52½ Kevin-street sent from five rooms nineteen persons in six weeks.

The spread of the disease was much aided by the ordinary annual migration of harvest labourers. It was the custom every year for cottiers in Connaught to shut up their cabins after the potatoes were planted, and to travel to the country round Dublin in search of work at the hay and corn harvests, leaving their families to beg; in the same way there was an annual migration from Clare to Kilkenny, from Cavan, Longford and Leitrim into Meath, and from Derry into Antrim, Down and Armagh[2]. In the summer of 1817 some parishes of Derry were left with only four or five families. The keeper of the bridge at Toome, over the Bann, counted more than a hundred vagrants every day passing into Antrim, from the middle of May to the

---

[1] The following is an instance, from Boyle, in Roscommon: "In the middle of June, 1817, or a little earlier, a soup-shop was established here by subscription, where soup was daily given out to one thousand persons, who, naturally anxious to procure it in time, crowded together during its distribution, though every pains was taken to keep order amongst them. From the 16th to the 23rd of that month the weather became suddenly and unusually hot, and the disease about that period spread rapidly among those persons, the greater number of whom attributed the origin of their complaint to attendance at the soup-shop; among that crowd, many of whom I have seen faint from absolute want during exposure to the sun, there were persons from houses where the disease existed." Report by Dr Verdon of Boyle, 26 June, 1818, in Barker and Cheyne, I. 325.

[2] Dr King of Tralee (Barker and Cheyne, I. p. 177) wrote as follows: "It is a custom in this country for very poor persons, living in the country parts, and possessing a miserable hovel with a small garden, after they have sowed their potatoes, to shut up their hut and carrying their families with them, to roam about the country, trusting to the known hospitality of the towns and villages for shelter and subsistence till the time for digging the potatoes shall have arrived."

beginning of July; and the same might have been seen at the other bridge over the Bann at Portglenone.

As the spread of contagion came to be realized, the ordinary hospitality to vagrants ceased. Rogan was struck with the apathy which at length arose towards sick or dead relatives; even parents became callous at the death of their children (of whom many died from smallpox). "For some time," he says, " it has been as difficult for a pauper bearing the symptoms of ill-health to procure shelter for the night, as it was formerly rare to be refused it." In Strabane they extemporised a poor's fund by voluntary contributions of £30 a month, by means of which eighty poor families were kept from begging in the streets. In Dublin there was so much alarm of infection from the number of beggars entering the shops that trade was checked. The following, relating to a town in the centre of Ireland, is an extreme instance of the panic which the idea of contagion at length caused :

" In Tullamore, when measures were proposed for arresting the progress of fever, by the establishment of a fever hospital, so little was the alarm that the design was regarded by most of the inhabitants as a well-intentioned project, uncalled for by the circumstances of the community. But when the death of some persons of note excited a sense of danger, alarm commenced, which ended in general dismay: military guards were posted in every avenue leading to this place, for the purpose of intercepting sickly itinerants. The town, from the shops of which the neighbouring country is supplied with articles of all kinds, was thus in a state of blockade. It was apprehended that woollen and cotton goods might be the vehicles of infection, and all intercourse between the shops and purchasers was suspended. Passengers who inadvertently entered the town considered themselves already victims of fever. No person would stop at the public inns, nor hire a carriage for travelling; in a word all communication between the town and the adjacent country was completely interrupted. Apprehension did not proceed in most other places to the same extent as in Tullamore[1]."

Several isolated places escaped the epidemic of typhus, either for a time or altogether. The island of Rathlin, seven miles to the west of Antrim, which was as famished as the mainland, had no typhus at the time when it was epidemic along the nearest shore; the island of Cape Clear, at the southernmost point of Ireland, had a similar experience. The whole county of Wexford, where the soil was dry and the harvest of 1816 had been fair, kept free from typhus until 1818, partly because it was out of the way of vagrants. The town of Dingle, at the head of a bay in Kerry, with old Spanish

---

[1] Barker and Cheyne, I. 60.

traditions, was totally free from typhus at a time when its near neighbour, Tralee, was full of it, the immunity being set down to the well-being of the population from their industry at the linen manufacture (and fisheries) and their thrifty habits.   But the counties of Wexford and Waterford, and other places more or less exempted in 1817, had a full share of the epidemic in 1818, which was the season of its greatest prevalence in most parts of Ireland except Ulster.   The harvest of 1817 had been little better than that of the year before, although the potato crop was hardly a failure.   The fine summer of 1818 brought out crowds of vagrants who slept in the open, and, when they took the infection, were placed in "fever-huts" erected near the roads[1]. The harvest of that year was abundant, and by the end of 1718 the epidemic had declined everywhere except in Waterford.

The most carefully kept statistics of the sickness and mortality were those by Rogan for the Strabane Dispensary district, and the adjoining manors of the Marquis of Abercorn, for each of which a private dispensary was established under the care of a physician.

Abstract of Returns of the Dispensary district of Strabane, shewing the numbers ill of fever from the commencement of the epidemic in the summer of 1817, till the end of September, 1818, the numbers labouring under the fever at that date, and the mortality caused by the disease (Rogan, p. 72).

	Population	Ill of Fever	Dead	Remaining ill
Town of Strabane	3896	639	59	13
Parish of Camus	2384	685	61	37
„ „ Leck	5092	1462	96	57
„ „ Urney	4886	1381	86	42
	16,258	4167	302	149

Similar return for those parts of the Marquis of Abercorn's estates not within the Dispensary district:

Manors	Population	Ill of fever (to Oct. 1818)	Dead
Magevelin and Lismulmughray }	5548	1666	101
Donelong	3126	1217	71
Derrygoon	2568	1215	90
Part of Strabane	2796	990	75
Totals	14,038	5088	337

[1] In Carleton's tale of 'The Poor Scholar,' it is related how the hay-mowers stopped in their work to erect a hut for the fever-stricken youth, and a much larger hut not far from the first for the numerous persons who ministered to his wants under a kind of quarantine arrangement.   The stealing of milk from rich men's cows for the sick youth is the subject of a dialogue between the Roman Catholic bishop and the leader of the kindly party of mowers, in which the latter shows a skill in casuistry creditable to his religious instructors.

The proportion of attacks in these tables for a part of Tyrone, one-third to one-fourth of the whole population, is believed to have been a fair average for the whole of Ireland. Each attack, with the weakness that it left behind, lasted about six weeks; cases would occur in a family one after another for several months; in some cottages, says Rogan, only the grandmother escaped.

One hundred thousand cases were known to have passed through the hospitals. Harty thought that seven times as many were sick in their cabins or houses, making 800,000 cases in all Ireland in two years; Barker and Cheyne estimated the whole number of cases at a million and a half (1,500,000). The mortality was comparatively small. It comes out greater in the tables for the Strabane district than anywhere else in Ireland except the hospital at Mallow. The following table, compiled by Harty, shows how widely the fatality ranged (if the figures can be trusted), from place to place and from season to season:

Proportions of fatal cases of typhus in the chief hospitals of Ireland 1817, 1818 and 1819 (Harty)[1].

	1817 One in	1818 One in	1819 One in	Average One in
Dublin	$14\frac{1}{2}$	24	$18\frac{1}{4}$	20
Kilkenny	$16\frac{1}{2}$	$14\frac{5}{6}$	$12\frac{2}{3}$	$14\frac{1}{4}$
Dundalk	$20\frac{5}{6}$	54	25	30
Belfast	$19\frac{2}{5}$	$15\frac{4}{5}$	19	$17\frac{1}{2}$
Newry	$21\frac{1}{10}$	$34\frac{1}{2}$	$13\frac{1}{2}$	26
Cork	29	35	35	$33\frac{1}{2}$
Limerick	$13\frac{1}{2}$	$15\frac{2}{3}$	$30\frac{2}{3}$	$16\frac{1}{2}$
Waterford	$27\frac{4}{5}$	25	$23\frac{3}{4}$	$24\frac{4}{5}$
Clonmel	27	18	$18\frac{1}{4}$	$19\frac{3}{4}$
Mallow	$22\frac{1}{2}$	$9\frac{2}{3}$		12
Killarney	74	67	33	62
Tralee	$20\frac{3}{4}$	69	43	39

What this meant to particular places will appear from some instances. In the parish of Ardstraw, Tyrone, with a population of about twenty thousand, 504 coffins are stated by the parish minister to have been given to paupers in eighteen months. The burials were about twice as many as in ordinary years,

[1] William Harty, M.D., *Historic Sketch of the Contagious Fever Epidemic in Ireland during* 1817–19. Dublin, 1820. This work contains information collected by a circular of queries addressed to practitioners in the several provinces. It was undertaken by Dr Harty at the instance of Sir John Newport, M.P. for Waterford. The work by Barker and Cheyne on the same epidemic took longer to prepare, having been published in 1821. See also Cheyne, *Dubl. Hosp. Rep.* II. 1—147.

according to the register of the Cathedral churchyard of Armagh :

1815	247 burials
1816	312 ,,
1817	571 ,,
1 May—25 Dec. 1818	463 ,,

Of the 463 burials in eight months of 1818, there were 165 from fever, 180 from smallpox, and 118 from other causes.

Barker and Cheyne make the whole mortality of the two years from fever and dysentery to have been 65,000; Harty makes it 44,300. But not more than a sixth part of the latter total were registered deaths, and the estimate of the whole may be wide of the mark. In the county of Kerry, ten Catholic priests died of it. Many medical men took it, as well as apothecaries and nurses, and several physicians died, of whom Dr Gillichan, of Dundalk, a young man of good fortune, made a notable sacrifice of his life. Everyone bore willing testimony to the devotion of the Roman Catholic clergy. Some harrowing incidents were reported, such as those from Kanturk, in county Cork :

Dr O'Leary visited a low hut in which lay a father and three children : "There were also two grown-up daughters who were obliged to remain for several nights in the open air, not having room in the hut till the father died, when the stronger of the two girls forced herself into his place. On the road leading to Cork, within a mile of this town, I visited a woman of the name of Vaughan, labouring under typhus ; on her left lay a child very ill, at the foot of the bed another child just able to crawl about, and on her right the corpse of a third child, who had died two days previously, and which the unhappy mother could not get removed. When the grant arrived from Government, I visited a man of the name of Brahill near the chapel gate, who with his wife and six children occupied a very small house, all of them ill of fever with the exception of one boy, who was so far convalescent as to creep to the door to receive charity from the passengers."

Infants rarely took the fever. Dr Osborne, of Cork, stated that in one instance a physician in attendance on the poor had to separate two children from the bed of their dead brother, the father and mother being already in a fever hospital; in another instance, he had to remove an infant from the corpse of its mother who had just expired in a hovel[1].

Nosologically the epidemic of 1817–18 presented several features of interest. It began with dysentery, and ended with the same in autumn, 1818. It was in great part typhus, but

---

[1] Barker and Cheyne, p. 65. A similar incident comes into Carleton's tale of 'The Clarionet': "At length, out of compassion, the few neighbours who feared not to attend a feverish death-bed, acting on the popular belief that children under a certain age are not liable to catch a fever, placed the boy in her arms." This popular belief was well founded.

towards the end of the epidemic, in Dublin, at Strabane, and doubtless elsewhere, it changed to relapsing fever, that is to say, the sick person "got the cool" about the fifth or seventh day instead of the tenth or twelfth, but was apt to have one or more relapses or recurrences of the fever. The relapsing type was milder in its symptoms and was more rarely fatal. The average fatality of typhus was much less than in ordinary years, while a good many of the fatal cases came from the richer classes, to whom the contagion reached, the proportion of fatalities among them being nôted everywhere as very high, up to one death in three or four cases[1]. The fatalities were most common, as usual, at ages from forty to sixty. A full share of the women and children took the fever, perhaps an excess of women, allowing for their excess in the population. The following were the numbers at each period of life among 18,891 cases treated in the hospitals of Dublin and Waterford:

Years of age	1—10	10—20	20—30	30—40	40—50	50 and over
Cases	2426	6116	5230	2476	1415	1228

The action of the English Government was thought by some to have been apathetic. Nothing was done to check the export of corn from Irish ports. Peel, who held the office of Irish Secretary in 1817, was probably actuated in this by the same constitutional and economic considerations which led him, as Prime Minister in 1845, to refuse O'Connell's demand for a proclamation against the export of corn.

Carleton says that there were scattered over the country "vast numbers of strong farmers with bursting granaries and immense haggards," and that long lines of provision carts on their way to the ports met or intermingled with the funerals on the roads, the sight of which exasperated the famishing people. Several carts were attacked and pillaged, some "strong farmers" were visited, and here or there a "miser" or meal-monger was obliged to be charitable with a bad grace; but on the whole there was little lawlessness, less indeed than in England in 1756 and 1766, or in Edinburgh in 1741. In September, 1817, Peel commissioned four Dublin physicians to visit the respective provinces and report on the causes and extent of the epidemic

[1] Accounts from various places in Barker and Cheyne, and in Harty. Rogan (u. s. p. 45) says: "The cases of typhus gravior were infinitely more numerous among the rich and well-fed than among the poor; and with them also the head was most frequently the seat of diseased action."

fever.   On 22 April, 1818, Sir John Newport, member for Waterford, for whom Dr Harty had been collecting information, raised a debate on the epidemic in the House of Commons, and moved for a Select Committee.   The debate, after the opening speech and a sensible brief reply by Peel, degenerated at once into irrelevant talk on the inadequacy of the fever hospital of London.   The Select Committee was named, and quickly reported on the 8th of May.

A Bill embodying the recommendations of the Committee received the royal assent on 30th May.   The Act provided for the extension of fever hospitals, the exemption of lodging-houses, under certain regulations, from the hearth-tax and the window-tax, and the formation of Boards of Health with powers to abate and remove nuisances.   The Boards of Health were found unworkable, partly by reason of expense, partly of excessive powers.   The epidemic having visited Waterford somewhat late in its progress, Sir John Newport again called attention to it on 6th April, 1819, and moved for the revival of last year's Committee.   Mr Charles Grant, afterwards Lord Glenelg, who was now Irish Secretary, gave much satisfaction to the patriotic members both by his sympathetic speech on the occasion and by his previous action at the Irish Office in the way of pecuniary help to the fever hospitals or Dispensary district officers.   The Second Report of the Committee re-marked that the rich absentee landlords had given nothing. Another Act, of June, 1819 (59 Geo. III. cap 41), defined the duties of officers of health, and contained an important clause (ix.) relating to the spread of contagion by vagrants.   By that time the epidemic was over ; nor can it be said that the action of the Government from first to last had made much difference to its progress.

Vagrancy was the principal direct cause ; and behind the vagrancy were usages and traditions, with interests centuries old, which made the landlords resolute not to pay poor-rates on their rentals.   It was not until twenty years after that the English Poor Law was applied to Ireland (in 1839), whereby the pauper class were dealt with as far as possible in their respective parishes.   How far that measure was effective in checking the spread of contagion will appear when we come to the great famine and epidemic of dysentery and fever in 1846–49.

It will not be necessary to follow with equal minuteness the successive famines and epidemics of typhus, relapsing fever and dysentery in Ireland, to the great famine of 1846–49. After 1817 distress became chronic among the cottiers and small farmers. Leases had been entered into at high rents during the years of war prices, and in the struggle for holdings tenants at will offered the highest rate. When peace came and prices fell, rents were found to be excessive, not to say impossible. But in Ireland with a rapidly increasing population it was easier to put the rents up than to bring them down. Other things helped to embarrass the poor cottager: he paid twice over for his religion, tithes to the parson, dues to the priest; and he paid all the more of the tithe in that the graziers, who were mostly of the established Church and the occupiers of the fertile plains, had taken care to make potato land titheable (at what date this innovation arose is not stated) but had used their power in the Irish Parliament to resist the tithe on arable pastures. Again the cottiers or cottagers paid, in effect, the whole of the poor rate in the form of alms; for the dogs of the gentry kept all beggars from their gates.

Famine and Fever in the West of Ireland, 1821–22.

The next famine in 1821–22 is remarkable for two things besides its purely medical interest. Owing to the number of desperate evicted tenants, it gave occasion to an increased activity of the secret associations, especially the Whiteboys of Tipperary and Cork[1]; and it called forth the first great dole of English charity in the form of princely subscriptions to a Famine Fund. The English charity in 1822 was prompt and large-hearted, contrasting with the tardy help from the exchequer in the much more serious famine of 1817–18. The true explanation of it is, doubtless, that England on the second occasion had more money to spare. The trouble in 1821–22 came from the total loss of the potato crop in Mayo, Galway, Clare and Kerry, and from a partial loss of it in some other counties of the south and west. There was no corn famine, and no general dearth. Accordingly it affected the poorest class only, and the most remote districts chiefly. The planting season of 1821 had

---

[1] *Report on the Present State of the Distressed District in the South of Ireland: with an Enquiry into the Causes of the Distresses of the Peasantry and Farmers.* Dublin, 1822.

not been favourable, and the yield of potatoes had been poor. But the autumn was so wet in the west that the floods in some places washed away the soil with the potatoes in it, and in other places drowned the potatoes after they had been pitted. The flooded state of the basin of the Shannon was a natural calamity on the great scale that touched the imagination and loosened the purse-strings. A Committee was formed at the London Tavern, which sat through the spring of 1822, and quickly raised an immense sum. The great mercantile firms of the City and of Liverpool gave each a thousand pounds; a ball at the Opera House under the patronage of the king (George IV.) brought six thousand, and from all sources the Committee found themselves with three hundred thousand pounds at their disposal (forty-four thousand of it from Ireland), while a fund at the Dublin Mansion House amounted to thirty thousand more. Much of this was sent to Galway, Mayo, Clare and Kerry, in time to save many thousands of families from starvation[1]; it was, no doubt, wastefully given away, and there was a balance of sixty thousand pounds sterling unused. More tardily in June, 1822, Parliament voted one hundred thousand "for the employment of the poor in Ireland," and in July two hundred thousand to meet contingencies of the famine. It was generally admitted that the Government grants were jobbed and misappropriated to a scandalous extent. The towns had to be made the centres of relief and the depôts of provisions; and yet the towns were not suffering from famine or fever but only from penury. The fever hospital at Ennis, the county town of Clare, was constantly filled by strangers, the townspeople remaining healthy. Kerry was one of the most afflicted counties, but Tralee and Killarney had no unusual sickness. Limerick town had hardly more fever than in an ordinary year. In Dublin the admissions for fever in 1822 were a good deal below the usual number. On the other hand, Sligo town had much fever, and Galway town had an altogether unique experience, the history of which, as related by Dr Graves, will be the best possible view of the peculiar circumstances of 1821–22[2].

---

[1] *Lachrymae Hiberniae, or the Grievances of the Peasantry of Ireland, especially in the Western Counties.* By a Resident Native. Dublin, 1822 (September). The author, a resident of the west coast, was concerned in the distribution of relief, and positively asserts the saving of thousands "from his own personal knowledge."

[2] Robert James Graves, M.D., "Report on the Fever lately prevalent in Galway and the West of Ireland." *Trans. K. and Q. Col. Phys.* IV. (1824), p. 408.

In Connemara, where the distress was acute, there were no roads over which the provisions from England could be carted to the famished districts. Accordingly a great store was made in Galway, to which crowds flocked from the country in boats and on foot. Many died a few days after they arrived, from exhaustion or from the surfeit of food after long hunger. Galway, a crowded place at best, with narrow streets and lanes, contained thousands of strangers, who slept about the quays and the fish-market, or in the lanes and entries, or in crowded lodging-houses four or five in a bed. The fever began in May, and quickly spread so much that the priests were kept fully employed by calls to the dying. In June and July the sixty beds of the fever hospital were filled, principally with the fugitives from Connemara. Sixty more beds were added, and these by the middle of September were insufficient. The infection had now spread to many good houses. When Dr Graves and three other Dublin physicians arrived, on 26 September, they found ropes stretched across the streets to stop the wheel traffic. The shops of tradesmen were avoided. The town was like a place in the plague ; people passing along the streets put their handkerchiefs to their noses when they came to a house with fever in it. Yet the number of cases was not remarkable ; on 3 ·October, there were 404 sick in a population of 30,000, of whom 130 were in the fever hospital and 274 at their homes, the new cases occurring at the rate of 29 per diem. At length it was found practicable to set up depôts of provisions in country places, and the crowd of strangers left Galway. The fever was mild but tedious among the poor, more violent and fatal among the well-to-do. In many country places dysentery and choleraic diarrhœa were prevalent, as well as fever. In Erris, county Mayo, dysentery and dropsy were more common than fever, many of the cottiers having subsisted on weeds, shell-fish, or new potatoes dug six weeks after the seed was planted. In this famine the people ate the flesh of black cattle dead of disease. Excepting in Connemara the county of Galway was not so soon affected as some other parts of Ireland ; but, as in 1818, the contagion of fever was spread abroad by vagrants. After Mayo, Galway, Clare and Kerry, the counties most affected were Roscommon and Sligo, and next to these Leitrim, Tipperary and Cork.

Dysentery and Relapsing Fever, 1826–27.

Fever and dysentery decreased to an ordinary level in 1823, but rose somewhat again in 1824, the summer of which was hot and moist. But it was in the hot and dry summers of 1825 and 1826 that dysentery became notably common in Ireland generally and in Dublin in particular. It began in the capital in June—among the richer class of people. About the middle of August admissions for dysentery were perceptibly raising the number of patients in the Cork Street Fever Hospital, and continued to do so throughout the autumn. At one dispensary three out of four applicants had dysentery. All those admitted to hospital were over twenty years of age; of thirty-five cases under Dr O'Brien, nine died, all of which had ulceration of the great intestine, in one case gangrenous. The mortality was not nearly so great among the richer classes, in which respect dysentery reversed the rule of typhus fever. O'Brien had one obvious case illustrating the curious connexion between dysentery and rheumatic fever, originally remarked by English observers in the 18th century. A hospital porter was admitted with "fever of a mixed catarrhal and rheumatic type." Having been blooded and subjected to free evacuations, his fever left him on the fourth day, but he was at once seized with dysentery, which ran its course[1].

It is to be noted that this epidemic of dysentery began in Dublin in the hot June weather of 1825 among the richer classes, and that there was no notable increase of fever while it lasted. It appears to have declined in Dublin in the early part of 1826. After a cold and dry spring there began one of the hottest and driest summers on record. The first rain for four months fell on the 15th of July, 1826, the thermometer rose as high as 86°, and was on a mean several degrees above summer temperature in Dublin. In the spring labour had become slack, and before long it was estimated that 20,000 artizans in the Liberties (weavers and others) were out of work. Early in May there began a most extraordinary epidemic of relapsing fever, with which some typhus was mixed. By the 9th of May, the 220 beds of the Cork Street Hospital were full,

---

[1] John O'Brien, M.D., "On the Epidemic Dysentery which prevailed in Dublin in the year 1825." *Trans. K. and Q. Col. Phys.* v. (1828) p. 221; Burke, *Ed. Med. Surg. Journ.* July, 1826, p. 56; Speer, *Med. Phys. Journ.* N. S. VI. 199.

and applicants were sent away daily. On 4 August, a temporary hospital of 240 beds was opened in the garden of the Meath Hospital; on the 18th, the Wellesley Hospital, in North King Street, was opened with 113 beds; on the 15th, tents to hold 180 patients were erected on the lawn of the Cork Street Hospital, raising its accommodation to 400; a warehouse in Kevin Street was furnished with beds for 230 patients, and some increase was made to the beds in Sir Patrick Dun's and Stevens's Hospitals. The whole number of fever-beds in Dublin hospitals at length reached 1400; but not half the number of cases was provided for. At a meeting in the Mansion House on 26 October, it was stated that there were at that date 3200 persons sick of the fever at their homes, besides the 1400 in the hospitals. Funds were subscribed, soup-kitchens and dispensaries opened in various districts of Dublin, and kept open most of the winter, "but they made little impression on the epidemic, which continued with unabated violence." In March, 1827, it began suddenly to decline, and fell rapidly until it was nearly extinct in May; and that, too, although "the complaints of distress and want are to the full as loud as at the commencement of the epidemic, and provisions are dearer[1]." The corresponding sicknesses in Edinburgh and Glasgow were later—the fever chiefly in 1828, the dysentery in 1827 and 1828.

This great epidemic was mainly one of relapsing fever. The patient "got the cool," or passed the crisis of the fever, usually on the evening of the fifth or seventh day, sometimes on the ninth, the evening exacerbation, which was to prove critical, being ushered in generally with a rigor, and passing off in profuse perspiration throughout the night. The five-day fever was more certain to relapse than that of seven days, the seven-day fever was more likely to relapse than that of nine days. The relapses might be one or two or three or more, prolonging the illness for weeks. The clear interval varied from twenty-four hours to fourteen days. There were some cases with jaundice which led Stokes and Graves to speak loosely of "yellow fever[2]." O'Brien saw only four cases with exquisite icterus in fifteen hundred cases of relapsing fever. There was a small proportion of cases of ordinary typhus of a severe kind,

[1] John O'Brien, "Med. Rep. of the H. of Recovery, Cork Street, Dublin, for the year ending 4 Jan. 1827." *Trans. K. and Q. Col. Phys.* v. 512.
[2] Graves, *Clinical Medicine*, 1843. Lect. XVIII.

marked by unusual delirium or phrensy and the absence of sordes on the teeth or petechiae on the skin ; the typhus cases became more numerous in the winter season, or, in other words, the original attack lasted to nine, eleven, or thirteen days, with little or no tendency to relapse. Gangrene was not uncommon in one part of the body or another, and in four cases the feet became gangrenous[1].

Even with the admixture of pure typhus cases, and with dysenteric complications in the autumn and winter, the mortality of the whole epidemic was small—not more than it would have been among a third part the number of fever cases in an ordinary year. At the Cork Street Hospital alone (including the tents) there were 8453 admissions from 4th August, 1826, to 4th April, 1827, with 332 deaths, or four deaths in a hundred cases. The proportion of recoveries was quite as remarkable in known instances in the squalid homes of the poor, where two or three would be found ill of fever on one pallet, or a father and six children in one room, shunned by the neighbours.

The strangest thing in this epidemic was the sequel of it. In the spring of 1827, intermittent fever, which had not made its appearance for several years in Dublin, began to prevail pretty generally; whilst the ordinary continued fever showed a strong tendency to assume the intermittent and remittent forms. It is not surprising, therefore, that Dr O'Brien, who had these varied experiences of epidemic dysentery in 1825, of epidemic relapsing fever and typhus in 1826, and of intermittent fever in 1827, should adopt Sydenham's language of epidemic constitutions, and revert to the old Sydenhamian doctrine of causes. While the sequence of epidemic diseases in Dublin was some dysentery in the autumn and winter of 1825 and relapsing fever on a vast scale during the excessively dry spring and summer of 1826, in country districts of Ireland, such as Skibbereen, dysentery became epidemic after the great drought and heat of 1826, while "fever disappeared altogether," and indeed all other prevalent forms of sickness gave way before it, so general was it. Such is the report from Skibbereen, county Cork, a district that became early notorious, in the great famine of 1846–47, and was perhaps a kind of barometer of Irish distress twenty years earlier. The epidemic dysentery of 1826 attacked all classes

[1] O'Brien, u.s.

C. II. 18

there, but chiefly the poorest; it was apt to begin insidiously, and, as it was often neglected, so it often became obstinate and hard to cure.   Dr McCarthy attributed it to the drought of 1826, the commercial distress of 1825, the lack of employment for labourers, the overgrowth of population, and the alarming rise in the prices of food[1].   He uses the same economic illustrations as O'Connell and Smith O'Brien in the Great Famine twenty years after, which were, indeed, as old as the time of Bishop Berkeley[2].

Although little is heard of the fever of 1826–27 except in Dublin, it is probable that the same causes which produced it there were operative in other large towns.   The admissions to the Limerick Fever Hospital rose rapidly in the end of 1826. Geary, who was appointed one of its physicians that year, estimates that about one in twelve of the population of Limerick (63,310) were treated for fever in 1827 at public institutions, besides those treated in private practice.   It was relapsing fever, as in Dublin[3].

Perennial Distress and Fever.

According to all the figures of Irish fever-hospitals, and the generalities of their physicians, fever was now constantly present in the towns.   After the relapsing epidemic of 1826–27 had subsided, there was no rise above the steady level until the years 1831 and 1832, when a considerable increase appears in the admissions to the hospitals of Dublin, Limerick and Belfast. But the fever of 1831–32 was totally eclipsed by the cholera, and little is heard of typhus in Irish writings until 1835–36, when an epidemic arose, purely of typhus fever, which is said to have been as severe upon some districts as that of 1817–18 had

[1] "Remarks on the Epidemic Dysentery of the Autumn of 1826 in the South of Ireland." By Alexander McCarthy, M.D. *Edin. Med. and Surg. Journ.* April, 1827, p. 289.
[2] "It is a melancholy picture of society to witness the increase of wealth and luxury on one side, and the greatest want and wretchedness on the other; to meet famine and exhaustion in the great body of the people, in a country that produces as much food as would afford a full supply for once and a half its present population; to see the granaries full of corn and flour, and the great body of the people scarcely existing on a half supply of bad potatoes.   Such is the miserable situation of the Irish, a race of people distinguished for their intellect, and above all for their resignation and patience under afflictions the most trying."
[3] *Dub. Quart. Journ. Med. Sc.* XI. 385.

been. This outbreak fell at the time of the Commission presided over by the Earl of Devon, the report of which is authoritative for the state of the Irish lower class and the causes of the same. The country cottiers and the poor of the towns were always on the verge of starvation. Dr Geary, of Limerick, in 1836 estimated as follows the proportion of poor to the whole population, "the poor" being taken to mean "those who would require aid if a Poor Law existed[1] : "

Proportion of "Poor" in the several Parishes of Limerick, 1836.

	St Nicholas and St Mary	St John and St Laurence	St Munchin	St Michael
Population	14,629	15,667	4,071	16,226
Number of Poor	7,000	6,400	930	2,500

Most of the poor lived in the old town of Limerick in lofty and closely-built houses which the better classes had abandoned. These dilapidated barracks were the abodes of misery and filth, two and often three families occupying a single room : " It is here, as in the decayed Liberties of Dublin[2], that the indigent room-keeper, the ruined artisan, the unemployed labourer, and the ejected country cottier, with their famishing families retreat." Their degradation, Dr Geary thought, was owing to the delay of Parliament in giving Ireland the Poor Law. The sanitary state of the old town was disgraceful. Heaps of manure were carefully kept in back yards, to be sold to farmers in the spring —"a very principal source of livelihood " for those who collected it. Certain houses near these depôts had always fever in them, dysentery was frequent, and Exchange-lane never free from it[3]. An extensive glue-mill in the Abbey poisoned the air with the effluvia of putrid animal matters. The following table shows the number of fever-cases admitted to the Hospital or attended from the Dispensary in 1827 and in four ordinary years thereafter :

[1] W. J. Geary, M.D., "Report of the St John's Fever and Lock Hospitals." *Dub. Quart. Journ. Med. Sc.* XI. 378 : XII. 94.
[2] Various descriptions of these exist, of which that by Carleton in the tale 'Barney Branagan,' is probably not overdone.
[3] The Report of the Roscrea Fever Hospital for 1827 says : " In March, when the dung is being removed from the back yards for the purpose of planting the potatoes, the number of patients becomes double in the Fever Hospital." *Dublin Medical Press*, Jan. 1846, p. 235.

Limerick:—Table of Hospital Cases of Fever and Cases at their Homes attended from the Dispensary.

	Hospital Cases			Dispensary Cases			
Year	Admitted	Died	Average mortality. One in	Attended	Died	Average mortality. One in	Total
1827	2781	137	20	2800	80	35	5581
1828	854	37	23	960	22	39	1714
1829	506	23	22	640	18	35	1146
1830	806	34	23½	910	25	36	1716
1831	1015	65	15½	920	31	29	1935
Totals	5962	296	20	6130	176	34	12092

From 1831 to 1836 the admissions to hospitals were as follows:

Year	Admitted	Died
1832	1028	57
1833	824	42
1834	906	55
1835	1484	121
1836	3227	235

The last lines show the epidemic increase, which began in the autumn of 1835. It will appear from the following (by Geary) that it was largely an epidemic of young people, and that the fatality was by far the greatest among the comparatively small number of persons attacked at the higher ages—a well-known law of typhus of which this Limerick demonstration was perhaps the first numerically precise:

Table of the Numbers admitted to Limerick Fever Hospital at stated ages of five years, with the deaths, from 6 Jan. 1836 *to* 6 *Jan.* 1837.

Ages in Years	Admitted	Died	Average mortality per cent.	Ages in Years	Admitted	Died	Average mortality per cent.
1—5	81	2	2¼	40—45	70	13	18½
5—10	489	13	2½	45—50	82	22	27
10—15	762	18	2¼	50—55	23	5	21½
15—20	701	37	5¼	55—60	36	12	33¼
20—25	362	22	6	60—65	2	1	50
25—30	304	27	8¾	65—70	10	5	50
30—35	100	12	12	Over 70	2	1	50
35—40	203	45	23¼	Total	3227	235	7¼

One-sixth of these Limerick hospital cases, to the number of 567, came from the county, chiefly from the damp, boggy districts five to sixteen miles from the city. The whole admissions were rather more than the same hospital received in the famine year, 1817. But, although 1836 was not a year of special scarcity, there must have been some cause at work to raise the perennial typhus to the height of an epidemic, not only in Limerick, but in Dublin, Cork, Waterford, Ennis, Belfast, and other towns. In the country, an epidemic outburst during the months of March, April and May, 1836, in the parish of Donoughmore, Donegal, is perhaps only a sample of others unrecorded: it was remarkable in that nine-tenths of the cases of fever had as a sequel large boils on various parts of the body, but principally on the limbs[1].

In Dublin, the influenza of the first months of 1837 seemed to check the prevalence of typhus for a time; but the latter increased greatly when the influenza was over, so that the admissions to the Cork Street Hospital until the end of 1838 nearly equalled those of the worst epidemics since the hospital was opened in 1804[2]. Females in typhus were admitted greatly in excess of males; a large proportion (1847 in two years) were under fifteen years of age; the fever rarely relapsed, so that it was mostly typhus, as in England and Scotland at the same time. In twelve months of the same period (Oct. 1837 to Sept. 1838) there were 1786 admissions for fever at Cork, 1840 at Limerick, and 1706 at Belfast[3].

In Dublin, as in London, Edinburgh and Glasgow, the continued fevers of the "thirties" were distinctively spotted typhus, which was a new constitution. Graves, lecturing at Dublin in November, 1836, said: "We are now at a point of time possessing no common interest for the reflection of medical observers. It is now nearly two years since my attention was first arrested by the appearance of maculated fever, of which the first examples were observed in some hospital cases from the neighbourhood of Kingstown. This form of fever has lasted ever since, prevailing universally, as if it had banished all other forms of fever, and being almost the only type noticed in our wards[4]."

[1] Babington, "Epidemic Typhous Fever in Donoughmore." *Dub. Quart. Journ.* X. 404.
[2] G. A. Kennedy, "Report of Cork St. Fever Hosp. 1837–38." *Ibid.* XIII. 311. Graves, *Ibid.* XIV. 363.
[3] Lynch, *Ibid.* N. S. VII. 388, gives some particulars of it also at Loughrea, Galway, in 1840.
[4] *System of Clinical Medicine.* Dublin, 1843, p. 57. The "change of type," with special reference to treatment, is discussed more fully in Lecture XXXIV. pp. 492–500. See also *Dub. Quart. Journ. Med. Sc.* XIV. 502, where a letter on the changed character of fever at Sligo is cited.

This increase of fever in Ireland, as well as the change in its type, corresponded closely to the great epidemic outburst in Scotland and England. The census of Ireland, taken in June, 1841, for the ten years preceding, gave a somewhat loose return of the causes of death in each year of the decennial period[1].

The worst years for fever were 1837 and 1840, the best year 1841. The deaths from fever in ten years were 112,072, being 1 in 10·59 of the deaths from all causes. The counties with highest fever mortality were Cavan, Mayo, Galway and Clare; the worst towns were Belfast, Kilkenny, Dublin, Limerick and Carrickfergus. Of these deaths from typhus-like fevers, 14,501 occurred in 86 fever-hospitals, which were open, or which kept records, for more or less of the decennial period. The following table shows the proportions of rural, urban and hospital fever-deaths in each of the four provinces:

Deaths from fever in ten years, 1831–41.

	Leinster	Munster	Ulster	Connaught
Rural fever-deaths	16,159	23,718	21,616	19,319
Urban	4,626	4,878	3,183	1,262
Hospital	9,030	5,465	2,439	386
	29,815	34,061	27,238	20,958
Rural population in 1841	1,531,106	2,009,220	2,160,698	1,338,635
Ratio of do. per sq. mile	247	332	406	386

The following detailed table for the province of Leinster shows the enormous preponderance of fever-deaths in the cottages or cabins[2]. Only Dublin and Kilkenny have most of the deaths in their fever hospitals or public institutions; it was not until near the end of this decennial period, the year 1839, that workhouses, with their infirmaries, began to be provided for all the poor-law unions:

---

[1] *The Census of Ireland*, 1841, Parl. Papers, 1843. "Report on the Table of Deaths," by W. R. Wilde. The deaths in the family, with their causes, &c., in each of the previous ten years were entered on the census paper by the head of the family, or by the parish priest for him. These returns were, of course, far from exhaustive or correct.

[2] Graves, *Clinical Medicine*, 1843, p. 46. Remarking on the much greater frequency of fever in Ireland than in England, he says (p. 47): "Nothing can be more remarkable than the facility with which a simple cold (which in England would be perfectly devoid of danger), runs into maculated fever in Ireland, and that, too, under circumstances quite free from even the suspicion of contagion—in truth, except when fever is epidemic, catching cold is its most usual cause."

Fever Mortality in Leinster, 1831–41.

Localities	Deaths from Fever in Hospitals and Public Institutions	Deaths from Fever at home	Total
Carlow County	202	891	1093
Drogheda Town	1	238	239
Dublin County	111	1248	1359
Dublin City	6393	2369	8762
Kildare County	276	1068	1284
Kilkenny County	114	2378	2492
Kilkenny City	487	204	691
King's County	126	1754	1880
Longford County	3	1265	1268
Louth County	1	1201	1202
Meath County	294	2151	2445
Queen's County	84	1763	1847
Westmeath County	54	1550	1604
Wexford County	637	1736	2373
Wicklow County	280	1002	1282
	9063	20,758	29,821

The Great Famine and Epidemic Sicknesses of 1846–49.

The great epidemic of relapsing fever, typhus, dysentery, anasarca and purpura, which arose in Ireland in the end of 1846 or spring of 1847 and lasted until the beginning of 1849, had for its direct antecedents the more or less complete loss of the potato-crop through blight in two successive autumns, 1845 and 1846, while the state of distress and sickness was prolonged by the potato disease in 1847 and 1848[1]. The potato-blight, which caused so much alarm in Ireland for the first time in September, 1845, had been seen in Germany several years before, in Belgium in 1842, in Canada in 1844, and in England about the 19th of August, 1845. Shortly after the last date, it attacked the Irish potato-fields, first in Wexford, and before the end of the year it was estimated that one-third to one-half of the yield, which was a fifth larger than usual from the greater breadth planted and the abundant crop, was lost by absolute rottenness or unfitness for food, the process of decay being of a kind to make great progress after the tubers were pitted. The loss to Ireland was estimated at about one pound sterling per head of the population. Sir Robert Peel was keenly alive to the magnitude of the calamity which threatened the Irish

[1] The principal work on the general circumstances of the Irish famine of 1846–47 is *The History of the Great Irish Famine of* 1847, *with notices of Earlier Irish Famines*. By Rev. John O'Rourke, P.P., M.R.I.A. Dublin, 1875.

peasantry. His first step was to summon to his aid a botanist, Dr Lindley, and a chemist, Dr Playfair; the latter went down to Drayton Manor, and joined the prime minister in examining samples of the diseased potatoes. The question was whether some chemical process could not be found to arrest the decay of the tubers. Sir Robert Peel, in a much talked-of address at the opening of the Tamworth Reading-Room in the winter of 1840, had hailed the rising sun of science and useful knowledge. It was only in reference to morals and religion that Peel's deliverance called forth criticism, more particularly the memorable series of letters to the *Times* by John Henry Newman. But one of Newman's gibes was in a manner prophetic of Peel's attitude in approaching the material distress of Ireland: "Let us, in consistency, take chemists for our cooks, and mineralogists for our masons." The two professors proceeded to Ireland, but could only confirm the fact, already known, that one-third, or one-half, of the potato-crop would be lost.

Botany and chemistry being powerless to stay the effects of the potato-blight, the appeal was next to economics. Ireland produced not only potatoes but also corn. But for the most part the cottiers and cottagers tasted little of the oats or wheat which they grew; as soon as the harvest was gathered, the corn was sold to pay the November rents, and was exported. Ireland was still in the paradoxical condition which Bishop Berkeley puzzled over a hundred years before: "whether our exports do not consist of such necessaries as other countries cannot well be without?" The industry and trade of Irish ports was largely that of corn-milling and shipping of oatmeal, flour and other produce; thus Skibbereen in the extreme south-west, where the horrors of famine were felt first, had several flour-mills and a considerable export trade in corn, meal, flour and provisions. The Irish corn harvest of 1845 had been abundant: O'Connell cited the *Mark Lane Express* for the fact that 16,000 quarters of oats from Ireland had arrived in the Thames in a single week of October; on the 23rd of the same month the parish priest of Kells saw fifty dray-loads of oatmeal on the road to Drogheda for shipment. Ireland paid its rent to absentee landlords in corn and butter, just as a century before it had paid it largely in barrelled beef, keeping little for its own use besides potatoes and milk. In the face of the potato famine, the measure approved by the Irish leaders of all parties, O'Connell and

Smith O'Brien as well as ducal proprietors, was to keep some of the oatmeal at home. A committee which sat at the Dublin Mansion House were of opinion, on 19 November, 1845, that the quantity of oats already exported of that harvest would have sufficed to feed the entire population of Ireland. O'Connell's plan was to raise a million and a half on the annual revenue of the Irish woods and forests (£74,000), and to impose a tax on landlords, both absentee and resident, and with the moneys so obtained to buy up what remained of the Irish corn harvest for use at home. In the ensuing session of Parliament, both he and Smith O'Brien protested that Ireland had no need of English doles, having resources of her own if the landlords were compelled to do their duty.

About the same time Lord John Russell, leader of the Opposition, was led by the danger of famine in Ireland to pronounce for the repeal of the Corn Laws of 1815; and at the meetings of the Cabinet in December, Peel urged the same policy upon his colleagues for the same reason. The political history does not concern us beyond the fact that the threatened Irish distress caused by the first partial potato-blight of 1845 was the occasion of the Corn and Customs Act of June, 1846, by which the Corn Laws were repealed, and that an Irish Coercion Bill, brought in on account of outrages following an unusual number of evictions, was made the occasion of turning out Peel's ministry at the moment of its Free Trade victory, by a combination of Tory protectionists, Whigs and Irish patriots.

The direct effects of the potato-blight of 1845 were not so serious as had been expected. The Government quietly bought Indian meal (maize flour) in America without disturbing the market, and had it distributed from twenty principal food-depots in Ireland, to the amount of 11,503 tons, along with 528 tons of oatmeal. This governmental action ceased on the 15th of August, 1846, by which time £733,372 had been spent, £368,000 being loans and the rest grants. The people were set to road-making, so as to pay by labour for their food, the number employed reaching a maximum of 97,000 in August. The Government, having been led by physicians in Dublin to expect an epidemic of fever, passed a Fever Act in March, 1846, by which a Board of Health was constituted. But no notable increase of sickness took place, and the Board was dissolved. There was a small outbreak of dysentery and diarrhoea at Kilkenny (and possibly elsewhere) in the spring of 1846, which the physician to the workhouse set down to the use of the Indian meal "and other substitutes for potatoes[1]."

It was the total loss of the potato crop in the summer and autumn following, 1846, together with a failure of the harvest in England and in other countries of Northern Europe, that brought the real Irish distress. A large breadth of potatoes had been planted as usual, but doubtless with a good deal of the seed tainted. An ordinary crop would have been worth, according to one estimate, sixteen millions sterling, according to another, twice as much. The crop was a total loss. The fields looked well in the summer, but those who dug the early potatoes found them unusually small. About the beginning of August the blight began suddenly and spread swiftly. A letter of the celebrated Father Mathew, the temperance reformer, brings this out:

"On the 29th of last month (July) I passed from Cork to Dublin, and this doomed plant bloomed in all the luxuriance of an abundant harvest. Returning on the 3rd instant (August) I beheld with sorrow one wide waste of putrefying vegetation. In many places the wretched people were seated on the fences of the decaying gardens wringing their hands and wailing bitterly the destruction that had left them foodless[2]."

The relief-works and distribution of Indian meal, which had been estimated by the Government to last only to August, 1846, at a cost of £476,000 (one-half of it being a free grant), were resumed under the pressure of public opinion, in the winter of 1846 and spring of 1847, at a cost of £4,850,000, one-half of the sum being again a free grant. Before the distress was over, other free grants and advances were made; so that, on 15 February, 1850, Lord John Russell summed up the famine-indebtedness of Ireland to the Consolidated Fund at £3,350,000, (which was to be repaid out of the rates in forty years from that date). Allowing an equal sum freely gifted from the national exchequer, the whole public cost of the famine would have been about seven millions sterling.

The short crops in Britain in 1846 were an excuse for not interfering with the export of oats from Ireland. The imports of Indian meal were left to the ordinary course of the market, and the distribution to retail traders. The corn merchants of Cork, Limerick and other ports made fortunes out of the

[1] Joseph Lalor, M.D., *Dub. Quart. Journ. Med. Sc.* N. S. III. 38.
[2] Cited by O'Rourke, p. 152.

American cargoes, and the dealers throughout the country made large profits.

To encourage the influx of foreign food-supplies, and to lower freights, the Navigation Laws were suspended for a few months, so that corn could be carried in other than British bottoms. When Parliament met in January, 1847, the distress in Ireland occupied the greater part of the Queen's Speech.

Lord George Bentinck proposed that sixteen millions should be advanced for the construction of railroads, so as to give employment and wages to the starving multitudes. The Government, however, objected that such relief would operate at too great a distance, in most cases, from the homes of the people; and it was urged by independent critics that a State loan for railways would really be for the relief of the landlords more than of the peasantry. The large sums actually voted were spent in road-making and in procuring food and medical relief. A Board of Works directed the relief-works. A Commissariat, with two thousand Relief Committees under it, directed the distribution of food. A Board of Health provided temporary fever-hospitals and additional physicians. It was not to be expected that this machinery would work well, and, in fact, the public relief was costly in its administration and often misdirected in its objects. Private charities, especially that of the Society of Friends, gave invaluable help, money being subscribed by all classes at home and sent from distant countries, including a thousand pounds from the Sultan of Turkey. On one day, the third of July, 1847, nearly three millions in Ireland received food gratuitously from the hands of the relieving officers. In March, 1847, the public works were employing 734,000. The number relieved out of the poor rates at one time reached 800,000. Workhouses were enlarged, and temporary fever-hospitals were built to the number of 207, which in the two years 1847 and 1848, received 279,723 patients.

Emigration to the United States and Canada, which had averaged 61,242 persons per annum from the last half of 1841 to the end of 1845, rose steadily all through the famine until it reached a total of 214,425 in the year 1849, the passage money to the amount of millions sterling having come largely from the savings of the Irish already settled in the New World.

The grand effect of the famine upon the population of Ireland was revealed by the census of 1851. The people in 1841

had numbered 8,175,124; in 1851 they numbered 6,515,794.
The decrease was 28·6 per cent. in Connaught, 23·5 per cent. in
Munster, 16 per cent. in Ulster, and 15·5 per cent. in Leinster.
In many remote parishes the number of inhabitants, and of
cabins, fell to nearly a half. The depopulation was wholly
rural, so much so that there was a positive increase of inhabitants
not only in the large county towns, but even in small towns
such as Skull and Kanturk, situated in Poor Law unions where
the famine and epidemics had made the greatest clearances all
over[1]. Our business here is with the epidemical maladies, which
contributed to this depopulation ; but a few words remain to be
said on the subject at large.

Malthus had been prophetic about this crisis in the history of
Ireland.   Criticizing Arthur Young's project to encourage the
use of potatoes and milk as the staple food of the English
labourer instead of wheat, so as to escape the troubles of
scarcity and high prices of corn, Malthus says:

"When, from the increasing population, and diminishing sources of
subsistence, the average growth of potatoes was not more than the average
consumption, a scarcity of potatoes would be, in every respect, as probable
as a scarcity of wheat at present; and when it did arrive it would be beyond

---

[1] *The Census of Ireland*, 1851.   Part V.   Table of deaths, vol. I.   Dublin, 1856,
p. 235.
The following are a few instances of depopulation between 1841 and 1851.

              Union of Loughrea, Co. Galway.
                  1841   65,636
                  1851   38,698
              Union of Clonakilty, Co. Cork.
                  1841   52,185
                  1851   31,473
              Union of Kanturk, Co. Cork.
                  1841   61,238
                  1851   41,801
              Parish of Kanturk.
                  1841   4,096
                  1851   6,754
              Union of Portumna, Co. Galway.
                  1841   30,714
                  1851   19,747
              Union of Skibbereen, Co. Cork.
                  1841   57,439
                  1851   37,283
              Parish of Skibbereen.
                  1841   9,557
                  1851   8,931
              Union of Skull, Co. Cork.
                  1841   26,620
                  1851   16,866
              Parish of Skull.
                  1841   2,895
                  1851   3,226

all comparison more dreadful. When the common people of a country live principally upon the dearest grain, as they do in England on wheat, they have great resources in scarcity; and barley, oats, rice, cheap soups and potatoes, all present themselves as less expensive, yet at the same time wholesome means of nourishment; but when their habitual food is the lowest in this scale, they appear to be absolutely without resource, except in the bark of trees, like the poor Swedes; and a great portion of them must necessarily be starved[1]."

The forecast of Malthus was repeated in his own way by Cobbett, although neither of them foresaw the potato-blight as the means.

"The dirty weed," said Cobbett in a conversation in 1834, "will be the curse of Ireland. The potato will not last twenty years more. It will work itself out; and then you will see to what a state Ireland will be reduced... You must return to the grain crops; and then Ireland, instead of being the most degraded, will become one of the finest countries in the world. You may live to see my words prove true; but I never shall[2]."

This is what has come to pass in a measure, and will come to pass more and more. Only in some remote parts do the Irish cottiers now live upon potatoes and milk. It has come to be quite common for them to grow an Irish half acre of wheat, and, what is more to the purpose, to consume what they thus produce instead of selling it to pay the rent. Doubtless the enormous imports of American, Australian and Black Sea wheat have made it easier for the Irish to have wheaten bread. But, whatever the reason, they have at length adopted the ancient English staff of life, a staple or standard which they were in a fair way to have achieved long ago, had not their addiction to "lost causes and impossible loyalties" given an unfavourable turn to the natural progress of the nation[3].

We come at length to the purely medical side of the great famine of 1846–47[4]. The distress in the latter part of the year

[1] *Essay on the Principle of Population.* Bk. IV. chap. XI. Thorold Rogers has in many passages emphasized the advantages of the English practice from medieval times of living on the dearest kind of corn; but he seems to have overlooked the priority of Malthus throughout the whole of the eleventh chapter of his fourth book. In *Six Centuries of Work and Wages* (p. 62), Rogers says: "Hence a high standard of subsistence is a more important factor in the theory of population than any of those checks which Malthus has enumerated."
[2] Cited in Thomas Doubleday's *Political Life of Sir Robert Peel.* London, 1856, II. 398 *note.*
[3] It is a doctrine of economics that the higher standard of living checks population. Thus Marshall says of England: "The growth of population was checked by that rise in the standard of comfort which took effect in the general adoption of wheat as the staple food of Englishmen during the first half of the 18th century." *Economics,* p. 230.
[4] Vol. VII. (1849) pp. 64–126, 340–404, and Vol. VIII. pp. 1–86, 270–339 of the *Dublin Quart. Journ. of Medical Science,* N.S. contain numerous reports collected

1846 was felt first in the west and south-west—in the districts to which the famine of 1822 had been almost confined. It happened that the state of matters around Skibbereen, the extreme south-western point of Ireland, was brought most under public notice; but it is believed that there were parts of the western sea-board counties of Mayo, Galway, Clare and Kerry from which equally terrible scenes might have been reported at an equally early period. It was in Clare that relief at the national charges was longest needed.

Dr Popham, one of the visiting physicians to the Cork Workhouse, wrote as follows:

"The pressure from without upon the city began to be felt in October [1846], and in November and December the influx of paupers from all parts of this vast county was so overwhelming that, to prevent them from dying in the streets, the doors of the workhouse were thrown open, and in one week 500 persons were admitted, without any provision, either of space or clothing, to meet so fearful an emergency. All these were suffering from famine, and most of them from malignant dysentery or fever. The fever was in the first instance undoubtedly confined to persons badly fed or crowded into unwholesome habitations; and as it originated with the vast migratory hordes of labourers and their families congregated upon the public roads, it was commonly termed 'the road fever'[1]."

It was the same in the smaller towns of the county, such as Skibbereen; in the month of December, 1846, there were one hundred and forty deaths in the workhouse; on one day there were fifteen funerals waiting their turn for the religious offices. Still farther afield, in the country parishes, the state of matters was the same. The sea-board parish of Skull was a typical poor district, populous with cabins along the numerous bays of the Atlantic, but with few residential seats of the gentry. On the 2nd of February, 1847, the parish clergyman, the Rev. Traill Hall (himself at length a victim to the contagion), wrote as follows:

"Frightful and fearful is the havock around me. Our medical friend, Dr Sweetman, a gentleman of unimpeachable veracity, informed me yesterday that if he stated the mortality of my parish at an average of thirty-five daily, he would be within the truth. The children in particular, he remarked, were disappearing with awful rapidity. And to this I may add the aged, who, with the young—neglected, perhaps, amidst the wide-spread destitution—are almost without exception swollen and ripening for the grave[2]."

by the editors from all parts of Ireland, and published either in abstract or in full. These are the chief medical sources. Some particulars are given also in the *Dublin Med. Press*, 1846 to 1849 in several papers on dysentery.

[1] John Popham, M.D., *Dub. Quart. Journ. Med. Sc.* N.S. VIII. 279.
[2] Cited by Dr Jones Lamprey, *Dub. Quart. Journ.* VII. 101.

They were "swollen" by the anasarca or general dropsy, which was reported from nearly all parts of Ireland as being, along with dysentery and diarrhoea, the prevalent kind of sickness before the epidemic fever became general in the spring of 1847. The same had been remarked as the precursor of the fever of 1817–18. In the end of March, Dr Jones Lamprey, sent by the Board of Health, found the parish of Skull "in a frightful state of famine, dysentery and fever." Dysentery had been by far more prevalent than fever in this district, as in many others. "It was easily known," says Dr Lamprey, "if any of the inmates in the cabins of the poor were suffering from this disease, as the ground in such places was usually found marked with clots of blood." The malady was most inveterate and often fatal. It must have had a contagious property, for the physician himself went through an attack of it[1].

In the Skibbereen district the dead were sometimes buried near their cabins; at the town itself many were carried out in a shell and laid without coffins in a large pit[2]. Along the coast of Connemara for thirty miles there was no town, but only small villages and hundreds of detached cabins; this district is said to have been almost depopulated[3].

Besides the dysentery and dropsy, which caused most of the mortality in the winter of 1846–47, another early effect of the famine was scurvy, a disease rarely seen in Ireland and unknown to most of the medical men. It was by no means general, but undoubtedly true scurvy did occur in some parts: thus in the Ballinrobe district, county Mayo[4], it was very prevalent in 1846 for some months before the epidemic fever appeared, being "evidenced by the purple hue of the gums, with ulceration along their upper thin margin, bleeding on the slightest touch, and deep sloughing ulcers of the inside of the fauces, with intolerable foetor"—affecting men, women, and children. In some places, as at Kilkenny early in 1846, there was much purpura[5]. These earlier effects of the famine (dysentery and diarrhoea, dropsy, scurvy and purpura), were seen in varying degrees before the end of 1846 in most parts of Ireland. The counties least touched by them were in Leinster and Ulster,

---

[1] Lamprey, *Dub. Quart. Journ.* VII. 101.
[2] O'Rourke.　　　　　　　　[3] Ormsbey, *Dub. Quart. Journ.* VII. 382.
[4] Pemberton, *ibid.* VII. 369.
[5] Lalor, u. s.

such as Down, Derry, Tyrone, Fermanagh and some others, where the peasantry lived upon oatmeal as well as on potatoes. But even these were invaded by the ensuing epidemic of fever, the only place in all Ireland which is reported to have escaped both the primary and the secondary effects of the famine having been Rostrevor, on the coast of Down, a watering-place with a rich population, which was also one of the very small number of localities that escaped in 1817–18.

According to the following samples of admissions to the Fever Hospital of Ennis in the several months, the summers were the season of greatest sickness, a fact which was noted also in the epidemic of 1817–18:

Year	Month	Patients	Year	Month	Patients
1846	November	93	1848	February	210
„	December	224	„	May	705
1847	June	757	„	November	400

The almost uniform report of medical men was that the epidemic of fever began in 1847, in the spring months in most places, in the summer in others. Relapsing fever was the common type. It was usually called the famine fever for the reason that it was constantly seen to arise in persons "recovering from famine," on receiving food from the Relief Committees[1]. It was a mild or "short" fever, apt to leave weakness, but rarely fatal. Dr Dillon, of Castlebar, reports that he would be told by the head of a family: "We have been *three times down* in the fever, and have all, thank God, got through it." Dr Starkey, of Newry, "knew many families, living in wretched poverty on the mountains near the town, who were attacked with fever, and who without any medical attendance, and but little attendance of any kind, passed through the fever without a single death." The doctor of Bryansford and Castlewellan, county Down, (where there was no famine), declared that the recoveries of the poor in their own cottages destitute of almost every comfort, were astonishing. In the Skibbereen district, Dr Lamprey was "often struck with the rarity of the ordinary types of fever among the thousands suffering from starvation." In some of the most famine-stricken places, such as the islands off the coast

---

[1] This epidemic called forth two pamphlets on the relation of famine to fever, one by Dominic Corrigan, M.D., *On Famine and Fever as Cause and Effect in Ireland* ("no famine, no fever"), and a reply to it by H. Kennedy, M.D., *On the Connexion of Famine and Fever.*

of Mayo and Galway, and in Gweedore, Donegal, not more than one in a hundred cases of relapsing fever proved fatal. In Limerick the mortality was "very small." In many places it is given at three in the hundred cases, in some places as high as six in the hundred. When deaths occurred, they were often sudden and unexpected,—more probable in the relapse than in the first onset. At Clonmel it was remarked that a certain blueness of the nose presaged death; in Fermanagh it was called the Black Fever, from the duskiness of the face. The report from Ballinrobe, Mayo, says that it was attended by rheumatic pains, which caused the patients to cry out when they stirred in bed[1]. It was mostly a fever of the first half of life, and more of the female sex than of the male. One says that it was commonest from five to fifteen years of age, another from ten to thirty years.

Relapsing fever was the most common fever of the famine years, in the cabins, workhouses and fever hospitals, in the country districts as well as the towns and cities. Dr Henry Kennedy says of Dublin: "Cases of genuine typhus were through the whole epidemic very rare, I mean comparatively speaking." But everywhere there was a certain admixture of typhus, and in some not unusual circumstances the typhus was peculiarly malignant or fatal—many times more fatal than the relapsing fever. The poor themselves do not appear to have suffered much from the more malignant typhus, unless in the gaols and workhouses. When the doors of the Cork workhouse were thrown open in December, 1846, five hundred were admitted pell mell in one week; the deaths in that workhouse were 757 in the month of March, 1847, and 3329 in the whole year. In the Ballinrobe workhouse, county Mayo, "men, women and children were huddled together in the same rooms (the probationary wards), eating, drinking, cooking, and sleeping in the same apartment in their clothes, without even straw to lie on or a blanket to cover them." Typhus at length appeared in that workhouse, said to have been brought in by a strolling beggar, and the physician, the master and the clerk died of it. Wherever the better-off classes caught fever, it was not relapsing but typhus, and a very fatal typhus. At Skibbereen the relapsing fever "was not propagated by contagion; but in persons so

---

[1] Pains resembling those of rheumatism were common in the fever of 1817–18 at Limerick. Barker and Cheyne, I. 432.

affected, when brought in contact with the more wealthy and better fed individuals, was capable of imparting fevers of different types[1]." There were many opportunities for such contact—in serving out food at the depôts, in superintending the gangs working on the roads, in attending the sessions, in visiting the sick. The crowds suffering from starvation, famine-fever or dysentery exhaled the most offensive smells, the smell of the relapsing fever and the anasarca being peculiar or distinguishable[2]. There appeared to be a scale of malignity in the fevers in an inverted order of the degree of misery. The most wretched had the mildest fever, the artizan class or cottagers had typhus fatal in the usual proportion, the classes living in comfort had typhus of a very fatal kind. This experience, however strange it may seem, was reported by medical observers everywhere with remarkable unanimity. One says that six or seven of the rich died in every ten attacks, others say one in three. Forty-eight medical men died in 1847 in Munster, most of them from fever; in Cavan county, seven medical men died of fever in twelve months, and three more had a narrow escape of death: two of the three physicians sent by the Board of Health to the coast of Connemara died of fever[3]. Many Catholic priests died as well as some of the Established Church clergy; and there were numerous fatalities in the families of the resident gentry, and among others who administered the relief. Yet a case of fever in a good house did not become a focus of contagion; the contagion came from direct contact with the crowds of starving poor, their clothes ragged and filthy, their bodies unwashed, and many of them suffering from dysentery. The greater fatality of fever among the richer classes had been a commonplace in Ireland since the epidemic of 1799–1801, and is remarked by the best writers[4]. At Loughrea, in Galway, Dr Lynch observed that "in the year 1840 the type of fever was very bad indeed, and

---

[1] Lamprey, u. s.

[2] Dr Kelly of Mullingar compared the smell of relapsing fever to that of burning musty straw. *Dub. Quart. Journ. Med.*, Aug. 1863, p. 341.

[3] Cusack and Stokes, *ibid.* IV. 134.

[4] Barker and Cheyne, Harty, and Rogan have been cited to this effect for earlier epidemics. Graves (*Clin. Med.* pp. 59–60) says: "In the epidemics of 1816, 1817, 1818 and 1819, it was found by accurate computation that the rate of mortality was much higher among the rich than among the poor. This was a startling fact, and a thousand different explanations of it were given at the time." He cites Fletcher (*Pathology*, p. 27) an Edinburgh observer, as follows: "The rich are less frequently affected with epidemic fevers than the poor, but more frequently die of them. Good fare keeps off diseases, but increases their mortality when they take place."

very many of the gentry were cut off by it." He reckoned that ordinarily one in six cases of fever among the richer class proved fatal, one in fifteen among the poor[1]. But in the great famine, six years after, the fever of the poor assumed the still milder type of relapsing, fatal perhaps to one in a hundred cases, or three in a hundred, while the fever which contact with them gave to those at the other extreme of well-being became a peculiarly malignant typhus, fatal to six or seven in ten cases, as Dr Pemberton of Ballinrobe found, or to three or four in ten cases, as many others found. Of course it was the peasantry who made up by far the greater part of the mortality in the years of famine; but they were cut off by various maladies, nondescript or definite, while the richer classes died, in connexion with the famine, of contagious typhus and here or there of contagious dysentery.

Even in the crowded workhouses and gaols, more deaths occurred from dysentery than from fever. But in some of the gaols great epidemics arose which cut off many of the poor by malignant infection. That was an old experience of the gaols, studied best in England in the 18th century; the worst fevers, or those most rapidly fatal, were caught by the prisoners newly brought to mix with others long habituated to their miserable condition. The gaols in Ireland during the famine were crowded to excess, not so much because the people gave way to lawlessness—their patience and obedience were matters of common complimentary remark—but because they committed petty thefts, broke windows, or the like, in order to obtain the shelter and rations of prisoners. The mortality in the gaols rose and fell as follows[2]:

Year	Deaths in gaol		Year	Deaths in gaol
1846	130		1849	1406
1847	1320		1850	692
1848	1292		1851	197

Most of the deaths in these larger totals came from two or three great prison epidemics in each of the series of years—at Tralee, Carrick-on-Shannon, Castlebar and Cork in 1847, at Galway in 1848, at Clonmel, Limerick, Cork and Galway in 1849, the highest mortality being 485 deaths in Galway county gaol in 1848. Descriptions remain of the state of the gaols at Tralee

---

[1] *Dub. Quart. Journ. Med. Sc.* N.S. VII. 388.
[2] *Census of Ireland,* 1851.

and Castlebar in 1847, from which it appears that they were frightfully overcrowded and filthy. Dr Dillon, of Castlebar, says that the county gaol there in March, 1847, had twice as many prisoners as it was built for, "those committed being in a state of nudity, filth and starvation." He expected an outbreak of typhus, and applied to the magistrates to increase the accommodation, which they declined to do. In due time, very bad maculated typhus broke out, of which the chaplain, matron and others of the staff died. This contagious fever is said to have proved fatal to forty per cent. of those attacked by it. The deaths for the year are returned at 83 in Castlebar gaol, those in Tralee gaol at 101, and in the gaol of Carrick-on-Shannon at 100.

No exact statistical details of the mortality in the great Irish famine of 1846–49 were kept. Ireland had then no systematic registration of deaths and of the causes of death, such as had existed in England since 1837. Information as to the mortality was got retrospectively once in ten years by means of the census, heads of families being required to fill in all the deaths, with causes, ages, years, seasons, &c., of the same, that had occurred in their families within the previous decennial period. This was, of course, a very untrustworthy method, more especially so for the famine years, when many thousands of families emigrated, leaving hardly a trace behind, many hamlets were wholly abandoned, and many parishes stripped of nearly half their inhabited houses. When a certain day in the year 1851 came round for the census papers to be filled up, a fourth part of the people were gone, and that fourth could have told more about the famine and the deaths than an equal number of those that remained. However, the Census Commissioners did their best with the defective, loose or erroneous data at their service. Much of the interest of the Irish Census of 1851 centered, indeed, in the Great Famine; and the two volumes of specially medical information compiled by Sir William Wilde, making Part V. of the Census Report, are a store of facts, statistical and historical, of which only a few can be given here[1].

---

[1] *The Census of Ireland of* 1851. Part V. Table of Deaths. 2 vols. Dublin, 1856. Upwards of two hundred pages are occupied with a chronological "Table of Cosmical Phenomena, Epizootics, Epiphitics, Famines and Pestilences in Ireland" from the earliest times. This retrospect, which is very replete but tedious and uncritical, is followed by a summary report of twenty pages on "The Last General Potato Failure, and the Great Famine and Pestilence of 1845-50," and by a long series of tabulated extracts from contemporary writings on all matters relating to the famine.

*Table of Workhouses and Auxiliary Workhouses in Ireland
during the Famine.*

Year	No. of Workhouses	Numbers relieved	Numbers that died	Ratio of deaths One in
1846	129	250,822	14,662	17·11
1847	130	332,140	66,890	6·92
1848	131	610,463	45,482	13·4
1849	131	932,284	64,440	14·47
1850	163	805,702	46,721	17·74

During the ten years from 6 June, 1841, to 30 March, 1851, the deaths from the principal infective or "zymotic" diseases in the workhouses were as follows:

Dysentery	50,019	Measles	8,943
Diarrhoea	20,507	Cholera	6,716
Fevers	34,644	Smallpox	5,016

Besides the workhouses, there were during the famine 227 temporary fever hospitals, which received 450,807 persons from the beginning of 1847 to the end of 1850, of whom 47,302 died.

According to the Census returns, the deaths from the several causes connected with the famine were as follows in the respective years:

Year	Fever	Dysentery (with Diarrhoea)	Starvation
1845	7,249	—	—
1846	17,145	5,492	2,041
1847	57,095	25,757	6,058
1848	45,948	25,694[1]	} 9,395
1849	39,316	29,446[2]	
1850	23,545	19,224	—

According to this table, fever caused more deaths than dysentery. But there are reasons for thinking that the deaths from dysentery, anasarca and other slow effects of famine and bad food really made up more of the extra mortality of the famine-years than the sharp fever itself. In the returns from the workhouses, dysentery is actually credited with about one-half more deaths than fever. It is known that most of the mortality at the beginning of the famine, the winter of 1846–47, was from dysentery and allied chronic forms of sickness. Dysentery also followed the decline of the relapsing-fever epidemic of 1847–48. Dillon, of Castlebar, says that many, who had gone through the fever in the autumn of 1847, fell into dysentery in 1848, during which year it was very prevalent.

---

[1] Of this total, 18,430 deaths were from dysentery and 7,264 from diarrhoea.

[2] The increase in 1849 was doubtless owing to choleraic diarrhoea during the epidemic of Asiatic cholera, the deaths from dysentery being one-half of the total.

Mayne says that dysentery often attacked those recovering from fever, and proved fatal to them[1]. In the General Hospital of Belfast the fatality of fever-cases was 1 in 8, "but this included dysentery." Probably the same explanation should be given of the high rates of fatality in the Fever Hospital of Ennis, the chief centre of relief for the greatly distressed county of Clare: 1846, 1 in 12½; 1847, 1 in 5¾; 1848, 1 in 5½.

It will be noticed that some thousands of deaths were put down to starvation in the Census returns. Perhaps a more technical nosological term might have been found for a good many of these, such as anasarca or general dropsy. But even if physicians had made the returns, instead of the priests or relatives, they would have put many into a nondescript class, for which starvation was a sufficiently correct generic name. Scurvy was another disease of malnutrition which was far from rare during the famine; the deaths actually set down to that cause were some hundreds over the whole period.

The deaths from all causes in the decennial period covered by the Census of 1851 were 985,366. But these returns were made, as we have seen, on a population which had been reduced by a fourth part in the course of ten years, so that they fall considerably short of the reality. If the population of Ireland had multiplied at the same rate as that of England and Wales from 1841 to 1851, namely, 1·0036 per cent. per annum, it should have been 9,018,799 in the year 1851; but it was only 6,552,385. Emigration beyond the United Kingdom had averaged 61,242 persons per annum from the 30th of June, 1841, to the 31st December, 1845; next year, 1846, it rose to 105,955, in 1847 it was "more than doubled," in 1848 it was 178,159, in 1849, 214,425, in 1850 it was 209,054, and in 1851 it touched the maximum, 249,721. Nearly a million emigrated in the six years preceding the date of the Census, and there was besides a considerable migration to Liverpool, Glasgow, London and other towns of England and Scotland. It is probable that emigration accounts for two-thirds of the decrease of inhabitants revealed by the Census of 1851; but the extra mortality of the famine years, or the deaths over and above the ordinary deaths in Ireland during a decennial period, can hardly be estimated below half a million.

---

[1] R. Mayne, M.D., "Observations on the late Epidemic Dysentery in Dublin." *Dub. Quart. Journ. Med. Sc.* VII. 294. See also papers in *Dubl. Med. Press*, 1849.

Decrease of Typhus and Dysentery after 1849.

The potato famines of 1845–48 were a turning-point in the history of Ireland. From that time the population has steadily declined and the well-being of the people steadily improved. By the Census of 1871 the population was 5,386,708, by that of 1881 it was 5,144,983, by that of 1891 it was 4,704,750. Registration of births and deaths, which began in 1864, shows the following samples:

Year	Births	Deaths
1867	144,318	98,911
1871	151,665	88,720
1880	128,010	102,955
1888	109,557	85,892

The enormous amount of pauperism which followed the great famine was at length brought within limits: from 1866 to the present time it has been marked by a steady increase of out-door relief, and by some increase in the numbers within the Union Workhouses; the out-door paupers have increased from 10,163 on 1 Jan., 1866, to 53,638 on 1 Jan., 1881, the absolute number of indoor paupers having remained, on an average of good and bad years, somewhat steady in a declining population.

The public health has been undisturbed by great epidemics since the potato famine, although the effects of that calamity did not wholly cease until some years after. It is best estimated by the mean annual average of deaths among a thousand inhabitants, a ratio which has been low for the provinces of Connaught and Munster, and not excessive for the provinces of Ulster and Leinster. The following tables are of the death rates in two sample years, 1880 and 1889 respectively[1]:

	1880	1889
Connaught	15·3	12·4
Munster	19·5	15·1
Ulster	20·0	16·8
Leinster	23·3	18·3

Four healthiest counties:

1880		1889	
Mayo	14·5	Galway	11·8
Sligo	15·3	Kerry	12·1
Galway	15·6	Leitrim	12·1
Roscommon	15·8	Cavan	12·2

[1] 17th and 26th Reports of the Regr.-Genl. Ireland.

Four unhealthiest counties :

1880		1889	
Dublin co.	31·7	Dublin co.	24·5
Waterford co.	24·9	Antrim	21·2
Louth	22·6	Down	18·6
Antrim	21·9	Armagh	17·0

The higher death rates of some counties are chiefly owing to their greater urban populations. The health of the cottier districts is remarkably good, and is rarely if ever disturbed by any *morbus miseriae*. The cabins, except in a few remote parts, are more comfortable than they used to be, the diet is better, the clothing is better, the education of the children is better. The present happier lot of the Irish peasantry can be measured not unfairly by the statistics showing the decrease in the number of cabins of the lowest class, and the increase of dwellings in the higher classes.

The history of fever and dysentery in Ireland subsequently to the great epidemics of 1846–49 has few salient points. Dysentery, the old "country disease," has steadily declined to about a hundred deaths in the year, while the considerable mortality from diarrhoea, nearly two thousand deaths in a year, is nearly all from the cholera infantum or summer diarrhoea of children in the large towns. The history of the continued fevers is made complex by the modern identification of typhoid or enteric fever. According to the testimonies of several, it played but a small part in the epidemics of 1846–49, even in Dublin itself[1], and it can hardly be doubted that its recent increase in that city is not apparent but real. The following table from the year 1880 to the present time will show how the deaths from continued fever are now divided in the registration returns :

Year	Typhus	Simple continued	Enteric
1880	934	1073	1087
1881	859	774	813
1882	744	657	844
1883	810	593	853
1884	628	572	693
1885	505	443	716
1886	394	380	772
1887	405	385	740
1888	362	330	741
1889	359	250	968
1890	391	231	855
1891	266	183	859
1892	268	210	714

[1] Review of Murchison in *Dub. Quart. Journ. Med. Sc.*, Aug. and Nov. 1863,

This decline of typhus in a country where for many generations it seemed to be a national malady is a remarkable testimony to the influence of the changed conditions which have made typhus rare everywhere.

There are some interesting points in connexion with Irish typhus since 1849. After the subsidence of the great epidemic of relapsing and typhus fevers (1847–49), says Dr Dennis O'Connor, of Cork, "intermittent fever made its appearance, and, as long as it lasted, scarcely a case of continued fever was seen. As soon as the last cases of intermittent disappeared, the present epidemic broke out (1864–65), and still rages with much severity. This alternation of continued and intermittent fever is remarkable. Indeed it might have been observed that the fever of 1847 passed first into a remittent form, and gradually into the intermittent which prevailed more or less for ten years subsequently[1]." The same succession of relapsing fever by intermittent fever was observed after the epidemic of 1826 by Dr John O'Brien, of Dublin[2]. The epidemic of fever which Dr O'Connor describes for Cork in 1864–65, appeared in Dublin about the same time—the latter half of 1864. It was of the nature of typhus in both cities, cerebro-spinal in part, but probably not typhoid[3]. At Cork it had some peculiarities—a croupous-like exudation on the tongue, resembling thrush in the mouth, and a dark mottled rash (rubeola nigra), or fiery red spots on a dark red ill-defined base. "The true typhoid rash has been seen but seldom, and the petechiae of genuine typhus, so frequent in former epidemics, have been equally rare. The latter I attribute to the improved condition of our poor in good clothing and the ventilation of their dwellings." The intellect was little disturbed in this fever, there was usually a crisis about the fourteenth day, and there were no relapses. The sequelae were peculiar—"great nervous debility, leading to a semi-paralysed state of the limbs," congestion of the lungs, sometimes solidification, or gangrene or suppuration of them. It occurred at a time "when the food of the people is most abundant and of the best quality." There

pp. 169 and 339: "We are able, from extensive opportunities of observing the epidemic [of 1846–48] in Dublin, to verify the statement of Dr H. Kennedy as to the infrequency of enteric fever."

[1] *Dub. Quart. Journ. Med. Sc.* Nov. 1865, p. 285.

[2] See p. 273, *supra.*

[3] O'Connor, u. s. p. 286, "Typhoid has scarcely appeared in this locality, which cannot boast of the excellence of its sewerage."

had been three bad harvests in succession from 1860, but it may
be inferred from a Dublin article of August, 1863, that no
epidemic of typhus had arisen in Ireland down to that date,
although there was much typhus in England, especially in
Lancashire owing to the "cotton famine." When the epidemic
did arise in Dublin, Cork, and doubtless elsewhere in Ireland,
in the latter part of 1864, to continue throughout 1865, it was
not connected with scarcity or distress among the common
people. On the other hand, Dr Grimshaw, of Dublin, found
that it was subject to influences of the weather, as if the infective principle had been a soil poison like that of plague, yellow
fever, cholera, or enteric fever. Taking the Cork Street Fever
Hospital for his study, he made out that there was a very close
correspondence, from the 29th of May to the 31st of December,
1864, between the fluctuating pressure upon its accommodation
and the periodic rises in the atmospheric moisture and heat,
the crowd of patients being always greater when a high temperature coincided with a large rainfall[1]. One would not have
been surprised to find some such law as that in enteric or
typhoid fever, although a correspondence from day to day is
subject to many sources of fallacy; but, by all accounts, the
disease was typhus, the last of the considerable outbreaks of it
in Ireland hitherto, and an outbreak that seemed to require,
both at Cork and Dublin, the language of Sydenham's epidemic
constitutions for its adequate description. For a good many
years, the continued fever of Dublin has been chiefly enteric or
typhoid. As late as 1862 a physician to the Fever Hospital,
unconvinced by the method of Sir William Jenner, believed that
he observed a transition from the old typhus into the new
enteric: "The change at first seemed to be to the gastric type;
to which was shortly added diarrhoea in nearly every instance;
and this latter, again, occurring in a large number of cases which
presented all the characters of typhus, including a dense crop of
petechiae[2]." Assuming that there had been a mixture of cases
of enteric and typhus fevers, the latter must have had diarrhoea
among the symptoms, as they often had in special circumstances
(as well as tympanitis). Since that time the species of typhus

[1] "On Atmospheric Conditions influencing the Prevalence of Typhus Fever."
Dub. Quart. Journ. Med. Sc., May, 1866, p. 309.
[2] H. Kennedy, M.D., "Further Observations on Typhus and Typhoid Fevers as
seen in Dublin." *Ibid.*, Aug. 1862, p. 50.

has greatly declined, and the species of typhoid has considerably increased. The remodelling which Dublin has undergone, like all other old cities, explains the one fact. The notorious Liberties have been in great part rebuilt, and the conditions of typhus, as well as its actual fomites, to that extent removed. On the other hand, something has happened to encourage the soil poison of enteric fever. It is not easy to say what are the conditions that have favoured the enteric poison in modern towns; but there can be little doubt about the fact in general, or that Dublin and Belfast are among the best fields for the study of the problem[1].

[1] Nearly one-half of all the enteric fever deaths in Ulster and Leinster come respectively from Belfast and Dublin:

Year	Belfast	Dublin
1889	236	231
1890	190	168

CHAPTER III.

INFLUENZAS AND EPIDEMIC AGUES.

EPIDEMIC agues are joined in the same chapter with influenzas for the reason that they can hardly be separated in the earlier part of the history. Until 1743 the name influenza was not used at all in this country. The thing itself can be identified clearly enough in certain instances from the earliest times. But there are periods, such as 1657–59, 1678–79, and 1727–29 when short waves of epidemic catarrhs or catarrhal fevers came in the midst of longer waves of epidemic agues, "hot agues," or intermittents, the whole being called by the people "the new disease," or "the new ague," while by physicians, such as Willis and Sydenham, they were taken to be the distinguishable constituent parts of one and the same epidemic constitution. The last period in which epidemic agues were so recognised and named in England was from 1780 to 1785; and in the midst of that also there occurred an epidemic catarrh—the "influenza" of the year 1782. It is possible that our own recent experience of a succession of influenzas, or strange fevers, from 1889 to 1893, in some respects the most remarkable in the whole history, would have seemed an equally composite group if they had fallen in the 17th century and had been described in the terminology of the time and according to the then doctrines or nosological methods. Without prejudice to the distinctness and unity of the influenza-type in all periods of the history, I am unable, after trying the matter in various ways, to do otherwise than take the epidemics of ague in chronological order along with the influenzas. As the history will require the frequent use of the name "ague," and, in due course, that of the name "influenza," it will be useful to examine at the outset their respective etymologies and the meanings that usage has given to them.

Originally the English name ague did not mean a paroxysmal or intermittent fever, or a fever with a long cold fit followed by a hot fit, or the malarial cachexia with sallowness, dropsy and enlarged spleen, or any other state of health arising from the endemic conditions which are known as malarial over so large a part of the globe in the tropical and sub-tropical zones. It meant simply *acuta*, the adjective of *febris acuta* made into a substantive. Thus Higden's reference in the *Polychronicon* (which is exactly in the words of Giraldus Cambrensis a century and a half before) to the *febris acuta* of Ireland is translated by Trevisa (14th cent.): "Men of that lond haue no feuere, but onliche the feuere agu, and that wel silde whanne"; and by an anonymous translator: "The dwellers of hit be not vexede with the axes excepte the scharpe axes, and that is but selde[1]." Again in the MS. English translation of the Latin essay on plague by the bishop of Aarhus, the acute fever which is described as the attendant or variant of bubo-plague proper (well known long after as the pestilential fever, a malignant form of typhus), is thus rendered:

"As we see a sege or prevy next to a chambre, or of any other particuler thyng which corrupteth the ayer in his substance and qualitee: whiche is a thing maye happe every daye. And therof cometh the ague of pestilence. And aboute the same many physicions be deceyved, not supposing this axes to be a pestilence...And suche infirmite sometime is an axes, sometime a postume or a swellyng—and that ys in many thinges."

The same use of ague is continued in the first native English book on fevers, Dr John Jones's 'Dyall of Agues,' which has chapters on plague as well as on pestilential fever and on all other fevers including intermittents. In Ireland the name of ague was applied until a comparatively late period to the indigenous typhus of the country, as if in literal translation of the *febris acuta* first spoken of by Giraldus in the 12th century. Ague in early English meant any sharp fever, and most .commonly a continued fever. The special limitation to intermittents appears to have followed the revival of the study of the Graeco-Roman writers on medicine, Galen above all, in the sixteenth century. But Jones, who was freer than the more academical physicians of his time from classical influences, is shrewd enough to see that it was a mistake to transfer the experiences of Greece verbatim to England and to make them our standard of

---

[1] Higden's *Polychronicon*. Rolls Series, I. 332.

authority: he is speaking, however, not of intermittents but of the simple ephemeral fever, or inflammatory fever of one day:

"Such as have the fever of heat or burning of the sun, sayeth Galen, theyr skin is drye and hot as that which is perched with the sun; of the which, in this orizon and countrye of oures, we have no great nede to entreate of, leaving it to the phisitions and inhabitantes that dwell nerer to the meridionall line and hoter regions, as Hispaine and Africke¹."

At a later date, when the Hippocratic tradition had displaced the Galenic, Rogers of Cork, perhaps the earliest writer on fevers whose observations are essentially modern, has occasion thus to reflect upon the extreme deference of Sydenham to his Greek model: "Again we learn from Hippocrates that fevers in the warmer climates of Greece, at Naxos, Thasos or Paros, ran their course in certain periods of time, which no ways answers in regions removed at a farther distance from the sun,"—Rogers himself having had no experience of intermittents among all the fevers and dysenteries that he saw from 1708 to 1734, although Cork was surrounded by marshes².

At the time of the Latin translations of Greek medical writings by Linacre and Caius in the Tudor period, there were in this country actual experiences of strange fevers, which were interpreted according to the Greek teaching of quotidians, tertians and quartans, with their several bastard or hybrid or larval forms. These, as I have said, were certainly not the endemic fevers of malarious districts; they were, on the contrary, widely prevalent all over the country during one or more seasons in succession and more occasional for a few years longer; then there would be a clear interval of years, and again an universal epidemic of "the new fever," "the new acquaintance," "the new ague" or the like.

Sydenham, for example, has much to say of agues or intermittents prevalent in town and country for a series of years, and then disappearing for as long a period as thirteen years at a stretch. But he does not count these as the agues of the marsh; his single reference to the latter is in his essay on Hysteria, where he interpolates a remark that, if one spends two or three days in a locality of marshes and lakes, the blood is in the first instance impressed with a certain spirituous

---

¹ *Dyall of Agues.* London, [1564].
² *Essay on Epidemic Diseases.* Dublin, 1734.

miasma, which produces quartan ague, and that in turn is apt to be followed, especially in the more aged, by a permanent cachectic state[1]. If Sydenham had intended to bring all the intermittents of his experience into that class, he would not have left the paludal origin of them to a casual interpolated remark. On the other hand, he refers the epidemic agues, which occupy his pen so much, to emanations from the bowels of the earth, according to a theory of his friend Robert Boyle, applied by the latter to epidemical infections in general and to epidemic colds or influenzas in particular. Sydenham and his learned colleagues were not ignorant of the endemic agues of marshy localities, but they made little account of them in comparison with the aguish or intermittent fevers that came in epidemics all over England.

In admitting the reality of such agues, we must be careful not to ascribe them to such conditions as Talbor, the ague-curer, found in one village in Essex. We must be careful not to do so, because there are plausible reasons for doing so. The ground is much better drained now than formerly; there is less standing water, fewer marshes, a much smaller extent of water-logged soil. But the malarious parts of England have been tolerably well defined at all times ; and at all times the greater part of the country was as little malarious as it is now. It is the frequent reference to agues in old medical writings that has led some modern authors to construct a picture of a marshy or water-logged England, for which there is no warrant. Cromwell died of a tertian ague which he caught at Hampton Court; therefore "the country round London in Cromwell's time" must needs have been "as marshy as the fens of Lincolnshire are now." The country round London was much the same then as now, or as in John Stow's time, or as in the medieval monk Fitzstephen's time, or as it has ever been since the last geological change. The ague of which Cromwell died in the autumn of 1658 was one of those which raged all over England from 1657 to 1659—so extensively that Morton, who was himself ill of the same for three months, says the country was "one vast hospital." Whatever was the cause of that great epidemic of "agues," and of others like it, we have no warrant to assume that "the country round London," or wherever else the epidemic

---

[1] *Dissert. Epistol.* § 93. Greenhill's ed. p. 378.

malady prevailed, was then as marshy as the fens of Lincoln-shire[1].

The other name in the title of this chapter, influenza, appeared comparatively late in the history. It is an Italian name, which is usually taken to mean the influence of the stars. It may have got that sense by popular usage, but the original etymology was probably different. As early as the year 1554 the Venetian ambassador in London called the sweating sick-ness of 1551 an *influsso,* which is the Italian form of *influxio.* The latter is the correct classical term for a humour, catarrh, or defluxion, the Latin *defluxio* itself having a more special limited meaning. It was not astrology, but humoral pathology, that brought in the words *influxio* and *influsso*; and I suspect that influenza grew out of the latter, but not out of the notion of an influence rained down by the heavenly bodies.

It was in 1743 that the Italian name of "influenza" first came to England[2], the rumour of a great epidemic, so called, at Rome and elsewhere in Italy having reached London a month or two before the disease itself. The epidemic of 1743 was soon over and the Italian name forgotten; so that when the same malady became common in 1762, some one with a good memory or a turn for history remarked that it resembled "the disease called influenza" nearly twenty years before. After the epidemic of 1782, the Italian name came into more general use, and from the beginning of the present century it became at once popular and vague. The great epidemics of it in 1833 and 1847 fixed its associations so closely with catarrh that an "influenza cold" became an admitted synonym for coryza or any common cold attended with sharp fever. Lastly, the series of epidemics

---

[1] One regrets to find the above mistake in the learned pages of Murchison (p. 8). The following by Dr Robert Williams (*Morbid Poisons,* II. 423) is absolutely erroneous: "In Sydenham's time, intermittent fever and dysentery were constantly endemic in London; and the mortality from the former cause alone averaged, in a comparatively small population, from one to two thousand persons annually." What Sydenham says is that dysentery was endemic in Ireland (on the authority of Boate, no doubt), that it was epidemic in London in the end of 1669 and in the three years following, and that for the space of ten years it had appeared quite sparingly (*quae per decennium jam parcius comparuerat*). As to intermittents, he says they were absent from London for thirteen years, from 1664 to 1677, except in sporadic or imported cases. In the London bills the deaths from "agues" are sometimes distinguished from "fevers," and are then seen to be only some dozen or twenty in two thousand.

[2] It is used in the Latin title of an Edinburgh graduation thesis, "De Catarrho epidemio, vel Influenza, prout in India occidentali sese ostendit," by J. Huggar, which is assigned in Häser's bibliography to the year 1703. Having been unable to find the thesis, I have not verified the date.

from 1889 to 1893 effectually broke the association with coryza or catarrh.

Before influenza became adopted as the common English name towards the end of last century, what were the names popularly given to the malady in this country? The earliest references to it are in the medieval Latin chronicles under the name of *tussis* or cough, or in some periphrasis. In the fifteenth century the English name was "mure" or "murre," which appears to be the same root as in murrain. Thus the St Albans Chronicle, under the year 1427, enters a certain "infirmitas rheumigata," which in English was called "mure"; and the obituary of the monks of Canterbury abbey has two deaths from "empemata, id est, tussis et le murra[1]." In the Tudor period there is no single distinctive name, unless it be "hot ague": in 1558 the name is "the new burning ague," in 1562 "the new acquaintance," in 1580 "the gentle correction," and at various times in the 17th century "the new disease," "the new ague," "the strange fever," "the new delight," "the jolly rant." Robert Boyle called one sudden outbreak "a great cold." Molyneux, of Dublin, mentions "a universal cold" in one year (1688), and "a universal transient fever" in another (1693). The earlier 18th century writers mostly use the word catarrh or catarrhal fever, either in Latin or in English, the popular names probably continuing fanciful as before, as for example Horace Walpole's "blue plagues." That which stands out most clearly in the English naming from the earliest times is the idea of something new or strange; but the newness or strangeness pertained quite as much to the agues as to the catarrhs. The notion of ague may be said to be uppermost in the 16th and 17th centuries, that of catarrh in the 18th and 19th; while our very latest experiences have once more brought a suggestion of ague to the front.

---

[1] *Annales Monastici* (St Albans), Rolls Series, No. 191, under the year 1427; *Hist. MSS. Commiss.* IX. pt. 1, p. 127, records of Canterbury Abbey.—An epidemic in Ireland a century before, in 1328, has been given by Sir W. R. Wilde, and by Dr Grimshaw following him, under the name of "murre," as if that had been its name at the time. The explanation seems to be that the contemporary Irish name *slaedan* was rendered by Macgeoghegan, in his translation of the Annals of Clonmacnoise, by the 15th century English term "murre." The "mure" of 1427 was a universal influenza; but the word was afterwards used for a common cold, along with poss, as in Gardiner's *Triall of Tabacco*, 1610, fol. 12 and 15: "stuffings in the head, murres and pose, coughs"; and "the poze, murre, horsenesse, cough" etc.

Retrospect of Influenzas and Epidemic Agues in the 16th and 17th centuries.

In the former volume of this history I have dealt with the various epidemics of "hot ague," "new disease" or the like down to the epidemic of 1657–59. It will be convenient to go over some of that ground again, with a view to distinguish, if possible, the catarrhal types from the aguish, and to illustrate the use of the word ague as applied to a universal epidemic. Two of the epidemic seasons in the 16th century, 1510 and 1539, are too vaguely recorded for our purpose; but I shall review briefly the seasons from 1557–58 onwards.

It is known from the general historians that there were two seasons of fever all over England in 1557 and 1558, of which the latter was the more deadly, the type according to Stow, being "quartan agues." In letters of the time the epidemic of 1557 is variously named: thus Margaret, Countess of Bedford, writes on 9 August from London to Sir W. Cecil that she "trusts the sickness that reigns here will not come to the camp [near St Quentin, where Francis, Earl of Bedford was]...As for the ague, I fear not my son." On the 18th of the same month, Sir Nicholas Bacon writes from Bedford to Cecil: "Your god-daughter, thanks be to God, is somewhat amended, her fits being more easy, but not delivered of any. It is a double tertian that holds her, and her nurse had a single, but it is gone clearly;" to which letter Lady Bacon adds a postscript about "little Nan, trusting for all this shrewd fever, to see her." On 21 September, it appears that the sickness had reached the English camp near St Quentin, for the Earl of Bedford writes: " Our general is sick of an ague, our pay very slack, and people grudge for want." As late as the 25th October the Countess of Bedford writes from London to Cecil that she "would not have him come yet without great occasions, as there reigns such sickness at London[1]."

Next year, 1558, the epidemic sickness returned in the summer and autumn, in a worse form than before. Stow calls it "quartan agues," which destroyed many old people and especially priests, so that a great number of parishes were unserved. Harrison, a canon of Windsor, says that a third part of the people did taste the general sickness. On the 6th September, sickness affected more than half the people in Southampton, Portsmouth, and the Isle of Wight. From the 20th October to the end of the year, no fewer than seven of the London aldermen died, a number hardly equalled in the first sweating sickness of 1485, and the queen (Mary) died of the lingering effects of an ague, which was doubtless the reigning sickness. On 17th October, the English commissioners being at Dunkirk to negotiate the surrender of Calais, one of them, Sir William Pickering, fell "very sore sick of this new burning ague: he has had four sore fits, and is brought very low, and in danger of his life if they continue as they have done." That year Dr Owen published *A Meet Diet for the New Ague,* and himself died of it in London on the 18th of October[2].

Fuller quaintly describes the ague of 1558 as "a dainty-mouthed disease, which, passing by poor people, fed generally on principal persons of greatest wealth and estate[3]." Roger Ascham wrote in 1562 to John

---

[1] *Cal. Cecil. MSS.* I. under the dates.
[2] Munk, *Roll of the College of Physicians,* I. 32.
[3] Cited in Southey's *Commonplace Book,* from Fuller's *Pisgah Sight,* p. 54.

Sturmius that, for four years past, or since 1558, "he was afflicted with continual agues, that no sooner had one left him but another presently followed; and that the state of his health was so impaired and broke by them that an hectic fever seized his whole body; and the physicians promised him some ease, but no solid remedy[1]." Thoresby, the Leeds antiquary of the end of the 17th century, found in the register of the parish of Rodwell, next to Leeds, a remarkable proof of the fatality of these agues, which fully bears out the general statements of Stow and Harrison. In 1557 the deaths in the register rose from 20 to 76, and in 1558, which the historians elsewhere say was the most fatal year, they rose to 124[2]. This was as severe as the sweating sickness of 1551, for example in the adjoining parish of Swillington, or in the parish of Ulverston, in Lancashire[3].

The English names of the epidemic sickness in the summers and autumns of 1557 and 1558 are all in the class of agues— "this new burning ague," "a strange fever," "divers strange and new sicknesses taking men and women in their heads, as strange agues and fevers," "quartan agues." One medical writer, Dr John Jones, says in a certain place that "quartans were reigning everywhere," and in another place, still referring to 1558, that he himself had the sickness near Southampton, that it was attended by a great sweat, and that it was the same disease as the sweating sickness of 1551. There were certainly two seasons of these agues, 1557 and 1558, the latter being the worst; and it is probable from Short's abstracts of a few parish registers in town and country that there was a third season of them in 1559. The year 1557 has been made an influenza year, perhaps because the Italian writers have emphasized catarrhal symptoms here or there in the epidemic of that year; while both the years 1557 and 1558 have been received into the chronology of epidemic or pandemic agues or malarial fevers[4]. There are perhaps a dozen English references in letters

---

[1] Southey, *Commonplace Book*, from Strype's *Memorials of Cranmer*, p. 284.
[2] Thoresby, *Ducatus Leodiensis*, ed. Whitaker, App. p. 152.
[3] Baines, *Lancashire*, II. 679: 39 deaths from 17 to 24 August, 1551, set down to "plague," i.e. sweat.
[4] Lest it may be supposed that there has been adequate discussion of the differences between epidemic agues and influenzas, I quote from Hirsch's *Handbuch der historisch-geographischen Pathologie* the passage in which these epidemics or pandemics of "malarial fever" are referred to : "These epidemics of malaria, which extend not unfrequently over large tracts of country, and sometimes even over whole divisions of the globe, forming true pandemics, correspond always in time with a considerable increase in the amount of sickness at the endemic malarious foci, whether near or distant; they either die out after lasting a few months, or they continue—and this applies particularly to the great pandemic outbreaks—for several years, with regular fluctuations depending on seasonal influences. On the very verge of the period to which the history of malarial epidemics can be traced back, we meet with a pandemic of that sort, in the years 1557 and 1558, which is said to have overrun all Europe (Palmarius, *De morbis contagiosis*. Paris, 1578, p. 322)...It is not until the years 1678–82 that we again meet with definite facts relating to an epidemic extending over a great part of Europe..." (Eng. Transl. I. 229.)

and chronicles to the sicknesses of those years, either to particular cases or to a general prevalence, but they do not enable us to distinguish a catarrhal type in 1557 from the aguish type which they assert for both 1557 and 1558.

Four years after, another very characteristic influenza was prevalent in Edinburgh.

> Randolph writes from Edinburgh to Cecil in the end of November, 1562: "Maye it please your Honer, immediately upon the Quene's (Mary's) arivall here, she fell acquainted with a new disease that is common in this towne, called here the newe acqayntance, which passed also throughe her whole courte, neither sparinge lordes, ladies nor damoysells, not so much as ether Frenche or English. It ys a plague in their heades that have yt, and a sorenes in their stomackes, with a great coughe, that remayneth with some longer, with others shorter tyme, as yt findeth apte bodies for the nature of the disease. The queen kept her bed six days. There was no appearance of danger, nor manie that die of the disease, excepte some olde folkes. My lord of Murraye is now presently in it, the lord of Lidingeton hathe had it, and I am ashamed to say that I have byne free of it, seinge it seketh acquayntance at all men's handes[1]."

It is not improbable that the interval between 1558 and 1562 may have been occupied with milder revivals of the original great epidemic, the one at Edinburgh counting in the series.

It appears from a Brabant almanack for the year 1561 that a sudden catarrhal epidemic was quite on the cards in those years: the astronomer foretells for the month of September, 1561: "Coughs innumerable, which shall show such power of contagion as to leave few persons unaffected, especially towards the end of the month[2]." There is an actual record from more

---

[1] *Queen Elizabeth and her Times.* Ed. Wright, 2 vols. Lond. 1838, I. 113. Sir W. Cecil writing from Westminster to Sir T. Smith on 29th December [1563] says: "The cold here hath so assayled us that the Queen's majestie hath been much troubled, and is yet not free from the same that I had in November, which they call a pooss, and now this Christmas, to keep her Majestie company, I have been newly so possessed with it as I could not see, but with somewhat ado I wryte this. We have had perpetuall frosts here sence the 16th of this month. Men doo now ordinarily pass over the Thamiss, which I thynk they did not since the 8th yere of the reign of King Henry the VIII." *Ibid.* I. 157. For "poss," see note p. 305.

[2] *Ephemer. Meteorol. anni* 1561 [for the latitude of Brabant]. Antwerp, 1561: "Tusses numero infinitae atque tanta contagionis vi praestabunt ut pauci immunes reliquant, praecipuè circa mensis finem." The almanacks of those times must have been constructed on the same principle as the weather forecasts of our own time—namely, that of using the experience of one year for the next, just as the weather of one day is an indication for the next. In 1575 Dr Richard Foster (who became president of the College of Physicians in 1601) issued an almanack in which he foretold "sweating fevers" for the month of July (*Ephemer. meteorol. ad ann.* 1575. Lond. 1575). Cogan says that Francis Keene, an astronomer, also prophesied the return of the sweating sickness in 1575, "wherein he erred not much, as there were many strange fevers and nervous sickness."

than one country (Italy, Barcelona, as well as Edinburgh) of such universal catarrhs and coughs a year later than the one foretold. The Italian writers assign the universal catarrhs and coughs to the autumn of 1562, the Barcelona writer to the winter solstice of that year, and the letter from Edinburgh to "the laste of November."

The next undoubted influenza, that of 1580, was compared abroad to the English sweat:

"In some places," says Boekel, "the sick fell into sweats, flowing more copiously in some than in others, so that a suspicion arose in the minds of some physicians of that English sweat which laid waste the human race so horribly in 1529;" and again, "the bodies were wonderfully attenuated in a short time as if by a malignant sudden colliquation, which made an end of the more solid parts, and took away all strength." The season of it was the summer.

The outbreak attracted much attention from its universality, and was described by many abroad.

Boekel says that it was of such fierceness "that in the space of six weeks it afflicted almost all the nations of Europe, of whom hardly the twentieth person was free of the disease, and anyone who was so became an object of wonder to others in the place...Its sudden ending after a month, as if it had been prohibited, was as marvellous as its sudden onset." It came up, he says, from Hungary and Pannonia and extended to Britain. The principal English account of this epidemic comes from Ireland[2]. In the month of August, 1580, during the war against the Desmonds, an English force had advanced some way through Kerry for the seizing of Tralee and Dingle; "but suddenlie such a sicknes came among the soldiers, which tooke them in the head, that at one instant there were above three hundred of them·sicke. And for three daies they laie as dead stockes, looking still when they should die; but yet such was the good will of God that few died; for they all recovered. This sicknesse not long after came into England and was called the gentle correction."

This outbreak among the troops in Ireland is said to have been in August, before the sickness came to England. But it can be shown to have been at its height in London in the month of July. The year 1580 was almost free from plague in London; the weekly deaths are at a uniform low level (a good deal below the births) from January to December, except for the abrupt rise shown in the following table,—the kind of rise which we shall see from many other instances to be the infallible criterion of an influenza[3]:

[1] Johan Boekel, Συνοψις *novi morbi quem plerique medicorum catarrhum febrilem, vel febrem catarrhosam vocant, qui non solum Germaniam, sed paene universam Europam graviss. adflixit.* Helmstadtii, 1580.

[2] Hoker's "Irish historie...to the present year 1587," p. 165 a in Holinshed's *Chronicles.*

[3] This very moderate increase of the deaths in London in 1580 may be compared with the probably fabulous figures which Webster (1. 163) gives for continental cities the same year: Rome, 4000 deaths, Lübeck, 8000 deaths, Hamburg, 3000 deaths. I have given the weekly deaths and baptisms in London for five years, 1578–82, in my former volume, p. 341.

Weekly Deaths in London.

1580.

Week ending	Deaths by all causes	Dead of plague	Baptised
June 23	55	2	59
„ 30	47	4	57
July 7	77	4	65
„ 14	133	4	66
„ 21	146	3	61
„ 28	96	5	64
Aug. 4	78	5	73
„ 11	51	4	53
„ 18	49	1	72

As in 1557–58, the English references are to agues, both before and after the Gentle Correction of July–August, 1580. Cogan says that for a year or two after the Oxford gaol fever (1577) "the same kind of ague raged in a manner all over England and took away many of the strongest sort in their lustiest age, etc." And he seems to have the name "gentle correction" in mind when he says: "This kind of sickness is one of those rods, and the most common rod, wherewith it pleaseth God to brake his people for sin." Cogan's dates are indefinite. But there is a letter of the Earl of Arundel to Lord Burghley, 19th October, 1582, which shows that "hot ague" was epidemic as late as the second autumn after the influenza proper: "The air of my house in Sussex is so corrupt, even at this time of the year, as when I came away I left twenty-four sick of hot agues."

Two such epidemics in England as those of 1557–8 and 1580–82, of hot agues or strange fevers, taking the forms of simple tertian or double tertian or quartan or other of the classical types, would have made ague a familiar disease, and its name a household word. For not only were there two or more aguish seasons (usually the summer and autumn) in succession, but to judge by later experience there would have been desultory cases in the years following, and in many of the seizures acquired during the height of the epidemic, relapses or recurrences would have happened from time to time or lingering effects would have remained. Hence it is unnecessary to assume that the agues that we hear casual mention of had been acquired by residence in a malarious locality. They may have been, and most probably were, the agues of some epidemic prevalent in all parts of the country. These epidemics were the great opportunities of the ague-curers, as we shall see more fully in the sequel. It is to the bargaining of such an empiric with a patient that Clowes refers in 1579: "He did compound for fifteen pound to rid him within three fits of his ague, and to make him as whole as a fish of all diseases."

There were more sicknesses of that kind, perhaps not without a sweating character, in the last ten years of the 16th century[1]. But they are indefinitely given as compared with earlier and later epidemics, and I shall pass to the next authentic instance.

The autumn of 1612 was undoubtedly a season of epidemic ague or "new disease" in England[2]. When Prince Henry, eldest son of James I., fell ill in November, in London, during the gaieties attending the betrothal of his sister the Princess Elizabeth to the Count Palatine of the Rhine, a letter-writer of the time said of his illness: "It is verily thought that the disease was no other than the ordinary ague that hath reigned and raged almost all over England since the latter end of summer[3]." The attack began in the end of October. The spirited and popular prince had been leading the gaieties in place of his father, who could not stand the fatigue, and was "seized by a fever that came upon him at first with a looseness, but hath continued a quotidian ever since Wednesday last [before the 4th of November], and with more violence than it began, so that on Saturday he was let blood by advice of most physicians, though Butler, of Cambridge, was loth to consent. The blood proved foul: and that afternoon he grew very sick.......I cannot learn that he had either speech or perfect memory after Wednesday night, but lay, as it were, drawing on till Friday between eight and nine of the evening that he departed. The greatest fault is laid on Turquet, who was so forward to give him a purge the day after he sickened, and so dispersed the disease, as Butler says, into all parts; whereas if he had tarried till three or four fits had been passed, they might the better have judged of the nature of it; or if, instead of purging, he had let him blood before it was so much corrupted, there had been more probability." At the dissection, the spleen was found "very black, the head full of clear water and all the veins of the head full of clotted blood. Butler had the advantage, who maintained that his head would be found full of water, and Turquet that his brains would be found overflown and as it were drowned in blood[4]." Butler, it appears, was "a drunken sot." When King James asked him what he thought of the prince's case, he replied "in his dudgeon manner" with a tag of verse from Virgil ending with "et plurima mortis imago." The Princess Elizabeth could not be admitted to see her brother "because his disease was doubted to be contagious[5]." It was at least epidemic, for in the same week alderman Sir Harry Row and Sir George Carey, master of the wards, died "of this new disease[6]." The earliest reference to it that I find is the death, previous to 11 September, of Sir Michael Hicks at his house Rackholt in Essex, "of a burning ague," which came, as was thought, by his

---

[1] There is a curious reference to "the sweat" in Shakespeare's *Measure for Measure*, Act I. scene 2, where the bawd, in an aside, says: "Thus, what with the war, what with the sweat, what with the gallows, and what with poverty, I am custom-shrunk." It is known that Shakespeare adapted and condensed his play from Whetstone's *Promus and Cassandra*, printed in 1578, who took it from an Italian romance. But Whetstone's dialogue, which is pointless and verbose beside Shakespeare's, gives an entirely different speech to the bawd at the same place in the action, making no reference to "the sweat." The date of *Measure for Measure* is not certain; but it seems to belong to the earlier period of Shakespeare's work, when he was adapting old plays most freely. Whatever its date, the war, the sweat, the gallows and poverty are evidently topical allusions pointed enough for the audience to have taken up.

[2] The year 1610 is mentioned by Short as a season of universal catarrhal fever abroad; but that epidemic is not in the modern chronologies of influenza.

[3] Chamberlain to Carleton in *Court and Times of James I.* 1.

[4] Same to same 4 Nov. 1612. *Ibid.* I. p. 201.

[5] *Court and Times of James I.* I. p. 206.   [6] *Ibid.* p. 208.

often going into the water this last summer, he being a man of years[1]; but much more probably was a case of "the ordinary ague that hath reigned and raged almost all over England since the latter end of summer." The next year was still more unhealthy, to judge by samples of parish registers; agues are mentioned also in letters; thus, one going on 25 March, 1613, to visit Sir Henry Savile, found him "in a fit, an ague having caught hold of him[2]."

The winter of 1613–14 was marked by most disastrous floods in Romney Marsh, in Lincolnshire, in the Isle of Ely, and about Wisbech, and most of all in Norfolk[3]; but the malarious conditions so brought about, being subsequent to, were not conceivably the cause of, the epidemics of ague in the autumn of 1612 and 1613, which made so great an excess of burials over christenings in the parish registers.

A curious record remains of an aguish sickness in a child, which had begun about January, 1614. On 18 March, of that year, the dowager Countess of Arundel wrote from Sutton, near Guildford, to her son Earl Thomas, who was making the grand tour to Rome and elsewhere with his wife, and had left the children to the care of their grandmother: " Your two elder boys be very well and merry, but my swett Will^(m.) continueth his tersion agu still. This day we expect his twelfth fitt. I assur myselfe teeth be the chefe cause. I look for so spedy ending of it, he is so well and merry on his good days, and so strong as I never saw old nor yonge bear it so well. I thank Jesu he hath not any touch of the infirmity of the head, but onely his choler and flushe apareth, but he is as lively as can be but in the time of his fits onely, which continueth some eight hours[4]."

The epidemic of ague or "new disease," which began to rage all over England in the end of the summer, 1612, had probably recurred in the years following, down to 1616. There is not a trace of plague during those years in any known record; and yet they are among the most unhealthy years in Short's abstracts of town and country parish registers[5].

The first half of the 17th century is a period which is almost a blank in the conventional annals of "influenza" in Europe. But that period, which was the period of the Thirty Years' War, had many widespread sicknesses. I do not wish to claim these as influenzas, or to contend that they were infections equivalent thereto in diffusiveness. We may, however, find a place for them in this context; for they were certainly as mysterious as any epidemics admitted into the canon of influenzas. So far as concerns Britain, the first was the epidemic ague, or "new disease," of 1612 and 1613, probably recurring until 1616. The second was the universal spotted fever of 1623 and 1624, of which I have given an account in the chapter on typhus. That was followed by the plague of 1625, and that again by a harvest ague in the country in the end of the same year. The next epidemic ague or "general sickness, called the new disease," fell mostly in England upon the two years 1638 and 1639. It was

---

[1] *Court and Times of James I.* p. 197.   [2] *Ibid.* p. 237.
[3] *Ibid.* Letter of 25 Nov. 1613.
[4] *Cal. Coke MSS.* I. 83.

in part a harvest ague, "a malignant fever raging so fiercely about harvest that there appeared scarce hands enough to take in the corn[1]"; but it was also a winter disease. I pass over the war-typhus of 1643, to which the name of "new disease" was also given, and the widespread fever of the year following. In 1651 we hear again of a strange ague, which "first broke out by the seaside in Cheshire, Lancashire and North Wales," eighty or a hundred being sick of it at once in small villages. Whitmore, who saw this epidemic in Cheshire, identified it with the Protean disease which he described in 1657–58, and hazarded the theory that the former was a diluted or "more remiss" infection carried by the wind from Ireland, where the plague was then raging, in Dublin, Galway, Limerick and other places, after their sieges or occupations by the army of the Commonwealth.

Thus in the first half of the 17th century we have more or less full evidence of epidemics of "new disease" in 1612–13, 1623–24, 1625, 1638–9, 1643–4 and 1651, not one of which was an influenza as we understand the term[2].

We come at length to the years 1657–59, in the course of which one catarrhal epidemic, or perhaps two, did prevail for a few weeks. The hot agues or "new disease" had been raging all over the country from the summer of 1657; then in April, 1658, there came suddenly universal coughs and catarrhs, "as if a blast from the stars"; they ceased, and the hot agues dragged on through the summer and autumn. A letter from London, 26 October, 1658, says: "A world of sickness in all countries round about London: London is now held to be the wholesomest place," and adds that "there is a great death of coach-horses almost in every place, and it is come into our fields[3]." It was after this, in the spring of 1659, if Whitmore has made no mistake in his dates, that coughs and catarrhs "universally infested London, scarce leaving a family where any store were, without some being ill of this distemper." The details have been

---

[1] Graunt, *Obs. upon the Bills of Mortality,* 1662.

[2] Robert Boyle did not attach much importance to the name of "new disease." "The term *new disease,*" he says, "is much abused by the vulgar, who are wont to give that title to almost every fever that, in autumn especially, varies a little in its symptoms or other circumstances from the fever of the foregoing year or season." (Boyle's *Works.* 6 vols. 1772, v. 66.) But it was the name commonly given to the epidemics of catarrhal fever among others, and it does not appear, when the history is examined closely, that it was ever given except to some epidemic separated by several years from the last of the kind.

[3] Sir R. Leveson's Letters. *Hist. MSS. Commiss.* v. 146.

given fully in the former volume[1]. I wish merely to remark here that the two catarrhal epidemics, or influenzas proper, in two successive springs, were sharply defined episodes in the midst of a period of epidemic agues, and that the "new disease" as a whole, during the two or three years that it lasted, had such an effect in the way of ill health and mortality that it was afterwards viewed as a "little plague" worthy of being set in comparison with the Great Plague of 1665.

Willis does not say that the epidemic agues lasted after 1658, perhaps because his essay was printed early in 1659; but Whitmore, whose preface is dated November, 1659, says, without distinguishing the hot ague from the catarrhal fever but speaking of them both as one Protean malady: "it now begins again, seizing on all sorts of people of different nature, which shows that it is epidemic." Sydenham does not appear upon the scene until 1661; but when his epidemic constitutions do begin, it is with intermittents or agues, which lasted, according to him, until 1664. Perhaps if Sydenham's experience had extended back to 1657 he would have made his aguish constitution to begin with that year, and to go on continuously until 1664. At all events it does not appear that the year 1660 was a clear interval between Willis's and Whitmore's period of 1657–59, and Sydenham's period of 1661–64; for it so happens that John Evelyn has left the following note of his own illness:

"From 17 February to 5 April [1660] I was detained in bed with a kind of double tertian, the cruell effects of the spleene and other distempers, in that extremity that my physicians, Drs Wetherburn, Needham and Claude were in great doubts of my recovery." Towards the decline of his sickness he had a relapse, but on the 14th April "I was able to go into the country, which I did to my sweete and native aire at Wooton." On the 9th of May he was still so weak as to be unable to accompany Lord Berkeley to Breda with the address inviting Charles II. to assume the crown.

Sydenham makes the "constitution" which began for him in 1661 to decline gradually, and to end definitely in 1664, after which he finds intermittents wholly absent for thirteen years, or until 1677. This clear interval will make a convenient break in the chronology, whereat we may bring in the popular and professional notions of ague then current, and the popular practice in that disease by empirics.

[1] Pp. 568–577.

The Ague-Curers of the 17th Century.

It is to be observed that all the respectable writers of the profession speak of agues or intermittents as epidemic over the country for a definite period, and as disappearing thereafter for years together. At the same time they say little or nothing of the endemic malarious fevers of marshy localities. Further, it appears that the professed ague-curers, although they would wish to represent ague as a perennial disease, are really basing upon the same experiences of occasional epidemics which Willis, Whitmore and Sydenham recorded as occasional. The best instance of this is the 'Pyretologia' by Drage of Hitchin. It was published for practice in 1665, being designed to show forth the author's skill as an ague-curer[1]. When we examine its generalities closely, we find that they all come from the sickly season of 1657, the first of those described by Willis.

The great autumnal epidemic of that year (and the following), which we know from other sources to have been reckoned a "little plague," he describes as "a malignant sickness," which was followed in the winter by quartans. He himself escaped the autumnal fever but he incurred the quartan later in the year. In his own case, while the original paroxysm of this ague was still going on, a new one arose towards evening, and again, on the following day, a new paroxysm gathered vigour and supplanted the old, becoming the substantive paroxysm. Many of those who died of the quartan in 1657 had either the paroxysms duplicated, or a total want of them, or, in another passage, "the quartan which followed the autumnal disease of hetero-geneous quality in 1657, cut off divers old people, the fever being erratic, duplicated or triplicated." It was a bad sign when the quartan became doubled or trebled; regularity of the paroxysm was a sign of a good recovery. The symptoms of a quartan are various; but it is not easy to pronounce that these all are the symptoms of an intermittent fever, or the prodromal signs thereof, unless intermittent fevers be epidemic at the time. He gives the case of a civil and pious priest who had a tedious quartan from being struck with lightning; he was confined to bed for two years, with loss of hearing, but, strangely enough, retaining the use of his eyes; sometimes he was vexed with convulsions, sometimes with quartan fever. The "plebs medicorum" say that a quartan fever comes of melancholy, a tertian of choler, a quotidian of putrefied pituitous matter. The "plebs plebis" think that the cause is wind or flatus, and that they get rid of the ague by belching. In his own case he observed that if he drank more cold ale than usual, he was seized with distension in the loins and with palpitation, and belched up "flatus and crass vapours infected with the quality of a quartan." He knew a man who, in the fourth or fifth month of a quartan, drank wine too freely, so that the paroxysms came every day, and that violently; after a week he had an especially severe paroxysm, and then no more for three weeks, when the fever returned under the type of an exquisite quartan. One case, which he mentions twice, led him to doubt whether quartans were not catching: a

[1] Πυρετολογια *sive Gulielmi Dragei Hitchensis* Ιατρου και Φιλοσοφου *Observationes ab Experientia de Febribus Intermittentibus.* Londini, 1665.

certain girl suffering from a quartan asked her father, who was skilled in the
art, to open a vein; her parent declared that during the blooding the morbid
smell of the flowing blood reached his nostrils, so that he was seized of his
daughter's fever at the proper time of her paroxysms, having three or four
ague fits in due order; meanwhile the girl was free from the paroxysms for a
whole week, but no longer. The singular nature of quartans is further
brought out in the fact that papules, pustules and exanthems breaking out on
the skin were quite common in the quartan fever which followed the malignant epidemic of the autumn of 1657. "In the fevers hardly any heat is
perceived; and so the unskilled vulgar say 'This is an ague' (Hoc est anglicè
Ague), and 'This is fever and ague' (Et hoc est febris et anglicè *Ague*) when
cold and heat are mixed equally or combined regularly." Peruvian bark does
not evacuate the morbific matter unless by chance it provokes vomiting; cases
treated by it often relapse, and are not well in the intervals. Bark does not
occur in his own prescriptions; but he had cured many with "pentaphyllum."
He knew several physicians in the epidemic of quartans in 1657 who trusted
to narcotics entirely.

Drage must have had a real experience of aguish distempers
of one kind or another during the sickly seasons of 1657–59.
But it is clear from the essays or advertisements of empirics
that agues were discovered in many forms of sickness that were
neither intermittent fevers nor fevers of any distinctive type.
One of these practitioners in the time of Charles I. claims to be
"the king's majesty's servant in ordinary[1]"; which is not incredible, as Sir Robert Talbor, whom Charles II. deigned to
honour, was an ague-curer of the same class.

"An ague, which hitherto amongst all sorts hath been accounted the
physitian's shame, both for definition and cure (thus farre hath ignorance
prevailed), but that the contrary is manifest appeareth sufficiently by this
following definition: and shall be cured whether *tertian*, *quartern* or
quotidian, by me Aaron Streater, physitian of Arts in Oxford, approved by
Authority, the King's Majesties servant in ordinary, and dwelling against the
Temple, three houses up in Chancerie Lane, next house to the Golden
Anchor." An ague, he goes on, is either interpolate (intermittent) or continual; it is either engendered of a melancholic humour or it is a splenetic
effect; the liver is obstructed by abundance of choler proceeding from a salt
rheum that cometh from the brain" etc. Agues are to be dreaded most for
their remote effects: "Say not therefore, 'It is but an ague, but a fever; I
shall wear it out.' Dally not with this disease;" and he adds a case to show
what people may come to if they neglect an ague at the beginning: "Being
carried downe from London to South-hampton by Master Thomas Mason,—
September 1640, word was brought me of a Mayd dead, 16 years of age: and
being requested to see what disease she dyed of, I took my chirurgion with
me and went. And after section or search, I found as followeth: a gallon
and a half of green water in the belly, that stunk worse than carrion; under
the lyver an impostume as bigg as my fist, full of green black corrupted
matter, and the lyver black and rot. The spleen and kidneys wholly
decayed, and the place as black as soot; the bowels they were fretted, ulcerated
and rotten. In the chesse was two great handfuls of black burnt blood in
dust or powder; the heart was all sound, but not a drop of blood in it; nor
one spoonfull in the whole body.

[1] His tract is dated 1641.

Here was an Annatomy indeed, skinne and bone; and I verily beleeve that there was no braine left, but that she lived while that was moyst: the sent was so ill, and I not well, that I forbore to search it.

God that knowes the secrets of all hearts knowes this is a truth, and nothing else here written. Arthur Fauset, chirurgion at Southampton, was the man I employed to cut her up, as many there can witness that were present.

And what of all this, may some say? Why this. An eight weeks' ague in the neglect of it breeds all these diseases, and finally death."

Let us take next the advertisement of an apothecary a generation after, who professed to cure Kentish agues,—" the description and cure of Kentish and all other agues...and humbly showing (in a measure) the author's judgment why so many are not cured, with advice in relation thereunto, whether it be Quotidian, Tertian or Quartan, simple, double or triple[1]." Before the Fire of London he had practised in Mark Lane, but after his house was destroyed he removed to Kent, attending Maidstone market every Thursday, and residing at Rochester, a city which, "besides being subject to diseases in common with others, hath two diseases more epidemical, namely, the Scurvey for one but the Ague in special." The symptoms of scurvy, as he gives them, cover perhaps the one moiety of disease, and those of ague the other.

Agues are of two sorts, curable and incurable; the curable are those that come in a common way of Providence, the incurable those that are sent more immediately from God in the way of special judgment, as instances adduced from Scripture show. What is an ague? Some think it is a strange thing, they know not what; the more ignorant think it is an evil spirit, but coming they know not whence. Agues have their seat in the humours either within the vessels or without them; those residing within are continual quotidians, continual tertians, continual quartans; those without are intermittent ditto. (This distinction of within and without the vessels is traditional, and is found in Jones's *Dyall of Agues* as well as in Dutch medical books a century later.) The paroxysms of the intermittents are really the uprising of the Archaeus [of van Helmont], or spirit, to oppose the rottenness of the humours. A quartan is harder to cure than any other ague; part of its cure is an old 14th-century rule of letting blood in the plague; "let blood in the left hand in the vein between the ring finger and the little finger, which said thing to my knowledge was done about sixteen years ago [to say nothing of three hundred years ago] by the empiric Parker in this country, with very good success and to his great honour and worldly advancement." This ague-curer says little of Peruvian bark; his specific is the powder of Riverius, "the preparation of which, as well as some of the powder itself is lately and providentially come to my hands." Three doses cost not above five shillings, "and I never yet gave more in the most inveterate of these diseases...My opinion is that he that will not freely part with a crown out of his pocket to be eased of such a disease in his body deserves to keep it."

[1] By Nicholas Sudell, licentiate in physick and student in chimistry. London, 1669.

The most celebrated ague-curer of the Restoration period was Sir Robert Talbor, who thus describes the high motives that made him a specialist[1]:

"When I first began the study and practice of Physick, amongst other distempers incident to humane bodies I met with a quartan ague, a disease that seemed to me the *ne plus ultra* of physic, being commonly called Ludibrium et Opprobrium Medicorum, folly and derision of my profession, did so exasperate my spirit that I was resolved to do what study or industry could perform to find out a certain method for the cure of this unruly distemper...I considered there was no other way to satisfy my desire but by that good old way, observation and experiment. To this purpose I planted myself in Essex near to the seaside, in a place where agues are the epidemical diseases, where you will find but few persons but either are, or have been afflicted with a tedious quartan. In this place I lived some years, making the best use of my time I could for the improving my knowledge."

Talbor's first chapter is a fluent account of how agues are produced by "obstructions" of the spleen. This was a matter of theoretical pathology which an empiric could make a show with as well as another. But the empiric betrays himself as soon as he comes to practice. The enlarged spleen of repeated agues, or of the malarial cachexia, is commonly known as the ague-cake. There is no doubt that much of the unhappiness of the aguish habit resides in the ague-cake, and that one of the best pieces of treatment is to apply counter-irritants or the actual cautery to the left side, against which the enlarged spleen presses as a cake-like mass. Talbor, however, desired to free the patient from his "ague-cake" altogether:

"I have observed these in four patients: two were cast out the stomach by nature, and the other two by emetic medicines. One of them was like a clotted piece of phlegm, about the bigness of a walnut, pliable like glue or wax, weighing about half an ounce; another about the bigness of the yolk of a pullet's egg, and like it in colour, but stiffer, weighing about five drachms; the other two of a dark colour, more tough, about the like bigness, and heavier. It is a general observation amongst them that their ague comes away when they see those ague-cakes[2]."

Having followed this "good old way of observation and experiment" for several years among the residents of the Essex

[1] Πυρετολογια. *A rational account of the Cause and Cure of Agues, with their signs, Diagnostick and Prognostick. Also some Specified Medicines prescribed for the Cure of all sorts of Agues, &c. Whereunto is added a short account of the Cause and Cure of Feavers and the Griping in the Guts.* Authore Rto. Talbor, Pyretiatro. Londini, 1672.

[2] Sir Thomas Watson (*Practice of Physic*, I. 725) has a story which shows how long these fancies, encouraged by quacks, may linger: "A coachman by whose side I sat while travelling from Broadstairs to Margate was speaking of the rarity of ague in that part of the Isle of Thanet. His father, he said, once had the complaint, and a fit came on while he was on a visit to him, the coachman, at Ramsgate. The son administered to his suffering parent a glass of brandy; whereupon 'he threw the agy off his stomach; and it looked for all the world like a lump of jelly.'"

marshes, Talbor came to London, and set up his sign next door to Gray's Inn Gate in Holborn. In 1672 (14th July) he issued a small work with a Greek title—the quacks were fond of the Greek character on their title-pages—" Πυρετολογια, a rational account of the cause and cure of agues, with their signs : whereunto is added a short account of the cause and cure of feavers." He made a bid also for practice in "scurvy," a disease of landsmen in those times which was more a bogey than ague itself—"a strange monster acting its part upon the stage of this little world in various shapes, counterfeiting the guise of most other diseases...sometimes it is couchant, other times rampant, so alternately chronic and acute."

Most of the agues which Talbor professed to have met with in London in those years must have been equally factitious : for Sydenham, who makes more of "intermittents" than other writers of repute, was of opinion that, for thirteen years from 1664 to 1677, fevers of that type had not been seen in London, except some sporadic cases or cases in which the attack had begun in the country. But the air was then full of talk and controversy about Peruvian bark, or Jesuits' powder (*pulvis patrum*), or "the cortex," which was cried up as a specific in agues by some, and cried down by others. Talbor had seized upon this specific, and claimed to have an original way of administering it, whereby its success was assured. We get a glimpse of his practice from Dr Philip Guide, a Frenchman who came to London and practised for many years as a member of the College of Physicians[1]. Talbor had cured the daughter of Lady Mordaunt of an ague, and the cure had reached the ears of Charles II. One of the French princesses having been long afflicted with a quartan ague,

" The king commanded Mr Talbor to take a turn at Paris, and as a mark of distinction he honoured him with the title of knight. He succeeded wonderfully. But he could not cure Lady Mordaunt's daughter a second time, whom he had cured once before at London, by whom he gained most of his reputation." He tried for two months, but did not relieve the symptoms. Dr Guide was called in, and being asked to give his opinion of the ague that the young lady was afflicted with, " after some inquiry I found her distemper was complicated and quite different from the ague, which made me lay the thought of the ague aside, and apply myself wholly to the complicated disease, which I effectually cured in twelve days, together with her ague, without having any further need of the infallible specific of Sir Robert Talbor."

[1] Philip Guide, M.D., *A Kind Warning*, &c. Lond. 1710.

The Peruvian Bark Controversy.

It can hardly be doubted that the conflicting opinions as to the benefit of Peruvian bark in ague, which have been often cited in disparagement of medicine and as an example of its intolerance, arose from the indiscriminate use of it in "agues" diagnosed as such by quacks and pushing practitioners. The bark had been brought first to Spain in 1632 and had been tried medicinally in 1639[1]. It was under the powerful patronage of the Jesuits, especially of Cardinal de Lugo, and most of it at that time found its way to Rome, the centre of a malarious district. In 1652 it failed to cure a "double quartan" in an Austrian archduke, and thereafter fell into some disrepute. A violent controversy on its specific use in agues arose in the Netherlands; it had failed in every case at Brussels, it had not failed in a single case at Delft. Meanwhile it remained very dear, sixty florins having been paid at Brussels in 1658 for as much as would make twenty doses, to be sent to Paris. The London 'Mercurius Politicus' of the week 9–16 December, 1658, contained an advertisement[2] that a supply of it had been brought over by James Thompson, merchant of Antwerp, and was to be had either at his own lodgings at the Black Spotted Eagle in the Old Bailey or at Mr John Crook's, bookseller, at the sign of the Ship in St Paul's Churchyard. The London physicians such as Prujean and Brady countenanced it, and Willis, in reprinting his essay on Fevers in 1660, spoke of it as coming into daily use. Sydenham, whose publisher was the same Crook at the sign of the Ship, made a brief reference to it in the first edition (1666) of his *Observationes Medicae*, in the section upon the epidemic constitution of intermittents during the years 1661–64. He admits that the bark could keep down fermentation for the time being; but the *materies* which the fermentation would have dissipated if it had been allowed its way, will remain in the system and quickly renew its power. He had known a quartan continue for several years under the use of bark. It had even killed some patients when given immediately before the paroxysm. Prudently and cautiously given, in the decline of such fevers, it had been sometimes

---

[1] The best summary of the "history of the use of Peruvian bark" is by Sir George Baker, in *Trans. Col. Phys.* III. (1785), 173.

[2] Cited by Baker, *l.c.* p. 190.

useful and had stopped the paroxysms altogether, especially if the aguish fits were occurring at a season when the malady was less epidemical. But it is clear that Sydenham in 1666 inclined strongly to non-interference with the natural depuratory action of the fever upon the *materies* of the disease. His teaching that the cortex, while it kept down the fermentation of the blood for a time, left the dregs of the fever behind, was thus popularly stated some years after by Roger North in relating the fatal illness of his brother the Lord Keeper Guilford in the summer of 1685[1].

The fever of Lord Guilford was not an intermittent at all, but a "burning acute fever without any notable remissions and no intermissions," a case of the epidemic typhus of that and the succeeding year, elsewhere described. The treatment was first in the hands of Dr Masters, pupil and successor of Dr Willis, whose cardinal doctrine of fevers was that they were a natural fermentation of the blood. He ordered phlebotomy. Next Dr Short, of another school, was sent for: "So to work with his cortex to take it off: and it was so done; but his lordship continued to have his headache and want of sleep. He gave him quieting potions, as they called them, which were opiates to make him sleep; but he ranted and renounced them as his greatest tormentors, saying 'that they thought all was well if he did not kick off the clothes and his servant had his natural rest; but all that while he had axes and hammers and fireworks in his head, which he could not bear.' All these were very bad signs; but yet he seemed to mend considerably; and no wonder, his fever being taken off by the cortex. And it is now found that, without there be an intermission of the fever, the cortex doth but ingraft the venom to shoot out again more perniciously." The Lord Keeper's illness dragged on, and at length the physicians "found he had a lent fever which was growing up out of the dregs which the cortex had left; and if it were not taken off, they knew he would soon perish. So they plied him with new doses of the same under the name of cordial powders, whereof the quantity he took is scarce credible; but they would not touch his fever any more than so much powder of port. And still he grew worse and worse. At length the doctors threw up[2]."

Sydenham having indicated in his edition of 1666 that bark was dangerous when given immediately before a paroxysm, but that it was sometimes useful in the decline of the fever, and that its benefits were greatest in those desultory agues which appeared at, or continued into, a season when agues had become less epidemical, he proceeded in his third edition of 1675 to enlarge these indications for giving bark in ague. He begins, as Talbor had begun in his essay of 1672, and as the empiric Streater had in his advertisement of 1641, by calling quartans the *opprobrium medicorum,* and he then lays down precisely how

[1] *Lives of the Norths.* New ed. by Jessopp. Lond. 1890, III. 188.
[2] He fell into a kind of decline and died at his country house on 5 September, Dr Radcliffe having been summoned from London without avail.

bark was to be given in those obstinate fevers, as well as in tertians of the aged or feeble: namely, after the fever had exhausted itself *suo Marte*, in the intervals between two paroxysms, an ounce of bark (in two ounces of syrup of roses) to be taken in the course of the two free days, a fourth part at a time morning and evening. The dosage may have been borrowed from Talbor, as Sir George Baker alleges[1]; it matters little for anyone's fame. Sydenham, however, in a letter of October, 1677, thus claimed to have been independent of Talbor so far as concerned the directions for giving bark which he inserted in his edition of 1675:

> "I have had but few trials, but I am sure that an ounce of bark, given between the two fits, cures; which the physicians in London not being pleased to take notice of in my book, or not believing me, have given an opportunity to a fellow that was but an apothecary's man, to go away with all the practice on *agues*, by which he has gotten an estate in two months, and brought great reproach on the faculty[2]."

Talbor was patronised by Charles II., who caused him to be made one of his physicians. On 2 May, 1678, a few months after the date of Sydenham's letter, Lord Arlington wrote to the president of the College of Physicians[3]: "His Majesty, having received great satisfaction in the abilities and success of Dr Talbor for the cure of agues, has caused him to be admitted and sworn one of his physicians." Next year, 1679, the king had an attack of the reigning ague, and a recurrence of it in 1680. It is probably to the occasion of one or other of these attacks that an undated letter belongs from the Marquis of Worcester to the marchioness: "The physicians came to the Council to acquaint them that they intend to give the king the Jesuit's powder five or six times before he goes to Newmarket, which they agreed to. He looks well, eats two meals of meat a day, as he used to do[4]." Evelyn has preserved a story told him by the Marquis of Normanby, which probably relates to the same aguish attack of Charles II.[5]:

---

[1] Baker, *l.c.*, "Had not physicians been taught by a man whom they, both abroad and at home, vilified as an ignorant empiric, we might at this day have had a powerful instrument in our hands without knowing how to use it in the most effectual manner." This was written at a time when physicians spoke of "throwing in the bark"—throwing it in "with a shovel," as an Edinburgh professor used to say.

[2] John Barker, M.D., of Sarum, and afterwards physician to the forces, says in 1742 (in his essay on the epidemic fever of 1741, u.s. p. 112) that he had Sydenham's letter in manuscript before him, and that it was written in October, 1677.

[3] Cited by Baker, *Trans. Col. Phys.* III. 208.

[4] Beaufort MSS. *Histor. MSS. Com.* XII. App. 9, p. 85.

[5] Evelyn's *Diary*, under the date of 29 Nov. 1694.

"The physicians would not give the *quinquina* to the king, at a time when, in a dangerous ague, it was the only thing that could cure him (out of envy, because it had been brought into vogue by Mr Tudor [Talbor] an apothecary), till Dr Short, to whom the king sent to know his opinion of it privately, sent word to the king that it was the only thing which could save his life, and then the king enjoined his physicians to give it to him, which they did, and he recovered. Being asked by this lord [Normanby] why they would not prescribe it, Dr Lower said it would spoil their practice, or some such expression."

What Dr Lower was most likely to have said was, that it went against his principles to give bark in fevers. He was a physiologist, in the sense of an anatomist, the pupil of Willis at Oxford and his successor in practice in London. It was the teaching of Willis that blood was like the juice of vegetables, particularly the juice of the grape, in respect of fermenting, just as it was like milk in respect of curdling. Fever was a sudden access of fermentation, apt to arise in spring and autumn, from internal or constitutional occasions, as well as to come at any time by infection; by this febrile ferment, ebullition or commotion, the blood was purged of certain impurities, comparable to the lees of wine, which were removed from the body in the sweat, the urine or other critical evacuation. Jesuit's bark was believed to check fermentation, or, in the later phrase of Pringle and others, it was antiseptic; and it was probably because he thought it would check the natural defaecating action of the blood in an ague that Lower refused to prescribe it. Sydenham was more tentative, pliant, empirical. He cavilled at Willis's doctrine of the ebullition or fermentation of the blood without actually rejecting it; for he held practically the same view of the salutary or depuratory nature of fever, which was indeed the Hippocratic view of it. Accordingly in his first reference to bark, in 1666, he sustains the objection to it, that it interfered with a natural depuratory action; and it was only in following the lead of Talbor, a more empirical person than himself, that Sydenham overcame his doctrinal scruples. Dr Short, to whom Charles II. sent privately for advice, was of Sydenham's party; soon after that occasion, the latter dedicated to Short his 'Tractate on Gout and Dropsy' (1683). It was Short who "went to work with his cortex" upon the Lord Keeper in 1685, after Dr Masters, of the school of Willis, had tried his hand with phlebotomy. The king's experiences, a few months before the Lord Keeper's death, had been just the same, and with the same result: the deathbed of Charles II., it is well known, was the scene of ecclesiastical rivalries; but the physicians at the bedside of the king had their rivalries too.

On Monday the 2nd of February, at eight in the morning, the king had a seizure of some kind in his bed-chamber, which was currently said to have been an "apoplectic fit[1]," although there is nothing said of paralysis. A letter of the 3rd February[2] says the king "was seized in his chair and bed-chamber with a surprising convulsion fit which lasted three hours." Dr King, an expert operator who had assisted Lower in the delicate operation before the Royal Society on 23 November, 1667, of transfusing blood from one body to another, happened to be at hand, and, at once drawing his lancet, bled the king. His promptitude in action, which probably left him little time for diagnosis, was much applauded, and the Privy Council voted him a reward of a thousand pounds, which Burnet says he never received.

"This rescued his Majesty for the instant," says Evelyn, (who came up from Wooton on hearing the news, and is probably correct in his narrative), "but it was only a short reprieve. He still complained, and was relapsing, often fainting, with sometimes epileptic symptoms, till Wednesday, for which he was cupp'd, let blood in both jugulars, had both vomit and purges, which so reliev'd him that on Thursday hopes of recovery were signified in the public Gazette; but that day, about noone, the physitians thought him feverish. This they seem'd glad of, as being more easily allay'd and methodically dealt with than his former fits; so as they prescribed the famous Jesuit's powder: but it made him worse, and some very able doctors who were present did not think it a fever, but the effect of his frequent bleeding and other sharp operations us'd by them about his head, so that probably the powder might stop the circulation, and renew his former fits, which now made him very weake. Thus he pass'd Thursday night with greate difficulty, when, complaining of a paine in his side, they drew 12 ounces more of blood from him; this was by 6 in the morning on Friday, and it gave him reliefe; but it did not continue, for being now in much paine, and struggling for breath, he lay dozing, and after some conflicts, the physitians despairing of him, he gave up the ghost at halfe an houre after eleven in the morning, being 6 Feb. 1685, in the 36th yeare of his reigne, and 54th of his age....Thus died King Charles II. of a vigorous and robust constitution, and in all appearance promising a long life[3]."

Whether the bark would have saved him if the aguish nature of the paroxysms (such as he had in 1679 and again in 1680) had been clear from the first, may be doubted. But his chances of recovery were certainly made worse by the halting

---

[1] Evelyn; Luttrell, I. 327.
[2] *Hist. MSS. Com.* v. 186. Sutherland correspondence.
[3] *The Diary of John Evelyn*, under the date 4 Feb. 1685.

and stumbling diagnosis, (according to Evelyn)—now apoplexy, now epilepsy, now fever[1].

The true value of cinchona bark in medicine was not seen until much that was vague in the use of the term "ague" had been swept away. In the last great epidemic period of agues in this country, as we shall see, from 1780 to 1786, bark was found, for some reason, to be ineffective. It is not in the treatment of epidemic agues, but of agues in malarious countries, that the benefits of Jesuits' bark have been from first to last most obvious.

The practice in so-called agues was long in the hands of empirics, who, like their class in general, made business out of ignorant or lax diagnosis. I shall add here what remains to be said of specialist ague-curers in later times. They are heard of in London in the Queen Anne period, and as late as 1745.

Swift writes in his Journal to Stella, 25 December, 1710, from Bury Street, St James's: "I tell you a good pun: a fellow hard by pretends to cure agues, and has set out a sign, and spells it *egoes*; a gentleman and I observing it, he said, 'How does that fellow pretend to cure agues?' I said, I did not know, but I was sure it was not by a *spell*. That is admirable." In 1745, Simon Mason, of Cambridge, published by subscription and dedicated to Dr Mead an essay, *The Nature of an Intermitting Fever and Ague considered* (Lond. 1745), in which he has the following on "charm-doctors":—"When one of these poor wretches apply to a doctor of this stamp, he enquires how many fits they have had; he then chalks so many strokes upon a heater as they tell him they have had fits, and useth some other delusions to strengthen the conceit of the patient" (p. 167). Francis Fisher, who had been upper hostler in a livery stable in Crutched Friars near forty years, "told me he seldom missed a week without several ague patients applying to him, and he cured great numbers by a charm they wore in their bosoms" (p. 239). Another, who kept a public-house near St George's Fields, Southwark, sold "febrifuge ale" at a shilling a pint. It was a small ale brewed without hops, but with bark, serpentery, rhubarb and cochineal mixed in the brewing. The receipt was given him by an old doctor who was a prisoner in the King's Bench. His customers came in the morning fasting, and drank their shilling's worth after the publican had given them faith by a cordial grip of the hand. "By this means," he told Mason, "I got a good trade to my house, and a comfortable maintenance too."

We may now return to the actual history of the epidemic fevers upon which the Peruvian bark was first tried on a large scale in England. The "intermittent" constitution which began in 1677 and lasted year after year until 1781 or even longer was

---

[1] The popular imagination at the time appears to have been most impressed by Dr King's promptitude in whipping out his lancet. Roger North must have had it incorrectly in his mind when he wrote: "About the time of the death of Charles II., it grew a fashion to let blood frequently, out of an opinion that it would have saved his life if done in time."

a very remarkable one.   It was called at the time the new fever, or the new ague, and it had at least one short interlude of influenza or epidemic catarrhal fever in the winter of 1679, just as the last epidemic of the kind, in 1657–59, had at least one, and probably two, short and swift epidemic catarrhs in spring. But before we come to that epidemic of 1678–81, there falls to be noticed an epidemic in the month of November, 1675, which has always been counted among the influenzas proper. After giving the particulars of it from Sydenham and from the London bills of mortality, I shall show from Sydenham and the bills of mortality that there was an exactly similar epidemic in the month of November, 1679, which has not been admitted into the conventional list of influenzas.   Thereafter I shall proceed to the epidemic constitution of 1678–81 as a whole, which has been reckoned among the epidemic agues or malarious epidemics.

The Influenza of 1675.

The first that we hear of the universal cold of 1675 is an entry which Evelyn makes in his diary under 15 October: " I got an extreme cold, such as was afterwards so epidemical as not only to afflict us in this island, but was rife over all Europe, like a plague.   It was after an exceeding dry summer and autumn."   It was not until November that the epidemic cold made an impression upon the death-rate in London ; the deaths mounted up from 275 in the week ending 2 November, to 420 and 625 in the two weeks following, and thereafter gradually declined to an ordinary level.   Part of the excess, but by no means the greater part of it, was set down under fevers, as the following section from the weekly bills of the year will show :

1675

Week Ending	Fever	Smallpox	Griping in the Guts	All causes
Nov. 2	42	9	29	275
9	60	12	42	420
16	130	13	43	625
23	99	2	28	413
30	61	6	29	349
Dec. 7	54	7	25	308
14	43	5	12	266

This shows the characteristic rise and fall of an epidemic

catarrh both in the article of fever deaths and in the column
of deaths from all causes.   The other excessive articles besides
fever in the two worst weeks are also characteristic of influenza
mortality :

	Week ending 9 Nov.	Week ending 16 Nov.
Consumption	68	99
Aged	40	67
Tissick	10	35

Sydenham's account bears out the figures[1].   At the end of
October, he says, the mild, warm weather turned to cold, while
catarrhs and coughs became more frequent than at any time
within his memory.   They lasted until the end of November,
when they ceased suddenly.   Afterwards he gives a special
chapter to the "Epidemic Coughs of the year 1675, with
Pleurisies and Pneumonias supervening."   The epidemic spared,
he says, hardly anyone of whatever age or temperament; it
went through whole families at once.   A fever which he calls
febris comatosa had been raging far and wide since the beginning
of July, with which in the autumn dysenteric and diarrhoeal
disorders were mingled (it was an exceedingly dry season).
This constitution held the mastery all the autumn, affecting
now the head, now the bowels, until the end of October, when
catarrhs and coughs became universal and continued for a
month.   Sydenham's view of the sequence of events was his
usual one, namely, that one constitution, by change of season,
passed by transition into another.   Whatever the constitution of
"comatose" fevers may have been, which prevailed "far and
near," it has left no trace upon the bills of mortality in London,
which are remarkably low until the beginning of November.
But as soon as the epidemic of coughs begins, the weekly
deaths mount up in an unmistakeable manner, so that for two
or three weeks in November, the mortality is nearly double that
of the weeks preceding or following.

The "severe cold and violent cough," of 1675, says Thoresby
of Leeds[2], who was then a boy, "too young or unobservant to

---

[1] *Obs. Med.* 3rd ed. 1675, V. 5.
[2] Ralph Thoresby, *Ducatus Leodiensis*, ed. Whitaker, App. p. 151.   Brand, *Hist.
of Newcastle*, under the year 1675, says that "the jolly rant" caused 724 deaths in
that town, the authority given being Jabez Cay, M.D., who left his papers to
Thoresby.   The number given is probably the mortality from all causes.

make such remarks as might be of use," was known in the north of England "profanely" by the name of the "jolly rant." Thoresby well remembered that it affected all manner of persons, and that so universally that it was impossible, owing to the coughing, to hear distinctly an entire sentence of a sermon. He gives December as the month of it in Leeds, and says that it affected York, Hull, and Halifax, as well as the counties of Westmoreland, Durham, and Northumberland. In Scotland also we find a trace of a strange epidemic sickness. It was the time of the persecution of the Covenanters, whose preachers moved hither and thither among the farm-houses. One of them, John Blackadder, was at the Cow-hill in the parish of Livingstown in August, 1675. He came in one evening from the fields very melancholy, and in reply to questions, he said he was afraid of a very dangerous infectious mist to go through the land that night. He desired the family to close doors and windows, and keep them closed as long as they might, and to take notice where the mist stood thickest and longest, for there they would see the effects saddest. "And it remained longest upon that town called the Craigs, being within their sight, and only a few families; and within four months thereafter, thirty corpses went out of that place[1]." The prophecy was fulfilled within four months, which would bring us to the date of the influenza, although the mortality for a small place is somewhat excessive.

The Influenza of 1679.

For the sake of comparison, I pass at once to an epidemic of coughs and colds in the month of November, 1679, which Sydenham has chronicled, but no one except Cullen[2] has thought of including among the influenzas. It produced the characteristic effect of influenza on the London weekly bills, and it came in the midst of epidemic agues, just as the epidemic catarrhs of 1658 and 1659 had done. The following rise and fall are just as distinctive of an influenza as on the last occasion in 1675:

---

[1] Patrick Walker's *Life of Cargill*, pp. 29, 30.
[2] *Synopsis Nosologiae.* 3rd ed. Edin. 1780, II. 173.

1679

Week ending	Fever	Smallpox	Griping of the Guts	All causes
Nov. 11	50	18	34	328
18	89	27	39	541
25	126	21	55	764
Dec. 2	82	27	38	457
9	63	12	38	388

Sydenham's account[1] of this remarkable November outburst of sickness in London, written within a few weeks of its occurrence, is almost exactly a repetition of his language concerning the epidemic coughs of November, 1675. The prevailing intermittent fevers, he says, gave place to a new epidemic depending upon a manifest crasis of the air. The new epidemic was one of coughs, which were so much more general than at the same season in other years that in nearly every family they affected nearly every person. In some cases of the cough, the aid of a physician was hardly needed; but in others the chest was so shaken by the violent convulsive cough as to bring on vomiting, and the head was affected with vertigo. For the first few days the cough was almost dry, and so purely paroxysmal as to remind Sydenham of the whooping-cough of children. Everyone was surprised, he says, at the frequency of these coughs in this season. His own suggestion was that the rains of October[2] had filled the blood with crude and watery particles, that the first access of cold had checked transpiration through the skin, and that Nature had contrived to eliminate this serous colluvies either by the branches of the "vena arteriosa" or (as some will have it) by the glands of the trachea, and to explode it by the aid of a cough. Phlebotomy and purging were the best cures; diaphoretics he considered less safe, and he ascribed to their abuse the fever into which some fell, and the pleurisies which were apt to attack patients with great violence during the subsidence of the epidemic catarrh.

The Epidemic Agues of 1678–80.

The other English writer on the epidemic constitution of 1678–79 is Dr Christopher Morley[3]. Like Sydenham, he is

---

[1] *Epist. respons. ad R. Brady*, § 42.

[2] Luttrell (*Diary*, I. 23) enters under Oct. 1629: "About the middle of this month vast great rains fell which have been very prejudiciall to many persons."

[3] Christopher Love Morley, M.D., *De Morbo Epidemico tam hujus quam superioris Anni, id est* 1678 *et* 1679 *Narratio*. Preface dated London, 31 Dec. 1679.

occupied almost exclusively with the epidemic agues; but he also records the extraordinary rise of the mortality in London for a few weeks in the last months of the year, and the causes thereof, although it did not occur to him to count that as a separate part of "the new disease," still less as the principal part, which it really was in London so far as concerned the death-rate. Dating his preface from London, the 31st of December, 1679, he says in the text: "Within the very days of my present writing, it happens that as many as four hundred deaths more than usual have taken place in a fortnight," the excessive mortality having been due to "coryza, bronchitis, catarrh, cough and fever," which were the effects of "most pernicious destillations."

I shall now go back to the beginning of the epidemic constitution in the midst of which this November interlude occurred, and I shall follow it season after season to the end, so as to set forth in historical prominence that which was regarded at the time as "the new disease." When Sydenham returned to London in the autumn of 1677, after six months' rest from practice, he was told by his professional friends that intermittents were being seen here and there (after a clear interval of thirteen years), being more frequent in the country than in the city. In the letter of October, 1677, cited above, he speaks of Talbor having made a fortune in two months by his cures of agues with bark.

The first particular notice of the "new fever" occurs in a London letter of 23 February, 16$\frac{77}{8}$: "Lady Katherin Brudenhall has been in great danger of death by the new feaver[1]." A severe aguish illness of Roger North, fully described in his 'Autobiography,' was probably another instance of the reigning malady; it came upon him in the hot weather of 1678, while he was residing with his brother, Lord Guilford, at Hammersmith[2]. In the autumn of 1678, the "new fever" came more into notice. On the 8th of September, a letter was brought to Evelyn in church, from Mr Godolphin (afterwards celebrated as the minister of William III.), to say that his wife was exceedingly ill and to ask Evelyn's prayers and assistance. Evelyn and his wife took boat at once to Whitehall, and found the young and much-beloved Mrs Godolphin "attacqu'd with the new fever then reigning this excessive hot autumn, and which was so violent that it was not thought she could last many hours." She died next day, in her twenty-ninth year; but, as she had been brought to bed of a son six days before, her fever may have been more from puerperal causes than from "the new fever then reigning." Other known cases of ague the next season were those of Sir James Moore, his majesty's engineer, who, in August, 1679, coming from Portsmouth "was seized with an ague, and had two or three violent fits, which carried him off[3];" and of the king, Charles II., who was congratulated on his recovery

[1] Lady Chaworth to Lord Roos, *Calendar of the Belvoir MSS.* II. 47.
[2] *Lives of the Norths. Ed. cit.* III. 143.
[3] Luttrell's *Historical Relation.* Oxford, 1857, I. 19.

by the lord mayor and aldermen, on 15 September, and had a recurrence of the aguish attack ("two or three fits") on 15 May, 1680[1]. There are also references to the agues of 1679 in the country, in the letters of Lady North[2].

Sydenham wrote his account of this epidemic of intermittents in compliance with a request from Dr Brady, Master of Gonville and Caius College, Cambridge, that he would continue the method of his 'Observationes Medicae' into the years following, and in particular give an account of his method of administering bark. He occupied most of his space with treatment; but he gives here and there the following epidemiological details. The agues were mostly tertians, or quotidians, or duplex forms of these, whereas on a former occasion they had been mostly quartans; after two or three intermissions they were apt to become continual fevers. The agues, which had occurred in the spring of 1678, became more common in the summer and autumn, when they raged so extensively that no other disease deserved the name of epidemic so much. In winter smallpox took the lead; but early in July, 1679, the agues began again, and so increased day by day that in August they were raging excessively and destroying many. It was in August that the king had his "great cold" at Windsor, which afterwards changed to an ague. Sydenham then comes to the November interlude of epidemic catarrhs, which was followed by "a fever without cough" (*non penitus deleta, sed manente adhuc in sanguine, malae crasis impressione*), lasting to the beginning of 1680. As that year wore on, the intermittent fevers began again, and continued more or less until 1685, becoming indeed less common in London, and less severe, than in the first four years of the constitution, but in other places, now here, now there, not less so than at first[3].

---

[1] Luttrell, *loc. cit.* 1. 20, 21, 44.

[2] On 16 March, the illness of "little Frank...hath made me suspect some kind of aguish distemper; but, if it be, it is so little that we neither perceive coming nor going." On 7 July, another child is recovered of her feverish distemper. On 5 October, "all my little ones are very well, but some of my servants have quartan agues." *Lives of the Norths*, Letters of Anne, Lady North.

[3] An authentic case of these lingering epidemic agues was that of John Evelyn in the beginning of 1683. On 7th February, 1687, he writes: "Having had several violent fits of an ague, recourse was had to bathing my legs in milk up to the knees, made as hot as I could endure it; and sitting so in a deep churn or vessel, covered with blankets, and drinking carduus posset, then going to bed and sweating. I not only missed that expected fit, but had no more, only continued weak that I could not go to church till Ash Wednesday, which I had not missed, I think, so long in twenty years"—in fact, since his "double tertian" in 1660, which kept him in bed from 17th February to 5th April.

I have kept to the last the special account of this epidemic written by Morley at the end of the second year of it, namely, in December, 1679. He had been a witness of this fever, first at Leyden in the autumn of 1678, and next in England in the autumn of 1679, and he made it the subject of a treatise at the request of an eminent physician in London. It was not so severe by half in England as in Holland, but the English made a great deal more of it, calling it the New Disease, the New Ague, the New Fever, the New Ague Fever, and, in Derbyshire sarcastically, the New Delight. In Holland they called it neither new nor old, neither intermittent nor continued, nor a conjunction of both, but simply *morbus epidemicus*, or *febris epidemica*. His master at Leyden, Professor Lucas Schacht, taught very decidedly that it was of a scorbutic nature, and as early as the month of June, 1678, had prophesied the arrival of such an epidemic fever because "tertians were becoming more and more scorbutic," just as they had done before the great epidemic of fever in Holland in 1669. Morley claims, however, that the fever of 1678 was in some respects different from that of 1669, as well as from that of the year immediately preceding, 1677, when "an incredible multitude of people all over Belgium, and in every city and town, fell sick." The Dutch, it appears, called these occasional outbreaks simply "the epidemic fever," neither intermittent nor continued ; and certainly that of 1669, which is sometimes counted among the epidemic agues, was a very remarkable "ague." (See Chapter I. p. 19.)

The epidemic fever of 1678, wherever it may have been bred or engendered, was prevalent in England at the same time as in Holland—in an exceedingly hot and dry autumn. The most constant symptoms, says Morley (and he writes both for Holland[1] in 1678 and for the country districts of England in the autumn of the following year), were nausea, severe vomiting, incredible tightness about the breast, weight in all the limbs, weariness, giddiness, vigils, thirst, restless tossing, and languor remaining after the disease was gone. Among the more remarkable symptoms were the following: Many had aphthae of the mouth, some twice or thrice, some being endangered by the severity and closeness of the patches of thrush. In some there

[1] Ralph Thoresby caught it at Rotterdam, suffered from it, in the tertian form, for several weeks of October and November, 1678, and brought it home with him to Leeds. He gives a good account of the illness in his *Diary* (2 vols. Lond. 1830).

occurred bleeding from the nose, or from piles, stranguary, etc. Round worms were observed, issuing both by the mouth and anus. In some few there were spots on the skin, but hardly ever petechiae or tumours near the ears. It affected all classes equally, all ages and both sexes. Some said it was easier to children than to adults, but others denied this. Some said it was more pernicious in the country than in the towns. In Leyden, the deaths never exceeded 150 in the week, being about twenty in a week above the ordinary level. More died from the coughs, anginas, peripneumonies and pleurisies that followed, than from the disease itself. Schacht says that the wind for nearly two years had been steadily from the North, or veering to the East or West. The Leyden faculty, and the Dutch generally, did not think the disease a malignant one ; it was very freely called so, however, in England, the chorus being led by empirics and illiterate persons : "Ac indicio est," says Morley, " libellus perexiguus nostra lingua ab Empirico conscriptus de hoc morbo." This seems to refer to the tract by one Simpson, which I shall notice briefly[1].

Simpson styles himself a Doctor of Physic, and denies that he is an empiric. One sign of his affinity to that order, however, is that he objects to the orthodox treatment—emetics, drenches, a too cooling regimen, and purges, while he thinks blood-letting of doubtful utility. The symptoms were chills at the outset, pains in the head and back (in some with shaking), then intense burning heat, thirst, profuse immoderate sweats and great debility, a general lassitude, dulness, and stupor which in many were followed by delirium and a comatose state. Sometimes the fever simulated a quotidian, sometimes a tertian. He calls it "this new fever so grassant in city and country" and says that in many it assumed "the guise of a morbus cholera, known by the much vomitings or often retchings to vomit ; and in others under the livery of the gripes with looseness, or, in some, looseness without gripes." This choleraic tendency concurring with other usual causes from the late season of fruit-eating etc., had swelled the bills of mortality. The morbus cholera and the gripes were to the new fever "like the circumjoviales that move in the same sphere with (but at some distance from) their master-planet."

The meaning of all this is obvious on turning to the London weekly bills of mortality. In the months of August and September for three years in succession, 1678–80, the deaths from "griping in the guts" and from "convulsions" rose greatly. These were, indeed, three successive seasons of fatal diarrhoea, mostly infantile, as I shall show in the chapter on that disease.

[1] *The History of this present Fever, with its two products, the Morbus Cholera and the Gripes.* By W. Simpson, Doctor in Physick. London, 1678.

The following extracts from the London weekly bills of mortality show how "fevers," as well as other diseases, contributed to the great rise in the autumns of 1678, 1679, and 1680.

Autumnal London Mortality in 1678.

1678

Week ending	Fever	Smallpox	Griping in Guts	All causes
Aug. 20	77	31	87	459
27	79	37	130	510
Sept. 3	82	37	121	530
10	103	27	164	621
17	82	23	178	580
24	83	20	152	528
Oct. 1	82	25	117	485
8	77	27	106	456

Summer and Autumnal London Mortality in 1679.

1679

Week ending	Fever	Smallpox	Griping in Guts	All causes
July 22	42	55	101	442
29	60	50	134	565
Aug. 5	78	63	143	531
12	62	43	161	579
19	55	64	149	545
26	68	53	112	514
Sept. 2	96	40	97	466
9	92	47	75	471
16	85	50	87	462

(For the Influenza weeks, see former Table.)

Autumnal London Mortality in 1680.

1680

Week ending	Fever	Smallpox	Griping in Guts	All causes
Aug. 10	70	17	108	427
17	90	6	132	494
24	98	17	127	552
31	140	18	228	816
Sept. 7	101	14	215	671
14	94	13	173	635
21	106	9	175	628
28	130	9	159	615
Oct. 5	125	16	138	597
12	121	10	94	530
19	109	14	68	488
26	93	5	58	407
Nov. 2	77	10	53	396

The last of the three autumnal seasons, 1680, is one of the few in the bills with high deaths from fever along with high deaths from choleraic disease; and that excess of fever mortality may have been due in part to the ague epidemic, then in its third season.

The following extracts from Short's summation of parish registers show the great excess of burials over baptisms in various parts of England during the years of the aguish epidemic constitution.

Country Parishes.

Year	Registers examined	Sickly parishes	Baptisms in do.	Burials in do.
1678	136	17	312	527
1679	137	44	800	1203
1680	137	54	1093	1649
1681	137	41	679	1156
1682	140	30	632	975

Market Towns.

Year	Registers examined	Sickly parishes	Baptisms in do.	Burials in do.
1678	22	5	578	789
1679	23	7	877	1371
1680	24	7	946	1494
1681	24	9	945	1333
1682	25	9	795	1092
1683	25	8	1109	1398
1684	25	8	865	1243
1685	25	4	741	1191

The Influenza of 1688.

The seasons continued, according to Sydenham, to produce epidemic agues until 1685, when the constitution radically changed to one of pestilential fevers, affecting many in all ranks of society and reaching a height in 1686. Sydenham records nothing beyond that date, having shortly after fallen into ill health and ceased to write or even to practise. One would wish to have known what he made of the "new distemper" in the summer of 1688, for it was a sudden universal fever and yet not a catarrh or a "great cold." It is thus referred to in a letter of the month of June, from Belvoir, Rutlandshire[1]: "The man that dos the picturs in inemaled is gon up to London for a weke ...I wish the man dos not get this new distemper and die before he comes agane." On turning to the London weekly bills of

---

[1] *Cal. Belvoir MSS.* II. 120. June, 1688. Bridget Noel to the Countess of Rutland.

mortality we find in the first weeks of June the characteristic rise of one of those sudden epidemic fevers or new diseases, of which the earliest with recorded figures was the "gentle correction" of July, 1580. The following are the weekly London figures corresponding to the "new distemper" of 1688:

Weekly London Mortalities.

1688

Week ending	Fevers	All causes
May 29	58	368
June 5	76	518
12	101	559
19	65	435
26	66	437

The contemporary London notice of this "influenza" comes from Dr Walter Harris, who mentioned it in a book written the year after[1]:

"From the middle of the month of May in the year 1688, for some weeks, a slight sort of fever became epidemical. It affected the joints of the patients with slight pains, and they complained of a pain in their heads, especially in the fore-part, and of a sort of giddiness. It was more rife than any that I ever observed before, from any cause whatsoever, or in any time of the year. A great many whole families were taken at once with this fever, so that hardly one out of a great number escaped this general storm. Now this so epidemical or febrile insult seemed plainly to me to depend upon the variety of the season of the year, the most intense heat of some days being suddenly changed to cold...Never were so many people sick together: never did so few of them die. They recovered under almost any regimen,—almost everyone of them."

It will be seen, however, that the bills rose very considerably for four weeks, and that, too, in the healthiest season of the year.

A somewhat fuller account of its symptoms is given by Molyneux for Dublin[2]. He had been informed by a learned physician from London that it had been as general there as in Dublin, which we know to have been the case from Harris's account. Both Molyneux and Harris call it a slight fever, without mentioning catarrhal symptoms. The spring months immediately preceding had been remarkable for drought.

At Dublin this "short sort of fever" was first observed about the beginning of July, or some six weeks later than in London. "It so universally seized all sorts of men whatever, that I then made an estimate not above one in fifteen escaped. It began, as generally fevers do, with a chilness and

[1] Walter Harris, M.D., *De morbis acutis infantum.* Lond. 1689. English transl. by Cockburn, 1693, p. 88.
[2] "Historical Account of the late General Coughs and Colds, with some Observations on other Epidemical Distempers." *Phil. Trans.* XVIII. (1694), p. 109.

shivering all over, like that of an ague, but not so violent, which soon broke
out into a dry burning heat, with great uneasiness that commonly confined
them to their beds, where they passed the ensuing night very restless; they
commonly complained likewise of giddiness, and a dull pain in their heads,
chiefly about the eyes, with unsettled pains in their limbs, and about the
small of their back, a soreness all over their flesh, a loss of appetite, with a
nausea or aptness to vomit, an unusual ill taste in their mouths, yet little or
no thirst. And though these symptoms were very violent for a time, yet
they did not continue long: for after the second day of the distemper the
patient, usually of himself, fell into a sweat (unless 'twas prevented by letting
blood, which, however beneficial in other fevers, I found manifestly retarded
the progress of this): and if the sweat was encouraged for five or six hours
by laying on more cloaths, or taking some sudorifick medicine, most of the
disorders before mentioned would entirely disappear or at least very much
abate. The giddiness of their head and want of appetite would often
continue some days afterwards, but with the use of the open fresh air they
certainly in four or five days at farthest recovered these likewise and were
perfectly well. So transient and favourable was this disease that it seldom
required the help of a physician; and of a thousand that were seized with it,
I believe scarce one dyed. By the middle of August following, it wholly
disappeared, so that it had run its full course through all sorts of people in
seven weeks time...This fever spread itself all over England; whether it
extended farther I did not learn."

This short fever of men was preceded by a slight but
universal horse-cold[1].

The Influenza of 1693.

Molyneux considered the strange transient fever of the
summer of 1688 to have been the most universal fever that
perhaps had ever appeared, and he thought the universal catarrh
of five years' later date (1693) to have been " the most universal
cold." We have thus a means of contrasting in the descriptions
of the same author a universal slight fever and a universal
catarrh, which happened within five years of each other, and
were neither of them called at the time by the name of influenza,
—a name not known in Britain until half a century later.
Before coming to Molyneux's description, it should be said that
the London bills of mortality bear no decided trace of an
influenza in the end of the year 1693, the following being the
highest weekly mortalities nearest to the date given for the
epidemic at Dublin[2]:

[1] "'Twas very remarkable that in England as well as this kingdom a short time
before the general fever, a slight disease, but very universal, seized the horses too: in
them it showed itself by a great defluxion of rheum from their noses; and I was
assured by a judicious man, an officer in the army of Ireland, which was then drawn
out and encamped on the Curragh of Kildare, there were not ten horses in a regiment
that had not this disease." Molyneux, u.s.
[2] Evelyn says nothing of a great epidemic cold in this season, but makes the
following remarks on the weather: " Oct. 31. A very wet and uncomfortable season.

1693

Week ending	Fever	All causes
October 10	43	353
17	62	353
24	53	384
31	69	457
November 7	68	455
14	48	365

Molyneux's account of the flying epidemic of 1693 is as follows[1]:

"The coughs and colds that lately so universally prevailed gave us a most extraordinary instance how liable at certain times our bodies are, however differing in constitution, age and way of living, to be affected much in the same manner by a spreading evil...'Twas about the beginning of November last, 1693, after a constant course of moderately warm weather for the season, upon some snow falling in the mountains and country about the town [Dublin], that of a sudden it grew extremely cold, and soon after succeeded some few days of very hard frost, whereupon rheums of all kinds, such as violent coughs that chiefly affected in the night, great defluxion of thin rheum at the nose and eyes, immoderate discharge of the saliva by spitting, hoarseness in the voice, sore throats, with some trouble in swallowing, whesings, stuffings and soreness in the breast, a dull heaviness and stoppage in the head, with such like disorders, the usual effects of cold, seized great numbers of all sorts of people in Dublin.

"Some were more violently affected, so as to be confined awhile to their beds; those complained of feverish symptoms, as shiverings and chilness all over them, that made several returns, pains in many parts of their body, severe head-aches, chiefly about their foreheads, so as any noise was very troublesome: great weakness in their eyes, that the least light was offensive; a perfect decay of all appetite; foul turbid urine, with a brick-coloured sediment at the bottom; great uneasiness and tossing in their beds at night. Yet these disorders, though they very much frightened both the sick and their friends, usually without help of remedy would abate of themselves, and terminate in universal sweats, that constantly relieved...When the cold was moderate, it usually was over in eight or ten days; but with those in whom it rose to a greater height, it continued a fortnight, three weeks, and sometimes a month. One way or other it universally affected all kinds of men; those in the country as well as city; those that were much abroad in the open air, and those that stay'd much within doors, or even kept close in their chambers; those that were robust and hardy, as well as those that were weak and tender—men, women and children of all ranks and conditions...Not one in thirty, I may safely say, escaped it. In the space of four or five weeks it had its rise, growth, and decay; and though from first to last it seized such incredible numbers of all sorts of men, I cannot learn that any one truly dyed of it, unless such whose strength was before spent by some tedious fit of sickness, or laboured under some heavier disease complicated with it...It spread itself all over England in the same manner it did here, particularly it seized them at London and Oxford as universally and with the same symptoms as it seized us in Dublin; but with this observable difference that

Nov. 12. The season continued very wet, as it had nearly all the summer, if one might call it summer, in which there was no fruit, but corn was very plentiful."

[1] Molyneux, *Phil. Trans.* XVIII. (1694), p. 105.

it appeared three or four weeks sooner in London, that is, about the beginning of October...Nor was its progress, as I am credibly informed, bounded by these Islands for it spread still further and reached the Continent, where it infested the northern parts of France (as about Paris) Flanders, Holland, and the rest of the United Provinces with more violence and no less frequency than it did in these countries."

Yet no other writer, English or foreign, appears to have mentioned it. Its existence rests on the authority of Molyneux alone, according to the above very circumstantial narrative.

The Influenza of 1712.

There were so many fevers from 1693 to the end of the century that it is not easy to distinguish epidemic agues or catarrhs among them. If we follow the continental writers, it is not until 1709 and 1712 that there is any concurrence of testimony for such widespread maladies. Evelyn, however, says that in the remarkably dry and fine months of February and March, 1705, "agues and smallpox prevail much in every place" (21st February). The very general coughs and catarrhs of 1709 seem to have been really caused by the severity of the memorable hard winter, the frost having begun in October, 1708 and lasted until March, 1709. The evidences of a truly epidemic infectious catarrh or influenza all over Europe in 1709 are scanty and ambiguous. It is probably to this "universal cold" that Molyneux refers under the year 1708[1]; but English writers have not otherwise mentioned an epidemic in 1709.

The next, in 1712, was a "new ague" of the kind without catarrhal symptoms, like that of 1688. One German writer called it the "Galanterie-Krankheit," another the "Mode-Krankheit," and it was about the same time that the French name "la grippe" came into use. These names all mean "the disease *a la mode*" or the reigning fashion[2]; they remind one of the earlier "trousse galante" and "coqueluche" (a kind of bonnet), and of the "grande gorre" of 1494. It appears to have made little or no impression on the mortality, and would hardly have been noticed but for its wide prevalence. In

---

[1] "An universal cold that appeared in 1708, and was immediately preceded by a very sudden transition from heat to cold in Dublin and its vicinity." Molyneux's *Memoirs*.

[2] *La Grippe* may, of course, be taken literally to mean seizure; but the common use of the word seems to have been figurative for some fancy that seized many at once and became the fashion.

England it was the subject of a brief essay by Dr John Turner under the title of "Febris Britannica Anni 1712[1]"—a certain epidemic fever, of the milder kind, fatal to none, but prevalent far and wide and leaving very few families untouched. It was marked by aching and heaviness of the head, burning or lancinating pains in the back, pains in the joints like those of rheumatism, loss of appetite, vomiting, pains of the stomach and intestines. The venom though not sharp, acted quickly. Turner ascribed it to malign vapours from the interior of the earth (*malignos terrae matris halitus*). Its season in England, as in Germany, was probably the summer or autumn. Turner begins his discourse with a reference to the plague in the East of Europe, which, he says, had been kept out of England by quarantine, to the murrain which was then raging in Italy (and appeared in England in 1714), and to fevers of a bad type which had traversed all France during the past spring, invading noble houses and even the royal palace. Having begun his discourse thus, he ends it by remarking that the slight British fever did not, in his opinion, forebode a plague to follow. It may have been a recurrence of this epidemic next year that Mead speaks of under the name of the "Dunkirk rant" (supposed to have been brought over from Dunkirk by returning troops after the Peace of Utrecht) in September, 1713; it was, he says, a mild fever, which began with pains in the head and went off easily in large sweats after a day's confinement[2]. The weekly bills of mortality in London are no help to us to fix the date of the one or more slight fevers or influenzas about 1712–13. The great fever-years of the period were 1710 and 1714; but the fever was typhus, probably mixed with relapsing fever, according to the evidence in another chapter. Even compared with the universal fever or influenza of 1688, that of 1712 must have been unimportant; for the former sent up the London mortality considerably, whereas there is no characteristic rise to be found in any month of 1712 or 1713.

---

[1] Joannes Turner, M.D., *De Febre Britannica Anni* 1712. Lond. 1713, pp. 3, 4.
[2] Mead, *Short Discourse concerning Pestilential Contagion.* Lond. 1720, p. 8. But Short, who wrote in 1749, places the "Dunkirk rant" under the year 1710: (*Air, Weather, &c.* I. 455).—"March 1, began and reigned two months an epidemic which missed few, and raged fatally like a plague in France and the Low Countries, and was brought by disbanded soldiers into England, namely a catarrhous fever called the Dunkirk rant or Dunkirk ague...It lasted eight, ten, or twelve days. Its symptoms were a severe, short, dry cough, quick pulse, great pain of the head and over the whole body, moderate thirst, and sweating. Diuretics were the cure."

Either to this period, or to the undoubted aguish years
1727–28, belongs a curious statement as to "burning agues,
fevers never before heard of to be universal and mortal," in
Scotland, the same having been a "sad stroke and great distress
upon many families and persons." The authority is Patrick
Walker, who traces these hitherto unheard of troubles to the
Union of the Crowns (1707)[1].

On other and perhaps better authority, it does appear that
Scotland before that period was reputed to be remarkably free
from agues; and it is probable that the universal and mortal
burning agues some time between 1707 and 1728, had come in
one of those strange epidemic visitations, just as the agues of
1780–84 did. It would be erroneous to conclude from such
references to ague that Scotland had ever been a malarious
country. Robert Boyle refers in two places to the rarity of
agues in Scotland in the time of Charles II.; the Duke of York,
he says[2], on his return out of Scotland, 1680, mentioned that
agues were very unfrequent in that country, "which yet that year
were very rife over almost all England"—to wit, the epidemic
of 1678–80. Again, agues, especially quartans, are rare in
many parts of Scotland, "insomuch that a learned physician
answered me that in divers years practice he met not with above
three or four[3]." However, Sir Robert Sibbald, while he admits
the rarity of quartans, does allege that quotidians, tertians and
the anomalous forms occurred, that agues might be epidemic
in the spring, with different symptoms from year to year, and
that certain malignant fevers, not called agues, were wont to
rage in the autumn[4].

Epidemic Agues and Influenzas, 1727–29.

The contemporary annalist of epidemics in England is
Wintringham, of York, who enters remittents and intermittents
almost every year from 1717 to the end of his first series of

[1] "The effects and evidences of God's displeasure appearing more and more
against us since the incorporating union [1707], mingling ourselves with the people of
these abominations, making ourselves liable to their judgments, of which we are deeply
sharing; particularly in that sad stroke and great distress upon many families and
persons, of the burning agues, fevers never heard of before in Scotland to be universal
and mortal." *Life and Death of Alexander Peden.* 3rd ed. 1728. *Biog. Presb.*
I. 140.
[2] Boyle's *Works.* Ed. 1772, V. 725.
[3] *Ibid.* v. 49.
[4] *Scotia Illustrata.* Edin. 1684. Lib. II. "De Morbis," p. 52.

annals in 1726; but none of his entries points very clearly to an epidemic of ague[1]. It is not until the very unwholesome years 1727–29 that we hear of intermittent fevers being prevalent everywhere, with one or more true influenzas or epidemic catarrhs interpolated among them. To show how unhealthy England was in general, I give a table compiled from Short's abstracts of the parish registers, showing the proportion of parishes, urban and rural, with excess of burials over christenings:

Country Parishes.

Year	Registers examined	Registers showing high death-rate	Births in ditto	Deaths in ditto
1727	180	55	1091	1368
1728	180	80	1536	2429
1729	178	62	1442	2015
1730	176	39	1022	1302

Market Towns.

Year	Registers examined	Registers showing high death-rate	Births in ditto	Deaths in ditto
1727	33	19	2441	3606
1728	34	23	2355	4972
1729	36	27	3494	6673
1730	36	16	2529	3445

It is clear from the accounts by Huxham, Wintringham, Hillary, and Warren, of Bury St Edmunds[2], that much of the excessive sickness in 1727–29 was aguish, although much of it, and probably the most fatal part of it, was the low putrid fever so often mentioned after the first quarter of the 18th century. At Norwich, where the burials for three years, 1727–29, were nearly double the registered baptisms, many were carried off, says Blomefield, "by fevers and agues, and the contagion was general." In Ireland also, a country rarely touched by true agues, Rutty enters intermittent fever as very frequent in May, 1728; and again, in the spring of 1729: "Intermittent fevers were epidemic in April; and some of the petechial kind. Nor was this altogether peculiar to us; for at that same time we were informed that intermittent and other fevers were frequent

---

[1] *Commentar. Nosolog.* Lond. 1727.

[2] *The Method and Manner of curing the late raging Fevers, and of the danger, uncertainty and unwholesomeness of the Jesuit's bark.* Dated 6 Dec. 1728: "You see that intermitting fevers, when they come to be chronical (and you may see it almost everywhere) make room for a great many distempers, and those very difficult to cure." p. 49.

in the neighbourhood of Gloucester and London; and very mortal in the country places, but less in the cities."

In the midst of this epidemic constitution of agues and òther fevers there occurred one or more horse-colds, and one or more epidemic catarrhs of mankind. The most definitely marked or best recorded of these was the influenza of 1729.

The universal cold or catarrh of 1729 fell upon London in October and November, and upon York, Plymouth and Dublin about the same time. It prevailed in various parts of Europe until March, 1730, its incidence upon Italy being entirely after the New Year. The rise in the London deaths was characteristic: the level was high when the epidemic began, but the epidemic nearly doubled the already high mortality during the worst week and trebled the deaths from "fever."

London Weekly Mortalities.

1729

Week ending		Fever	All causes
October	21	88	564
	28	118	603
November	4	213	908
	11	267	993
	18	166	783
	25	124	635

The high mortalities of the weeks following may be taken as due to the sequelae of the epidemic (pneumonias, pleurisies, malignant fevers) and are indeed so explained in one contemporary account:

Week ending		Fever	All causes
December	2	92	678
	9	132	779
	16	116	707
	23	123	710
	30	109	628

The influenza of October and November, 1729, was the occasion of a London essay[1], which appears to treat solely of the epidemic catarrh and its after-effects, and not of the two years' previous sicknesses, which are the subject of another essay, by Strother, written before the influenza began. London, says

[1] *An Enquiry into the Causes of the Present Epidemical Diseases, viz. Fevers, Coughs, Asthmas, Rheumatisms, Defluxions, &c.* By the author of "The Family Companion for Health." London, 1729, pp. 6, 7.

this author, as well as Bath, and foreign parts, have been on
a sudden seized universally with the disorders named in his
title (fevers, coughs, asthmas, rheumatisms, defluxions etc.).
These had come in the course of an unusually warm and wet,
or relaxing, winter; "we have for some time past dwelt in fogs,
our air has been hazy, our streets loaden with rain, and our
bodies surrounded with water." So many different symptoms
attend the "New Disease" that a volume, he says, would not
suffice to describe them, but he thus summarizes them:

> Sudden pain in the head, heaviness or drowsiness, and anon their noses
> began to run; they coughed or wheezed, and grew hoarse; they felt an
> oppression and load on their breasts, and turned vapourish, either because
> they apprehended ill consequences, or because their spirits were oppressed
> with a load of humours. The victims of the epidemic, he says again, were
> very subject to vapours; they are, upon the least fatigue or emotion of mind,
> dispirited, and flag upon every emergency. Among other symptoms were,
> quick pulse, thirst, loss of appetite and vertigo: the mouth and jaws hot,
> rough and dry, the thrush raising blisters thereon; the throat hoarse; a
> fierce brutal cough, which weakens by bringing on profuse sweats; the
> urine, muddy and white, "if they who are seized have been old asth-
> maticks."

He speaks of cases that had proved suddenly fatal and says
that all who died of "epidemical catarrhs" had been found
to have polypuses in their hearts. If reference be made to the
Table, it will be seen that the high mortality continued in
London for at least a month after the epidemic had passed
through its ordinary course of rise, maximum and decline; and
it is probably to that post-epidemic mortality that the author
refers in the following passages:

> "Numbers, as appears by our late bills, are taken with malignant fevers,
> or malignant pleurisies or with pleuritic fevers....Whosoever, then, would
> prevent a defluxion from turning into a fever, or from anything yet worse, if
> worse can be, must keep warm and observe a diluting regimen so long as till
> their water subsides and the symptoms are vanquished...I am convinced by
> experience that many poor creatures have perished under these late epi-
> demical fevers, from the fatal mistake of never retiring from their usual
> employments till they have rivetted a fever upon them, and till they have
> neglected twelve or fourteen days of their precious time." This was fully
> endorsed by Huxham for the influenza of 1733: "Morbus raro lethalis, quem
> tamen, multi, vel ob ipsam frequentiam, temeri spernentes, seras dedêre
> poenas stultitiae, asthmatici, hectici, tabidi."

Hillary's account for Ripon is very brief[1]:

> "The season continuing very wet, and the wind generally in the southern
> points, about the middle of November [1729] an epidemical cough seized

---

[1] "Variations of the weather and Epid. Diseases, 1726–34 at Ripon." Appendix
to *Essay on the Smallpox.* Lond. 1740, p. 35.

almost everybody, few escaping it, for it was universally felt over the kingdom; they had it in London and Newcastle two or three weeks before we had it about Ripon."

Wintringham, of York, says the epidemic in the early winter of 1729 was "a febricula with slight rigors, lassitude, almost incessant cough, pain in the head, hoarseness, difficulty in breathing, and attended with some deaths among feeble persons, from pleuritic and pulmonary affections[1]." There was a tradition at Exeter as late as 1775 that two thousand were seized in one night in the epidemic of 1729. Huxham, of Plymouth, says of the epidemic in November:

"A cartarrhal febricula, with incessant cough, slight dyspepsia, anorexia, languor, and rheumatic pains, is raging everywhere. When it is more vehement than usual, it passes into bastard pleurisy or peripneumony; but for the most part it is easily got rid of by letting blood and by emetics." In December, the coughs and catarrhal fever continued, while mania was more frequent than usual, and in January, 1730, the cartarrhal fever still infested some persons.

Rutty, of Dublin, merely says: "In November raged an universal epidemic catarrh, scarce sparing any one family. It visited London before us[2]."

These references to the unusual catarrhal febricula in November, 1729, are all that occur in the epidemiographic records kept by some four British writers who recorded the weather and prevalent diseases of those years. The epidemic catarrh made a slight impression upon them beside some other epidemics, and hardly a greater impression than another of the same kind, which seems to have occurred in the beginning of 1728. Thus, Rutty says, under November, 1727: "In Staffordshire and Shropshire their horses were suddenly seized with a cough and weakness. In December, it was in Dublin and remote parts of Ireland; some bled at the nose." On December 25th, he enters: "The horses growing better, a cough and sore throat seized mankind in Dublin[3]." Huxham, for Devonshire, under Oct.–Nov. 1727 confirms this: "a vehement cough in horses, which lasted to the end of December; the greater number at length recovered from it." He does not say in that context

[1] *Comment. Nosol.* p. 142.
[2] This epidemic appears to have made a much greater impression in Italy. The *Political State of Great Britain* for 1730, p. 172, under the date of 12th January, N.S. speaks of "the influenza, a strange and universal sickness and lingering distemper," as causing thirty deaths a day in the public hospital of Milan, as well as fatalities at Rome, Bologna, Ferrara and Leghorn, including the deaths of two cardinals.
[3] *Chronological History*, p. 10.

that an epidemic cough followed among men, as Rutty does say for Dublin; but in a subsequent note upon horse-colds, he says: "In 1728 and 1733 it [the precedence of the horse-cold] was most manifest; in which years a most severe cough seized almost all the horses, one or two months earlier than men." From which it would appear that the influenza of Nov.–Dec. 1729, was not the only one during the aguish years 1727–29.

In the weekly London bills the other series of mortalities that look most like those of an influenza are in the month of February, 1728 (748, 889, 850 and 927 in four successive weeks, being more than double the average).

The Influenza of 1733.

The next influenza was three years after that of 1729—in January, 1733. In London, it raised the weekly deaths for a couple of weeks to a far greater height than the preceding had done. Also the purely catarrhal symptoms of running from the eyes and nose are more prominent in the accounts for 1733 than for the influenza of 1729. The first notice of it comes from Edinburgh. The horses having been "attacked with running of the nose and coughs towards the end of October and beginning of November," the same symptoms began suddenly among men on the 17th December, 1732[1]. By the 25th the epidemic was general in Edinburgh, very few escaping, and it continued in that city until the middle of January, 1733. In a great many it began with a running of lymph at the eyes and nose, which continued for a day. Generally the patients were inclined to sweat, and some had profuse sweats. It was noted as remarkable that the prisoners in the gaol escaped; also the boys in Heriot's Hospital, as well as the inhabitants of houses near to that charity. The Edinburgh deaths rose as in the following table; the bulk of these extra burials are said to have been at the public charges, the epidemic having swept away a great number of poor, old, and consumptive people:

---

[1] *Edinburgh Medical Essays and Observations*, II. p. 22, Art. 2. "An Account of the Diseases that were most frequent last year in Edinburgh" (June, 1832 to May, 1833): There had been tertian agues throughout the month of June, 1732, and from August to October an epidemic in the suburbs and villages near Edinburgh, of a slow fever, having symptoms like the "comatose" fever of Sydenham, or the remittent of children.

Buried in November, 1732   89
„   „ December, 1732   109
„   „ January, 1733   214
„   „ February, 1733   135

Hillary[1] fixes the date of its beginning at Leeds on 3 February, one week later than at York, three weeks later than at Newcastle, or than in London and the south of England generally. At Leeds in three days' time about one-third part of the people were seized with chills, catarrh, violent cough, sneezing and coryza; the epidemic lasted five or six weeks in the town and country near. Dr John Arbuthnot, who was then living in Dover Street, is clear that the outbreak in London was later than in Edinburgh, which indeed appears also from the paragraph in the *Gentleman's Magazine*, dated Wednesday the 11th January, and from a comparison of the dates of highest mortalities in London (p. 349) and Edinburgh. It was in Saxony from the 15th November to the 29th of that month, and in Holland before it broke out in England. But it had begun in New England in the middle of October, and had broken out soon after in Barbados, Jamaica, Mexico and Peru. Its outbreak in Paris was at the beginning of February, 1733, and at Naples in March. The symptoms, says Arbuthnot, were uniform in every place—small rigors, pains in the back, a thin defluxion occasioning sneezing, a cough with expectoration. In France the fever ended after several days in miliary eruptions, in Holland often in imposthumations of the throat. In some, the cough outlasted the fever six weeks or two months. The horses were seized with the catarrh before mankind[2].

The account of the influenza of 1733 in London in the *Gentleman's Magazine* is under the date of 11 January: "About this time coughs and colds began to grow so rife that scarce a family escaped them, which carried off a good many, both old and young. The distemper discovered itself by a shivering in the limbs, a pain in the head, and a difficulty of breathing. The remedies prescribed were various, but especially bleeding, drinking cold water, small broths, and such thin liquids as dilute the blood[3]."

Huxham says that it was in Cornwall and the west of Devon in February, 1733, and that at Plymouth, on the 10th of that

[1] *Op. cit.* p. 47.
[2] John Arbuthnot, M.D., *Essay concerning the Effects of Air on Human Bodies.* London, 1733, p. 193. His remarks upon the "hysteric" maladies that were common after the wave of influenza in Jan.–Feb. 1733, are referred to in the chapter on Continued Fevers, along with the corresponding information from Hillary, of Ripon.
[3] *Gent. Magaz.* 1733, Jan. p. 43.

month, some were suddenly seized: "the day after they fell down in multitudes, and on the 18th or 20th of March, scarce anyone had escaped it."

It began with slight shivering, followed by transient erratic heats, headache, violent sneezing, flying pains in the back and chest, violent cough, a running of thin sharp mucus from the nose and mouth. A slight fever followed, with the pulse quick, but not hard or tense. The urine was thick and whitish, the sediment yellowish-white, seldom red. Several had racking pain in the head, many had singing in the ears and pain in the meatus auditorius, where sometimes an abscess formed: exulcerations and swelling of the fauces were likewise very common. The sick were in general much given to sweating, which, when it broke out of its own accord and was very plentiful, continuing without striking in again, did often in the space of two or three days carry off the fever. The disorder in other cases terminated with a discharge of bilious matter by stool, and sometimes by the breaking forth of fiery pimples. It was rarely fatal, and then mostly to infants and old worn out people. Generally it went off about the fourth day, leaving a troublesome cough often of long duration, "and such dejection of strength as one would hardly have suspected from the shortness of the time." The cough in all was very vehement, hardly to be subdued by anodynes: and it was so protracted in some as to throw them into consumption, which carried them off within a month or two[1].

Huxham is unusually full on the coughs and anginas of horses for several months before the influenza of men. In August, 1732, coughs were troubling some horses; in September, a coughing angina (called "the strangles") everywhere among horses which almost suffocates most of them; in October the disease of horses is raging at its worst; and in December it is still among them.

The Influenza of 1737.

After several years, unhealthy in other ways, the influenza came again in the autumn of 1737. In Devonshire, according to Huxham, the horses began to suffer from cough and angina, and some of them to die, as early as January, 1737, the epizootic being mentioned again in February, but not subsequently. The same observer says the influenza began at Plymouth in November and lasted to the end of December, 1737, seizing almost everyone, and proving much more severe than the epidemic catarrhal febricula of 1733[2]. In London it must have begun in the end of August, to judge by the characteristic rise in the weekly bills, and in the item of "fevers" more especially; and

---

[1] Huxham, *Obs. de aere et morbis epidemicis*, 1728–52, *Plymuthi factae.*
[2] *De Aere, &c.* pp. 3, 136–8.

although the deaths kept high for a longer period than in 1733, yet no single week of 1737 had much more than half the highest weekly mortality of the preceding influenza season.

London Weekly Mortalities.

1733			1737		
Week ending	Fevers	All causes	Week ending	Fevers	All causes
January 16	69	531	August 30	117	611
23	83	783	September 6	161	720
30	243	1588	13	201	837
February 6	170	1166	20	229	861
13	110	628	27	167	770
20	66	591	October 4	143	687
			11	114	551

In Dublin the worst week's mortality in 1737, in the month of October, was 144, whereas in the influenza of 1733 the highest weekly bill had been only 98[1]. Hardly any particulars of the influenza of 1737 remain, although it appears to have been widely diffused, being recorded for Barbados and New England. The only source of English information is Huxham of Plymouth, who mentions some symptoms which should serve to characterize this outbreak, namely : violent swelling of the face, the parotids and maxillary glands, followed by an immense discharge of an exceedingly acrid pituita from the mouth and nose; toothache and, in some, hemicrania ; " in multitudes," wandering rheumatic pains ; in others violent sciatics; in some griping of the bowels. Huxham makes one interesting statement: "This catarrhal fever has prevailed more or less for several winters past;" or, in other words, the interval between the severe influenza of 1733 and the milder influenza of 1737 was not altogether clear of the disease. He adds that it put on various forms, according to the different constitutions of those it attacked.

The Influenza of 1743.

Six years after, in 1743, came another influenza, which presents some interesting points. A writer in the *Gentleman's Magazine* for May, 1743, says that the epidemic began in September last in Saxony, that it progressed to Milan, Genoa, and Venice, and to Florence and Rome, where it was called the Influenza ; in February last (1743) no fewer than 80,000 were

---

[1] Rutty, *Chronol. Hist. of Diseases in Dublin.* Lond. 1770.

sick of it [? in Rome] and 500 buried in one day. At Messina it was suspected to be the forerunner of a plague—which did, indeed, ensue. It is now (May) in Spain, depopulating whole villages. The outbreak in Italy is authenticated by many notices collected by Corradi, Brescia having had the epidemic in October, 1742, Milan and Venice in November, Bologna in December, Rome, Pisa, Leghorn, Florence and Genoa in January, 1743, Naples and the Sicilian towns in February. The English troops, in cantonments near Brussels, were little touched by it when it reached that capital about the end of February, but, strangely enough, "many who in the preceding autumn had been seized with intermittents then relapsed[1]."

In London the epidemic appears to have begun in the end of March, and had trebled the deaths in the week ending 12th April; by the beginning of May it was practically over.

London Weekly Mortalities.

1743

Week ending	Fevers	All causes
March 29	94	579
April 5	189	1013
12	300	1448
19	223	1026
26	115	629
May 3	82	537

The familiar view of the influenza in London is given in a letter by Horace Walpole from Arlington Street, 25 March, 1743[2]:

"We have had loads of sunshine all the winter: and within these ten days nothing but snows, north-east winds and *blue plagues*. The last ships have brought over all your epidemic distempers; not a family in London has scaped under five or six ill; many people have been forced to hire new labourers. Guernier, the apothecary, took two new apprentices, and yet could not drug all his patients. It is a cold and fever. I had one of the worst, and was blooded on Saturday and Sunday, but it is quite gone; my father was blooded last night; his is but slight. The physicians say there has been nothing like it since the year thirty-three, and then not so bad [the bill of mortality almost the same]; in short our army abroad would shudder to see what streams of blood have been let out! Nobody has died of it [as yet, but later some 1000 in a week above the usual bill] but old Mr Eyres of Chelsea, through obstinacy of not bleeding; and his ancient Grace of York; Wilcox of Rochester succeeds him, who is fit for nothing in the world but to die of this cold too."

[1] Pringle, *Diseases of the Army*, p. 16.
[2] *Letters of Horace Walpole*, ed. Cunningham, I. 235.

The account in the *Gentleman's Magazine* confirms the vast shedding of blood: "In the last two months it visited almost every family in the city; so that the surgeons and all the phlebotomists had full employment. Bleeding, sweating and blistering were the remedies usually prescribed. All over the island it cut off old people. At Greenwich upwards of twenty hospital men and boys were buried in a night[1]." In Edinburgh, as in London, the weekly burials were trebled. On Sunday, May 6th, fifty sick persons were prayed for in the Edinburgh churches, and in the preceding week there had been seventy burials in the Greyfriars, being three times the usual number[2]. It reached Dublin in May, proving milder and less fatal than in London (perhaps that is why the writer in the *Gentleman's Magazine* says it did not visit Ireland at all); it visited, also, the remote parts of Ulster and Munster, scarce sparing a family[3].

It had reached Plymouth in the end of April. Huxham, who is again the chief witness to its symptoms, says that it was much less severe there than in the south of Europe or even than in London.

Innumerable persons were seized at once with a wandering kind of shiver and heaviness in the head; presently also came on a pain therein, as well as in the joints and back; several, however, were troubled with a universal lassitude. Immediately there ensued a very great and acrid defluxion from the eyes, nostrils and fauces, and very often falling upon the lungs, which occasioned almost perpetual sneezings, and commonly a violent cough. The tongue looked as if rubbed with cream. The eyes were slightly inflamed; and, being violently painful in the bottom of the orbit, shunned the light. The greater part of the sick had easy, equal and kindly sweats the second or third day, which, with the large spitting, gave relief. Great loss of strength, however, remained. Frequently towards the end of this "feveret," several red angry pustules broke out: often, likewise, a sudden, nay a profuse, diarrhoea with violent griping. In many cases Huxham was astonished at the vast sediment (yellowish white), which the urine threw down, "than which there could not be a more favourable symptom[4]." One remarkable feature of the epidemic of 1743 was recalled by W. Watson in a letter to Huxham on the epidemic of 1762: "In the disorder of 1743 the skin was very frequently inflamed when the fever ran high; and it afterwards peeled off in most parts of the body[5]."

---

[1] *Gent. Magaz.* XIII. May 1743, p. 272.

[2] R. Chambers, *Domestic Annals of Scotland*, III. 610.

[3] Rutty, u. s. under the year 1743. In an earlier passage, he says that the influenza of 1743 raised the Dublin weekly bills to a highest point of 67, so that it must have been very slight in that city.

[4] Huxham, *Obs. de aere etc.*, 2nd ed. 3 vols. Lond. 1752–70, II. 99.

[5] W. Watson, *Phil. Trans.* LII. 646.

Some Localized Influenzas and Horse-colds.

For the space of nineteen years, from 1743 to 1762, there occurred no universal cold common to all the countries of Europe; the convergence of positive testimony, which is so remarkable on many occasions from the 16th century onwards, is found on no occasion during that interval. And yet the period is not wanting in instructive notices of epidemic catarrh, which I shall take from English writings only. British troops occupied Minorca during some of those years, and the epidemics of the island were carefully noted by Cleghorn. Under the year 1748 he writes:

> "About the 20th April there appeared suddenly a catarrhal fever, which for three weeks raged so universally that almost everybody in the island was seized with it. This disease exactly resembled that which was so epidemical in the year 1733. For in most part of the sick the feverish symptoms went off with a plentiful sweat in two or three days; while the cough and expectoration continued sometime longer. In a few athletic persons, who were not blooded in time, it terminated in a fatal pleurisy or phrensy[1]."

Another English epidemiographist, Hillary, who had begun his records at Ripon, was in those years resident in Barbados; and in that island, as in Minorca, we hear of unmistakeable universal colds, although none of them at the same time as the one recorded by Cleghorn. The Barbados annalist records a general catarrhous fever in September, 1752[2], and a recurrence of the same in the end of December, lasting until February 1753 (catarrh and coryza, cough, hoarseness, a great defluxion of rheum, some having fever with it). As it ceased in February, 1753, a slow nervous fever began, and continued epidemic for eighteen months, until September, 1784, when it totally disappeared, and was not seen again so long as Hillary remained in the island (1758). In 1755 there was another epidemic catarrhal fever, first in February and again in the end of the year. In the earlier outbreak, few escaped having more or less of it, the symptoms being cold ague for a few hours, followed by a hot fever with great pain in the head, or pains in the back and all

---

[1] Cleghorn, *Observations on the Epidemical Diseases in Minorca*, 1744–49, p. 132.
[2] This influenza was observed in the North American Colonies. It is noteworthy that Huxham, of Plymouth, records under October, 1752, that hundreds of people at once had cough, sore throat, defluxions from the nose, eyes and mouth, attended with a slight fever, and more or less of a rash, several having a great flux of the belly.—*On Ulcerous Sore Throat*, 1757, p. 13.

over the body, which lasted two or three days, or longer, and then went off in some by a critical sweat.   In the October outbreak it affected children mostly.   Once more, in 1757, the same catarrhous fever returned, with almost the same circumstances[1]. That year there was a universal catarrh in North America.

Not less remarkable than the epidemic catarrhal fever in Minorca in 1748, or those in Barbados in 1752–3, 1755 and 1757, was the epidemic of 1758 in Scotland[2].   It was first noticed with east winds from the 16th to 20th September, several children having taken fever like a cold.   In the last week of September thirty out of sixty boys at the Grammar School of Dalkeith were seized with it in two or three days.   In October it became more general, among old and young, and increased till about the 24th, when it began to abate.   In Edinburgh not one in six or seven escaped.   It was in most parts of Scotland in October—Kirkaldy, St Andrews, Perthshire (where many died of it), Ayrshire, Glasgow, Aberdeenshire, Rossshire (end of October).   A gentleman told Dr Whytt that in the Carse of Gowrie, in September, "before this disease was perceived, the horses were observed to be more than usually affected with a cold and a cough."

The symptoms in Scotland were of the Protean kind of "influenza": there might be fever with no cold; or a coryzal attack with little or no fever; or some had bleeding at the nose for several days, which might be profuse; or the soreness and pains in the bones might be in all parts of the body, or confined to the cheekbones, teeth and sides of the head.   Others had a fever without any distinctive concomitant, but a cough when the fever subsided[3].   One of Whytt's patients, a lady aged thirty, had been feverish for four days, when a scarlet rash

---

[1] W. Hillary, M.D., *Obs. on...Epid. Diseases in Barbadoes.* Lond. 1760.
[2] It is not described for England, unless a reference by Bisset for Cleveland, Yorkshire, should apply to it.   Short says, under the year 1758 (*Increase and Decrease of Mankind in England, &c.* 1767): A healthy year in general, "only in the harvest was a very sickly mortal time among the poor, of a putrid slow fever, which carried off many.   An epidemic catarrh broke out in November, and made a sudden sweep over the whole kingdom."   Barker, of Coleshill, says, in his *Putrid Constitution of* 1777 (Birmingham, 1779, p. 49): "In the remarkable intermittents of 1758 or 9... the early and consequently injudicious use of the bark was attended with such fatal effects that a few doses only sometimes totally oppressed the head, brought on a most rapid delirium, and cut off persons in half-an-hour."
[3] Robert Whytt, M.D., "On the Epidemic Disorder of 1758 in Edinburgh and other parts of the South of Scotland." *Med. Obs. and Inq. by a Society of Physicians*, 6 vols. Lond. II. (1762), p. 187.   With notices by Millar, of Kelso, and Alves, of Inverness.

appeared, but did not come fully out; the fall of the pulse and fever coincided with the beginning of a troublesome tickling cough, "so that the cough might be said to have been truly critical." Those who exposed themselves too soon frequently relapsed. Few died of the disease, except some old people. "In some parts of the country, when the disease was not taken care of in the beginning, as being attended with no alarming symptoms, it assumed the form of a slow fever, which sometimes proved mortal."

The year after the localised influenza of Scotland there was an epidemic of the same kind in Peru and Bolivia, that year, 1759, being one in which no universal fever or catarrh is reported from any other country. It extended from south to north, along the coast as well as over the high table-lands of Bolivia and the sierra region of Peru, invading, among others, the populous towns of Chuquisaca, Potosi, La Paz, Cuzco and Lima. In five or six days hardly one inhabitant of a place had escaped it, although some had it very slightly. As it was swift in its attack, so it was soon over, lasting about a month in each place. Its symptoms were great dizziness and heaviness of the head (vertigo and gravedo), feebleness of all the senses, deafness, strong pains over all the body, moderate fever, weariness, great prostration, complete loss of appetite, bleeding from the mouth and nostrils (this had been noted in Scotland the year before), and a long convalescence. Dogs shared the disorder, and might have been seen lying stretched out in the streets, unable to stand. It will be observed that the symptoms given do not include catarrh[1].

Before we come to the next general influenza in Britain, that of 1762, there are some facts to be mentioned as to agues and horse-colds in the interval since 1743. In Rutty's Dublin chronology, agues are entered as prevalent in 1745. In 1750, about the middle or end of December, the most epidemic and universally spreading disease among horses that anyone living remembered made its appearance in Dublin, and in Ulster and Munster almost as soon. It had been in England in November, and was like that which preceded the universal catarrhs of mankind in 1737 and 1743. In 1751, irregular agues were

---

[1] Archibald Smith, M.D., "Notices of the Epidemics of 1719–20 and 1759 in Peru," &c. from the Medical Gazette of Lima, on the authority of Don Antonio de Ulloa. *Trans. Epid. Soc.* II. pt. 1, p. 134.

frequent in March, as were also tumours of the face, jaws and throat. Agues also continued to be frequent in April, both in Dublin and in several parts of the country. In December, 1751, and January, 1752, there was another horse-cold, the same as a twelvemonth before. In 1754 the spring agues were frequent in Kilkenny and Carlow, though rare in Dublin. In 1757, "intermittent fevers, which had not appeared since April, 1746," came in the end of February. In 1760, a great catarrh among horses became general in Dublin in April. Coughs and tumours about the fauces and throat, with a slight fever, often occurred in March ; and regular intermittents, tertians or quotidians, were more frequent than for some years past. These, according to Sims, of Tyrone, abated after 1762, so that he had not seen an intermittent since 1764 until the date of his writing, 1773.

The horse-cold of 1760 was observed in London in January. The *Annual Register* says under date 27 Jan.: "A distemper which rages amongst horses makes great havock in and about town. Near a hundred died in one week." In a letter a day later (28 Jan.) Horace Walpole writes : "All the horses in town are laid up with sore throats and colds, and are so hoarse you cannot hear them speak....I have had a nervous fever these six or seven weeks every night, and have taken bark enough to have made a rind for Daphne[1]." This same horse-cold is reported from the Cleveland district of Yorkshire : "In February, [1760] horses were invaded by the most epidemic cold or catarrh that has ever happened in the remembrance of the oldest men living[2]." The same authority for Cleveland says that intermittents were frequent and obstinate in the spring of 1760.

Among these miscellanies of the history may be mentioned an outbreak of "violent pleuritic fever or peripneumene" in the spring of 1747, which was fatal to a comparatively large number in the parish of George Ham, North Devon. Thirteen died of it from the 20th to the 31st March, four in April, four in May, and one in June, "most of them in four or five days after the first seizure." The same family names recur in the list[3].

[1] Horace Walpole's *Letters*, ed. Cunningham, III. 281.
[2] C. Bisset, *Essay on the Medical Constitution of Great Britain*, 1 *Jan.* 1758, *to Midsummer* 1760. Lond. 1762, p. 279.
[3] Extract from the parish register printed by Dr G. B. Longstaff in an appendix to his *Studies in Statistics*. Lond. 1891, p. 443.

The Influenza of 1762.

The universal slight fever or catarrhal fever of 1762 was, in London, much less mortal than those of 1733 and 1743.

London Weekly Mortalities.

1762

Week ending	Fevers	All causes
May 4	72	467
11	104	626
18	159	750
25	162	659
June 1	121	516
8	85	504

It began in London about the 4th of April, and by the 24th of that month "pervaded the whole city far and wide, scarcely sparing anyone." It was in Edinburgh by the beginning of May, and in Dublin about the same time, but did not reach some parts of Cumberland until the end of June. Short, who was then living at Rotherham, says that it "continued most of the summer[1]." It had the usual variety of symptoms in the individual cases, of which only a few need be again particularized. Where the fever was sharp, it usually remitted during the day, having its exacerbation in the night. Sometimes it proved periodical, and of the tertian type: "it usually returned every night with an aggravation of the feverish symptoms" (Rutty). Perspiration was a constant symptom; the tongue was as if covered with cream (Baker repeats this figure of Huxham's in 1743). "Depression of mind and failure of strength were in all cases much greater than was proportionate to the amount of disease. A great number of those affected were very slowly restored to health, languishing for months, and some even for a whole year with cough and feverishness—relics of the disease which it was difficult to shake off. Some, after struggling long with impaired health, fell victims to pulmonary consumption. In some there were pains in all the joints and in the head, with lassitude and vehement fever, but with little signs of catarrh." Rutty, of Dublin, says that in some a measly efflorescence or a red rash was seen, attended by violent itching[2]. Among

---

[1] *Increase and Decrease of Mankind in England &c.* London, 1767.
[2] Rutty, *op. cit.* p. 275. Compare Watson, *supra*, p. 351.

labourers in the country, the pestilence was so violent as to destroy many within four days, from complications of pneumonia, pleurisy and angina. Sometimes it took the form of a slow fever, "and approximated to that form of malady which the ancients denominated 'cardiac'[1]."

The mortality is said to have varied much. White, of Manchester, declared that fewer died there than in ordinary while the epidemic lasted. On the other hand Offley, of Norwich, said there were more victims there than by the epidemic of 1733 "or by the more severe visitation called influenza in 1743"—the two visitations which were incomparably the worst in the whole history, according to the London bills. Baker says that it infested cities and the larger towns crowded with inhabitants earlier than the surrounding villages, and is inclined to think that it was mostly brought by persons coming from London[2].

The progress of this epidemic over Europe had been peculiar. It was seen in the end of February, 1762, at Breslau, where the deaths rose from 30 or 40 in a week to 150. It was in Vienna at the end of March, and in North Germany about the same time as in England—April and May. There were at that time British troops in Bremen, among whom the epidemic appeared shortly after the 10th April[3].

" It looked at first as if they were going to have agues, but soon they were attacked with a cough and a difficulty of breathing and pain of the breast, with a headache, and pains all over the body, especially in the limbs. The first nights they commonly had profuse sweats. In several it had the appearance of a remitting fever for the two or three first days." The cough in many was convulsive. The epidemic seized most of the people in the town of Bremen: very few of the British escaped, but none of them died, except one or two, from a complication of drunkenness and pneumonia.

It is said to have been nowhere in France except in Strasburg and the rest of Alsace, in June. Baker says, "Whilst

---

[1] G. Baker, *De Catarrho et de Dysenteria Londinensi epidemicis*, 1762, Lond. 1764; W. Watson, "Some remarks upon the Catarrhal Disorder which was very frequent in London in May 1762, and upon the Dysentery which prevailed in the following autumn." *Phil. Trans.* LII. (1762), p. 646.

[2] Professor Alexander Monro, *primus*, of Edinburgh, describes his own attack in a letter to his son, Dr Donald Monro, 11 June, 1766 (*Works of Alex. Monro, M.D. with Life*, Edin. 1781, p. 306): "My case is this: in May, 1762, I had the epidemic influenza, which affected principally the parts in the pelvis; for I had a difficulty and sharp pain in making water and going to stool. My belly has never since been in a regular way, passing sometimes for several days nothing but bloody mucus, and that with considerable tenesmus" &c. Dysentery was epidemic in 1762 as well as influenza.

[3] Donald Monro, M.D., *Diseases of the British Military Hospitals in Germany, &c.* Lond. 1764, p. 137.

it raged everywhere else, it did not reach Paris or its vicinity, a fact which I learned from trustworthy persons." On board British ships of war in the Mediterranean it occurred in July. Its severity appears to have varied greatly in different cities of the same country. Rutty, for Ireland, agrees with Baker, for England, that it was more fatal in the country than in the towns.

The Influenza of 1767.

The next influenza, that of 1767, was so unimportant that its existence in England would hardly have been known but for Dr Heberden's paper, "The Epidemical Cold in June and July 1767[1]." Those few who were affected by a cold in London early in June observed that it differed from a common cold, and resembled the epidemical cold of the year 1762, on account of the great languor, feverishness, and loss of appetite. It became more common, was at its height in the last week of June or beginning of July, and before the end of July had entirely ceased. It was less epidemical and far less dangerous than the cold of 1762, so much so that the London bills of mortality hardly witness at all to its existence. The attack began with several chills; then came a troublesome and almost unceasing cough, very acute pains in the head, back, and abdomen under the left ribs, occasioning want of sleep. Many of the symptoms hung upon several for at least a week, and sometimes lasted a month. The fever might be great enough to bring on deliriousness, yet had plain remissions and intermissions. The same disorder was reported to be common about the same time in many other parts of England, and more fatal than it was in London. Heberden did not anticipate from it the lingering effects in the individual, for months or years, which marked so many of the cases in 1762[2].

---

[1] *Med. Trans. published by the College of Physicians in London,* I. 437. Heberden's paper was read at the College, Aug. 11, 1767.

[2] The nearest approach to Heberden's London influenza of 1767 is an epidemic that Sims observed in Tyrone in the autumn of 1767; a season remarkable for measles and acute rheumatism. At the same time that the acute rheumatism prevailed, a fever showed itself, like it; the patients for two or three days were languid, chilly, with pains in the bones, headache, stupor, dry tongue, costiveness. It was marked by remissions, was by no means mortal, and usually ended by a sweat from the 14th to the 17th day, followed by a copious deposit in the urine. James Sims, *Obs. on Epidemic Disorders,* Lond. 1773, p. 84.

The Influenza of 1775.

Heberden invited physicians in the provinces to send in accounts of the epidemic of June and July, 1767, but no one seems to have responded. However, the next epidemic catarrh, of November and December, 1775, was made the subject of many communications from all parts of Britain, in response to a circular drawn up by Dr John Fothergill. This was a distinctly catarrhal epidemic, running of the nose and eyes, cough and (or) diarrhoea, being commonly noted.

At Northampton some had "a severe pain in one side of the face, affecting the teeth and ears, and returning periodically at certain hours in the evening, or about midnight, attended with vertigo, delirium and limpid urine during the exacerbation. Some whose cases were complicated with the above symptoms had a general rash, but without its proving critical...Many of those who escaped the catarrh have been more or less sensible of giddiness, or pains in the head or face," with limpid urine, etc., as if they had a full attack[1]. The epidemic began in London about the 20th October, and made a slight impression upon the bills of mortality in some weeks of November and December[2]. Grant says that it lasted nearly five months in London, having been attended by the same "comatose" fever which Sydenham associated with the epidemic catarrh of 1675. The fatalities in Grant's practice occurred late in the epidemic :

"On the 23rd December [1775] I had lost one patient, and soon after two others; all died comatous, owing, as I then imagined, to the remains of the comatose fever of Sydenham, which had raged all the autumn, was complicated with the catarrhous fever, and continued by the wet, warm uncommon weather for the season of the year; and I still [1782] am of opinion that this complication is the reason why the epidemic catarrh of 1775 proved much more fatal than it did in 1782—a fact known to all of us[3].'

[1] Anthony Fothergill, *Mem. Med. Soc.* III. 30. This paper is not included in John Fothergill's series. There is also a separate Dublin essay, *Advice to the People upon the Epidemic Catarrhal Fever of Oct. Nov. Dec.* 1775. By a Physician.

[2] I have not found the weekly bills for this year in London; but the following averages, taken from the four-weekly or five-weekly totals in the *Gentleman's Magazine*, will show how slight the rise was:

1775.	October	weekly average	323 births	345 deaths
	November	,, ,,	334 ,,	447 ,,
	December	,, ,,	369 ,,	449 ,,

[3] W. Grant, M.D., *Observations on the late Influenza as it appeared at London in* 1775 *and* 1782. Lond. 1782. Also, by the same, *A Short Account of the Present Epidemic Cough and Fever, in a letter &c.* First printed at Bath, and afterwards at London, 1776.

A Liverpool writer also says that the catarrh of 1782 "distinguished by the same title," was a much slighter complaint than the "influenza" of 1775. The latter, however, was a summer epidemic, and was naturally less complicated with pneumonia and bronchitis, whatever the "comatose" fever of 1775 may have been. Grant's statement that the influenza of 1775 lasted five months in London is borne out by the Foundling Hospital records: on 11 November, there were 16 in the Infirmary with "epidemic fever and cough," next week 22 with "fevers, coughs and colds," and so on week by week under the same names until the 9th of March, 1776[1]. At Dorchester it was general after 10th November; about the same time it was in Exeter, where within a week it seized all the inmates, but two children, in the Devon and Exeter Hospital, to the number of 173 persons. The middle of November is also the date of its decided outbreak at Birmingham, at Worcester, and at Chester, where Howard found the prisoners suffering from it. At York in the north, as at Blandford in the south, it is claimed to have begun earlier than in London. At Lancaster it was not seen until three weeks after the accounts of its prevalence in London began to come in, but only three days after it was first heard of in Liverpool. At Aberdeen it was fully a month later than in London. It did not visit Fraserburgh, though there was a putrid fever there very fatal at that time[2].

In many cases the disease assumed the type of an intermittent towards its decline, but bark was not useful (Fothergill, Ash, while Baker says that bark did good when the fever was spent). All the observers agree both as to its slight fatality and its universality. At Chester it attacked 73 out of 97 affluent persons, neighbours in the Abbey Square; at the Cross, inhabited by people in trade, 109 had the disease out of 144; in the House

[1] MS. Infirmary Book.

[2] The reports collected by Dr John Fothergill (*Med. Obs. and Inquir.* VI. 340) were by himself, and by Pringle, Baker, Heberden and Reynolds, of London; Cuming, of Dorchester; Glass, of Exeter (long account): Ash, of Birmingham; White, of York; Haygarth, of Chester; Pulteney, of Blandford; Thomson, of Worcester; Skene, of Aberdeen; and Campbell, of Lancaster. The papers of this collective inquiry, as well as the two collections in 1782, the collection of Simmonds in 1788, that of Beddoes in 1803 (in a digest) and the Report of the Provincial Medical Association in 1837, together with some other extracts from books or papers, were brought together in a volume, without much editing, by Dr Theophilus Thompson, under the title of *The Annals of Influenza in Great Britain from* 1510 *to* 1837. London, 1852. This has been reprinted and brought down to date by Dr Symes Thompson, 1891.

of Industry, not one escaped out of 175 ; it attacked people in the country rather later than in the town, and less generally, but it was in villages and even in solitary houses.

The unusual prevalence of catarrh among horses (and dogs) is asserted by John Fothergill ("during this time"), Cuming ("after the middle of August very generally in Yorkshire"), Glass (in September), Haygarth (in North Wales, about August and September), Pulteney ("before we heard of it among the human race"). The fullest statement is by Dr Anthony Fothergill, of Northampton:

"This distemper prevailed some time among horses before it attacked the human species. The cough harassed them severely and rendered them unfit for work, though few died. About the same time also it infested the canine species and with great fatality, especially hounds. An experienced huntsman informed me that it ran through whole packs in many parts of England and that several dogs died[1]."

The progress of influenza from other countries towards Britain was so much a matter of rumour or vague statement in the earlier periods that it has not seemed worth while to make a point of it under each epidemic. It happens, however, that there is good evidence of the line of progress of the epidemic of 1775. The afterwards celebrated Professor Gregory, of Edinburgh, encountered it in Italy in the autumn, and followed it all the way home to Scotland. He saw it successively in Genoa, in the south of France, in the north of France, in London, and last of all in Edinburgh, where he himself at length fell ill with it, several of his travelling companions having taken it in Italy two or three months before. In his lectures long after (as reported by Christison, who heard them about 1817) he traced the influenza of 1775 from south to north: "It appears to have broken out somewhere on the north and west coast of Africa, whence it spread not only north into Europe, but likewise eastward to Arabia, Egypt, Syria, Palestine, Asia Minor, Hindostan, China, and was ascertained to have spread over the whole immense empire of the Chinese. From China it returned westward by a northern route through the extensive dominions of Russia and from that country it was sent again over Europe in 1782[2]."

[1] *Mem. Med. Soc.* III. 34.
[2] *Life of Sir Robert Christison*, 2 vols. Edin. 1885, vol. I. (Autobiography), p. 82.

The Influenza of 1782.

Seven years after, in the early summer of 1782, there came another swift and brief wave of catarrhal fevers over England, Scotland and Ireland, in the midst of a great "constitution" of epidemic agues which continued for several years. This was the occasion when the Italian name of "influenza" was formally adopted by the College of Physicians. Perhaps the first appearance of the name in English was in an account of the epidemic in Italy in 1729, given by a London periodical devoted to political news from foreign countries, and called, "The Political State of Great Britain[1]." In 1743 the news of the Italian epidemic under its native name reached London before the infection itself, the Italian name being frequently given to it while it lasted that season in England. When the next epidemic came, in 1762, it was not called the influenza as a matter of course, but was compared to the disease in 1743 "called the influenza." In the epidemic of 1775, "influenza" came more into use, and in 1782 it was the name usually given to the epidemic malady. The adoption of this name put an end at length to the ambiguity between epidemic agues and influenzas, leaving the curious correspondences between them in time and place, or the nosological affinities between them, as interesting as ever.

As late as the very fatal aguish years 1727–29, there was no clear separation of the epidemic agues from the influenzas, of which latter there were two or more, the one in the end of 1729 being easy to identify. In the great aguish constitution of 1678–81, Sydenham distinguished the epidemic coughs and catarrhs in Nov. 1679; but Morley made no such distinction, describing the whole series of agues for two seasons (and he might have done so for two seasons more) as the "new fever," "new ague," or "new delight," as in Derbyshire, without a suspicion that the universal coughs, catarrhs and fevers in November, 1679, were something nosologically distinct, which the future would identify as "influenza." In like manner Whitmore, in the great aguish period immediately preceding, that of 1658–59, had described the "new disease" as one single Proteus. In the still earlier epidemic seasons of 1557–58 and 1580–82, everything was "ague," although we now discover influenza mixed therewith.

[1] For the year 1730, under the date 12 January, p. 172.

I do not say that this inclusive naming was the better scientifically; nor do I uphold Willis and Sydenham in their teaching that the intermittent constitution passed into the catarrhal, in 1658 and 1679 respectively. But it is necessary to bear in mind the matter of fact, namely, that those agues, amidst which the "great colds" occurred, were epidemic agues, and not the endemic fevers of malarious places; and I have now to show that the "influenza" of 1782 was in like manner a brief episode in the midst of several successive seasons of agues, which were as much "new" or "strange" as any of those in the earlier history. Whether the epidemic agues of 1780–85 were the last of the kind in Britain had better be left an open question until our most recent and most strange experiences in 1890–93 are read in the light of history.

The influenza of 1782 was a very definite incident of a few weeks—*teres atque rotundus*. It is easily discoverable in the weekly bills of mortality in London to have fallen in the month of June:

London Weekly Mortalities.

1782

Week ending	Fevers	All causes
May 21	45	336
28	49	390
June 4	57	385
11	121	560
18	110	473
25	89	434
July 2	49	296

The sudden rise and fall of the deaths and the height reached are much the same as in other such epidemics in the summer— the "gentle correction" of 1580, the "transient slight fever" of 1688, and the epidemic catarrh of 1762. On the other hand the epidemics of autumn, winter or spring in 1729, 1733, 1737 and 1743 were far more severe, while the winter epidemics of 1675 and 1679 had figures almost the same as the summer epidemics.

The influenza of 1782 was not remarkable, whether in its fatality or in its characters; but it received far more attention than any that had preceded it. Two collective inquiries were held upon it, one by a Society for promoting Medical Knowledge[1], the other by a committee of the College of

---

[1] "An Account of the Epidemic Catarrh of the Year 1782; compiled at the request of a Society for promoting Medical Knowledge." By Edward Gray, M.D., F.R.S., *Medical Communications*, I. (1784), p. 1.

Physicians of London[1], many physicians all over England, Scotland and Ireland contributing to one or other. There were also three or more separate essays[2].

The epidemic appeared in 1782 at Newcastle in the end of April, and raged there all May and part of June. In London it appeared between the 12th and 18th of May, in the Eastern Counties about the middle of May, in Surrey and at Portsmouth, Oxford and Edinburgh, also about the third week of May, but not in Musselburgh until the 9th or 10th of June. It was at Chester on the 26th of May, at Plymouth on the 30th, at Ipswich, Yarmouth, York, Liverpool and Glasgow in the first week of June. In Northumberland it was raging in July, and did not cease until the third week of August. In Scotland it was at a height in July, during the haymaking[3]. The most curious fact in its incidence comes from North Devon; it was prevalent in Barnstaple at the usual time, the month of June; but the neighbouring town of Torrington was not then affected by it, having previously gone through the epidemic, it is said, from a date as early as the 24th of March[4]. In all places it spread quickly, affecting from three-fourths to four-fifths of the adult inhabitants, but children not so much. At Christ's Hospital, London, only fourteen out of seven hundred boys had it. Wherever it attacked children, it did so mildly. It lasted under six weeks in each place that it came to. There were some strange attacks of it in London in September, "two months after the late epidemical catarrh had entirely disappeared from England." The king's ships 'Convert' and 'Lizard' arrived in the Thames from the West Indies in September. Their crews were perfectly healthy till they reached Gravesend, where they took on board three custom-house officers; and in a very few hours after that the influenza began to make its appearance. Hardly a man in either ship

---

[1] "An Account of the Epidemic Disease called the *Influenza*, of the Year 1782, collected from the observations of several physicians in London and in the Country; by a Committee of the Fellows of the Royal College of Physicians in London." *Medical Transactions published by the Coll. of Phys. in London*, III. (1785), p. 54. Read at the College, June 25, 1783.

[2] John Clark, M.D., *On the Influenza at Newcastle*. Dated 26 May, 1782; Arthur Broughton, *The Influenza or Epid. Catarrh in Bristol in* 1782. London, 1782; W. Falconer, *Account of the Influenza at Bath in May-June*, 1782. Bath, 1782.

[3] Gregory, cited by Christison, *Life &c.* 1. 84: "I have been told of the haymakers attempting to struggle with the sense of fatigue, but being obliged in a few minutes to lay down their scythes and stretch themselves on the field."

[4] Gray, u. s. p. 107.

escaped it; and many both of the officers and common seamen had it in a severe degree[1]. Others who came to London from the West Indies in merchantmen in the end of September were attacked by influenza in their lodgings in the beginning of October[2]. To this epidemic belong also the strange experiences of the Channel Fleet in its two divisions under Howe and Kempenfelt; but I postpone for the present the whole question of influenza at sea.

Gray thus sums up the great variety of symptoms as related by his numerous correspondents:

Chilliness and shivering, sometimes succeeded by a hot fit, the alternation continuing for some hours; languor and lassitude, sneezing, discharge from the nose and eyes, pain in the head (particularly between or over the eyes), cough, sometimes dry, sometimes accompanied with expectoration, inflammation in one or both eyes, oppression and tightness about the praecordia, difficulty of breathing, pain in the breast or side, pain in the loins, neck, shoulders or limbs, sense of heat or soreness in the throat and trachea, hoarseness, bleeding from the nose, spitting of blood and loss of smell and taste, nausea, flatulence. Also watery blisters about the upper parts of the body, and swellings in the face and other parts, attended with considerable soreness, apparently erysipelatous. In some the catarrhal symptoms were very slight, or entirely wanting, the disorder in those cases being like a common fever.

The committee of the College of Physicians said that "the universal and almost pathognomonic symptom was a distressing pain and sense of constriction in the forehead, temples, and sometimes in the whole face, accompanied with a sense of soreness about the cheek-bones under the muscles," reminding one of the *fierro chuto* or "iron cap" of the South American epidemic in 1719. Sometimes no catarrhous affection followed these strange head pains. The languor of body and depression of spirits were thought to be more protracted than in 1762, but the fatalities at the time were fewer than in the earlier epidemic, and there were fewer consumptions following. Sweating, also, was said by some to be less remarkable than in 1762; but Carmichael Smyth said: "The late influenza [1782] might very properly have been named the sweating sickness, as sweating was the natural and spontaneous solution of it[3]." One distinctive

---

[1] *The London Medical Journal*, III. (1783), 318.
[2] College of Physicians' Report: "A family which came in the Leeward Islands fleet in the end of September, 1782, was attacked by it in the beginning of October. This family afterwards told the physician who attended them that several of their acquaintances, who came over in the same fleet with them, had been attacked at the same time and in the same manner as themselves."
[3] He had another experience not quite the rule: "Children and old people either escaped this influenza entirely, or were affected in a slight manner."

thing in the epidemic of 1762 was missed by most in 1782, namely, the peculiar constriction of the breast, with heat and soreness of the trachea, as if excoriated; but Hamilton describes that very thing for 1782 in Bedfordshire[1]. As in other epidemics of the kind, especially those which have been least catarrhal, there were hardly two cases quite the same.

The Epidemic Agues of 1780–85.

Let us now take up the strange history of epidemic agues for two or three years preceding and following the influenza of June, 1782. Sir George Baker begins his account of them thus[2]: "The predominance of certain diseases observable in some years, and the total or partial disappearance of the same in other years, constitute a subject worthy of our contemplation."

These agues were first noticed in London in the spring and autumn of 1780, but they infested various parts of England a little earlier. In the more inland counties the agues were "often attended with peculiarities extraordinary and alarming. For the cold fit was accompanied by spasm and stiffness of the whole body, the jaws being fixed, the eyes staring and the pulse very small and weak." When the hot fit came on the spasms abated, and ceased in the sweating stage; but sometimes the spasm was accompanied by delirium, both lasting to the very end of the paroxysm. Even in the intermissions a convulsive twitching of the extremities continued to such a degree that it was not possible to distinguish the motion of the artery at the wrist. "This fever had every kind of variety, and whether at its first accession it were a quotidian, a tertian or a quartan, it was very apt to change from one type to another. Sometimes it returned two days successively, and missed the third day; and sometimes it became continual. I am not informed that any died of this fever whilst it intermitted. It is, however, certain that many country people whose illness had at its beginning put on the appearance of intermission, becoming delirious, sank under it in four or five days."

Reynolds, another London physician, in a letter to Sir George Baker confirms all that the latter says of these singular epidemic agues: "No two cases resembled each other except in very few circumstances[3]"—the remark commonly made about the influenza itself. If these descriptions of the epidemic ague had not been given by physicians living as late as 1782, and altogether modern in their methods, we might have

---

[1] R. Hamilton, M.D., "Some Remarks on the Influenza in Spring, 1782," *Mem. Med. Soc.* II. 422. This author had some difficulty in deciding where the influenza ended and the epidemic ague began.
[2] *Trans. Col. Phys.* "On the late Intermittent Fevers," III. 141. Read at the College, 10 Jan., 1785.
[3] *Ibid.* p. 168.

supposed that they were confusing influenzas with agues, or using the latter term inexactly. "The ague with a hundred names" is the striking phrase of Abraham Holland, in his poem on the plague of 1625. Whitmore, describing the fatal epidemic ague (with an episode of influenza) in 1658–59, does not say that it had a hundred names, but that it assumed a hundred shapes, "which render it such a hocus-pocus to the amazed and perplexed people, they being held after most strange and diverse ways with it....So prodigious in its alterations that it seems to outvie even Proteus himself[1]."

As farther showing the anomalous character of these epidemic agues, or their difference from the endemic, Baker adds :—

"It is a remarkable fact, and well attested, that in many places, whilst the inhabitants of the high grounds were harassed by this fever, in its worst form, those of the subjacent valleys were not affected by it. The people of Boston and of the neighbouring villages in the midst of the Fens were in general healthy at a time when fever was epidemic in the more elevated situations of Lincolnshire." Women were nearly exempt, but few male labourers in the fields escaped it.

Baker heard from all parts that the same constitution continued through 1781 and 1782 ; and that since that time, though it seemingly abated, yet agues had been much more prevalent than usual, and had even been frequent in places where before that period they were uncommon. They were very noticeable in London from 1781 to 1785, not least so during the very severe cold of the winter and spring of 1783–84. We hear of great numbers attacked at Hampstead with common inter-mittents in February and the following months of 1781, during which time even the measles, in the greater number of cases, "ended in very troublesome intermittents[2]"—just as they were apt to end often in troublesome coughs.

The annals of Barker, of Coleshill, are full of references to agues, among other fevers, from 1780 onwards. Under 1781 he writes :—

"This spring that very peculiar, irregular, dangerous and obstinate disease, the burning, or as the people in Kent properly enough called it, the Plague-ague, made its appearance, became very epidemical in the eastern part of the kingdom, and raged in Leicestershire, the lower part of Northamptonshire, Bedfordshire, and in the fens throughout the year...This

---

[1] *Febris Anomala, or the New Disease.* Lond. 1659, p. 1.

[2] "Remarks on the Treatment of Intermittents, as they occurred at Hampstead in the Spring of 1781." By Thomas Hayes, Surgeon. *Lond. Med. Journ.* II. 267.

strongly pestilential disease had such an effect upon them that the complexion of their faces continued for a time as white as paper, and they went abroad more like walking corpses than living subjects."

As many as five persons in an evening were buried from it in some large towns in Northamptonshire; and about Boston it was so general and grievous that out of forty labourers hired for work in harvest, half of them, it was said, would be laid up in three days[1]. In 1783 the "pestilential agues" were as bad in Northamptonshire and eastern parts as the year before. A Liverpool writer says:

"In the autumn of 1782 the quartan ague was very prevalent on the opposite shore of the river in Cheshire: it was universal in the neighbourhood of Hoylake, where many died of it. Yet it was scarcely heard of in Liverpool, although from the uncommon wetness of the season it prevailed throughout the kingdom[2]."

On October 25, 1783, a correspondent of the *Gentleman's Magazine* offered an explanation of the "present epidemic disorder, which has so long ravaged this country, and that in the most healthy situations of it," namely, "the putrescent air caused by the number of enclosures, and the many inland cuts made for navigation[3]." Next year, 1784, appears to have been the principal season of epidemic agues on both sides of the Severn valley, one practitioner at Bridgenorth making them the subject of a special essay[4].

It was at this time that Fowler brought into use his solution of arsenic as a substitute for bark in agues, the latter having notably failed in the epidemics since 1780.

Baker says: "The distinguishing character of this fever was its obstinate resistance to the Peruvian bark; nor, indeed, was the prevalence of the disease more observable than the inefficacy of the remedy:" in that respect the epidemic agues had belied the experience with bark in ordinary agues. Again, it is

---

[1] *Epidemicks* (1777-95), pp. 58, 72, 75, &c.   Barker's annals from 1779 to 1786 are full of references to agues, "bad burning fevers" and the like, but are on the whole too confused to be of much use for history.   See the Boston bills under Small-pox.

[2] W. Moss, *Familiar Medical Survey of Liverpool*.   Liverpool, 1784, p. 117. This writer's object is to show that Liverpool escaped most of the epidemic diseases that troubled other places, including typhus fever.   As to the influenzas he says: "The influenza of 1775, so universal and very fatal in many parts, was less fatal here; and also that much slighter complaint, distinguished by the same title, which appeared in the spring of 1783."

[3] *Gent. Magaz.* LIII. pt. 2, p. 920.   Letter dated from "Pontoon."

[4] William Coley, *Account of the late Epidemic Ague in the neighbourhood of Bridgenorth, Shropshire, in 1784...to which are added some observations on a Dysentery that prevailed at the same time.*   Lond. 1785.

singular that bark had failed most, and arsenic been especially useful in those parts of England where ordinary malarious agues were never seen. One practitioner in Dorset laid in a large stock of arsenic, wherewith he "hardly ever failed to stop the fits soon[1]." Another, at Painswick, in Gloucestershire, used it successfully in two hundred cases of epidemic agues from 1784 onwards. He gives the following account of these unusual agues at Painswick:

"This town, which is situated on the side of a hill, and is remarkable for the purity of its air, is very populous. In the year 1784 the epidemic ague, that prevailed in many parts of the kingdom, made its appearance in this place, and has continued till the present time [Nov. 1787], although previously to that period the disease was hardly ever seen here, unless a stranger came with it for the recovery of his health, on account of the healthy situation of the place. It affected whole families, and appeared to be most violent in spring and autumn. In the summer of 1786 it was followed by a fever of the kind called typhus, or low nervous fever, which not unfrequently degenerated into a putrid fever and proved very fatal[2]." In May, 1785, at a general inoculation of smallpox, "many had been afflicted with intermittents of several months' duration attended with anasarcous swellings[3]."

It will be seen from the following table of cases treated at the Newcastle Dispensary, under the direction of Dr John Clark, during twelve years from 1 October, 1777, to 1 September, 1789, that influenza makes the smallest show among them, being far surpassed by the intermittent fevers and dysenteries, while all three together are greatly exceeded by the perennial typhus fever:

	Cases treated
Putrid fever	1920
Intermitting fever	313
Epidemic dysentery in 1783 and 1785	329
Influenza of 1782	53

In Scotland, also, agues became epidemic about the year 1780. There is no reason to suppose that their prevalence in these years was less exceptional there than in England and Ireland. It will be seen, indeed, from the following table compiled from the books of the Kelso Dispensary that the only years of their considerable prevalence were the same as the years of epidemic ague in England.

---

[1] Baker, u. s.
[2] "An Account of the Effects of Arsenic in Intermittents." By J. C. Jenner, surgeon at Painswick, Gloucestershire. *Lond. Med. Journ.* IX. (1788), p. 47.
[3] *Ibid.* VII. (1786), p. 163.

Kelso Dispensary[1].

Year	All cases	Cases of Ague	Year	All cases	Cases of Ague
1777	302	17	1792	570	16
1778	306	33	1793	666	19
1779	460	70	1794	447	9
1780	675	161	1795	513	23
1781	510	103	1796	355	12
1782	440	61	1797	318	9
1783	510	73	1798	415	7
1784	459	40	1799	558	2
1785	573	62	1800	665	4
1786	563	48	1801	433	9
1787	525	24	1802	377	5
1788	577	25	1803	308	2
1789	546	48	1804	422	5
1790	640	18	1805	469	0
1791	715	13	1806	318	1

It was doubtless the recollection of these epidemic agues that led the parish ministers who wrote in the 'Statistical Account of Scotland' from 1791 to 1799 to remark upon a supposed progressive decline of endemic ague, which they set down to drainage of the land[2]. It is probable, however, that each tradition of ague in Scotland dated from one of its epidemic periods; it has been shown, indeed, in the foregoing that Scotland in the end of the 17th century was reputed tolerably free from ague, and that the severe agues previous to 1728, which belonged to the epidemical kind, were thought to be something new.

The Influenza of 1788.

According to Barker, of Coleshill, who kept systematic notes of the epidemic maladies from year to year, there were several recurrences of the influenza of 1782[3]. But there is only one of

[1] Table compiled by Dr Mackenzie, and printed by Christison, *Trans. Soc. Sc. Assoc.* Edin. Meeting, 1863, p. 97. Christison pointed out very fairly the difficulties in the way of accepting the drainage-theory for the decline of ague (p. 98), but he had not realized the fact that the disease used to come in epidemics at long intervals.

[2] e.g. parish of Dron, Perthshire (IX. 468): "The return of spring and autumn never failed to bring along with them this fatal disease [ague], and frequently laid aside many of the labouring hands at a time when their work was of the greatest consequence and necessity." That had now ceased, owing to drainage. See also Cramond parish, I. 224, and Arngask, Perthshire, I. 415.

[3] The following extracts are from Barker's book, *Epidemicks*, Birmingham [1795]: 1782. Influenza in the latter end of spring. Nine out of ten in Lichfield and other towns had violent defluxions of the nose, throat and lungs, bringing on violent sneezings, soreness of the throat, coughs, &c. attended with a pestiential fever, of which many were relieved by perspiration...Some had swelled faces, and violent pains

these seasons, the summer of 1788, that other English writers
have singled out as a time of influenza. It was undoubtedly of
a very mild type, producing hardly any effect upon the bills of
mortality; but it attracted the notice of several. Dr Simmons,
the editor of the *London Medical Journal*, became the recorder
of it, collecting reports from various parts, as others had done
in 1782. He himself treated 160 cases at the Westminster
General Dispensary, and 65 more elsewhere. It was most
prevalent in London from the second to the fourth week of
July, but the mortalities for those weeks show no abrupt rise.
It was at Chatham, Dover, Plymouth and Bath about the same
time, at Manchester in the beginning of August, in Cornwall in
the middle of August, and at Montrose about the end of August,
or perhaps most certainly in October. On 5 August, a physician
at York wrote: "We have not had the slightest appearance of a
catarrh in our city or neighbourhood during the year." The
epidemic was undoubtedly a partial one in Britain, and so slight
as to have made little impression where it did occur. It is said
to have been very general at Warsaw in April or May, at
Vienna in April (20,000 cases before the 20th), at Munich in
June, at Paris in the end of August and still continuing on the
24th October, at Geneva on the 10th October. Its most
constant symptom in England was pain in the fore-part of
the head, with vertigo; next most constant was a pain at the
pit of the stomach and along the breast-bone; cough was
wanting in perhaps a third of the cases and was always slight,
diarrhoea was somewhat general, running from the eyes exceptional, sore-throat in perhaps one-sixth of the cases[1]. At
Plymouth where it was seen earliest and clearest among the

in the teeth...Some, giddiness and violent headaches, accompanied with a slow fever,
and even loss of memory...By its running through whole families it appeared also to
be communicable by infection.
    1783. The influenza also began to appear again; and those who had coughs last
year began now to be afflicted with them again, the disorder at length frequently
ending in a consumption. Also dogs in this year and the next had running at the
eyes and a loss of the use of their hind legs, which in the end killed most of those that
were seized with it. Horses also suffered.
    1786. In the middle of this season the influenza returned, and colds and coughs
were epidemical.
    1788 [spring]. A species of influenza of the pestilential kind, akin to that of
1782, has almost constantly returned in spring and autumn since that time...[summer]
A species of influenza, as in the spring, and it is also at Edinburgh,
    1789 [spring]. Influenza returned. Even dogs affected.
    1791. Influenza very bad, especially in London.
    [1] Samuel Foart Simmons, M.D., F.R.S., "Of the Epidemic Catarrh of the year
1788." *Lond. Med. Journ.* IX. (1788), p. 335.

regiment of artillery and in the guardships, the symptoms were
pain in the head and limbs, soreness of the throat, pain in the
breast, a feeling of coldness all over the skin, and these
followed by cough, a great discharge from the nose and eyes,
and slight nausea. It was much less noticeable among the
townspeople than among the troops and sailors[1]. It occurred
chiefly among soldiers or sailors also at Dover and Chatham.
At Bath it was marked by chills, headache, swelling of the
throat, difficult swallowing, quick pulse, hot, dry skin (but not
pungent as in malignant fever), ending in a sweat; no delirium,
but broken sleep or vigil; the eyes scarcely affected, cough in
some, but not vehement; in some, sublingual swellings which
suppurated[2]. At Manchester it looked as if it had been brought
in by travellers who had acquired it in London[3].

At Portsmouth a singular thing happened two or three
months after the epidemic had passed. The frigate 'Rose'
arrived on 4 November from Newfoundland; within a short
time all the dogs on board were seized with cough and catarrh,
and soon after the whole ship's company were affected in the
same way[4]. Simmons says of the epidemic of 1788 in general:
"During the progress of the influenza, a complaint which was
evidently an inflammatory affection of the mucous membrane of
the fauces, etc. was frequently observed among horses and other
cattle, and was generally as violent among them as it was mild
among their rational neighbours"—many dying after four or six
days.

The very slight and partial influenza of July and August,
1788, happened at a time when there was much fever of a more
serious kind in the country. The history of the latter belongs
to another chapter; but there was in Cornwall, in the same
season as the influenza, an epidemic fever which might in
former times have been described as a part, and the most fatal
part, of the "new disease," and may be taken in this context

[1] Vaughan May, surgeon to H. M. Ordnance, "Observations on the Influenza as
it appeared at Plymouth, in the summer and autumn of the year 1788." Duncan's
Med. Commentaries, Decade 2, vol. iv. p. 363.
[2] Falconer, "Influenzae Descriptio, uti nuper comparebat in urbe Bathoniae,
mensibus Julio, Augusto et Septembri A.D. 1788." *Mem. Med. Soc.* III. 25.
[3] George Bew, M.D., physician at Manchester, "Of the Epidemic Catarrh of the
year 1788." *Lond. Med. Journ.* IX. (1788), p. 354. "The influenza has been *very*
prevalent," writes Withering, of Birmingham, to Lettsom, 19 Aug. 1788. *Mem. of
Lettsom*, III. 133.
[4] Related to Dr Simmons (l. c. p. 346), by Mr Boys, surgeon, of Sandwich, who
was told it by his son, a lieutenant on board the 'Rose.'

rather than in the chapter on typhus. The same physician, Dr William May, of Truro, gave an account of the influenza first[1] and of the other fever afterwards[2].

The latter began at Truro in the end of April, 1788, and was also at St Ives and other small towns in various parts of the county. A malignant fever had for near two years before been exceedingly rife among the poor (owing to distress from loss of pilchard fishing), and had carried off a great number of them; but this was something new. Yet it was "truly a fever of the typhus type," one of its symptoms being constant wakefulness. It passed through whole families, affecting all ages and constitutions. It ended on the 17th day, whereas the influenza (says May in his other paper) ended with a sweat on the fourth or fifth day. In one small neighbourhood this epidemic fever affected chiefly the aged, who were blooded owing to dyspnoea: out of ten or eleven so affected, not one recovered, an experience that reminded May of what Willis said of the village elders being swept off by the "new fever" of 1658. Surgeons at St Austel, East Looe and Falmouth are cited as having seen much of the same fever. In like manner the Manchester chronicler of the influenza of 1788 says: "Fevers of different kinds, but chiefly of the type now distinguished by the appellation of typhus, were exceedingly prevalent after the epidemic catarrh had in great measure ceased to be general; but from which, by tracing the symptoms, the fever might usually be found to have originated[3]."

For a good many years after the period last dealt with, nothing is heard in Britain either of epidemic agues or of influenza[4]. Writing in 1800, Willan said that intermittents had not, to his knowledge, been epidemic in London at any time within twenty years. He explains this by "the practice of draining, and the improved modes of cultivating land in Essex, Kent, and some other adjoining counties, from which either agues were formerly imported, or the effluvia causing them were conveyed by particular winds"—the latter being the doctrine of Lancisi for the country round Rome. But he forgets that their appearance nearly twenty years before was a strange phenomenon to the practitioners of that generation, and that Sydenham, whom he cites to prove agues in London in former times, had also remarked their absence, except in occasional cases, for as long a period as thirteen years. Of such occasional agues

---

[1] In a note to Simmons' paper, u. s., p. 342.

[2] "An Account of an Epidemic Fever that prevailed in Cornwall in the year 1788." *Lond. Med. Journal*, X. p. 117 (dated Truro, Jan. 26, 1789).

[3] Bew, u. s., p. 365. Carmichael Smyth has a similar remark on the influenza of 1782: "This epidemic distemper very soon declined. But it seemed to leave behind it an epidemical constitution which prevailed during the rest of the summer; and the fevers, even in the end of August and beginning of September, assumed a type resembling, in many respects, the fever accompanying the influenza."

[4] A solitary reference occurs to an influenza in 1792, which I have not succeeded in verifying :—B. Hutchinson, "An Account of the Epidemic Disease commonly called the Influenza, which appeared in Nottinghamshire and most other parts of the kingdom in the months of November and December, 1792." *New. Lond. Med. Journ.*, Lond. 1793, II. 174. Cited in the Washington Medical Catalogue.

acquired in London, Willan and Bateman had each one or two examples in the autumn of 1794, and the spring of 1805.

As in the case of epidemic agues, so also in the case of influenzas, there was immunity in Britain for a good many years after 1788; and, as the slight epidemic catarrh of 1788 was something less than universal, the clear interval may almost be reckoned from the summer of 1782, a space of over twenty years. Willan's monthly reports of the weather and diseases in London from March, 1796, to December, 1800, twice mention epidemic catarrhs,—in February and March, 1797, and in February, 1800, the latter chiefly among children. But to neither of them will he concede the name of "influenza," as the complaint was merely epidemical from a particular state of the atmosphere, and not propagated by contagion, nor quite general.

The symptoms, however, were headache, sometimes attended with vertigo, a thin acrid discharge from the nostrils, slight inflammation of the throat, a sense of constriction in the chest, with a frequent dry cough, pains in the limbs, a white tongue, a quick and small pulse, with a sensation of languor and general debility. These symptoms, fairly complete for influenza of the correct type, lasted about eight days and ended in a gentle sweat or in a diarrhoea. Coughs had been remarkably severe and obstinate; they were frequently attended with painful stitches and spitting of blood[1].

The Influenza of 1803.

The number of the *Medical and Physical Journal* for March, 1803, announced that "a cold attended by symptoms of a very alarming nature has been general in the city of Paris for some time"; but it said nothing of the alarming disorder being in London. It is in the next number, under the date of Soho Square, March 11th, that a correspondent identifies the Paris epidemic with "the complaint now general in this metropolis, and called by some the Influenza." In a report upon the diseases "in an Eastern District of London from February 20 to March 20, 1803," the "catarrhal fever" is thus described:

"This disease has been so general as to claim the title of the reigning epidemic, and is very similar to one which prevailed a few years ago, and was denominated Influenza. It has generally been introduced by chilliness and shivering, which have been succeeded by violent pains in the head, with some discharge from the eyes and nostrils, as in a common catarrh, together with hoarseness and cough. The pains in the head have in some cases been the first symptoms and have been succeeded by giddiness, sickness and vomiting" &c. There were also rheumatic pains in the limbs, intercostals &c.

[1] Robert Willan, M.D., *Reports on the Diseases in London, particularly during the years* 1796, '97, '98, '99 *and* 1800. London, 1801, pp. 76, 253.

Meanwhile the information from various sources showed that the old influenza was once more really in this country. Two collective inquiries were made on the influenza of 1803: one by Dr Beddoes of Bristol, who issued a circular of five queries, and received answers to them (with other information) from one hundred and twenty-four correspondents[1]; the other by the Medical Society of London[2]. The *Medical and Physical Journal* and Duncan's *Annals* each received a few independent papers on it; and several pamphlets were issued, mostly devoted to treatment—two in London[3], one at Edinburgh[4], one at Bath[5], and one at Bristol[6].

In these abundant data there is little novelty and not much variety.

The attack began with chills and severe pain in the head, along with slight running of the eyes and nose, as typhus fever might have begun. After the slightly catarrhal onset the malady was mostly a fever, with dry cough, dry and hot skin, pain in the forehead and about the eyeballs, pains in the limbs, "spontaneous" weariness and extreme prostration—a group of symptoms which led Hooper to find a rheumatic character in the malady. Among other symptoms were vertigo, nausea, vomiting and diarrhoea. Much sweating is not reported; but there was often a gentle sweat in recovering after about a week, less or more. There was the usual range from mildness to severity. Pneumonia and pleurisy were not rare, and were commonly the cause of fatalities.

The deaths were for the most part among the phthisical, the asthmatic and the aged; but these were not many, certainly not so many as in 1729, 1733 and 1743, and probably in about the same proportion as in 1762, 1775 and 1782. In the London bills the weekly deaths rose in March, to an average of 537 from an average of 429 in February, and of 375 in January, falling to an average of 417 in April. In Ireland the epidemic is said to have been seen among the troops in garrisons as early as December, 1802; it became universal in spring and summer. In Edinburgh the rise in the burials at Greyfriars churchyard was in the weeks ending 5th and 12th April, making them about a half more than usual for the brief period. When the wave of influenza was

---

[1] Published in the *Med. and Phys. Journal* from August to December, 1803.

[2] *Memoirs of the Medical Society*, vol. VI.

[3] R. Hooper, M.D., *Obs. on the Epidemic Disease now prevalent in London.* London, 1803. R. Pearson, M.D., *Obs. on the Epid. Catarrhal Fever or Influenza of* 1803. Lond. 1803.

[4] J. Herdman, *The prevailing Epid. Disease termed Influenza.* Edin. 1803.

[5] W. Falconer, M.D., *The Epidemic Catarrhal Fever commonly called the Influenza, as it appeared at Bath &c.* Bath, 1803.

[6] John Nott, M.D., *Influenza as it prevailed in Bristol in Feb.–April,* 1803. Bristol, 1803.

past, the public health in nearly all places became unusually good, as had happened immediately after the influenza of 1782.

The question most to the front in the influenza of 1803 was its manner of spreading. Beddoes, who believed in personal contagion, had this in view in his five queries:

1. When did the influenza appear and disappear with you?
2. Was its date different in remote places within your reach?
3. After being general, did it occur for some time in single instances?
4. Did it ever seem to pass from person to person?
5. If so, is it likely that clothes or fomites conveyed it in any case?

The dates of commencement were earlier or later according to no rule of direction or of distance from London. In some large towns of Yorkshire it appeared to be unusually late, in Chester unusually early; Edinburgh, certainly, was as long behind London as London was behind Paris. Haygarth, who took the most narrow view of contagion, made out the incidence thus: London first, then the towns which have the greatest intercourse with London, such as Bath and Chester, then smaller towns, and last of all the villages around each of the more populous centres. Several towns had the brunt of the epidemic in the same weeks (of March) as London; in very few was it later than the first weeks of April. In some towns it attracted little notice. In North Devon, it was said to have been at Hartland and Clovelly a fortnight before it was seen in Bideford; the first of it seen by one of the doctors of that town was in a solitary potter's house four miles to the eastward, on a peninsula made by the confluence of a small stream with the Torridge, all the inmates of the house being attacked; in the town itself from first to last he saw but few cases, whereas there were many in the adjacent country[1].

The general rule seems to have been that the more sparse populations had it later, the nearer they were to the extremities of the kingdom, as in Cornwall, the north of Scotland, and in Ireland. Opinion was divided as to the part played by persons in carrying contagion from place to place, some holding that the facts of diffusion could be explained on no other hypothesis, while most held that the influenza was in the air. Beddoes got as many answers favouring the doctrine of personal contagion as made a respectable show for it; but when these had all been set forth to the best advantage, a practitioner wrote to say that, after all, nine-tenths of professional opinion was against the con-

---

[1] *Med. and Phys. Journ.* x. 104.

tagiousness of influenza. The practical question for Haygarth, Beddoes, and other contagionists was whether influenza was not a disease, like smallpox or scarlet fever, which could be kept from spreading by means of isolation, disinfection (with the fumes of mineral acids) and other precautions.

Some curious facts came out, showing the effect of influenza upon other epidemic diseases, or the effect of other epidemic diseases upon influenza. One writer applied to influenza what used to be said of the plague or pestilential fever, that these Leviathan constitutions swallowed up all other reigning epidemics. Holywell, a town in Flintshire, with a large cotton-weaving industry, had not been free from a bad kind of typhus for two years. "On the appearance of the influenza the typhus entirely ceased, and only one case of fever has occurred since. I have not for many years known this country so healthy as since the influenza disappeared[1]." The influenza was said also to have superseded typhus fever at Navan, in Meath[2]. At St Neots typhus was peculiarly prevalent for three months before the influenza, but ceased thereafter[3]. Another relation to typhus was seen at Clifton: " In the low, confined, and ill-ventilated houses in the Hot Well road, where typhus often abounds, the influenza was very unfrequent; while in the exposed high-lying buildings on Clifton Hill it was almost universal[4]." As to ague, which had often before stood in a remarkable relation to epidemics of catarrhal fever, there is one possibly relevant fact related from the Lincolnshire fens. A Wisbech physician writes :

"The influenza which ceased here about the middle of April made its appearance again in May; the leading symptoms were the same as in the first attack. About the same time also a most malignant fever, having some symptoms in common with the influenza, began to rage in that part of Lincolnshire contiguous to us, which has proved fatal to hundreds[5]."

From 1803 to 1831, nothing is heard in England of a universal influenza, although there was one such in the end of 1805 and beginning of 1806 in Russia, Germany, France and

---

[1] Dr Currie of Chester, *Med. and Phys. Journ.* X. 213.
[2] *Ib.* X. 527, quoted by Beddoes from memory, the letter from Navan having been lost.
[3] Alvey, *Mem. Med. Soc.* VI. 462.
[4] Dr Carrick, of Bristol, in Duncan's *Annals of Med.* III. Compare the report for Fraserburgh in 1775, supra, p. 360.
[5] Frazer, *Med. and Phys. Journ.* X. 206, dated 12 June, 1803.

Italy; and there were four great influenzas in the Western Hemisphere (1807, 1815–16, 1824–25, and 1826). Catarrhs were perhaps commoner than usual in England and Scotland in the winter of 1807–8, but they cannot be reckoned an epidemic of influenza[1]. The summer following (1808) was unusually hot and agues became more epidemic in the fens than at any time since the great aguish period of 1780 and following years[2]. Agues were again unusually rife in England in 1826, 1827 and 1828, at the same time as the remarkable epidemics of them, from inundations and subsequent drought, in Holland and along the German coast of the North Sea. Dr John Elliotson, of London, met with cases of agues in his practice in those years in the following scale:

Year	Cases		Year	Cases
1823	8		1827	53
1824	14		1828	27
1825	15		1829	8
1826	44			

They had increased, he says, throughout the country as well as in London, owing, as he thought, in agreement with Macmichael, to the higher mean temperature of the respective years; and he would apply the same law of increase to the epidemic periods of ague in Britain in former times[3]. Christison saw his first case of ague at Edinburgh in the autumn of 1827, in a labourer who had caught it working at the harvest in the fen-country of Lincolnshire.

[1] Hirsch cites authorities for influenza in Edinburgh, London, Nottingham and Newcastle in the winter of 1807-8. In Roberton's monthly reports from Edinburgh (*Med. and Phys. Journ.* XXI.), and Bateman's quarterly reports from London, I find only common colds recorded. Clarke for Nottingham (*Ed. Med. Surg. Journ.* IV. 429) says catarrh was so general "as to have acquired the name of influenza; but there was no reason to suppose it contagious."

[2] W. Royston, "On a Medical Topography," *Med. and Phys. J.* XXI. 1809, (Dec. 1808), p. 92: "After the unusual heat of the last summer, the frequency of intermittents in the autumn was increased in the fens of Cambridgeshire to an almost unprecedented degree; and even quadrupeds were not exempt, for distinctly marked cases of *tertian* were observed in horses. In the year 1780 a similar prevalence of this disease occurred in the same part; and though in an interval of 28 years many and frequent sporadic cases have arisen, yet its universality during that period was suspended. We have to regret that a correct record of the constitution of the year 1780, as applying to this particular district, has not been preserved in such a manner as to admit of a direct comparison with that of 1808. If it were possible, from authentic documents to compare the history of these two seasons, much light might be thrown on the obscure cause of intermittents." Clarke, of Nottingham, (l. c.) says there were some cases of irregular ague among a few privates of the regiment there, who had all come from a marshy quarter, some of them with the fever on them. The paroxysms came at unusually long intervals. Bark increased the fever.

[3] Lecture on Agues, in the *Lond. Med. Gaz.* IX. 923-4, 24 March, 1832.

The Influenza of 1831.

The next influenza in Britain fell in the early summer of 1831. It was a mild epidemic of the catarrhal type, which attracted hardly any notice in England. In one of the London medical journals there is no other notice of it but this, dated 2 July, 1831[1]: "In consequence of the sudden variations of temperature which have prevailed since the last fortnight of May an epidemic bronchitis has shown itself in Paris." Another London journal[2], on the very same day, wrote: "Influenza in a severe form is at present prevailing in London and some of the provincial towns. It commences like a common cold, but is soon discovered to be more serious, &c." The physician to the public dispensary in Chancery Lane found that more than half of the seventy applicants on 23 June came with the symptoms of influenza—severe, harsh, dry cough, in paroxysms, pain behind the sternum, a fixed pain in one side, congested state of the throat, nose and eyes, heaviness of the head, languor, debility, hot skin, foul tongue, impaired sense of taste. The symptoms went off after three or four days with a sweat in the night and a discharge from the nostrils[3].

This epidemic hardly affected the London bills of mortality, according to the following figures:

Four weeks, 25 May to 21 June, 1579 births, 1430 deaths.
Five weeks, 22 June to 26 July, 2153 births, 2010 deaths.
Four weeks, 27 July to 23 Aug., 1997 births, 1652 deaths.

The rise in the last four weeks was due to summer diarrhoea, or choleraic diarrhoea, which was unusually common in 1831. This slight influenza was also reported from Plymouth by a surgeon who had seen the disease, and suffered from it, at Manilla in September, 1830[4], and by a Plymouth practitioner, who wrote, on 14 July, that it had been extensively prevalent there and in the neighbouring towns and villages[5]. It is recorded also from the Isle of Man, Glasgow[6], and Ayr[7], and it is supposed to have been in Aberdeen[8]. But, while there are many

---

[1] *Lancet*, s. d., p. 438.   [2] *Lond. Med. Gazette*, 2 July, 1831.
[3] John Burne, M.D., *Ibid.* VIII. (1831), p. 430.
[4] G. Bennett, *Lond. Med. Gaz.* 23 July, 1831.   [5] Bellamy, *Ibid.*
[6] "Report of Diseases among the Poor of Glasgow," *Glas. Med. Journ.* IV. 444.
[7] McDerment, *ibid.* v. 230: "In June and July to an extent unequalled " etc.
[8] During the last general election before the passing of the Reform Bill, which was held in the month of June, 1831, a number of the Aberdeen radicals went out on a

accounts of this epidemic in Germany in May and June, and undoubted evidence of it in France and Italy, as well as in Sweden, and in Poland and Russia earlier in the year, the accounts of it in Britain are so meagre and casual as to make one doubt whether it really was an influenza worth reckoning.

The Influenza of 1833.

The next year, 1832, which was the first great season of Asiatic cholera in Britain, is absolutely free from records of influenza in all Europe. It was in the spring of the year following, 1833, that the really serious influenza came. The continental literature of the epidemic of 1833 is immense, the English literature of it is all but non-existent: and yet it was a very severe influenza with us, just as with other European peoples. There was no collective inquiry in Britain on this occasion, such as had been made first by Fothergill in 1775, by the College of Physicians and another Society in 1782, by Simmons in 1788, and by Beddoes and the Medical Society of London in 1803, or such as was made in the next influenza, that of 1837, by a committee of the Provincial Medical Association. But enough is known of it to place it among the severer influenzas. In London the bills of mortality, which relate only to a part of London, showed the characteristic sudden rise and fall:

			Baptisms	Burials
Four weeks,	20 Feb. to 16 March		2310	2352
Five „	17 March to 23 April		1955	2105
Four „	24 April to 21 May		2016	3350
Four „	22 May to 18 June		2070	1685

For a whole month the burials in London were nearly doubled, and for the two worst weeks they were nearly quadrupled. This mortality, by all accounts, fell most on the richer classes, to whom it was a much more serious calamity than the Asiatic cholera of the year before. The president of the Medical Society said, on the 22nd April, that he had "heard of nine lords or ladies who had been carried off by it or by its indirect agency, in the course of last week[1]." Its type in the

hot and dusty day to meet the candidate of their party who was posting from the south. It was remarked that all those who had been of this company "caught cold," unaccountably but as if from some common cause. The date would correspond to the prevalence of influenza elsewhere.

[1] Mr Kingdon, reported in the *Lancet*, s. d.

month of May was worse than in April[1]. When it was first seen it was a somewhat short catarrhal attack, ending in a sweat after two, three or four days, with the usual head-pains, soreness of the ribs and limbs, languor and prostration. Later, it became a more "adynamic" illness, beginning indeed with slight catarrhal symptoms, but soon passing into subacute nervous fever which might last for three weeks, involving much risk to life[2]. Hence arose the warnings, just as in 1890–92, that the influenza was a much more serious thing than it had been thought when the epidemic began, and hence the delay, as it were, in the bills of mortality to show the effects of the epidemic until it had been two or three weeks prevalent. It is to the month of April, before the highest death-rate was reached in London, that the following, in the *Gentleman's Magazine*, applies[3]:

"During the month a severe form of catarrhal epidemic, generally termed influenza, has been extremely prevalent in London. It has laid up at once all the members of many large households, and has attacked great numbers in several public offices, particularly the Bank of England and some divisions of the new police. The performers at the theatres have much suffered, and their houses have been closed for several nights. It commences suddenly with headache and feeling of general discomfort, attended or soon followed by cough, hoarseness, or loss of voice; oppression, and sometimes severe pain in the chest, tenderness about the ribs, and sense of having been bruised about the limbs or muscles...The disease is generally attributed to the constant north-east winds; but by some of the learned is regarded as the epidemic influenza which has lately prevailed in the eastern parts of Europe, and that is travelling, like many of its predecessors, to the west."

It would have been in this earlier stage of the epidemic, when it was laying up whole households, thinning workshops and closing theatres, that a practitioner was heard to say (as reported by the *Lancet*): "Best thing I ever had! Quite a god-send! Everybody ill, nobody dying!" The seriousness of the disease was, however, at length recognized, so that the members of the Medical Society debated the subject at three successive meetings. One of the questions was, whether the malady called for blooding—a question that had divided opinion as long ago as 1658[4]. On 13 May, the following passed at the Medical Society:

[1] Venables, *Lancet*, 11 May, 1833.
[2] Hingeston, *Lond. Med. Gaz.* XII. 199.
[3] *Gent. Magaz.*, April, 1833, p. 362.
[4] Whitmore, *Febris anomala, or the New Disease, etc.*, London, 1659, p. 109 :—
"And for a plethora or fulness of blood, if that appears (though this may seem a paradox yet 'tis certain) that it is so far in this disease from indicating bleeding that it

Mr Williams remembered the similar influenza of 1803, and said that depletion was then regarded as an injurious plan of treatment.

Mr Proctor :—Yes, but the Brunonian doctrines were then in full fling, and practitioners had not learned the full use of the lancet.

Graves states very fairly the reasons that induced them to take blood in the influenza of 1833, as well as the results of the practice[1]:

"The sudden manner in which the disease came on, the great heat of skin, acceleration of pulse, and the intolerable violence of the headache, —together with the oppression of the chest, cough, and wheezing—all encouraged us to the employment of the most active modes of depletion; and yet the result was but little answerable to our expectations; for these means were found to induce an awful prostration of strength, with little or no alleviation of the symptoms."

The prostration, be it said, was probably as great and as frequent in the epidemics of 1890–93, when bleeding had gone out altogether; still it was not understood that all these signs of sthenic action in the attack were really paradoxical, as Whitmore, in the passage cited in the note, saw clearly two centuries before.

The epidemic became rapidly prevalent all over England, Scotland and Ireland in April and May, following no very definite order of progression. The Liverpool newspapers asserted that ten thousand were down with it in that town in one week. A doctor at Lincoln wrote, on 13 May, that few families there had escaped it[2]. Other towns in which it is said to have been "more or less" prevalent were Portsmouth, Sheffield, Birmingham, Leeds, York, Halifax, Glasgow, Edinburgh[3], Dublin and Armagh; so that we may fairly assume, although we are without the detailed evidence available for earlier epidemics, that it was ubiquitous in town and country.

At Birmingham[4], among the outpatients of the Infirmary, the cases of influenza were as follows, the 25th and 26th April being the days when cases came first in rapid succession, while the middle of May was practically the limit:

stands absolutely as a contradiction to it and vehemently prohibits it. And whereas they think the heat, by bleeding, may be abated and so the feaver took off, they are mistook, for by that means the fermentation through the motion of the blood is highly increased, so as sad experience hath manifested in a great many: upon the bleeding they have within a day or two fallen delirious and had their tongues as black as soot, with an intolerable thirst and drought upon them....Petrus a Castro, who rants high for letting blood, at last as if he had been humbled with the sad success, saith etc."

[1] *A System of Clinical Medicine*, Dublin, 1843, pp. 500–501. Lecture delivered in the session 1834–35.

[2] Rawlins, *Lond. Med. Gaz.* s. d.

[3] *Ed. Med. Surg. Journ.* XLIII. 1835, p. 26.

[4] Parsons, "Report of Outcases, Birmingham Infirmary, 1 Jan. to 31 Dec. 1833." *Trans. Provin. Med. Surg. Assoc.* II. 474.

	Cases of Influenza	Males	Females
April	151	52	99
May	464	159	305
June	28	9	19
	643	220	423

The great excess of females is remarkable, but was probably due to some local circumstances. Of the 643 cases, 122 were under ten years of age. Of the females, 9 died, of the males 3. But the deaths in Birmingham caused by the epidemic directly or indirectly were many; the burial registers of four churches and chapels showed a marked increase of burials above those of the corresponding months of 1832:

	1832	1833
April	205	245
May	211	434
June	193	230
	609	909

Medical opinion in 1833 was decidedly adverse to the contagiousness of influenza. The common remark was that it was just as little contagious as the cholera of the year before had proved to be. As in 1837 and 1847, when the doctrine of contagiousness was equally out of favour, the disease was observed to spread rapidly, in no very definite line, affecting most parts of the country in the same two or three weeks, affecting the population within a considerable radius almost at once, and the inmates of houses all together. These, it was said, are not the marks of a disease that persons hand on one to another, *quasi cursores.*

The Influenza of 1837.

Between the influenza of April–May, 1833, and that of January–February, 1837, it seems probable that there were minor catarrhal outbreaks, distinguishable from ordinary colds. One writer on the influenza of 1837 refers to those " who had it in 1834 or in the intervening period between the two epidemics." The table of diseases of the outpatients at the Birmingham Infirmary for the year 1836 contains a large total of catarrhs, and, in another line, 24 cases of " epidemic catarrh" in the summer months. The *Gentleman's Magazine* begins its notice of the epidemic of 1837 by calling it "an influenza of a peculiar character," which shows that influenza of the ordinary kind was a familiar thing. Probably the name was a good deal mis-applied in the years following every great epidemic from 1782 onwards: thus in 'St Ronan's Well,' which was written in 1823, or twenty years from the last general influenza, a tradesman's widow in easy circumstances and given to good living comes to the Spa on account of a supposed malady which she calls the *influenzy*. But our recent experiences of four great influenza seasons in succession from 1889–90 to 1893, although it is without precedent in the history, will incline us the more to credit what is recorded of influenza cases in the intervals between the years of great historical epidemics[1]. However that may be for the years following 1833, the influenza of January, 1837, was sudden, simultaneous, universal.

The first cases, which Watson compares to the first drops of a thunder-shower, were seen earlier in some places than in others; but from all parts of England it was reported that the influenza was at its height from the middle of January to the end of the first week of February. Possibly it was a few days earlier in London than in most other towns, inasmuch as the great increase of the deaths that is shown in the following table, in the second and third weeks of January, would imply a prevalence of the epidemic for at least a fortnight before.

Weekly Mortalities in London (by the old Bills).

1837

Week ending	Influenza	All causes
Jan. 10	0	284
17	13	477
24	106	871
31	99	860
Feb. 7	63	589
14	35	558
21	20	350
28	8	321
March 7	4	262

This sudden rise in the deaths from all causes is a character-istic influenza bill, comparable with those already given from

[1] In the report upon the influenza of 1837 by a Committee of the Provincial Medical Association, the preceding epidemic is uniformly referred to the year 1834. Graves, in a clinical lecture upon that of 1837, speaks two or three times of the last as that of 1834, and, in another place, he calls it the epidemic of 1833–34. But these, I think, are mere laxities of dating, of which there are many other instances where the date is recent and not yet historical.

1580 onwards. But the bill is far from showing the whole of the mortality in London in 1837. The London bills of mortality compiled by the Parish Clerks' Company had fallen into the last stage of inadequacy, and were on the eve of being superseded by the general system of registration for all England and Wales[1].

The London bills, so long as they existed, never took in the great parishes of St Pancras, Marylebone, Kensington and Chelsea. The area "within the bills of mortality" was that of London about the middle of the 18th century. But, instead of becoming more and more crowded as time went on, it had actually become much less populous, especially in the old City and Liberties, owing to the erection of warehouses, workshops, counting-houses and other non-residential buildings where dwelling houses used to be ; so that the decrease of mortality "within the bills" in the 19th century is in part due to the decrease of population within the same area. This has to be kept in mind when the above table is compared with one of those for former influenzas, such as that of 1737, exactly a hundred years before.

It was thought that the 1837 influenza in London was worse than that of 1833, but the figures show the contrary as regards the number of deaths from all causes[2]. Both of them, however, were in the first rank of severity, finding their nearest parallels in the three great influenzas of the 18th century, in 1733, 1737 and 1743, when the deaths from all causes during the influenza rose, indeed, to a much larger total within the bills, but rose from a much higher mean level.

In Dublin the great increase of burials from the influenza of

---

[1] As early as 1612 a proposal had been made to James I. for "a grant of the general registrarship of all christenings, marriages and burials within this realm." *State Papers*, Rolls House, Ja. I. vol. LXIX. No. 54. It was a device for raising money.

[2] The account in the *Gentleman's Magazine* for February, 1837, p. 199, is almost identical with the paragraph in the number for April, 1833: "An influenza of a peculiar character has been raging throughout the country, and particularly in the Metropolis. It has been attended by inflammation of the throat and lungs, with violent spasms, sickness and headache. So general have been its effects that business in numerous instances has been entirely suspended. The greater number of clerks at the War Office, Admiralty, Navy Pay Office, Stamp Office, Treasury, Post-Office and other Government Offices have been prevented from attending to their daily avocations....Of the police force there were upwards of 800 incapable of doing duty. On Sunday the 13th the churches which have generally a full congregation presented a mournful scene &c....the number of burials on the same day in the different cemeteries was nearly as numerous as during the raging of the cholera in 1832 and 1833. In the workhouses the number of poor who have died far exceed any return that has been made for the last thirty years."

1837 fell at the same time as in London, according to the following comparison with the year before for Glasnevin Cemetery[1]:

1835–36		1836–37	
Dec. 1835	355	Dec. 1836	413
Jan. 1836	392	Jan. 1837	821
Feb. „	362	Feb. „	537
Mar. „	392	Mar. „	477
	1501		2248

At Glasgow the deaths from influenza were as follows[2]:

1837

	Males	Females	Total
January	111	118	229
February	37	62	99
March	9	20	29
	157	200	357

But the heading of "influenza" did not nearly show the full effects of the epidemic upon the mortality, which was enormous in Glasgow in January, as compared with the same month of 1836:

	All causes	Catarrh	Aged	Asthma	Fever	Decline
Jan. 1836	790	4	73	31	45	124
Jan. 1837	1972	229	274	185	201	247

There was also a great increase in the deaths of infants by bowel complaint. The only period of life which did not show a great rise of mortality was from five to twenty; the greatest rise was between the ages of forty and seventy, corresponding to the London experience in the epidemic of 1847.

At Bolton, Lancashire, the great rise in the deaths, as compared with the average of five years before, was in February:

	Average of five years 1831–36	1837
January	111·2	115
February	79·0	205
March	97·8	100
	288·0	420

At Exeter, the burials in the two chief graveyards were 227

[1] Graves, u. s., p. 545.
[2] Robert Cowan, M.D., *Journ. Stat. Soc.* III. 257.

in January and February, 1837, as compared with 125 in the same months of 1836. These mortalities, although large, were but a small ratio of the attacks. In 2347 cases enumerated in the collective inquiry, there were 54 deaths, a ratio of two deaths in a hundred cases being considered a full average. The attacks were mostly in middle life, and the deaths nearly all among the asthmatic, the consumptive and the aged. The ages of one hundred persons attacked at Birmingham were as follows[1]:

Ages	1—	5—	10—	20—	30—	40—	50—	60—	70—	80—90
Cases	3	2	12	23	21	19	12	7	0	1

At Evesham only five out of 93 were under five years. At Leamington, in a list of 170 cases, there were 26 under fourteen years, 119 from fourteen to sixty-five years, and 25 above the age of sixty-five[2]. In some places males seemed to be most attacked, just as at Birmingham in 1833 there was a great excess of female cases; but the collective inquiry showed that the sexes shared about equally all over. The type of the malady was on the whole catarrhal, as in 1833. Nearly all the cases had symptoms of sneezing, coughing, and defluxions; many cases had nothing more than the symptoms of a severe feverish cold; the more dangerous cases had dyspnoea, pneumonia and the like; while all had the languor, weariness, and soreness in the bones which mark every influenza, whether it incline more to the moist type of catarrhal fever or to the dry type of the old "hot ague."

The influenza of 1837 having been remarkably simultaneous, sudden and brief, the doctrine of personal contagiousness found little favour, just as in 1833. The 12th query sent out by the committee of the Provincial Medical Association was: "Are you in possession of any proof of its having been communicated from one person to another?" The answers are said to have been nearly all negative; namely, that there was "no proof of the existence of any contagious principles by which it was propagated from one individual to another." Shapter, a learned physician at Exeter, inclined to a certain modified doctrine of

---

[1] Peyton Blakiston, *A Treatise on the Influenza of* 1837, *containing an analysis of one hundred cases observed at Birmingham between* 1 *Jan. and* 15 *Feb.* Lond. 1837.
[2] These and some former particulars are from the "Report upon the Influenza or Epidemic Catarrh of the winter of 1836–37," compiled by Robt. J. N. Streeten, M.D. for the Committee of the Provincial Medical Association. *Trans. Prov. Med. Assoc.* VI. 501.

contagion by persons. Blakiston, of Birmingham, an exact mathematician, declared that the question as ordinarily stated did not admit of an answer.

At Liverpool there was an interesting observation made, exactly parallel with those made at Gravesend in 1782 and Portsmouth in 1788. The influenza of 1837 was practically over by the first or second week of March; but "that the atmosphere of Liverpool was still contaminated by the epidemic influence up to the middle and latter end of April was apparent from the fact that many of the officers and men of the American ships, and generally the most robust, were violently attacked shortly after their arrival in port,"—the same being the case also with black sailors on ships arriving from the Brazils and the West Coast of Africa[1]. At the naval stations of Sheerness, Portsmouth, Plymouth and Falmouth, every one of the ships of war had been attacked in January, the ships cruising on the south coast of Spain, or lying at Barcelona, in February, the ships at Gibraltar in April, and those at Malta in May. The 'Thunderer,' on the passage from Malta to Plymouth, had the first cases of influenza at sea on the 3rd of January, four days before reaching Plymouth[2], as if she had sailed into an atmosphere of it somewhere near the coast of Brittany.

For fully ten years, from March or April 1837 to November 1847, there was no great and universal influenza in England. But there were several undoubted minor, and perhaps localized, outbreaks of an epidemic malady which was in each case judged to be truly the influenza, and not a common cold. The earliest of these was in the spring of 1841. It was recognized by the Registrar-General to have been in London from 20 February to 24 April, the mortality having been little affected by it. It was also recognized in Dublin in March, and remarked upon by two physicians to the Cork Street Fever Hospital; it was characterized by the usual languor, weariness, and pains in the head, by defluxions of the eyes, nose and throat, but not by any affection of the lungs, and was in all respects mild[3]. Exactly a year after, in March, 1842, influenza was described as epidemic

[1] Streeten's Report, u.s., p. 505.
[2] *Statist. Report on Health of Navy*, 1837–43.
[3] Jackson, *Dubl. Med. Press*, VIII. 69; Brady, *Dubl. Journ. Med. Sc.* XX. (1842), 76.

at York[1]: it was noted also in London in March[2], and is mentioned as having been again in Ireland in 1842[3]. The next undoubted influenza is reported from a rural part of Cheshire (Holme Chapel) in January, 1844, in the wake of an epidemic of scarlatina; it continued in all kinds of weather until June, and had a remarkable intercurrent episode, for some weeks from the middle of March, in the form of an epidemic of pneumonia among young children, which passed into mild bronchitis in the cases last attacked[4]. Coincidently with the influenza in Cheshire, there is a report of a series of catarrhal cases in Dublin about the beginning of January, 1844, in which the sense of constriction and suffocation under the sternum and the paroxysmal character of the attacks seemed to point to influenza[5]. Two years after, a Dublin physician in extensive practice among the rich wrote, at the request of a medical editor, an account of an epidemic of influenza in January and February, 1847; he had sixty cases among children under fourteen in his private practice, usually several children in one house, and sometimes the adults in the house[6]. This was in the midst of the great epidemic of relapsing fever in Dublin and all over Ireland, due to the potato famine. The same prevalence of influenza to a slight extent is recorded also for London at the end of 1846 and beginning of 1847[7]. It is easy to object that these "influenzas" between 1837 and 1847 were but the ordinary catarrhal maladies of the seasons. But the physicians who took the trouble to record them—probably more might have done so—were, of course, aware of the distinction that had to be made between many common feverish colds concurring in the ordinary way, and a truly epidemic influenza, however slight.

The Influenza of 1847–48.

The great influenza of 1847 began in London about the 16th or 18th of November, was at its height from the 22nd to the

---

[1] Laycock, *Dubl. Med. Press*, VII. 234. Several cases of sudden and great enlargement of the liver and of suppression of urine were judged to be part of the epidemic.
[2] Ross, *Lancet*, 1845, I. p. 2.
[3] Report of Holywood Dispensary for 1842, *Dublin Med. Press*, IX. 204.
[4] Hall, *Prov. Med. Journ.* 1844, p. 315.
[5] M'Coy, *Med. Press*, XI. 133.
[6] Fleetwood Churchill, *Dubl. Quart. Journ.*, May, 1847, p. 373.
[7] Farr, in *Rep. Reg.-Gen.*

30th, had "ceased to be very prevalent" by the 6th or 8th of December, but affected the bills of mortality for some time longer, as in the following table:

Weekly Mortalities in London.

1847

Week ending	All causes	Influenza	Pneumonia	Bronchitis	Asthma	Typhus
Nov. 20	1086	4	95	61	12	86
27	1677	36	170	196	77	87
Dec. 4	2454	198	306	343	86	132
11	2416	374	294	299	78	136
18	1946	270	189	234	52	131
25	1247	142	131	107	14	83
Jan. 1	1599	127	148	138	26	74

In the thirteen weeks of the first quarter of 1848 the influenza deaths declined as follows: 102, 102, 89, 56, 59, 47, 27, 33, 18, 11, 10, 16, 8.

This was the first great epidemic of influenza under the new system of registration. According to the Superintendent of Statistics, it caused an excess of 5000 deaths during the six weeks that it lasted, of which about a fourth part only were set down to influenza, and the rest to pneumonia, bronchitis, asthma, etc. During the three worst weeks it raised the deaths in the age of childhood 83 per cent., in the age of manhood 104 per cent., in old age 247 per cent., whereas the deaths between fifteen years and twenty-five were but little raised by it, and those between ten and fifteen hardly at all. It raised the deaths during six weeks in St George's-in-the-East to a rate per annum of 73 per 1000 living: in some other parishes it increased the death-rate very little. But it had the usual effect of lengthening enormously the obituary columns of the newspapers, which shows that it fell, as usual, to a large extent upon the richer classes. It went all over England in a short time, the month of December being the time of excessive mortality in the towns, according to the following sample totals of deaths from all causes:

1847

	Manchester (Ancoats)	Sheffield (West)	York (Walmgate)	Places in Scotland
October	169	27	61	521
November	135	27	52	728
December	270	85	99	1001

In some parts of England, as in Kendal, a district of Anglesea and in the Isle of Wight, the mortality of the last quarter of 1847 was actually lower than that of the year before. From St Albans the sub-registrar reported that there had been "no epidemic." In most parts of the country, including the medium-sized towns, the mortality directly or indirectly due to influenza was lower than in London. The principal returns did not come in from the country until after the new year, the effects of the epidemic having been, as usual, later in rural districts. Hence, while London had 1253 deaths put down to "influenza" in 1847 (nearly all in December), and 659 in 1848 (nearly all in the first quarter), the rest of England had 4881 influenza deaths before the New Year, and 7963 after it[1]. This influenza in the mid-winter of 1847–8 made a great impression everywhere[2]. As regards its range and its fatality, it was like those of 1833 and 1837; and it had once more so much of the catarrhal type, that the name of influenza became still more firmly joined to the idea of a feverish cold or defluxion.

By the year 1847, agues had almost ceased to be written of in England, although they still occurred in the Fens. But Peacock begins his account of the influenza of that winter with an enumeration of prevailing diseases, which reads somewhat like an old "constitution" by Sydenham or Huxham. The summers and autumns of 1846 and 1847, he says, were both highly choleraic, and dysentery (as well as enteric fever) was unusually common in the former year. Fatal cases of "ague and remittent fever" were also more numerous than usual. Then came much enteric fever, "not unfrequently complicated with catarrhal symptoms." Throughout the spring and early summer of the influenza year, 1847, "intermittent fevers were common, and in March, April and May, purpura was frequently met with, either as a primary or secondary disease. Scurvy also, owing to the deficiency of fresh vegetables, and from the general failure of the

[1] Farr, in the *Report of the Registrar-General for* 1848. He cites (p. xxxi) Stark for Scotland, that it "suddenly attacked great masses of the population twice during November"—on the 18th, and again on the 28th.

[2] A curious trace of the temporary interest excited by influenza in 1847–8 remains in a great book of the time, Carlyle's *Letters and Speeches of Cromwell*, the third edition of which, with new letters, was then under hand. One of the new letters related to the death of Colonel Pickering from the camp-sickness among the troops of Fairfax at Ottery St Mary in December, 1645. Carlyle's comment is: "has caught the epidemic 'new disease' as they call it, some ancient *influenza* very prevalent and fatal during those wet winter operations." "New disease" was the name given by Greaves to the war-typhus in Oxfordshire and Berkshire in 1643, but neither that nor the sickness at Ottery (which is not called "new disease" in the documents) had anything of the nature of influenza.

potato crop in the previous year was occasionally seen." Then follows much concerning a fever called remittent, which reads more like relapsing fever than anything else[1]. "The remittent form of fever was frequent in the course of the epidemic [of influenza], though seldom registered as the cause of death." Peacock says truly that the rather unusual concurrence of so many sicknesses was "not peculiar to the recent influenza alone;" and he can "scarcely refrain from acknowledging that these several affections are not merely coetaneous but correlative, and types and modifications of one disease, with which they have a common origin. Assuming this inference to be admitted, we may advance to the solution of the further question of what is the essential nature or proximate cause of the disease." But the inquiry led him to no result: the precise cause he leaves "involved in the obscurity that veils the origin of epidemics generally"—which are surely not all equally obscure[2].

Influenza having continued epidemic for a few weeks in the beginning of 1848, ceased thereafter to attract popular notice in Britain during a period of more than forty years. But a certain number of "influenza" deaths continued to appear steadily year after year in the registration tables. In 1851 this number was nearly doubled, in 1855 it was more than trebled; and those two years were undoubtedly seasons (about January and February) of real influenza epidemics in Europe, recorded by several but not by English writers. A slight epidemic was described for Scotland in 1857, and one for Norfolk in 1878, neither of which seems to have influenced the registration returns in an obvious degree. After the undoubted influenza of 1855, the annual total of deaths in England set down to that cause steadily declined from four figures, to three figures, and then to two figures, standing at 55 in the bill of mortality for 1889. It is improbable that those small annual totals of deaths in all England and Wales were caused by the real influenza; the name at that

---

[1] But Dr Rose Cormack, who had known relapsing fever well in Edinburgh, wrote from Putney, near London, in October, 1849: "For some months past the majority of cases of all diseases in this neighbourhood have...presented a well-marked tendency to assume the remittent and intermittent types." "Infantile Remittent Fever," *Lond. Journ. of Med.*, Oct. 1849, reprinted in his *Clinical Studies*, 2 vols., 1876.

[2] T. B. Peacock, M.D., *On the Influenza, or Epidemic Catarrhal Fever of 1847–8.* London, 1848.

time was synonymous with a feverish cold, and would have been given here or there to fatalities from some such ordinary cause. An epidemic ague was reported from Somerset in 1858[1].

The Influenzas of 1889–94.

More than a generation had passed with little or no word of epidemic influenza in this country, when in the early winter of 1889 the newspapers began to publish long telegrams on the influenza in Moscow, St Petersburg, Berlin, Paris, Madrid and other foreign capitals. This epidemic wave, like those immediately preceding it in the Eastern hemisphere, in 1833, 1837 and 1847, and like one or more, but by no means all, of the earlier influenzas, had an obvious course from Asiatic and European Russia towards Western Europe[2]. In due time it reached London, and produced a decided effect upon the bills of mortality for the first and second weeks of January, 1890, but a moderate effect compared with that of 1847, which was the first to be recorded under the same system of registration. It spread all over England, Scotland and Ireland in the months of January and February, 1890, proving itself everywhere a short and sharp influenza of the old kind, but with catarrhal symptoms on the whole a less constant feature than in the epidemics of most recent memory. At the end of February it looked as if Great Britain and Ireland had got off lightly from the visitation which had caused high mortalities in many countries of Continental Europe. But this epidemic in the beginning of 1890 was only the first of four, and less severe than the second and third. It returned in the spring and early summer of 1891, in the first weeks of 1892, and in the winter of 1893–94. To understand this influenza prevalence as a whole, its four great seasons should be compared. The following tables show its incidence upon London on each occasion:

---

[1] Haviland, *Journ. Pub. Health*, IV. 288, (94 cases in June—Aug. in a village).

[2] See F. Clemow, M.D., of St Petersburg, "The Recent Pandemic of Influenza: its place of origin and mode of spread." *Lancet*, 20 Jan. and 10 Feb. 1894. These papers bring together and discuss the Russian opinions, official and other. The Army Medical Report favoured the view that the birthplace of this pandemic in the autumn of 1889 was an extensive region occupied by nomadic tribes in the northern part of the Kirghiz Steppe. There is evidence of its rapid progress westwards over Tobolsk to the borders of European Russia. Influenza is said to be constantly present in many parts of the Russian Empire; but the circumstances that have, on four or five occasions in the 19th century, set the infection rolling in a great wave westwards from the assumed source are wholly unknown.

Four epidemics of Influenza in London, 1890–94.

1890

Week ending	Annual death-rate per 1000 living	Deaths from all causes	Influenza	Bronchitis	Pneumonia
Jan. 4	28·0	2371	4	530	215
11	32·4	2747	67	715	253
18	32·1	2720	127	630	281
25	26·3	2227	105	468	193
Feb. 1	21·8	1849	75	339	145
8	20·6	1749	38	369	117

1891

Week ending	Annual death-rate per 1000 living	Deaths from all causes	Influenza	Bronchitis	Pneumonia
April 25	21·0	1809	10	240	179
May 2	23·3	2006	37	280	241
9	25·6	2069	148	302	230
16	27·7	2245	266	352	207
23	27·6	2235	319	337	219
30	28·9	2337	310	353	189
June 6	27·0	2189	303	320	176
13	23·3	1886	249	255	166
20	23·0	1865	182	248	159
27	19·0	1538	117	151	113
July 4	16·8	1363	56	108	103

1891–92

Week ending	Annual death-rate per 1000 living	Deaths from all causes	Influenza	Bronchitis	Pneumonia
Dec. 26	21·9	1771	19	355	131
Jan. 2	42·0	3399	37	927	256
9	32·8	2679	95	740	246
16	40·0	3271	271	867	285
23	46·0	3761	506	1035	317
30	41·0	3355	436	844	255
Feb. 6	30·6	2500	314	492	215
13	24·6	2010	183	368	140
20	20·7	1693	79	259	137

1893–94

Week ending	Annual death-rate per 1000 living	Deaths from all causes	Influenza	Bronchitis	Pneumonia
Nov. 4	20·2	1695	8	191	125
11	21·4	1679	20	220	137
18	24·4	2016	22	318	228
25	26·5	2190	36	384	215
Dec. 2	27·1	2235	74	426	248
9	31·0	2556	127	491	266
16	29·1	2401	164	421	232
23	26·3	2170	147	387	203
30	23·3	1920	108	306	157
Jan. 6	24·5	2040	87	342	169
13	29·5	2462	75	490	211
20	23·7	1975	69	320	172
27	19·8	1655	41	232	152

It will· be seen that the third epidemic, that of Jan.–Feb. 1892, had the highest maximum weekly mortality from influenza (506) as well as the highest maxima from bronchitis and pneumonia not specially associated in the certificates with influenza; that the second epidemic, of 1891, had the next highest maxima, and that the first and last of the four outbreaks were both milder than the two intermediate ones. All but the second, which fell in early summer, are strictly comparable as regards season (mid-winter). But although the second, in 1891, had the advantage of falling in some of the healthiest weeks of the year, it was more protracted than the original outbreak, much more fatal than it in the article influenza, more fatal also in the article pneumonia, and less fatal only in the article bronchitis. The third outbreak was not only more protracted than the first, in the same season of the year, but much more fatal in all the associated articles. As to the deaths referred to influenza (whether as primary or secondary cause), the numbers are not strictly comparable in all the outbreaks; they are probably too few in the first table, more nearly exact in the second, third, and fourth, the diagnosis having at length become familiar and the fashion of nomenclature established. It is undoubted that many of the deaths from bronchitis and pneumonia in January, 1890, were due to the epidemic; for, "while the ordinary rise of mortality in cold seasons is mainly among the very aged, the increased mortality in this fatal month was mainly among persons between 20 and 60 years " (Ogle).

While the first epidemic of the series was universal and of short duration all over the kingdom, the second and third were more partial in their incidence and more desultory or prolonged. The second, which began in Hull (and at the same time on the borders of Wales), produced the following highest weekly death-rates per annum from all causes among 1000 persons living :

Highest Weekly Death-rates in the Second Influenza.

1891

	Week ending	Annual death-rate from all causes per 1000 living		Week ending	Annual death-rate from all causes per 1000 living
Hull	Apr. 11	42·5	Huddersfield	May 16	54·5
Sheffield	May 2	70·5	Leicester	,, 16	44·6
Halifax	,, 2	42·1	Oldham	,, 23	50·4
Leeds	,, 9	48·5	London	,, 30	28·9
Manchester	,, 9	43·6	Salford	,, 30	45·9
Bradford	,, 16	56·7	Blackburn	June 6	48·5

The third was heard of first in the west of Cornwall and in the east of Scotland, in the last quarter of 1891. It was in the following English towns that it produced the maximum weekly death-rates per annum from all causes :

Highest Weekly Death-rates in the Third Influenza.

1892

Town	Week ending	Annual death-rate from all causes per 1000 living
Portsmouth	Jan. 16	57·0
London	,, 23	46·0
Norwich	,, 23	44·7
Brighton	,, 23	60·9
Croydon	,, 30	47·2

These highest death-rates in the third successive season of influenza were all in the southern or eastern counties; in the latter, Colchester also had a maximum death-rate during one week of about 80 per 1000 per annum. Liverpool, among the northern great towns, appears to have had most of the third influenza. The fourth outbreak, in the end of 1893, was noticed first in the Midlands (Birmingham especially), and was afterwards heard of in the mining and manufacturing districts of Stafford-shire, South Wales, Lancashire, Yorkshire and Durham, as well as in Scotland and Ireland, London, as in the table, having a share of it. The tables given of the London mortality in each of the four outbreaks, from influenza and the chest-complaints which were its most usual secondary effects, are a fair index both of the period and of the severity of the disease all over the kingdom in each of its successive appearances[1]. Everywhere the first and the fourth were the mildest, the second and third the most fatal. Deaths from "influenza" were reported from all the counties of England and Wales in the first and second epidemics, the highest rates of mortality per 1000 inhabitants in the corresponding calendar years having been in the following counties, while in all the counties the greater fatality of the second epidemic is equally marked:

---

[1] The collective inquiry on the epidemics was made by the medical department of the Local Government Board, the result being given in two reports : *Report on the Influenza Epidemic of* 1889–90, *Parl. Papers*, 1891, and *Further Report and Papers on Epidemic Influenza*, 1889–92, *Parl. Papers*, Sept. 1893. By H. Franklin Parsons, M.D. Statistical tables comparing the epidemics in London with those in some other capitals were published by F. A. Dixey, M.D., *Epidemic Influenza*, Oxford, 1892.

1890		1891	
Cumberland	·35	Rutland	1·36
North Wales	·28	Lincolnshire	1·19
Herefordshire	·28	North Wales	1·09
Salop	·28	Westmoreland	1·02
Wilts	·28	Monmouth	1·00
Somerset	·26	E. Riding Yorks	·98
Dorset	·25	Herefordshire	·98
Bucks	·25	Northamptonshire	·95

In London the entry of influenza is in the weekly bills of mortality throughout the whole period, with the exception of a few weeks; but the deaths were often reduced to unity, and there was perhaps only one occasion, besides the four great outbursts, namely the months of March and April, 1893, when cases were so numerous or so close together in households or neighbourhoods as to constitute a minor epidemic.

The type of the influenza of 1890–93 was not quite the same as on the last historical occasions. When it was announced as approaching from the Continent, everyone looked for "influenza colds"; but the catarrhal symptoms, although not wanting, were soon found to be unimportant beside the nameless misery, prostration and ensuing weakness. Some, indeed, contended that the disease was not influenza but dengue, so pronounced were the symptoms of break-bone fever[1]. Many cases had a decided aguish or intermittent character. The name of ague itself was once more heard in newspaper paragraphs, and more freely used in private talk; but, as we have long ceased to write of epidemic agues, equally as of marsh intermittents, in this country, it is not probable that there will remain any record of agues in Britain accompanying the influenzas of the years 1890–94. On the other hand the complications and after-effects of our latest influenza, more especially as affecting the nervous system, have been very fully studied[2].

That which chiefly distinguishes the influenza of the end of the 19th century from all other invasions of the disease is the

[1] The notable difference between the type of this epidemic and that of the epidemics of 1833, 1837 and 1847, from which the conventional notion of "influenza cold" was derived, is perhaps the explanation of the following apt and erudite remark by Buchanan, on "influenza proper," in his introduction to the first departmental report, 1891: "It would be no small gain to get more authentic methods of identifying influenza proper from among the various grippes, catarrhs, colds and the like—in man, horse, and other animals—that take to themselves the same popular title" (p. xi).

[2] The volume by Julius Althaus, M.D., *Influenza: its Pathology, Complications and Sequelae*, 2nd ed., Lond. 1892, includes a summary and bibliography of recent observations.

revival of the epidemic in three successive seasons, the first recurrence having been more fatal than the original outbreak, and the second recurrence more fatal (in London at least) than the first.   The closest scrutiny of the old records, including the series of weekly bills of mortality issued by the Parish Clerks of London for nearly two hundred years, discovers no such recurrences of influenza on the great scale in successive seasons.   It is true that several of the old influenzas came in the midst of sickly periods of two or more years' duration, such as the years 1557–58, 1580–82, 1657–59, 1678–80, 1727–29 and 1780–85. But in those periods the bulk of the sickness was aguish, the somewhat definite episodes of catarrhal fever having been distinguished from the epidemic agues by Willis in 1658, by Sydenham in 1679, by several in 1729, and by Baker, among others, in 1782.   It is probable, indeed, that there were two strictly catarrhal epidemics in successive years in the periods 1657–59 and 1727–29, just as we know that, in New England, there was a catarrhal epidemic in the autumn of 1789 and an equally severe influenza, less catarrhal in type, in the spring of 1790[1].   But history does not appear to supply a parallel case to the four successive influenzas in the period 1889–94, unless we count the seasonal epidemic agues of former "constitutions" as equivalent to influenzas for the purpose of making out a series.

The Theory of Influenza.

Influenza is not an infection which lends itself to a simple theory of its nature or a neat formula of its cause.   All that one can do is to indicate the direction in which the truth lies. Something broad, comprehensive, steady from age to age, telluric if not cosmic, must be sought for.   Some have thought that the legendary or representative universal sickness at the siege of Troy was influenza, because it began upon the horses and dogs, as so many historical influenzas have done.   But it will be sufficient to show that influenza was the same in the Middle Ages as now; for what circumstances make a broader contrast than medieval and modern?   The first writer in England to mention influenza—of course not under that name—was a dean of St Paul's in the reign of Henry II., Radulphus de

---

[1] Noah Webster, *Brief History of Epidemick Diseases*, I. 288 ; Warren, of Boston, to Lettsom, 30 May, 1790, *Lettsom's Memoirs*, III. 238: "whether this [the second] is a variety of influenza, or a new disease with us, I am at a loss to determine."

Diceto[1]. He is narrating the journey to Rome of the arch-bishop-elect of Canterbury: his election in England was in June, 1173, he had got as far as Placentia by Christmas, whence he turned aside to Genoa, and at length reached Rome, to have his election confirmed by the pope in the nones of April, 1174. It is in the midst of this account of the archbishop's journey, that reference is made to an influenza, otherwise known, from German and Italian chronicles, to have happened in December, 1173: "In those days the whole world was infected by a nebulous corruption of the air, causing catarrh of the stomach and a general cough, to the detriment of all and the death of many"—*universus orbis infectus ex aeris nebulosa corruptione.* What kind of infection can that be which has befallen men on both sides of the Alps within the same short time in the 12th century as in the 19th? And what kind of infection is it which has outlived so many changes in the great pestilences of mankind, has seen the extinction of plague and the rise of cholera, and all other variations, most of them for the better, in the reigning types of epidemic sickness? To have lasted unchanged through so many mutations of things, from medieval to modern, and from modern to ultra-modern, and to have become more in-veterate or protracted at the end of the 19th century than it had ever been, is unique in this history. Influenza appears to correspond with something broadly the same in human life at all times. Or is it rather a thing telluric, of the crust of the earth or the bowels of the earth? Or is it perhaps cosmic, affecting men as the vintage is affected by a comet, or as if it came from the upper spheres? My belief is that we need not transcend the globe to look for its source, and that, upon the earth, we need not go deeper than the surface, nor beyond the inhabited spots. I shall come back to this from giving the history of English opinion upon it.

The best known influenzas of the 16th century all came in summer, as some of the later ones have done, so that no one thought of them as exaggerated common colds. But it hap-pened that the influenzas observed by Willis in 1658, and by Sydenham in 1675 and 1679, came in spring or winter and in such weather as to suggest to each of those physicians that the catarrhal symptoms corresponded to the season. Robert Boyle, their great philosophical contemporary, was also a witness of

[1] In Twysden's *Decem Scriptores*, col. 579.

one or more of these influenzas, and it appeared to him that there was more than season and weather in them.

"I have known a great cold," he says, "in a day or two invade multitudes in the same city with violent, and as to many persons, fatal symptoms; when I could not judge (as others also did not), that the bare coldness of the air could so suddenly produce a disease so epidemical and hurtful; and it appeared the more probable that the cause came from under ground, by reason that it began with a very troublesome fog[1]."

I am unable to say whether Boyle was the first to apply the doctrine of telluric or subterranean emanations to influenza; he was certainly not the first to apply it to pestilences in general, for it is found in Seneca among the ancients[2], and it is clearly stated in Ambroise Paré's essay "Sur les Venins," having been probably a familiar notion of the sixteenth century, although a mystical and undefined one. Sydenham also, who must have discussed these questions with Boyle, referred all the more obscure or "stationary" epidemic constitutions to effluvia discharged into the air from "the bowels of the earth": those hypothetical miasmata were for him the τὸ θεῖον of Hippocrates, the mysterious something which had to be assumed so as to explain plague, pestilential fever, intermittent and remittent fevers, the "new fever" of 1685–6, and all other epidemic constitutions which were not caused by obvious changes of season and weather. But it does not appear, and it is not probable, that he ascribed to that mysterious cause the two transient waves of influenza which fell within his own experience, those of November, 1675, and of November, 1679. On the other hand, Boyle certainly did so; he included influenza in his hypothesis explicitly; and if one examines its general terms, it will appear as if it had been made specially for influenza.

Boyle's general expression, for both endemial and epidemic maladies, is that they are due to subterranean effluvia sent up into the air. As a chemist, and as dealing with the new knowledge then most in vogue, he assumed the sources of these miasmata to be for the most part mineral deposits in the crust of the globe, especially "orpimental and other mischievous fossiles"; but later in his writing he says:

[1] Boyle's *Works*, 6 vols., London, 1772, V. 52.
[2] Seneca, *Nat. Quaest.* § 27, cited by Webster. After earthquakes, "subitae continuaeque mortes, et monstrosa genera morborum ut ex novis orta causis." The passage cited from Baglivi (p. 530) looks like a repetition of this: "imo nova et inaudita morborum genera...post terraemotus."

"To speak candidly I do not think that these minerals are the causes of even all those pestilences whose efficients may come from under ground"; there were many mischievous fossils of which physicians and even chymists had no knowledge, and "the various associations of these, which nature may, by fire and menstruums, make under ground and perhaps in the air itself, may very much increase the number and variety of hurtful matters."

He makes provision, also, for the hurtful matters multiplying in their underground seats, according to a principle which we know now to be true for organic, instead of mineral matters, and to be true for them above ground, or in the air, as well as under ground :

"I think it possible that divers subterraneal bodies that emit effluvia may have in them a kind of propagative or self-multiplying power. I will not here examine whether this proceeds from some seminal principle, which many chymists and others ascribe to metals and even to stones; or (which is perhaps more likely) to something analogous to a ferment, such as, in vegetables, enables a little sour dough to extend itself through the whole mass, or such as, when an apple or pear is bruised in one part, makes the putrefied part by degrees to transmute the sound into its own likeness; or else some maturative power...as ananas in the Indies, and medlars...after they are gathered, acquire (as it were spontaneously) in process of time a consistence and sweetness and sometimes colour and odour, and, in short, such a state as by one word we call maturity or ripeness."

Other of Boyle's fruitful principles (I am separating them out from amidst much other matter not specially related to influenza) are these :

"It is possible that these effluvia may be, in their own nature, either innocent enough, or at least not considerably hurtful, and yet may become very noxious if they chance to find the air already imbued with certain corpuscles fit to associate with them."

Again, the effluvia sent up into the air may pass by certain places without causing an epidemic, because these "are not inhabited enough to make their ill qualities taken notice of; but, more frequently, because by being diffused through a greater tract of air, they are more and more dispersed in their passage, and thereby so diluted (if I may so speak) and weakened as not to be able to do any notorious mischief."

Again, the effluvia may not produce epidemic disease at the part of the globe where they had emerged from under ground; an illustration of which may be intended in the case of the Black Death, which, as he says, came from China, yet plague is little heard of in that country, a Jesuit, Alexander de Rhodes, who spent thirty years in those parts, testifying that the plague is not so much as spoken of there. Again, why are some epidemics of so short duration at a given place? Either, he answers, because the morbific expiration from under ground had ascended almost at once, and been easily spent; or the subterraneal commotion which sends up the miasmata "may pass from one place to another and so cease to afford the air incumbent on the first place the supplies necessary to keep it impregnated with noxious exhalation; and it agrees well with this conjecture that sometimes we may observe certain epidemical diseases to have, as it were, a progressive motion, and leaving one town free, pass on to another" —as notably in the case of sweating sickness and influenza.

Lastly there are ever new forms of epidemic disease appearing, not to count every variation of an autumnal ague "which the vulgar call a New Disease." Of the really new types Boyle offers the following explanation : "Some among the emergent variety of exotick and hurtful steams may be found capable to disaffect human bodies after a very uncommon way, and thereby to produce new diseases, whose duration may be greater or smaller according to the lastingness of those subterraneal causes that produce them. On which account it need be no wonder that some new diseases have but a short duration, and vanish not long after their appearing, the sources or fumes being soon destroyed or spent; whereas some others may continue longer upon the stage, as having under ground more settled and durable causes to maintain them."

As a chemist, Boyle sought for the source of the pestilential emanations in underground minerals, in the new combinations of these under the action of "fire and menstruums," in their self-multiplying power as if by subterraneous fermentation ("which many chymists and others ascribe to metals and even to stones"), and in their meeting with suitable "corpuscles" in the air of an inhabited spot wherewith to combine for their morbific effects. He assumed, also, their discharge into the air at particular spots of the globe (where they might not be directly morbific in their effects), or in a series of localities from the wave-like progress of the underground commotion ; in which assumption he seems to be applying the very old idea of classical times that earthquakes and volcanic eruptions were a cause or antecedent of epidemics. Sometimes his mineral fossils were deep in the crust of the globe, touched only by the greater cataclysms ; and then we might expect novelties in the forms of epidemic disease. But he does not exclude emanations from the earth's surface proceeding more gently or insensibly.

It would be a mistake to set aside Boyle's hypothesis of epidemical miasmata as made altogether void by his choosing strange minerals to be the source of them, and by his assuming a kind of fermentation in these inorganic matters so as to explain the continuance and spreading of the infections. Substitute organic matters in the soil for minerals in the crust of the earth, and read a modern meaning into the doctrine of underground or aërial fermentation or leavening, and we shall find Boyle's hypothesis, especially as applied to influenza, far from obsolete. Some such adaptation of the doctrine of miasmata was made two generations later by Dr John Arbuthnot in his 'Essay concerning the Effects of Air upon Human Bodies,' the immediate occasion of which was the London influenza of 1733. There is nothing to note between Boyle and Arbuthnot ; for

Willis and Sydenham, using the Hippocratic language of "constitutions," explained, as we have seen, the epidemic catarrhs of the spring or winter as the reigning febrile constitution modified to suit the season and weather.

Arbuthnot's essay makes more modern reading than Boyle's. He assumes emanations from the ground, but they are no longer from the bowels of the earth, or from deposits of strange minerals requiring earthquakes to set them free, or "fire and menstruums" to give potency to them. Of all the things that pass into the atmosphere, he makes most of the various steams and other volatile decomposing matters of men and animals; and when he brings in the earth, it is as the storehouse or receptacle of such matters, in a surface stratum no deeper than the effects of drought and rainfall could reach. While he accepts the Hippocratic doctrine of epidemic constitutions, and recognizes the air with its ·various organic contents as the τὸ θεῖον, the *quid divinum* or mysterious something of epidemical causation, he does not forget that the earth is inhabited by creatures, human and other, who befoul the atmosphere by "their own steams"; again, he lays stress upon alternations of drought and moisture in the soil and subsoil as a cause of morbific emanations, not, indeed, stating the matters of fact in the very terms of Pettenkofer's law, but assuming the presence of special organic matters in the soil as much as that does. Although Arbuthnot was hardly a serious epidemiologist, any more than Boyle, yet in the growth of opinion on the subject of morbific matters in the air, he may be said to have shifted the interest from inorganic or mineral substances and gases, to organic matters chiefly of human or animal origin, and from the deeper regions of the globe, such as only earthquakes reach, to the surface stratum of soil and subsoil which is affected by every rise and fall of the ground-water. I shall now give a few extracts, to bear out the above summary, from Abuthnot's essay.

"Air," he says, "is the τὸ θεῖον in diseases, which Hippocrates takes notice of. Air is what he means by the powers of the universe, which, he says, human nature cannot overcome; and he lays it down as a maxim 'that whoever intends to be master of the art of physick must observe the constitution of the year; that the powers and influence of the seasons (what are seldom uniform) produce great changes in human bodies.'" He then pays a compliment to Sydenham as "endowed with the genius of Hippocrates," and passes on to his own analytic method. "Many great effects must follow, and many sudden changes may happen in human bodies by absorbing outward air with all its qualities and contents.

Nothing accounts more clearly for epidemical diseases seizing human creatures inhabiting the same tract of earth, who have nothing in common that affects them except air : such as that epidemical catarrhous fever of 1728 and of this present year [1733]...It seems to be occasioned by effluvia, uncommon either in quantity or quality, infecting the air...It is likewise evident that these effluvia were not of any particular or mineral nature, because they were of a substance that was common to every part of the surface of the earth : and therefore one may conclude that they were watery exhalations, or, at least, such mixed with other exhalable substances that are common to every spot of ground."

In his account of the qualities and contents of the air, he enumerates them, not so much as detected in the air on analysis, but as having of necessity passed into it, and in some instances been deposited again from it, as in strange dews. One class of substances that pass into the air are the oils, salts, seeds and insensible abrasions of vegetables. Also all excrements and all the carcases of animals vanish into air. Another ingredient of the air is the perspirable matters of animals, the amount of which for human beings he works out by a curious calculation of a column of their own steams raised so many feet high in so many days. Perhaps there are insects in the air invisible to human eyes: one may observe, in that part of a room which is illuminated with the rays of the sun, flies sometimes darting like hawks as if it were upon a prey. Some have imagined the plague to proceed from invisible insects: this system agrees with many of the appearances in the progress or manner of propagation of that disease, but is altogether inconsistent with others. Air replete with the steams of animals, especially such as are rotting, has often produced pestilential fevers in that place : of which there are many instances.

But why should certain years or seasons have a pestilential atmosphere, for example the season of the catarrhous fever of 1733? There had been, he says, an unusual drought for these two years past, the best estimate of the dryness of the surface of the earth being taken from the falling of the springs, "the consequence of which has been unusual diseases amongst several animals, and a great mortality amongst mankind. It is true, this did not happen during the dry weather...The previous great drought must have been particularly hurtful to mankind. Great droughts exert their effects after the surface of the earth is again opened by moisture, and the perspiration of the ground, which was long suppressed, is suddenly restored. It is probable that the earth then emits several new effluvia hurtful to human bodies : this appeared to be the case by the thick and stinking fogs which succeeded the rain that had fallen before."

Arbuthnot knew the progress of the influenza of 1732–33. Its worst week in London was from the 23rd to the 30th January, 1733 ; but he tells us that it had been at a height in Saxony from the 15th to the 29th November, 1732, had been earlier in Holland than in England, earlier in Edinburgh than in London, in New England before Great Britain. Again, it appeared in Paris in February, somewhat later than in London, and in Naples in March. This progress, he says, was often against the wind. Nor does he assume a progressive infection of regions of atmosphere. The effluvia, he says, were of a substance that was common to every part of the surface of the earth ; they were exhalable substances that were common to every spot of ground ; the excessive drought of two years, followed by heavy rains in the end of 1732, is also assumed to have been common, for, in Germany and France, especially in November, 1732, the air was filled with frequent fogs. It is clear that Arbuthnot traced the universality of influenza, the uniform symptoms of which he recognized, to certain conditions of soil and atmosphere common to all the countries visited by the epidemic.

Throughout the rest of the 18th century there were numerous and varied experiences of influenza, in summer and winter, spring and autumn, coming up from the south as if from Africa, or from the east as if from Central Asia, or appearing in America sooner than in Europe—experiences which made a theory of the disease difficult. Some inclined to Arbuthnot's view of unusual seasons and weather producing the same effects everywhere ; others favoured the hypothesis of contagion from a remote source, which might be China or might be some other territory. Geach, a surgeon at Plymouth who was a Fellow of the Royal Society, actually went back to the astrological cause, pointing out that Jupiter and Saturn were in a certain con-junction during the influenza of 1775. The only elaborate theory of the strange disease that calls for notice, besides those of Boyle and Arbuthnot, is that of Noah Webster, the famous lexicographer of Hartford, Connecticut.

While Webster was a journalist in New York about the years 1794–6, the subject of yellow fever, which was then of great practical moment, set him reading and speculating about pesti-lences in general. Writing to Priestley, he said that in the course of his inquiries he found the American libraries ill supplied with books[1]; but he certainly made diligent and skilful use of his literary materials, and produced in his 'Brief History of Epidemic and Pestilential Diseases,' a work which was better than any before it in the chronological part, and remains to the present time unique in its philosophical part for the boldness of its generalities[2]. He saw that influenza was the crux of epidemiology, and paid special attention to it.

In looking for the antecedents of influenza, he kept in view the greater telluric changes and convulsions, such as earthquakes and volcanic eruptions. He did not regard these as the cause of

[1] Cited by Horace E. Scudder, in *Noah Webster*. New York and London, 1881, p. 105.
[2] *Brief History of Epidemic and Pestilential Diseases.* 2 vols., Hartford, 1799.

influenza, but as the index of some hidden cause to which both they and the universal catarrh were due.

"It is probable to me," he says, "that neither seasons, earthquakes, nor volcanic eruptions are the causes of the principal derangements we behold in animal and vegetable life, but are themselves the *effects* of those motions and invisible operations which affect mankind. Hence catarrh and other epidemics often appear *before* the visible phenomena of eruptions and earthquakes[1]." As to influenza, he found "reason to conclude the disease to be the effect of some access of stimulant powers to the atmosphere by means of the electrical principle. No other principle in creation, which has yet come under the cognizance of the human mind, seems adequate to the same effects."

And again: "It is more probable that it is to be ascribed to an insensible action of atmospheric fire, which is more general and violent about the time of eruptions, and which fire is probably agitated in all parts of the globe, although it produces visible effects in explosions in some particular places only." It is due to Webster to give his reason for preferring a physical force to an organic poison: "If a deleterious vapour were the cause, I should suppose its effects would be speedy, and its force soon expended, the atmosphere being speedily purified by the winds. But if stimulus is the cause, it may exist for a long time in the atmosphere, and the human body not yield to its force in many weeks or months. This would better accord with facts. For, although diseases appear soon after an earthquake, yet the worst effects are often many months or years after[2]."

Dr Blagden also saw a difficulty in "the prodigious quantity of matter required in the air to infect the space not only of the Chinese land, but to a hundred leagues of the coast, or, as in this instance [1782] all Europe and the circumjacent sea," and was accordingly driven to Arbuthnot's view of an origin in the unusual weather of each locality.

Webster drew up a chronological table of influenzas in either Hemisphere, with the volcanic eruptions, earthquakes, comets, etc., to suit[3]. A few instances from near the beginning may serve as samples:

1647. First catarrh mentioned in American annals, in the same year with violent earthquakes in South America, and a comet.

1655. Influenza in America, in the same year with violent earthquakes in South America and an eruption of Vesuvius. It began about the end of June.

1658. Influenza in Europe after a severe winter: the summer cool.

---

[1] *Brief History of Epidemic and Pestilential Diseases,* II. 15.

[2] *Id.* II. 34, 84. Dr Robert Williams, in his work on *Morbid Poisons* (II. 670) argues for Webster's electrical theory of influenza without knowing, or at least without saying, that it was Webster's. The much-advertised writings of Mr John Parkin on *The Volcanic Theory of Epidemics* (or other title) follow Webster very closely both in the main idea and in its ramifications, but without acknowledgment to the American *philosophe.* Milton's rule was that one might take from an old author if one improved upon him; but neither Williams nor Parkin has improved upon Webster.

[3] *Ibid.* II. 30.

1675. Influenza in Europe while Etna was still in a state of explosion: the winter mild.

1679–80. Influenza in Europe during or just after the eruption of Etna: the season wet: a comet.

1688. Influenza in Europe in the same year with an eruption of Vesuvius, after a severe winter, and earthquakes: it began in a hot summer.

1693. Influenza in Europe in the same year with an eruption in Iceland and great earthquakes : the season cool.

1697–98. Influenza in America after a great earthquake in Peru: a comet the same year: the winter severe.

In most instances the region of the earthquake is not specified in the table; but it is sometimes named in the text of the annals under the respective years. Volcanoes are on the whole made more of than earthquakes, Webster's object being to find evidence of "electrical stimulus," and not of material miasmata discharged into the air. Etna and Hecla are much in request. Any earthquake suits, as if "earthquake" and "volcano" were like algebraic symbols, always a and b, and never anything but a and b, "influenza" being always x. One begins to realize the difficulties of the volcano or earthquake theory of influenza on turning to Mallet's Catalogue of Earthquakes[1]. Here, indeed, is an embarrassing choice between China and Peru, Asia Minor and North Africa, Portugal and Sicily or Calabria, Iceland and Jamaica, the Azores and the Philippines, Caracas or Acapulco and Valparaiso, Hungary and Savoy, Kamtschatka and Amboina; between earthquakes great and small ; between earthquakes and volcanoes. Any influenza year might be suited with one or more earthquakes, perhaps in either Hemisphere ; but there are some long clear intervals between the greater influenzas in Europe, for example the interval from 1803 to 1831, which seem to occupy as many pages of the catalogue of earthquakes as the years wherein influenzas came thickest, for example from 1729 to 1743, or from 1831 to 1847.

None the less, Webster, like Boyle, obeyed a true impulse when he looked for the cause of influenzas in something telluric, occasional, phenomenal. A wave of influenza comes up unexpectedly from a particular point of the compass, passes quickly over many degrees of latitude and longitude, lasting a few weeks at any given place, disappears in the distance, and does not return again perhaps for a whole generation. Influenza has the qualities of suddenness, swiftness, transitoriness; it has a certain

---

[1] "Catalogue of Recorded Earthquakes from 1606 B.C. to A.D. 1850." *British Assocn. Reports*, 1852–54.

sameness in its symptoms; it can be identified as certainly in the brief phrases of medieval chronicles as in elaborate modern descriptions; it has had no season for its own, as plague and cholera have had the summer and autumn, but has reached a height in Europe sometimes in midsummer, sometimes in midwinter. No other epidemic malady can compare with it in these respects; all the rest seem to have been provoked more or less by the turns and changes in human affairs, some being of a medieval colour, others of a modern, each in its own way admitting of explanation from unwholesome living, or from famine, or from over-population, or from something more recondite but still within the sphere of things insanitary in an intelligible sense. Other plagues besides influenza were, it is true, once reckoned mysterious, or associated in the popular mind with earthquakes and comets. But several such plagues have disappeared from among us, while their alleged causes, the earthquakes or comets, continue as before. Influenza alone returns at intervals as of old, untouched by civilization, by sanitation, by the immense differences between medieval and modern, making the same impression upon England in the year 1890 as it did in 1173, or 1427, or 1580, or, if changed at all, then changed for the worse inasmuch as the epidemic came back more severely in 1891, and still more severely in 1892. It is not surprising that for such a disease something telluric or even cosmic should have been assigned as the cause, something as occasional as itself, phenomenal, if not cataclysmic. It may be proper, therefore, that we should try over again the philosophic generalities of Boyle, Arbuthnot and Webster, peradventure a combination of them may yield a true theory. From Boyle we may take the great principle of a progressive infection through regions of air (or leagues of ground), which was expressed once for all by Lucretius in the sixth book of the 'De Rerum Natura':

> ...atque aer inimicus serpere coepit;
> Ut nebula ac nubes paulatim repit, et omne
> Qua graditur, conturbat et immutare coactat;
> Fit quoque ut in nostrum quum venit denique coelum
> Corrumpat reddatque sui simile atque alienum.

From Arbuthnot we may take the organic source and nature of the influenzal miasmata, and the association with changes in the level of the water in the soil. From Webster we may take the idea that the historic influenzas, having been sudden, occasional or phenomenal, must have had phenomenal causes somewhere in either Hemisphere. Instead of sketching a theory in the abstract, and safeguarding it by following all its ramifications, I shall proceed by the way of instances, choosing them so as to bring out particular points in order.

The only generality which may be indicated at starting is one that has presented itself time after time in the foregoing history, namely that there is something more than accident in the association between epidemics of influenza and epidemics of ague. So close was this association in former times that both the influenza and the widely prevalent ague were included together under such names as "the new ague," "the new fever," "the new distemper." As late as 1679, Morley did not distinguish the epidemic of influenza from the epidemic agues in the midst of which it was set, although the distinction was real, and was actually made by Sydenham on that occasion, as it had been made by Willis and in a manner by Whitmore on the occasion immediately preceding, and as it was made by everyone on the last great occasion when an influenza made an interlude among epidemic agues in the year 1782. It has often been suspected that influenza was related to some other infection: at one time it was taken for a volatile emanation of plague, in our own time it has been regarded as a volatile emanation of Asiatic cholera. In a wider historical view the question may arise, whether the real relation is not rather to those remarkable agues which have been epidemic in company with influenza when there was no plague and no cholera.

I come now to certain influenzas, as illustrating particular points of theory, in order.

I.

It is probable that Webster's theory of influenza as related to earthquakes and volcanoes, first published in 1799, was suggested to him by a communication to the Royal Society on the volcanic waves seen at Barbados on the 31st of March, 1761, and on the epidemic of influenza thereafter ensuing all over the island. At Bridgetown, in the afternoon of the 31st of March, 1761, the water in the bay and harbour ebbed and flowed to the extent of eighteen inches or two feet at intervals of eight minutes, and continued to do so for the space of three hours, the oscillation regularly decreasing till night when it was no more observable. These tidal waves were due to volcanic upheavals somewhere; and it was found that the centre of disturbance had been in the Atlantic near the coast of Portugal, and the time some hours earlier than the waves were felt at Bridgetown. The Barbados chronicler proceeds :

"It is very remarkable that since that time the island has been in a very deplorable condition, having suffered under the severest colds that have been ever known. The distress has been so general that I may venture to assert (with confidence) that nineteen twentieths of the inhabitants of the island have felt the effects of the contagion; and to some it has been repeated several times. It has puzzled all the adepts in pharmacy to find out the cause and cure of it. One favourable circumstance has attended it, viz. few have died with it. The Leeward Islands have not escaped, it having raged there more violently and more fatal. His Majesty's ships have severely felt the effects of it, some of them not being capable of keeping the seas for want of men fit for service. This happening at a season of the year remarkably the healthiest, makes it the more surprising[1]."

This is as good an instance as we shall find, of explaining something sudden, swift, and phenomenal, by something else sudden, swift, and phenomenal, in a purely empirical way and without pausing to ask whether the latter could have been a *vera causa* of the former. That the influenza came to Barbados in the wake, as it were, of the volcanic waves, had been a common subject of talk among the residents; and that common opinion of the colony had found expression in the paper sent to the Royal Society. The influenza was not only in Barbados, in the Leeward Islands, and in the ships on the West Indian Station, but also in New England and "over the whole country" of the North American Colonies. Dr Tufts, of Weymouth, New England, wrote to Webster that "it began in April, and in May ran into a malignant fever which proved fatal to aged persons. It spread over the whole country and the West India Islands[2]." It was not until some nine months after that influenza appeared in Europe, at first in the east of that continent,—Hungary, Vienna, Breslau, Copenhagen—in February and March, 1762, in central Germany and Scotland in April, in London about the first of May and all over England and Ireland thereafter, but not in France until June and July.

Precisely the same order was followed by the influenza twenty years after : it began in North America in March, 1781, and, says Webster, spread over that continent ; it appeared in

[1] Abraham Mason, *Phil. Trans.* LII. Part 2, p. 477.
[2] Webster, I. 150.

the East Indies in October and November, 1781, and on the eastern confines of Europe in January, 1782, having been traced from Tobolsk, made a slow progress westwards, and was at its height in London about the end of May or beginning of June. Assuming, says Webster, that the American influenza of 1781 had been continuous with the European of 1782, it must have " passed the Pacific in high northern latitudes," traversed Siberia and Tartary, and so reached Russia in Europe. In like manner, if the European influenza of 1762 were continuous with the American of 1761, it must have made the circuit of the globe in the same order, as if it were following the first impulse of the volcanic waves across the Atlantic from the coast of Portugal westwards, and so round the earth until it came back to Europe on its eastern frontier. So much may be fairly advanced on the ground of a particular set of facts. But then there were many other facts, both in 1761–62, and in 1781–82. Meanwhile let us take another instance of volcanic waves felt at Barbados six years before, on the same afternoon as the great earthquake of Lisbon.

II.

At Bridgetown, on the 1st November, 1755, Dr Hillary saw the peculiar flux and reflux of the water in the harbour from 2.20 p.m. to 9 p.m. and pronounced that there must have been an earthquake somewhere. The waves came at first at intervals of five minutes, and at last at intervals of twenty minutes. The day was calm, and the ships in the bay were not touched ; but small craft lying in the channel over the bar were driven to and fro with great violence. There was no motion of the earth, and no noise. The distance from Lisbon was 3400 miles, the vibrations having taken seven and a half hours to reach Barbados. The one notable effect in the harbour of Bridgetown was that the water flowed in and out with such a force that it tore up the black mud in the bottom of the channel, so that a great stench was sent forth and the fishes caused to float on the surface, many of them being driven a considerable distance on to the dry land where they were taken up by the negroes[1].

It so happened that there was an epidemic catarrh prevalent at that very time all over the island of Barbados, chiefly among

---

[1] Hillary, *Changes of the Air, etc.*, p. 82.

children, few or none of whom, white or black, escaped it. It had begun in October, says Hillary[1] (who chronicled the epidemiology very exactly), and continued into November, so that it both preceded and followed the great convulsion in the bed of the Atlantic, which destroyed Lisbon and tore up the mud in the harbour of Bridgetown, disengaging a great stench therefrom and poisoning the fish. Webster's theory of a relation between earthquakes and influenzas provides for such discrepancies in the dates of each : it is probable, he says, that seasons, earthquakes and volcanic eruptions are themselves the effects of those motions and invisible operations which affect mankind, so that catarrh and other epidemics often appear *before* the visible phenomena of eruptions and earthquakes. In like manner, the chronicler of the earthquake of Lisbon in the *Philosophical Transactions* drew attention to the fact that there had been a remarkable drought for several years before, and that some of the springs near Lisbon were actually dried up at the time. That droughts precede earthquakes is perhaps the most instructive generality that has yet been reached as to the cause of the latter.

Let us see, then, whether any such remote antecedents, in a possible relation to the influenza epidemics, hold good for the island of Barbados. Hillary's chronicle is sufficiently full to let us answer the question.

Following the seasons and prevalent maladies backwards from the influenza of children in October–November, 1755, we find a catarrhal fever all over Barbados in February of the same year, which "few escaped having more or less of." The immediate precursor of that influenza had been a very definite constitution, eighteen months long, of a "slow nervous fever," from February, 1753 to September, 1754, which corresponds in every respect to the "remittent" fever of nearly the same period in England and Ireland, described by Fothergill, Rutty, Huxham and Johnstone, and to the famous Rouen fever described by Le Cat. Hillary is clear that the "slow nervous fever" was not seen again so long as he remained in the colony (1758). Just before it began, there had been an influenza so general in December, 1752, and January, 1753, "that few people, either white or black, escaped having it," and that, in turn, was preceded by a season of agues, which, says Hillary, "are never seen in Barbados now [1758], unless brought hither from some place of the Leeward Islands."

So many influenzas in Barbados, and so many things possibly relevant to them among their antecedents. So also in New England, the influenza which seemed to follow the earthquake

---

[1] Hillary, *Changes of the Air, etc.*, p. 80.

along the coast of Portugal on the 31st of March, 1761, had the same remittent and intermittent fevers among its antecedents.

In the winter and spring of 1760–61 there had been much fever in New England, which was believed to be malarious. Webster, however, says : "There is no necessity of resorting to marsh exhalations for the source of this malady. The same species of fever [as at Bethlem] prevailed in that winter and the spring following in many other parts of Connecticut where no marsh existed. In Hartford it carried off a number of robust men, in two or three days from the attack...In North Haven it attacked few persons, but everyone of them died. In East Haven died about forty-five men in the prime of life, mostly heads of families. The same disease prevailed in New Haven among the inhabitants and students in college." In Bethlem the sickness began in November, 1760, and carried off about forty of the inhabitants in the winter following. This was the fever, generally reckoned malarious, which preceded the influenza of April and May, 1761[1].

III.

The next great influenza, twenty years after, which was in America in the spring of 1781 and in Europe in the winter and spring following, will repay the same kind of scrutiny. There had been influenza here or there in Europe since the beginning of 1780, but no great epidemic of it ; and in England, as elsewhere, there had been epidemic agues and dysenteries since that year, or the autumn before. The epidemic agues became worse in England in 1783, 1784, and 1785, appearing in places which had never been thought malarious. The whole period from 1780 to 1784 was remarkable for hot and dry summers and great earthquakes. Italy and Sicily were troubled by earthquakes to an unusual extent in 1780, 1781, 1782, and 1783 ; they were so frequent in 1781 that the pope ordered public prayers. The great earthquake of the period was in Calabria at half an hour after noon of the 5th of February, 1783, about six months after the great influenza of the period was over. Sir William Hamilton, the British ambassador at Naples, visited the numerous scenes of the earthquake in Calabria and Sicily in the first fortnight of May, 1783, and sent to the Royal Society an account of what he saw. At several places he found fever epidemic, part of it from the overcrowding and filth of the temporary barracks in which the people were living, part of it malarious from the damming of water by changes in the river beds. At Palmi the spilt oil mixed with the corn of the overthrown granaries, and the corrupted bodies, had a sensible effect on the

---

[1] Webster, I. 250.

air, which threatened an epidemic; at the village of Torre del Pezzolo an epidemical disorder had already manifested itself[1].

But the most striking effect of the earthquake was that a dry fog began in Calabria in February, and overspread until autumn the greater part of Europe, extending even to the Azores. This fog, though not consisting apparently of moisture, was so dense that the sky was quite obscured, appearing a light grey colour instead of blue, while the sun became a blood-red disc. In Calabria the darkness was so great that lights were needed in the houses, and ships came into collision at sea. There was a most disagreeable odour[2]. The fog spreading over all Europe from Calabria was not at all mythical, as we are apt to suppose that similar recorded phenomena of the wonder-loving Middle Ages may have been. The phenomenon was independently re-produced in Iceland the same year, from the 1st to the 11th of June, causing the same darkness at sea, the same atmospheric effects at a distance, but not to so great a distance, and some amount of sickness, but seemingly not aguish or febrile, among the population[3].

Those two great convulsions of the year 1783, each of them the cause of a widely spreading dry fog, may have been con-ceivably the cause of pestiferous miasmata in the air, such as the corresponding hypothesis of influenza requires; but how little comparable or equivalent were the miasmata—in the one case from the ancient and well-peopled soil of Southern Italy, in the other from the inhospitable Danish colony just without the Arctic Circle! In any case, the earthquakes of 1783 were both too late for the great influenza of the period. The antecedent common alike to the influenza and the earthquakes was the extraordinary droughts, which caused famine and famine-fever in Iceland, and, according to old experience, was probably related to the epidemic prevalence of agues in Britain and on the continent of Europe.

---

[1] Hamilton, *Phil. Trans.* LXXIII. 176.   [2] Mallet's Catalogue, u. s.
[3] Holm, *Vom Erdbrande auf Island im Jahre* 1783, Kopenhagen, 1784, says: "Since the outbreak began, the atmosphere of the whole country has been full of vapour, smoke and dust, so much so that the sun looked brownish-red, and the fishermen could not find the banks....Old people, especially those with weak chests, suffered much from the smell of sulphur and the volcanic vapours, being afflicted with dyspnoea. Various persons in good health fell ill, and more would have suffered had not the air been cooled and refreshed from time to time by rains," pp. 57, 60. The real sickness of Iceland in those years had been before the volcanic eruptions, in 1781 and 1782, when some parts of the island were almost depopulated by the famine and pestilential fevers that followed the unusual seasons.

IV.

What kind or kinds of epidemic sickness earthquakes may produce as an effect immediate and at the place, will appear from other instances. One of the most remarkable of earthquakes was that which destroyed Port Royal and nearly all the planters' houses and sugar-works throughout the island of Jamaica on the 7th of June, 1692. Jamaica had been an English colony for little more than thirty years, during which time it had passed from its state of lethargy under the Spaniards into an emporium of commerce with a rapidly growing population of slaves and whites. The business capital was at Port Royal, wholly built since the British occupation. The site of it was a sandy key or shoal which was said to have risen perceptibly within the memory of original settlers ; a writer in September, 1667, said of it: "wherever you dig five or six feet, water will appear which ebbs and flows as the tide. It is not salt, but brackish[1]." A quay had been built along this spit of land, at which vessels of 700 tons could lie afloat. It was here that the havoc of the earthquake was most complete.

Sloane, who had visited Jamaica a few years before, said that the inhabitants expect an earthquake every year, and that some of them were of opinion that they follow their great rains[2]. The year 1692 began in Jamaica with very dry and hot weather which continued until May: then came gales and heavy rains until the end of the month, and from that time until the day of the earthquake, the 7th of June, the weather was excessively hot, calm and dry. The shakes began at 11.40 a.m., and at the third shake, the ground of nearly all Port Royal fell in suddenly, so that in the course of a minute or two most of the houses were under water and the whole wharf was covered by the sea to the depth of several fathoms. The loss of life was, of course, greatest where population was densest ; but in the interior of the island the effects on the soil were greater than at the shore : in the north a thousand acres of land sank and thirteen people with it ; mountains on either side of a narrow gorge came together and blocked the way ; wide chasms appeared in the

[1] *Phil. Trans.* II. (1667), p. 499.
[2] *Ibid.* March–Apr. 1694, p. 81. Sloane had himself felt several shocks at Port Royal on the 20th October, 1687, between four and six o'clock in the morning, which were due to the same earthquake that destroyed Lima in Peru.

ground, and on one mountain side there were some dozen
openings from which brackish water spouted forth.   The first
effect in the streets of Port Royal was that men and women
seemed all at once to be floundering up to the neck in the wet
shifting sand, and were speedily drowned or floated away by
the inrushing water.   The shakes ceased for days at a time, and
then began again, five or six perhaps in twenty-four hours; so
that those who had escaped to ships in the bay remained on
board for two months, being afraid to come ashore.   The
weather was hotter after the earthquake than before, and mos-
quitoes swarmed in unheard of numbers.

During the upheavals or subsidences in Port Royal, and
the rushing of water into or from the gapings in the ground, " ill
stenches and offensive smells " arose, so that " by means of the
openings and the vapours at that time belcht forth from the
earth into the air, the sky, which before was clear and blue, was
in a minute's time become dull and reddish looking (as I have
heard it compared often) like a red-hot oven."   A very great
mortality followed among those who had escaped the earthquake.   Some of them settled at Leguanea, others at the place
on the bay which became the Kingston of later history, enduring many hardships in their hastily built shelters, from the
heavy rains that followed the earthquake, and from want of
clothes, food and comforts.

One writes: " Our people settled a town at Leguanea side; and there is
about five hundred graves already [20th September, 1692], and people every
day is dying still.   I went about once to see it, and I had like to have tipt
off."   Another says: " Almost half the people that escaped upon Port
Royal are since dead of a malignant fever": and another, referring to the
hasty settlement on the bay at Kingston, says " they died miserably in
heaps."   But the most interesting information is his next sentence : " Indeed
there was a general sickness (supposed to proceed from the hurtful vapours
belched from the many openings of the earth) all over the island, so general
that few escaped being sick: and 'tis thought it swept away in all parts of
the island three thousand souls, the greatest part from Kingstown, only yet
an unhealthy place[1]."

That great mortality from a malignant fever after the earthquake of 7th June, 1692, is usually counted an epidemic of the
yellow fever which became established at Kingston and Port
Royal from that time for at least a century and a half.   I have
not found any contemporary medical account of it, but all the

[1] *Phil. Trans.* XVIII. p. 83 (March–April, 1794).   Series of reports from Jamaica
collected by Sloane.

later writers on yellow fever at Kingston and Port Royal have accepted the tradition that it was yellow fever. But there was one peculiarity, which marks it off from all subsequent epidemics of yellow fever—the sickness was all over the island, so general that few escaped being sick, and was supposed to proceed from the hurtful vapours belched from the many openings of the ground in and near Port Royal. In all subsequent experience yellow fever has been almost confined to the shore or to the ships in the bay[1]. Certainly it has never been all over the island as in 1692, "so general that few escaped being sick": that is rather in the manner of influenza, although there is nothing to show that the sickness of the interior was so different from that of the shore as to be counted an influenza, or that the mortality of the sick was other than that of a "malignant fever."

The earthquake at Port Royal in 1692 produced "ill stenches and offensive smells." The tidal waves, or the subterranean vibrations which caused them, in tearing up the mud at the bottom of the channel at Bridgetown, Barbados, in 1755, had in like manner sent forth a great stench which poisoned the fish. Such offensive vapours were supposed in former times to come, as in a figure, from "the bowels of the earth"; and undoubtedly the sulphurous fumes which have overhung the region of Sicilian earthquakes must have had a source as deep as the strange minerals or "fossils" of Boyle's hypothesis. But, while the commotion of an earthquake is deep, it is also superficial; whatever miasmata issue from the ground in the ordinary alternations of wet and drought, would be discharged into the atmosphere in unusual quantity and with unusual force in such disturbances of soil as sunk Port Royal in 1692 or were felt at Barbados across the whole width of the Atlantic in 1755. Nor is that effect upon miasmata instantaneous or quickly past; in Jamaica the rumblings and shakes lasted for nearly two months, during which time the pressure upon the gases in the subsoil must have been such as to make them pass into the atmosphere in stronger ascending currents than the mere alternations of moisture and drought would have done. And just as the ordinary seasonal changes in the level of the ground-water are

[1] A few cases have been exceptionally seen at Spanish Town, six miles from the head of the bay, the infection of which was supposed to have been brought from the shore by sailors, and it has also prevailed in the barracks on the high ground of Newcastle not far from the shore.

of little or no account for miasmatic-infective disease unless the soil in which they occur be full of organic impurities from human occupancy, so one may reason that the great cataclysmic changes of the earth's crust are, in this hypothesis of influenza, of most account as touching the stratum of soil wherein lie organic impurities, and as touching those areas of the surface,— the sites of cities, the populous plains, the shores of bays, the bottoms of harbours or any other definite spots—in which the products of organic decomposition are present in largest amount and, perhaps, of somewhat special kind.   Such impurities of the soil are indeed a *vera causa* of infective disease, known to be capable of the effect which has to be accounted for; and, as discharged into the air in great volume and with great force by some upheaval, they would make a local beginning of that "aer inimicus" which the Roman poet figures as creeping like a mist from one region of the heavens to another so that it corrupts each successive tract of air with its own baleful qualities, "reddatque sui simile atque alienum."

But, as soon as we begin to apply this formula to particular historic cases, difficulties and ambiguities arise[1].   To come back to the instance of Jamaica in 1692, did the general sickness of the island, manifestly miasmatic as it was, and due to disturbances of soil, become an influenza for other regions of the globe?   About fifteen months after there was, indeed, a universal catarrh in Britain and Ireland, of no great fatality, which is said by Molyneux, of Dublin, to have prevailed also in the northern parts of France, Flanders, and Holland, but is not reported in the usual way from Europe generally nor from America.   Let us suppose a miasmatic cloud formed over the

---

[1] Without seeking to argue for the connexion between particular earthquakes and influenzas, but merely to illustrate the possibilities, I append here an instance that ought not to be overlooked. On the 1st of November, 1835, there was a great earthquake in the Moluccas, which so completely changed the soil of the island of Amboina, that it became notably subject to deadly miasmatic or malarious fevers from that time forth. For three weeks before the earthquake the atmosphere had been full of a heavy sulphurous fog, so that miasmata were rising from the soil by some unwonted pressure before the actual cataclysm. There is no doubt at all that Amboina became "malarious" in a most marked degree from the date of the earthquake; it is a classical instance of the sudden effect of great changes in the earth's crust upon the frequency and malignity of remittent and intermittent fevers, according to the testimony of physicians in the Dutch East Indian service. The influenza nearest to the earthquake was about a year after, at Sydney, Cape Town, and in the East Indies, during October and November, 1836. The epidemic appeared about the same time in the north-east of Europe, spread all over the continent, and reached London in January, 1837. There was again influenza in Australia and New Zealand in November, 1838, two years after the last outbreak in that region.

island of Jamaica in June, July, August and September, a cloud of infective particles which might produce influenza at a distance from its place of origin, whatever disease the miasmata after the earthquake may have produced in Jamaica itself. Let this invisible cloud, or emanation, get into the warm atmosphere over the great oceanic current that sets out from the Gulf of Mexico. The vehicle lies ready to hand,—to receive the miasmata not far from their place of origin, to carry them far into the Atlantic, and to bring them, perhaps, to the shores of Britain. This may seem a sufficiently plausible source of the influenza of October and November, 1693, which appears to have been felt only in the British Isles and on the opposite shores of the North Sea. But Webster's own choice is the volcanic eruption in Iceland in the same year as the influenza; and if we prefer, in this hypothesis, an earthquake to an active volcano, there is a rival source for the British influenza of 1693, nearer both in place and time than that of Jamaica in 1692, and not less important in respect of miasmatic disease in its own locality. This was the disastrous series of earthquakes in Calabria and Sicily, culminating on the 9th of January, 1693. The following extracts from the account sent to the Royal Society will show how great was the commotion of soil, of underground water, and of atmosphere, and how close the connexion of these with the sickness ensuing[1]:

"In the plain of Catania, an open place, it is reported that from one of the clefts in the ground, narrow but very long and about four miles off the sea, the water was thrown forth altogether as salt as that of the sea, [as in Jamaica the year before]. In Syracuse and other places near the sea, the waters in many wells, which at first were salt, are become fresh again... The fountain Arethusa for the space of some months was so brackish that the Syracusans could make no use of it, and now that it is grown sweeter the spring is increased to near double. In the city of Termini all the running waters are dried up...It was contrary with the hot-baths, which were augmented by a third part.

Darkness and obscurity of the air has always been over us, but still inferior to that on the 10th and 11th of January; and often these clouds have been thin and light, and of a great extent, such as the authors call *rarae nubeculae*. The sun often and the moon always obscured at the rising and setting, and the horizon all day long dusky...

The effects it has had on humane bodies (although I do not believe they have all immediately been caused by the earthquake) have (yet) been various : such as foolishness (but not to any great degree), madness, dulness, sottishness, and stolidity everywhere : hypochondriack, melancholick and cholerick distempers. Every-day fevers have been common, with many continual and tertian : malignant, mortal and dangerous ones in a great

[1] *Phil. Trans.* for the year 1694, p. 5.

27—2

number, with deliria and lethargies. Where there has been any infection caused by the natural malignity of the air, infinite mortality has followed. The smallpox has made great destruction among children."

Thus we find in Sicily a great disturbance of soil followed, as in Jamaica, by a great increase of local sickness, and by an atmosphere visibly charged with products of the earthquake for months after. This is a nearer source than the Jamaican for the British influenza of Oct.-Nov. 1693,—nearer in time, if that be any advantage for the theory, nearer also in place. There are, however, no intermediate stages to connect the influenza on the northern edge of the European continent with the disturbance of soil and the miasmata arising therefrom in Sicily and Calabria. If there had been any such dry fog as spread all over Europe from the Calabrian earthquake of January, 1783, it would have been a help at least to the imagination in bridging over a gulf of space and time.

As to the interval of time, it should at all events be kept in mind that the same difficulty has to be reckoned with in any hypothesis of influenza and in every great historic instance. In the instance still before us, the infection began in England, according to Molyneux, in October, 1693, and was in Dublin a month later. But we must assume it to have been in the air for some time before it became effective upon mankind. Influenza has been observed, with curious uniformity, to attack the horses, say of London, of Plymouth, of Edinburgh, or of Dublin (as on the occasion before this, 1688) two months or more in advance of the inhabitants of the respective places; and if it had waited, so to speak, for two months before it showed its effects upon men, it may have waited equally long, or longer, before it showed its effects upon horses. That would give at least four months; and then we know, from such an influenza as that of 1743, that there may be weeks, perhaps months, between its prevalence in Naples, Rome or Milan, and its prevalence in London or Edinburgh, and, from the influenza of 1693 itself, that it was a month later in Dublin than in London. An earthquake in Sicily on the 9th of January, 1693, with effects there for months after upon the water, the air, and the prevalent diseases, is not excluded by lapse of time from being a *vera causa* of an influenza in England in October of the same year, and in Ireland in November. The sort of proof which most men desire, a proof such as we rarely get, and one that is suspiciously neat when we do get it, would be to find an influenza in Sicily and Calabria following the earthquake, and to trace the same step by step over Europe. But the miasmatic sickness in the countries of the earthquakes was not influenza, so far as is known; and there was no epidemic catarrh, so far as is known, in any other part of Europe but the British Isles and the neighbouring shores of the North Sea.

V.

Molyneux, who recorded with a good deal of circumstance the influenza of 1693, is the principal authority, along with Dr Walter Harris, of London, for another influenza in 1688, seemingly peculiar to the British Isles. Its effects can be discovered with the utmost certainty in the London bills of mortality for two or three weeks at the end of May and beginning of June, and it is mentioned as "the new distemper" in letters of the time. Is it possible to find an earthquake for it? Webster's note is: "in the same year with an eruption of Vesuvius, after a severe winter and earthquakes"—which is somewhat general. Turning to Evelyn's diary, where these matters are often recorded, we find, in the very weeks when the influenza was at a height in London, this entry: "News arrived of the most prodigious earthquake that was almost ever heard of, subverting the city of Lima and country in Peru, with a dreadfull inundation following it"—as if the influenza and the news of the earthquake had reached London at the same time. This was the earthquake of 20th October, 1687, which destroyed Lima, Callao and an immense district along the coast of Peru. The rocking of the earth was most violent, the sea retreated like a sudden immense ebb and filled again like a sudden immense flood, the effect of the commotion being felt on board ships a hundred and fifty leagues out in the Pacific. It was remarked that wheat and barley would not thrive in Peru after that earthquake[1]. Here was undoubtedly a great disturbance of soil and of subsoil, almost certainly attended with the discharge of effluvia or miasmata into the air, as in other great earthquakes. But the universal slight fever of the British Isles in the months of June and July, 1688, is remote from the earth-

---

[1] Mallet, "First Report on the Facts of Earthquake Phenomena." *Trans. Brit. Assoc. for* 1850, Lond. 1851. Cited from von Hoff.

quake of Lima in place ; and, if it be a question of earthquakes at all, there are others nearer to it both in place and time, such as that in the Basilicata province of Naples in January, 1688, and the Jamaica earthquake, felt through all the island, on the 1st of March, 1688. The greatest of them all, that of Smyrna, on the 10th of July, was a few weeks too late for the hypothesis.

VI.

A continent so subject to earthquakes as South America might be expected, in this hypothesis, to have had some corresponding influenzas. It has indeed had influenzas, some of them peculiar to itself. The Western Hemisphere as a whole has, on several great occasions, had influenzas which were not felt in the Old World. Again, there are one or two instances in which the infection, while it spread widely over the table-lands of Bolivia and Peru, does not appear by existing testimony to have been carried north of the Isthmus. One of these was the influenza of 1720, as special to a region of South America as that of 1688 was to the British Isles. The account of it was given in an essay by Botoni 'On the Circulation of the Blood,' published at Lima in 1723[1]. He calls it *catarro maligno*; it was popularly known as *fierro chuto* or "iron cap." It appeared at Cuzco in the end of March, or beginning of April, 1720, and was over about November. Four thousand are said to have died of it in the diocese of Cuzco, and it is said to have made so great a scarcity of hands that the first harvest after it was imperfectly gathered. It had all the marks of an influenza, with the addition of bleeding from the nose and lungs. It had also the grand characteristic common to influenza and epidemic ague: "the symptoms were so diverse and even contradictory that no correct diagnosis, or curative plan, could be fixed." The Lima writer of 1723 says that it followed an eclipse of the sun on the 15th of August, 1719, having begun on the eastern side of the Andes, in the basin of La Plata, about that time, and travelled northwards and westwards, as the South American influenza of 1759 did.

This is a localized influenza in a country of earthquakes. But the two great earthquakes in 1719 are not South American.

---

[1] Archibald Smith, M.D., "Notices of the Epidemics of 1719–20 and 1759 in Peru," etc.   *Trans. Epid. Soc.* II. pt. I, p. 134.   From the *Medical Gazette of Lima,* 15 March, 1862.

They both happened in July: one along the coast of Fez and Morocco, which ruined many villages and a part of the city of Morocco (there is also a later disturbance in the Azores in December, followed by the upheaval of a new island), the other in North China. Here we have the choice of following the "aer inimicus" of Lucretius either from China or from the African coast; and if it be the case that the influenza began in the latter part of the year 1719 in the basin of the La Plata, to cross the Andes next year, it may seem, in this hypothesis, that a course from east to west, bringing the infection across the Atlantic from Africa, is to be preferred to a course from west to east, bringing it across the Pacific from North China. In either case there need be no difficulty in finding local clouds of miasmata. Some traces of the corresponding great earthquake in China were found in November of the following year, by Bell, an English traveller who crossed from Moscow to Peking:

"Jumy," he says, "suffered greatly by the earthquakes that happened in the month of July the preceding year [1719], above one half of it being thereby laid in ruins. Indeed more than one half of the towns and villages through which we travelled this day had suffered much on the same occasion, and vast numbers of people had been buried in the ruins. I must confess it was a dismal scene to see everywhere such heaps of rubbish[1]."

The atmospheric effects of Chinese earthquakes have been pictured since medieval times, in obviously superstitious colours; and there are reasons why a great disturbance of soil in that country should produce remarkable miasmata. The surface soil of China is peculiar in having the bodies of the dead dispersed at large in it, insomuch that excavations for the foundations of houses, or for roads and railway cuttings, can hardly be made without the constant risk of exposing graves[2].

If the soil of China is peculiar in one way, that of the West Coast of Africa is peculiar in another. Without entering on the large question of "malaria" in each of them, I shall take an old illustration of the miasmata of the West Coast of Africa as a

---

[1] Bell's Travels, in Pinkerton, VII. 377.
[2] See an article "Railways—their Future in China," by W. B. Dunlop, in *Blackwood's Magazine*, March, 1889, pp. 395–6. A letter in the *Pall Mall Gazette*, dated 23 May, 1891, and signed "Shanghai," recalled the outbreak of Hongkong fever, "the symptoms of which bore a curious resemblance to the influenza epidemic," at the time when much building was going on upon the slope of Victoria Peak: "It was said at the time—I do not know with what truth—that in this turning-up of the soil, several old Chinese burying-places were included."

cause of dengue-fever, a disease curiously like influenza in its symptoms, and like it also in its occasional wave-like dispersion over wide regions. The authority is Dr Aubrey, who resided many years on the coast of Guinea, saw much of the slave-trade, and wrote a very sensible book in 1729, called 'The Sea Surgeon, or the Guinea Man's Vade Mecum.' He describes quite clearly the fever which was long after described by West Indian physicians as dengue, or three-days' fever, or break-bone fever, including in his description the characteristic exanthems of it and the penetrating odour of the sweat. He gives also, in clinical form, a series of cases on board the galley 'Peterborough' in December, 1717, which are exquisite examples of break-bone fever. This disease, he says, " many times runs over the whole ship, as well negroes as white men, for they infect one the other, and the ship is then in a very deplorable condition unless they have an able man to take care of them." But the original source of infection, he believed, was the fogs that hung at nightfall over the estuaries of the rivers; and he gives an experimental proof, remarkable but not quite incredible, of the poisonous nature of the miasmata :

" But to let you see the evil, malevolent, contagious, destructive quality of those fogs that fall there in the night, and how far they are inimical to human nature, I will tell you of an experiment of my own. I made a lump of paste with oat-meal somewhat hard, and about the bigness of a hen's egg, which was exposed to the fog from twilight to twilight, i.e. from the dusk of the evening till daybreak in the morning; after which I crumbled it, and gave it to fowls, which we had on board, and soon after they had eaten it, they turned round and in a kind of vertigo dropt down and expired."

A great mortality in Guinea in 1754 or 1755 was ascribed by Lind, the least credulous in such matters, to "a noxious stinking fog[1]."

What the alternations of heat and chill, of moisture and drought, produce ordinarily in the way of miasmata, the same, we may suppose, is produced on the great scale, as a pheno-menon at some particular time and place, by one of those cataclysms which break the surface of the earth or the bed of the sea, lower or raise the level of wells and springs, and fill the air with particles of dust or vapour which may overhang the locality for months and visibly disperse themselves to a great distance. Nothing relating to miasmata in the air need be hard

[1] *Essay on the Most Effective Means of preserving the Health of Seamen in the Royal Navy.* London, 1757, p. 83.

for belief after the wonderful diffusion and permanence in the atmosphere of the whole globe, for two years or more, of finely divided particles shot up by the earthquakes and eruptions of Krakatoa in the Straits of Sunda on the 27th and 28th of August, 1883[1].

A theory of influenza constructed from such generalities as those of Boyle, Arbuthnot and Webster will have attractions for many over the theory that influenza is always present in some remote country and becomes dispersed now and then over the world by contagion from person to person: it will have superior attractions, for the reason that influenza is a phenomenal thing which needs a phenomenal cause to account for it. But if anyone were to attempt to fit each historic wave of influenza with its particular earthquake, or to find the precise locality where clouds of infective matter had arisen, or the particular circumstances in which they arose, he would certainly find his fragile structure of probabilities pulled to pieces by the professed discouragers and depravers. I make no such attempt; but I am not the less persuaded of the direction in which the true theory of influenza lies.

Influenza at Sea.

There is no point more essential to a correct theory of influenza than to find out in what circumstances it has occurred among the crews of ships on the high seas. If it be true that a ship may sail into an atmosphere of influenza, just as she may sail into a fog, or an oceanic current, or the track of a cyclone, then the possible hypotheses touching the nature, source, and mode of diffusion of influenza become narrowed down within definite limits.

One of the first observations was made in the case of a Scotch vessel in the influenza of 1732-33[2]. The epidemic was earlier in Scotland than in England; it began suddenly in Edinburgh on 17 December, 1732, the horses having been attacked with running of the nose towards the end of October. About the time when the disease began among mankind, in December, a vessel, the 'Anne and Agnes' sailed from Leith for Holland. One sailor was sick on this voyage. She sailed on the return voyage to Leith, with the other ten of her crew in perfect health. Just as she made the English coast at Flamborough Head on the 15th of January, 1733, six of the sailors fell ill together, two more the next day, and one more on the day after

---

[1] See *The Eruption of Krakatoa and subsequent phenomena.* Report of the Krakatoa Committee of the Royal Society....Edited by G. J. Symons, London, 1888.
[2] *Edin. Med. Essays and Obs.* II. 32.

that, so that when the vessel anchored in Leith Roads there was only one man well, and he fell ill on the day following the arrival. The symptoms were the common ones of the reigning epidemic. The dates are not given more precisely or fully than as above. Influenza was prevalent in Germany and Holland somewhat earlier than in Scotland or England; the men may, of course, have imbibed the infection when they were in the Dutch port, just as it is almost certain that the crews of Drake's fleet in 1587 had received during a ten days' stay upon the island of St Jago, of the Cape de Verde group, the miasmatic infection of which they suddenly fell sick in large numbers together in mid-Atlantic some six days after sailing to the westward.

This early case of the 'Anne and Agnes' in 1733 may pass as an ambiguous one. The next occasion when influenza on board ship attracted much notice was the epidemic of 1782.

On the 6th of May, Admiral Kempenfelt sailed from Spithead with seven ships of the line and a frigate, on a cruize to the westward; on the 18th May, he came into Torbay, and sailed again soon after; on the 30th May he came again into Torbay with eight sail of the line and three frigates, and on 1 June sailed again to the westward. Sometime before his squadron put into Torbay for the second time, influenza had appeared among them at sea, it is said in the 'Goliath' on the 29th of May[1]. A letter from Plymouth, of the 2nd June, after referring to the violence of influenza in that town, at the Dock, and on board the men-of-war lying there, says that the 'Fortitude' of 74 guns, and 'Latona' frigate came in that afternoon with 250 sick men from the fleet under Admiral Kempenfelt, mostly with fevers. Another Plymouth letter two days later (4 June) says: "Kempenfelt is returning to Torbay: he could keep the sea no longer, on account of the sickness that rages on board his fleet. More than 400 men have been brought to the hospital this morning. Our men drop down with it by scores at a time. The 'Latona' frigate, that sailed the other day is returned, the officers being the only hands that could work the ship[2]."

This outbreak on board ships in the Channel was fully as early as the great development of influenza in 1782 on shore, whether in London or Plymouth; but there were almost certainly cases of it at the latter port before the 'Latona' sailed to join Kempenfelt's squadron. Robertson, however, who was surgeon on the 'Romney' in the Channel service at that time, says that "hundreds in different ships, towns, and counties, which had *no* communication with one another, were seized nearly as suddenly and so nigh the same instant as if they had been electrified.... The companies of many of the ships were very well at bed-time, and in the morning there were hardly enough able to do the common business of the ship[3]." This is confirmed by McNair, surgeon of the 'Fortitude,' who told Trotter that two hundred

[1] *Trans. Col. Phys.* III. 62.   [2] *Gent. Magaz.* 1782, p. 306.
[3] R. Robertson, M.D., *Observations on Jail, Hospital or Ship Fever from the 4th April, 1776, to the 30th April, 1789.* Lond. 1789, New ed., p. 411.

of her men, as she lay in Torbay, were seized in one night and were unable to come on deck in the morning[1].

There was another English fleet in the North Sea at the same time, under Lord Howe, watching the Dutch fleet or seeking to intercept the Dutch East Indiamen.

Howe sailed from St Helen's on the 9th May, with twelve ships of the line. Towards the end of that month he had his fleet in the Texel; the men were in excellent health, "when a cutter arrived from the Admiralty, and the signal was given for an officer from each ship [to come on board the admiral]. An officer was accordingly sent with a boat's crew from every vessel, and returned with orders, carrying with them also, however, the influenza"—which soon prostrated the crews to the same extraordinary extent as in the ships under Kempenfelt at the other end of the Channel. This was the oral account given to Professor Gregory of Edinburgh, by a lieutenant on board a sixty-four gun ship[2]. Another account says that the disorder first appeared in Howe's fleet on the Dutch coast about the end of May, on board the 'Ripon,' and in two days after in the 'Princess Amelia'; other ships of the same fleet were affected with it at different periods, some indeed, not until their return to Portsmouth about the second week of June. "This fleet, also, had no communication with the shore until their return to the Downs, on their way back to Portsmouth, towards the 3d and 4th of June[3]."

But, apart from the story of the Admiralty despatch-boat carrying the influenza to Howe's squadron, it appears that both Kempenfelt and Howe were joined from time to time by additional ships, which might have carried an atmosphere of influenza with them[4]. Still, it was an influenza atmosphere that they had carried, and not merely so many sick persons. The doctrine of contagion from person to person would have to be so widened as to become meaningless, if all those experiences of the fleet in 1782 were to be brought within it. In the history both of sweating sickness and of influenza, there are instances of the disease breaking out suddenly in a place after someone's arrival ; but the new arrival may not have had the disease, it was enough that he came from a place where the disease was[5]. That was, perhaps, the reason why Beddoes, in his inquiry of 1803, framed one of his questions so as to elicit information about the dispersal of influenza by *fomites*.

[1] Trotter, *Medicina Nautica*, I. 1797, p. 367.
[2] Notes of a lecture on Influenza, by Gregory, taken by Christison about the year 1817, in the *Life of Sir Robert Christison*, I. 82.
[3] College of Physicians' Report, *Trans. Col. Phys.* III. 63.
[4] This is inferred from the varying number of ships in the two fleets in the several notices of their movements in the *Gentleman's Magazine*, for May and June, 1782.
[5] Brian Tuke to Peter Vannes, 14 July, 1528 : "For when a whole man comes from London and talks of the sweat, the same night all the town is full of it, and thus it spreads as the fame runs." *Cal. State Papers, Henry VIII.* IV. 1071.

It is not easy to prove that a ship may meet with an atmosphere of influenza on the high seas; but many have believed that ships have done so. Webster says: " The disease invades seamen on the ocean in the same [western] hemisphere, when a hundred leagues from land, at the same time that it invades people on shore. Of this I have certain evidence from the testimony of American captains of vessels, who have been on their passage from the continent to the West India Islands during the prevalence of this disease[1]." There are several instances of this, authenticated with times, places, and other data of credibility.

The best known of these is the voyage of the East Indiaman 'Asia' in September, 1780, through the China Sea from Malacca to Canton: " When the ship left Malacca, there was no epidemic disease in the place; when it arrived at Canton it was found that at the very time when they had the *Influenza* on board the Atlas (*sic*) in the China seas, it had raged at Canton with as much violence as it did in London in June, 1782, and with the very same symptoms[2]."

In the present century, the cases nearly all come from the medical reports of the navies of Great Britain, France, Germany and the Netherlands, and they relate to ships on foreign service —in the East Indies, the Pacific, Africa, or other foreign stations. In some of the instances influenza went through a ship's company in port or in a roadstead, others are examples of outbreaks at sea:

1837: " The ship's company of the ' Raleigh,' were attacked by epidemic catarrh—influenza—first in March, while at sea between Singapore and Manilla, and again, although less severely, in June and July while on the coast of China...Influenza also made its appearance amongst the crew of the ' Zebra' in April while she lay at Penang; it was supposed to have been contracted by infection from the people on shore, as they were then suffering from it. No death occurred under this head[3]."

1838: In the ' Rattlesnake,' at Diamond Harbour, in the Hooghly River, a large proportion of the men were suffering from epidemic catarrh. Intermittent fever made its appearance; " the change from the catarrhal to the febrile form was sudden and complete, the one entirely superseding the other[4]."

1842: In the ' Agincourt' on a voyage from the Cape of Good Hope to Hongkong in August and September, the greater part of 102 cases of catarrh occurred; many of these were accompanied with inflammation of tonsils and fauces, and in some there was deafness with discharge from the ear. This is not claimed as an instance of epidemic influenza, but as an aggregate of common colds, due to cold weather in the Southern Ocean and to wet decks[5].

---

[1] Webster, II. 63.

[2] College of Physicians' Report. *Trans. Col. Phys.* III. (1785), p. 60–61. " Information has been received " of the incident.

[3] *Statist. Report of Health of Navy*, 1837–43. Parl. papers, 1 June, 1853, p. 8.

[4] *Ibid.* p. 14.   [5] *Ibid.* s. d.

1857: "Influenza broke out in the 'Monarch' while at sea, on the passage from Payta [extreme north of Peru] to Valparaiso. She left the former place on the 23d August, and arrived at the latter on the last day of September. About the 12th of the month [twenty days out], the wind suddenly changed to the south-west, when nearly every person in the ship began to complain of cold, although the thermometer did not show any marked change in the temperature. On the 12th and 13th seven patients were placed on the sick list with catarrhal symptoms; and during the following ten days, upwards of eighty more were added, but by the end of the month the attacks ceased. [She carried 690 men, and had 191 cases of "influenza and catarrh," in the year 1857.] Some of the cases were severe, ending either in slight bronchitis or pneumonia, accompanied with great prostration of the vital powers. On the arrival of the ship at Valparaiso, the surgeon observes : ' We found the place healthy, but in the course of a few days some cases of influenza made their appearance, and very soon afterwards the disease extended over the whole town. It was generally believed that we imported it, and the authorities took the trouble to send on board a medical officer to investigate the matter.' He further observes that the whole coast, from Vancouver's Island southward to Valparaiso was visited by the epidemic." It made its appearance on board the 'Satellite' at Vancouver's Island in September, and among the residents ashore, both on the island and mainland, at the same time[1].

1857 : Catarrh "assumed the form of influenza in the 'Arachne' [149 men, 114 cases] while the vessel was cruizing off the coast of Cuba, "with which, however, she had no communication. There was nothing in the state of the atmosphere to attract special attention. A question therefore arises whether it might not have been caused by infection wafted from the shore." It was prevalent at the time at Havana[2].

1857 : "Australian Station :—An eruption of epidemic catarrh occurred in the 'Juno' [200 men, 131 cases], but long after she left the station[3]."

Whilst the influenza was on the American Pacific coast in September, 1857, it was on the coast of China three months earlier—on board the 'Inflexible' at Hongkong on the 18th of May, and in the 'Amethyst' and 'Niger' in a creek near Hongkong early in June[4]. But it had been on the Pacific coast of South America the year before, according to the following :

" 1856 : Epidemic catarrh broke out in the 'President' when lying off the island of San Lorenzo in the bay of Callao, first on the 20th October, and the last cases were placed on the sick list on 1st November,—the usual period which influenza takes to pass through a frigate ship's company. About sixty required to be placed on the sick list." It had occurred on board English ships of war at Rio de Janeiro, on the other side of the continent, some two months before, in August, 1856[5].

1863: The following, in the experience of the French navy, has been elaborately recorded[6] : The frigate 'Duguay-Trouin' left Gorée, Senegambia, for Brest, in February. There were no cases of influenza in Gorée when she left; but four days out, an epidemic of influenza began on board, the weather being fine and the temperature genial at the time. Another French frigate, which had left Gorée, on the same voyage to Brest, two days earlier, did not have a single case.

The following instance, here published for the first time, belongs to the most recent pandemics of influenza, 1890–93. It

---

[1] *Report on Health of Navy*, 1857, p. 69.   [2] *Ibid.* p. 41.
[3] *Ibid.* p. 131.   [4] *Ibid.* p. 112.   [5] *Report for* 1856, p. 100.
[6] Chaumezière, *Fievre catarrhals épidemique, observée à bord du vaisseau 'Le Duguay-Trouin' aux mois de Fevr. et Mars*, 1863. Paris, 1865. Cited by Hirsch.

relates to only a single case of influenza, in the captain of a merchantship ; it would have been a more satisfactory piece of evidence, if there had been several cases in the ship ; but among the comparatively small crew of a merchantman, the same groups of cases are not to be looked for that we find on board crowded men of war ; and in this particular case the only other occupants of the quarter-deck were the first mate and the steward.

The ship 'Wellington,' sailed from the Thames, for Lyttelton, New Zealand, on the 19th December, 1891. The epidemic of influenza in London in that year had been in May, June and July ; the mate of the 'Wellington' had had an attack of it ashore, on that occasion, but not the captain nor the steward. On the 2nd of March, 1892, when seventy-four days out and in latitude 42° S., longitude 63 E., near Kerguelen's Land, the captain began to have lumbago and bilious headaches, for which he took several doses of mercurial purgative followed by saline draughts. The treatment at length brought on continual purging, which, together with three days' starving from the 22nd to the 24th of March, caused him a loss of weight of eight pounds. The navigation had meanwhile been somewhat difficult and anxious, owing to a long spell of easterly head winds. Quite suddenly, on the 26th March, when the ship was in latitude 44 S., longitude 145 E., or about two hundred miles to the south of Tasmania, he had an aguish shake followed by prolonged febrile heat, which sent him to his berth. The symptoms were acute from the 26th to the 30th March,—intense pain through and through the head, as if it were being screwed tight in an iron casing, pain behind the eyeballs, a perception of yellow colour in the eyes when shut, a feeling of soreness all over the body, which he set down at the time to his uneasy berth while the ship was ploughing through the seas at about twelve knots, and a pulse of 110. The head pains were by far the worst symptom, and were so unbearable as to make the patient desperate. This acute state lasted for four days, and suddenly disappeared leaving great prostration behind. The captain, who had long experience with crews and passengers, and a considerable amateur knowledge of medicine, summed up his illness as a bilious attack, passing into "ague" with "neuralgia of the head." While the acute attack lasted the ship had covered the distance from Tasmania to the southern end of New Zealand, and on the 31st of March the captain by an effort came on deck to navigate the vessel in stormy weather up the coast to Lyttelton, which was reached on the 2nd of April. The pilot coming on board found the captain ill in his berth, and on being told the symptoms, at once said, " It is the influenza: I have just had it myself." The doctor who was sent for found the captain " talking foolishly," as he afterwards told him, and had him removed to the convalescent home at Christchurch, where he remained a fortnight slowly regaining strength. The doctor[1] could find no other name for the illness but influenza, although he had not supposed such a thing possible in mid-ocean. They had just passed through an epidemic of it in New Zealand, and it is reported about the same time in New South Wales, afterwards in the Tonga group, and still later in the summer in Peru. The symptoms of this case are sufficiently distinctive: the intense constricting pain of the head is exactly the "*fierro chuto*" or "iron cap" of South American epidemics ; the pain in the eyeballs, the soreness of the limbs and body, and the unparalleled depression and despair, are the marks of influenza without catarrh. The

[1] Dr Guthrie, of Lyttelton.

patient was of abstemious habits, and had made the same voyage year after year for a long period without any illness that he could recall. He had reduced himself by purging and starving, on account of a bilious attack during a fortnight of foul winds from the eastward, and had doubtless become peculiarly susceptible of the influenza miasm before the ship came into the longitude of Tasmania on the 26th March.

The Influenzas of Remote Islands.

The full and correct theory of influenza will not be reached by the great pandemics only. On the other hand some very localized epidemics may prove to be signal instances for the pathology, although they do not bear upon the source of the great historic waves of influenza. The instances in view are the influenzas started among a remote community on the arrival of strangers in their ordinary health. This phenomenon has been known at the island of St Kilda, in the Outer Hebrides of Scotland, since the year 1716, when it was recorded in the second edition of an essay upon the island by Martin. Some thought these "strangers' colds" mythical, so much so that Aulay Macaulay, in preparing a work upon St Kilda, was advised to leave them out; he declined to do so, and Dr Johnson commended him for his magnanimity in recording this marvel of nature. There is now no doubt about the fact. H.M.S. 'Porcupine' visited the island in 1860; a day or two after she sailed again, the entire population, some 200 souls, were afflicted with "the trouble," and another visitor, who landed ten days after the 'Porcupine's' visit, saw the epidemic of influenza in progress. The same thing happened in 1876, on the occasion of the factor landing, and again in 1877 on the occasion of a crew coming ashore from a wrecked Austrian ship. A medical account of this epidemic catarrh was given in 1886: The patient complains of a feeling of tightness, oppression and soreness of the chest, lassitude in some cases, pains in the back and limbs, with general discomfort and lowness of spirits. In severe cases there is marked fever, and great prostration. A cough ensues, at first dry, then attended with expectoration, which may go on for weeks[1].

In the remote island of Tristan d'Acunha, in the South Atlantic midway between the River Plate and the Cape of Good Hope, the same thing happens "invariably" on the arrival

[1] Macdonald, *Brit. Med. Journ.*, 14 July, 1886.

of a vessel from St Helena[1]. It is reported also as a common phenomenon of the island of Wharekauri, of the Chatham Group, about 480 miles to the eastward of New Zealand. Residents, both white and coloured, suddenly fall into an illness, one symptom of which is that they feel "intensely miserable." It lasts acutely for about four days, and gradually declines. It resembles influenza in all respects, and is known by the name of *murri-murri*, which is curiously like the old English name of *mure* or *murre*. "The mere appearance of murri-murri is proof to the inhabitants, even at distant parts of the island, which is thirty miles long, that a ship is in port, insomuch that, on no other evidence, people have actually ridden off to Waitangi to fetch their letters[2]."

About equally distant in the Pacific from Brisbane, as Wharekauri from Christchurch, lies Norfolk Island, originally colonized by the mutineers of the 'Bounty.' A writer in a newspaper says:

"During a seven years' residence in Norfolk Island, I had opportunities of verifying the popular local tradition that the arrival of a vessel was almost invariably accompanied by an epidemic of influenza among the inhabitants of the island. In spite of the apparent remoteness of cause and effect, the connexion had so strongly impressed itself on the mind of the Norfolk Islanders that they were in the habit of distinguishing the successive outbreaks by the name of the vessel during whose visit it had occurred[3]."

Something similar has long been known in connexion with the Danish trade to Iceland, the first spring arrivals from the mother country bringing with them an influenza which the crews did not suffer from during the voyage, nor, in most cases, during the progress of the epidemic in Reikjavik. The experience at Thorshaven, in the Faröe Islands, has been the same[4].

These are important indications for the pathology of influenza in general. They point to its inclusion in that strange class of infections which fall most upon a population, or upon those orders of a population, who are the least likely to breed disease by anything that they do or leave undone. Veterinary as well

[1] *Cruise of H.M.S. 'Galatea' in* 1867–8.
[2] R. A. Chudleigh, in *Brit. Med. Journal*, 4 Sept. 1886. The experiences are not altogether recent, for they were noted for "the Chatham Islands and parts of New Zealand" by Dieffenbach, in his German translation of Darwin's *Naturalist's Voyage round the World.* See English ed. 1876, p. 435 *note.*
[3] *Pall Mall Gazette*, 11 Dec. 1889.
[4] Hirsch, *Geograph. and Histor. Pathol.* i. 29. Engl. Transl.

as human pathology presents instances of the kind[1]. In seeking for the source of such an infectious principle, we are not to look for previous cases of the identical disease, but for something else of which it had been an emanation or derivative or equivalent, something which may have amounted to no more than a disparity of physical condition or a difference of race. And as the countries of the globe present now as formerly contrasts of civilized and barbarous, nomade and settled, rude and refined, antiquated and modern, with the aboriginal varieties of race, it may be said, in this theory of infection, that mere juxtaposition has its risks. But, in the theory of influenza, the first requisite is an explanation of its phenomenal uprisings and wave-like propagation, at longer or shorter intervals, during a period of many centuries.

[1] See the chapter on Sweating Sickness in the first volume of this History, p. 269, and the author's other writings there cited.

CHAPTER IV.

SMALLPOX.

THE history of smallpox in Britain is that of a disease coming gradually into prominence and hardly attaining a leading place until the reign of James I. In this respect it is unlike plague and sweating sickness, both of which burst upon the country in their full strength, just as both made their last show in epidemics which were as severe as any in their history. In the former volume of this work I have shown that smallpox in the first Tudor reigns was usually coupled with measles, that in the Elizabethan period the Latin name *variolae* was rendered by measles, and that smallpox, where distinguished from measles, was not reputed a very serious malady[1]. From the beginning of the Stuart period, smallpox is mentioned in letters, especially from London, in such a way as to give the impression of something which, if not new, was much more formidable than before; and that impression is deepened by all that is known of the disease later in the 17th century, including the rising figures in the London bills of mortality.

An early notice of a particular outbreak of smallpox is found in the Kirk Session records of Aberdeen in 1610, under the date of 12 August: "There was at this time a great visitation of the young children with the plague of the pocks[2]."

---

[1] See the first volume, pp. 456–461. I shall add here a reference to smallpox among young people in Henry VIII.'s palace at Greenwich in 1528. Fox, newly arrived from a mission to France, writes to Gardiner, 11 May, 1528 (Harl. MS. 419, fol. 103): The king "commanded me to goe unto Maystress Annes chamber, who at that tyme, for that my Lady prynces and dyvers other the quenes maydenes were sicke of the small pocks, lay in the gallerey in the tilt yarde."

[2] *Selections from the Records of the Kirk Session, Presbytery and Synod of Aberdeen.* Edited by John Stuart, for the Spalding Club, Aberd. 1846, I. 427.

In 1612 there are various references to deaths from smallpox in London in rich houses. In 1613, the Lord Harrington, who is said in a letter of Dr Donne's to be suffering from "the pox and measles mingled," died of smallpox (probably haemorrhagic) on the Sunday before 3 March, at which date also the Lady Burghley and two of her daughters were sick of the same disease. Those two years were probably an epidemic period. Another epidemic is known from a letter of December, 1621 : " The smallpox brake out again in divers places, for all the last hard winter and cool summer, and hitherto we have had no sultry summer nor warm winter that might invite them. The Lord Dudley's eldest son is lately dead of them, and the young Lady Mordaunt is now sick." On 28 January, 1623, "the speech that the smallpox be very rife there [Newmarket] will not hinder his [James I.'s] journey." The years 1623 and 1624 were far more disastrous by the spotted fever all over England ; but smallpox attended the typhus epidemic, as it often did in later experience, the two together having "taken away many of good sort as well as mean people."

The first epidemic of smallpox in London, from which some figures of the weekly mortalities have come down, was in 1628 : this was the year before the Parish Clerks began to print their annual bills, but they had kept the returns regularly since 1604, and appear to have made known in one way or another the weekly mortality and the chief diseases contributing thereto. The smallpox deaths in London in the week ending 24 May, 1628, were forty-one, in the following week thirty-eight, and in the third week of June fifty-eight[1]. Such weekly mortalities in a population of about 300,000 belong to an epidemic of the first degree; and it is clear from letters of the time that the London smallpox of 1628 made a great impression. Lord Dorchester, in a letter of 30 August, calls it "the popular disease[2]." Several letters relating to a fatal case of smallpox in June in the house of Sir John Coke in the city (Garlick Hill) bear witness to the dread of contagion through all that circle of society[3]. One of the letters may be cited :

[1] Mead to Stutteville, in *Court and Times of Charles I.*, I. 359. Joan, Lady Coke to Sir J. Coke, 26 June, 1628. *Cal. Coke MSS.*

[2] Lord Dorchester to the Earl of Carlisle, 30 Aug. 1628, in *C. and T. Charles I.* : "Your dear lady hath suffered by the popular disease, but without danger, as I understand from her doctor, either of death or deformity."

[3] Gilbert Thacker to Sir J. Coke at Portsmouth, 9 June, 1628; Thomas Alured to the same, 21 June ; Richard Poole to the same, 23 June. *Cal. Coke MSS.*, I.

"It pleased God to visit Mrs Ellweys [Coke's stepdaughter] with such a disease that neither she nor any other of her nearest and dearest friends durst come near her, unless they would hazard their own health. The children and almost all our family were sent to Tottenham before she fell sick, and blessed be God are all in health. Mrs Ellweys was sick with us of the smallpox twelve days or thereabouts." Before she was out of the smallpox, she was taken in labour on 15 June, and died the next morning at five o'clock, being buried the same night at ten, with only Sir Robert Lee and his lady of her kindred at the funeral. The letter proceeds : "God knows we have been sequestered from many of our friends' company, who came not near us for fear of infection, and indeed we were very circumspect, careful, and unwilling that any should come to us to impair their health." Lady Coke was fearful to go to Tottenham because of the children who had been removed thither.

All the indications, whether from letters of the time, from poems and plays, or from statistics, point to the two first Stuart reigns as the period when smallpox became an alarming disease in London among adults and in the upper class. The reference to smallpox at Aberdeen in 1610 is to the disease among children ; and so also is an unique entry, opposite the year 1636, on the margin of the register of Trinity parish, Chester : "For this two or three years, divers children died of smallpox in Chester[1]." In London, the disease had not yet settled down to that steady prevalence from year to year which characterized it after the Restoration. On the other hand, the periodic epidemics were very severe while they lasted. The epidemic of 1628 was followed by three years of very slight smallpox mortality in London ; then came a moderate epidemic in 1632 and a severe one in 1634, with again two or more years of comparative immunity, as in the following table from the earliest annual printed bills :

Smallpox deaths in London, 1629–36[2].

Year	Smallpox deaths	Deaths from all causes
1629	72	8771
1630	40	10554
1631	58	8532
1632	531	9535
1633	72	8393
1634	1354	10400
1635	293	10651
1636	127	23359

Thomas Alured's house "hath been visited in the same kind, once with the measles and twice with the smallpox, though I thank God we are now free ; and I know not how many households have run the same hazard."

[1] Harl. MS., No. 2177.

[2] The original heading in the Bills of Mortality was "flox and smallpox." "Flox" meant flux, or confluent smallpox, which was so distinguished, as if in kind, from the ordinary discrete form, seldom fatal. Huxham, in 1725, *Phil. Trans.* XXXIII. 379,

For the next ten years, 1637–46, the London figures are lost[1], excepting the plague-deaths and the totals of deaths from all causes, but it is known from letters that there was a great epidemic of smallpox in one of them, the year 1641 : the deaths were 118 in the week ending 26 August, and 101 in the week ending 9 September[2], totals seldom reached a century later, when the population had nearly doubled. In those weeks of 1641, it was second only to the plague as a cause of dread, and was, along with the latter, the reason that "both Houses grow thin," for all the political excitement of the time. The next London epidemic was in 1649, when the annual bill gives 1190 deaths from smallpox. Willis says that the epidemic was also at Oxford that year, not so very extensive, "yet most died of it" owing to the severe type of the disease[3]. Five years after, in 1654, "at Oxford, about autumn, the smallpox spread abundantly, yet very many escaped with them." The London deaths from smallpox for a series of years were as follows:

Year	Smallpox deaths		Year	Smallpox deaths
1647	139		1655	1294
1648	401		1656	823
1649	1190		1657	835
1650	184		1658	409
1651	525		1659	1523
1652	1279		1660	354
1653	139		1661	1246
1654	832			

Smallpox after the Restoration.

The period which must now concern us particularly, from the Restoration onwards, opens with two deaths from smallpox in the royal family within a few months of the return of the

still used these terms: "When the pustules broke out in less than twenty-four hours from the seizure, they were always of the flux kind, as is commonly observed ... Pocks which at first were distinct would flux together during suppuration." Dover, *Physician's Legacy*, 1732, p. 101, has "the flux smallpox, or variolae confluentes," as one of the varieties: and again, pustules "fluxing in some parts, in others distinct."

[1] Having been omitted by Graunt in his table. *Op. cit.* 1662.

[2] *Cal. State Papers*, under the dates. The epidemic seems to have revived in 1642. An affidavit among the papers of the House of Lords, excusing the attendance of a witness, states that Thomas Tallcott has recently lost his wife and one child by smallpox, and that he himself, six of his children and three of his servants are now visited with the same disease. 13 July, 1642, *Hist. MSS. Com.* v. 38. The Mercurius Rusticus, 1643, says that Bath was much infected both with the plague and the smallpox. Cited in Hutchins, *Dorsetshire*, III. 10.

[3] *Remaining Works.* Transl. by Pordage. Lond. 1681. "Of Feavers," p. 142. In one of his cases Willis was at first uncertain as to the diagnosis, because "the smallpox had never been in that place."

Stuarts. When Charles II. left the Hague on 23 May, 1660, to assume the English crown, his two brothers, the Duke of York and the Duke of Gloucester, accompanied him in the fleet. In the first days of September, the Duke of Gloucester was seized at Whitehall with an illness of which various accounts are given in letters of the time[1]. On 4 September, "the duke hath been very sick, and 'tis thought he will have the smallpox." On the 8th "the doctors say it is a disease between the smallpox and the measles; he is now past danger of death for this bout, as the doctors say"; or, by another account, "the smallpox come out full and kindly, and 'tis thought the worst is past." On the 11th the duke is "in good condition for one that has the smallpox." But a day or two afterwards his symptoms took an unfavourable turn; the doctors left him, apparently with a good prognosis, one evening at six o'clock, but shortly after he bled at the nose three or four ounces, then fell asleep, and on awaking passed into an unconscious state, in which he died. When his body was opened, the lungs were full of blood, "besides three or four pints that lay about them, and much blood in his head, which took away his sense." Pepys says his death was put down to the great negligence of the doctors; and if we can trust a news-letter of the time, their negligence was such as would have been now approved, for "the physicians never gave him anything from first to last, so well was he in appearance to everyone[2]." Three days after his funeral, the king and the Duke of York went to Margate to meet their sister, the princess Mary of Orange, on her arrival from the Hague. Her visit to the Court extended into the winter, and about the middle of December she also took smallpox, of which she died on the 21st. Pepys, dining with Lady Sandwich, heard that "much fault was laid upon Dr Frazer and the rest of the doctors for the death of the princess." Her sister, the princess Henrietta, who had come on a visit to Whitehall with the Queen-mother in October, was removed to St James's on 21st December, "for fear of the smallpox"; but she must have been already sickening, for on the 16th January it is reported that she "is recovered of the measles."

These deaths at Whitehall of a brother and sister of Charles II. happened in the autumn and winter of 1660; but

---

[1] *Histor. MSS. Commis.* v. 156–184. Sutherland Letters.
[2] Sutherland Letters, u. s. Andrew Newport to Sir R. Leveson at Trentham.

it was not until next year that the smallpox rose to epidemic height in London, the deaths from it having been only 354 in 1660, rising to 1246 in 1661, and 768 in 1662. In 1661 it appears to have been epidemic in other parts of England: Willis, who was then at Oxford, says that smallpox began to rage severely before the summer solstice (adding that it was "a distemper rarely epidemical"), and there are letters from a squire's wife in Rutlandshire to her husband in London, which speak of the disease raging in their village in May and June[1].

There was much fever of a fatal type in London in 1661, which is more noticed than smallpox itself in the diary of Pepys. The town was in a very unhealthy state; and it would have been in accordance with all later experience if the "pestilential constitution" of fevers, which continued more or less until the plague burst forth in 1665, had been accompanied by much fatal smallpox. The occasion was used by two medical writers to remark upon the fatality of smallpox as something new. The second of the two essays (1663), was anonymous, and bore the significant title of *Hactenus Inaudita*, the hitherto unheard of thing being that smallpox should prove so fatal as it had been lately. The author adopts the dictum of Mercurialis, with which, he says, most men agree: "Smallpox and measles are wont for the most part to terminate favourably"; and he makes it clear in the following passage that the blame of recent fatalities was laid, justly or unjustly, at the door of the doctors, as, indeed, we know that it was from the gossip of Pepys:

"And I know not by what fate physicians of late have more lost their credit in these diseases than ever: witness the severe judgment of the world in the cases of the Duke of Gloucester and the Princess Royal: so that now they stick not to say, with your Agrippa, that at least in these a physician is more dangerous than the malady[2]."

The other essay was by one of the king's physicians, Dr Tobias Whitaker, who had attended the Court in its exile at

---

[1] Mary Barker to Abel Barker, 26 May and 2 June, 1661. *Hist. MSS. Com.* v. 398: "There is many dy out in this town, and many abroad that we heare of"; the squire's mother is living "within a yard of the smallpox, which is also in the house of my nearest neighbour"; her own children had whooping cough, but do not appear to have taken smallpox.

[2] *Hactenus Inaudita, or Animadversions upon the new found way of curing the Smallpox.* London, 1663. Dated 10 July, 1662. The burden of his own complaint is of a prominent personage in the smallpox who was killed, as he maintains, by enormous doses of diacodium, an opiate with oil of vitriol, much in request among the partisans of the cooling regimen.

St Germain and the Hague. He was by no means an empiric, as some were whom Charles II. delighted to honour; and, although he protests warmly against the modish injudicious treatment of smallpox by blooding and cooling, he has little of the recriminating manner of the time, which Sydenham used from the one side and Morton from the other. He is, indeed, all for moderation : "upon this hinge of moderation turneth the safety of every person affected with this disease." His moderation is somewhat like that of Sir Thomas Browne (whose colleague he may have been for a few years at Norwich), and is apt to run into paradox. In 1634 he wrote in praise of water, including the waters of spas and of the sea, and in 1638 he wrote with even greater enthusiasm in praise of wine[1]. He says of his "most learned predecessor" at Court, Harvey, that his demonstration of the circular motion of the blood was a farther extension of what none were ignorant of "though not expert in dissection of living bodies." On his return to London in 1660, he seemed to find as great a change in smallpox as in the disposition of the people towards the monarchy. His statement as to the change for the worse that had come over smallpox within his memory would be of the highest historical importance if we could be sure it was not illusory ; it is difficult to reconcile with the London experiences of smallpox in 1628 and 1641, but, such as it is, we must take note of it :

"It is not as yet a complete year since my landing with his Majesty in England, and in this short time have observed as strange a difference in this subject of my present discourse as in the variety of opinions and dispositions of this nation, with whom I have discoursed." This disease of smallpox, he proceeds, "was antiently and generally in the common place of *petit* and *puerile*, and the cure of no moment....But from what present constitution of the ayre this childish disease hath received such pestilential tinctures I know not ; yet I am sure that this disease, which for hundreds of yeares and before the practice of medicine was as exquisite, hath been as commonly cured as it hapned, therefore in this age not incurable, as upon my own practice I can testifie....Riverius will not have one of one thousand of humane principles to escape it, yet in my conjecture there is not one of one thousand in the universe that hath any knowledge or sense of it, from their first ingress into the world to their last egress out of this world ; which could

---

[1] His first book was Περὶ ὑδροποσίας, or *A Discourse of Waters, their Qualities and Effects, Diaeteticall, Pathologicall and Pharmacuiticall.* By Tobias Whitaker, Doctor in Physicke of Norwich. Lond. 1834. In 1638, being then Doctor in Physick of London, he published *The Tree of Humane Life, or the Bloud of the Grape. Proving the Possibilitie of maintaining humane life from infancy to extreame old age without any sicknesse by the use of wine.* An enlarged edition in Latin was published at Frankfurt in 1655, and reprinted at the Hague in 1660, and again in 1663. The passages cited in the text occur in his *Opinions on the Smallpox.* London, 1661.

not be, if it were so inherent or concomitant with maternal bloud and seed," referring to the old Arabian doctrine, which Willis adhered to, that every child was tainted in the womb with the retained impure menstrual blood of the mother, and that smallpox (or measles) was the natural and regular purification therefrom. "But smallpox," he continues, "is dedicated to infants more particularly which are moist, and some more than others abounding with vitious humours drawn from maternal extravagancy and corrupt dyet in the time of their gestation; and by this aptitude are well disposed to receive infection of the ayre upon the least infection[1]."

When Whitaker calls smallpox a "childish disease," a disease that was "antiently and generally in the common place of *petit* and *puerile,* and the cure of no moment," he says no more than Willis and others say of smallpox as it affected infants and children. Says Willis: "there is less danger if it should happen in the age of childhood or infancy"; and again: "the sooner that anyone hath this disease, the more secure they are, wherefore children most often escape"; and again: "the measles are so much akin to the smallpox that with most authors they have not deserved to be handled apart from them," although he recognizes that measles is sooner ended and with less danger. Nor was Willis singular among seventeenth-century physicians in his view—"the sooner that anyone hath this disease the more secure they are." Morton in two passages remarks upon the greater mildness of smallpox in "infants": "For that they are less anxious about the result, infants feel its destructive force more rarely than others"; and again: "Hence doubtless infants, being of course ἀπαθεῖς, are afflicted more rarely than adults with the severe kinds of confluent and malignant smallpox[2]."

In the very first treatise written by an English physician specially on the Acute Diseases of Infants, the work by Dr Walter Harris, there is a statement concerning the mildness of "smallpox and measles in infants" (who are defined as under four years of age), which goes even farther than Morton's:

"The smallpox and measles of infants, being for the most part a mild and tranquil effervescence of the blood, are wont to have often no bad character, where neither the helping hands of physicians are called in nor the abounding skill of complacent nurses is put in requisition[3]."

[1] His only reference to the deaths in the royal family, which were currently set down to professional mismanagement, comes in where he opposes the prescription of Riverius to bathe the hands and feet in cold water: "this hath proved fatall," he says, "in such as have rare and tender skins, as is proved by the bathing of the illustrious Princess Royal. Therefore I shall rather ordain aperient fomentations in their bed, to assist their eruption and move sweat."

[2] *Pyretologia,* II. 94, 112.

[3] Walter Harris, M.D., *De morbis acutis infantum,* 1689. There were several editions, some in English.

It has to be said, however, that Morton's statement about infants is made to illustrate a favourite notion of his that apprehension as to the result, which infants were not subject to, made smallpox worse; and that Harris's assertion of the natural mildness of the "smallpox and measles" of infants comes in to illustrate the evil done by the heating regimen of physicians and nurses, who are mentioned in obviously sarcastic terms. So also Sydenham says that "many thousands" of infants had perished in the smallpox through the ill-timed endeavours of imprudent women to check the diarrhoea which was a complication of the malady, but was in Sydenham's view, although not in Morton's, at the same time a wholesome relieving incident therein. If we may take it that infants and young children had smallpox in a mild form, or more rarely confluent than in adults, we may also conclude that many of them died, whether from the alexipharmac remedies which Morton advised and Sydenham (with his follower Harris) denounced, or from the attendant diarrhoea which Sydenham thought a natural relief to the disease and Morton thought a dangerous complication.

Making every allowance for motive or recrimination in the statements, from their several points of view, by Willis, Sydenham, Morton, Harris (Martin Lister might have been added), as to the naturally mild course of smallpox in infants, or when not interfered with by erroneous treatment, it cannot but appear that infantile smallpox at that time was more like measles in its severity or fatality than the infantile smallpox of later times. It is perhaps of little moment that Jurin should have repeated in 1723 the statements of Willis and others ("the hazard of dying of smallpox increases after the birth, as the child advances in age")[1], for he had little intimate knowledge of epidemics, being at that time mainly occupied with mathematics, and with smallpox from the arithmetical side only. But it is not so easy to understand why Heberden should have said the same a generation after[2]; or how much credit should attach to the remark of "an eminent physician from Ireland," who wrote to Dr Andrew, of Exeter, in 1765: "Infants usually have the natural pock of as benign a kind as the artificial[3]."

[1] Jurin, *Letter to Cotesworth.* Lond. 1723, p. 11.
[2] Speaking of malignant sore-throat, he says: "The younger the patients are, the greater is their danger, which is contrary to what happens in the measles and small-pox." *Commentaries on Diseases,* p. 25.
[3] Andrew's *Practice of Inoculation impartially considered.* Exeter, 1765, p. 60.

Whatever may have been its fatality or severity among infants and children, it was chiefly as a disease of the higher ages that smallpox in the Stuart period attracted so much notice and excited so much alarm. The cases mentioned in letters and diaries are nearly all of adults; and these were the cases, whatever proportion they may have made of the smallpox at all ages, that gave the disease its ill repute. About the middle of the 18th century we begin to have exact figures of the ages at which deaths from smallpox occurred: the deaths are then nearly all of infants, so much so that in a total of 1622, made up from exact returns, only 7 were above the age of ten, and only 92 between five and ten; while an age-incidence nearly the same continued to be the rule until after the great epidemic of 1837–39, when it began gradually to move higher[1]. But we should err in imagining that state of things the rule for the 17th century, just as we should err in carrying it forward into our own time. Not only are we told that smallpox of infants was like measles in that the cure was of no moment (which is strange), but we do know from references to smallpox in the familiar writings of the Stuart period that many of its attacks, with a high ratio of fatalities, must have happened to adults. Thus, to take the diary of John Evelyn, he himself had small-pox abroad when he was a young man, his two daughters died of it in early womanhood within a few months of each other, and a suitor for the hand of one of them died of it about the same time. Medical writings leave the same impression of

---

[1] Duvillard (*Analyse et Tableaux de l'Influence de la Petite Vérole sur la Mortalité à chaque Age.* Paris, 1806) gives the ages at which 6792 persons died of smallpox at Geneva from 1580 to 1760, according to the registers of burials:

Total at all ages.	0—1,	—2,	—3,	—4,	—5,	—6,	—7,	—8,	—9,	—10,	—15,	—20,	—25,	—30.
6792	1376	1300	1290	898	603	381	301	189	109	78	126	54	39	31

The public health of Geneva altered very much for the better in the course of two centuries from 1561 to 1760. From 1561 to 1600, in every hundred children born, 30·9 died before nine months, on an annual average, and 50 before five years. From 1601 to 1700 the ratios were 27·7 under nine months, and 46 before five years. From 1701 to 1760 the deaths under nine months had fallen to 17·2 per cent., and under five years to 33·6 per cent. (Calculated from a table in the *Bibliothèque Britannique*, Sciences et Arts, IV. 327.) Thus, with an increasing probability of life, the age-incidence of fatal smallpox may have varied a good deal within the period from 1580 to 1760. It is given by Duvillard separately for the years 1700–1783 (inclusive of measles): during which limited period a smaller ratio died under nine months, and a larger ratio above the age of five years, than in the aggregate of the whole period from 1580 to 1760. Whatever may have been the rule at Geneva, it cannot be applied to English towns; for, while some 30 per cent. of the smallpox deaths were at ages above five in the Swiss city (1700–1783), only 12 per cent. were above five in English towns such as Chester and Warrington in 1773–4.

smallpox attacking many after the age of childhood. Willis gives four cases, all of adults. Morton gives sixty-six clinical cases of smallpox, the earliest record of the kind, and one that might pass as modern : twelve of the cases are under six years of age, nine are at ages from seven to twelve, eleven from thirteen years to twenty, seven from twenty-two to forty, and all but two of the remaining twenty-four clearly indicated in the text, in one way or another, as adolescents or adults, the result being that 23 cases are under twelve and 43 cases over twelve[1].

That ratio of adults to children may have been exceptional. Morton was less likely to be called to infants than to older persons, even among the middle class ; and no physician in London at that time knew what was passing among the poorer classes, except from the bills of mortality. But if Morton had practised in London two or three generations later, say in the time of Lettsom, when "most born in London have smallpox before they are seven," his casebook would not have shown a proportion of forty-three cases over twelve years to twenty-three under that age. Whatever things contributed to the growing evil repute of smallpox among epidemic maladies, there is so much concurrent testimony to the fact itself that we can hardly take it to have been wholly illusion. In some parts the mildness of smallpox was still asserted as if due to local advantages. Thus Dr Plot, who succeeded Willis in his chair of physics at Oxford, wrote in 1677 : "Generally here they are so favourable and kind that, be the nurse but tolerably good, the patient seldom miscarries[2]."

The reason commonly assigned for the large number of fatalities in smallpox after the Restoration was erroneous treatment. That is the charge made, not only in the gossip of the town, as Pepys reported it, but in Sydenham's animadversions on the heating regimen, in Morton's on the cooling regimen, and in the sarcasms of both physicians upon the practice of "mulierculae" or nurses. One may easily make too much of this view of the matter; it is certain that the incidence of smallpox, its fatality and its frequency in general, were determined in the Stuart period, as at other times, by many things besides. Still, the treatment of smallpox has always had the first place in its epidemiological history. The fashion of it that concerns us at

---

[1] *Pyretologia*, 2 vols. Lond. 1692–94, vol. II.
[2] *Natural History of Oxfordshire.* Oxford, 1677, p. 23.

this stage was the famous cooling regimen, commonly joined with the name of Sydenham.

Sydenham's Practice in Smallpox.

Sydenham occupied his pen largely with smallpox, and gained much of his reputation by his treatment of it. At the root of his practice lay the distinction that he made between discrete smallpox and confluent. His practice in the discrete form was to do little or nothing, leaving the disease to get well of itself. Whether the eventual eruption were to be discrete or confluent, he could not of course tell for certain until two or three days after the patient sickened; but in no case was the sick person to be confined to bed until the eruption came out. If the latter were sparse or discrete, the patient was to get up for several hours every day while the disease ran its course, the physician having small occasion to interfere with its progress: "whoever labours under the distinct kind hardly needs the aid of a physician, but gets well of himself and by the strength of nature." One may see how salutary a piece of good sense this was at the time, by taking such a case as that of John Evelyn, narrated by himself[1]. He fell ill at Geneva in 1646, and was bled, leeched and purged before the diagnosis of smallpox was made. "God knows," he says, "what this would have produced if the spots had not appeared." When the eruption did appear, it was only the discrete smallpox; the pimples, he says, were not many. But he was kept warm in bed for sixteen days, during which he was infinitely afflicted with heat and noisomeness, although the appearance of the eruption had eased him of his pains. For five whole weeks did he keep his chamber in this comparatively slight ailment. When he suggested to the physician that the letting of blood had been uncalled for, the latter excused the depletion on the ground that the blood was so burnt and vicious that the disease would have turned to plague or spotted fever had he proceeded by any other method[2].

As there were many such cases, Sydenham's radical distinction between discrete and confluent smallpox, with his

[1] In his *Diary*, under the year 1646, homeward journey from Rome.
[2] The physician was "a very learned old man," Dr Le Chat, who had counted among his patients at Geneva such eminent personages as Gustavus Adolphus and the duke of Buckingham.

advice to leave the former to itself, was of great value, and is justly reckoned to his credit. But in the management of confluent smallpox he advised active interference. If there were the slightest indication that the disease was to be confluent (that is to say, the eruption copious and the pocks tending to run together), he at once ordered the patient to receive a vomit and a purge, and then to be bled, with a view to check the ebullition of the blood and mitigate the violence of the disease. Even infants and young children were to have their blood drawn in such an event. This heroic treatment at the outset was according to the rule of *obsta principiis*; by means of it he thought to divert the attack into a milder course. The initial depletion once over, Sydenham had resort to what is known as the cooling regimen. He set his face against the "sixteen days warm in bed," which Evelyn had to endure even in a discrete smallpox. It was usually a mistake for the patient to take to bed continually before the sixth day from his sickening or the fourth day from the appearance of the eruption; after that stage, when all the pustules would be out, the regimen would differ in different confluent cases, and, of course, in some a continuance in bed would be inevitable as well as prudent. In like manner cardiac or cordial remedies, which were of a heating character, were indicated only by the patient's lowness. The more powerful diaphoretic treacles, such as mithridate, were always a mistake. The tenth day was a critical time, and then paregoric was almost a specific. In the stage of recovery it was not rarely prudent to prescribe cordial medicines and canary wine. Thus, on a fair review of Sydenham's ordinances for smallpox in a variety of circumstances, it will appear that he did not carry the cooling regimen to fanatical lengths and that he was sufficiently aware of the risks attending a chill in the course of the disease[1].

Apart from his rule of leaving cases of discrete smallpox to recover of themselves, Sydenham's management of the disease

---

[1] Dr Dover has left us an account of Sydenham's practice in the smallpox as he himself experienced it: "Whilst I lived with Dr Sydenham, I had myself the small-pox, and fell ill on the twelfth day. In the beginning I lost twenty ounces of blood. He gave me a vomit, but I find by experience purging much better. I went abroad, by his direction, till I was blind, and then took to my bed. I had no fire allowed in my room, my windows were constantly open, my bedclothes were ordered to be laid no higher than my waist. He made me take twelve bottles of small beer, acidulated with spirit of vitriol, every twenty-four hours. I had of this anomalous kind to a very great degree, yet never lost my senses one moment." *The Ancient Physician's Legacy.* London, 1732, p. 114.

was neither approved generally at the time, nor endorsed by posterity. His phlebotomies in confluent cases, usually at the outset, but sometimes even after the eruption was out if the patient had been under the heating regimen before, were an innovation borrowed from the French Galenists. The earlier writers had, for the most part, excepted smallpox among the acute maladies in which blood was to be drawn. But the Galenic rules of treatment were made more rigorous in proportion as they were challenged by the Paracelsist or chemical physicians, and it was among the upholders of tradition that blood-letting was extended to smallpox. Whitaker says that, when he was at St Germain with the exiled Stuarts, the French king was blooded in smallpox ten or eleven times, and recovered; "and upon this example they will ground a precept for universal practice."

The ambiguity of the diagnosis at the outset, and the desire to lose no time, may have been the original grounds of this indiscriminate fashion of bleeding. Evelyn's doctor at Geneva in 1646, "afterwards acknowledged that he should not have bled me had he suspected the smallpox, which brake out a day after," but eventually he defended his practice as having made the attack milder. In like manner Sir Robert Sibbald, of Edinburgh, (1684) took four ounces of blood from a child of five, who was sickening for some malady; when it turned out to be smallpox, the mother expressed her alarm that blood should have been drawn; but Sibbald pointed to the favourable character of the eruption as justifying what he had done : "Optime enim eruperunt variolae, et ab earum eruptione febris remissit[1]."

The ill effects of blood-letting, says Whitaker, may be observed in French children, which by this frequent phlebotomizing are "withered in *juvenile* age." Therefore, he concludes, blooding in smallpox should not be a common remedy, "but in such extremity as the person must lose some part of his substance to save the whole." He calls it the rash and inconsiderate practice of modish persons; "and if the disease be conjunct [confluent], with an undeniable plethory of blood, which is the proper indication of phlebotomy, yet such bleeding ought to be by scarification [upon the arms, thighs or back] and cupping-glasses, without the cutting of any major vessel." Another English physician of the time, Dr Slatholm, of Buntingford in Hertfordshire, who wrote in 1657[2], says that he had known physicians in Paris not to abstain from venesection in children of tender age, even in sucklings. He had never approved the

[1] *Scotia Illustrata.* Lib. II., cap. 10.
[2] *De Febribus &c.*, Lond. 1657 : cap. ix. "De Variolis et Morbillis," p. 141.

letting of blood in such cases, lest nature be so weakened as to be unable to drive the peccant matter to the skin. For the most part, he says, an ill result follows venesection in smallpox; and although it sometimes succeeds, yet that is more by chance than by good management. As to exposing the sick in smallpox to cold air, he declares that he had known many in benign smallpox carried off thereby, instancing the case of his brother-in-law, the squire of Great Hornham, near Buntingford, whose death from smallpox in November, 1656, in the flower of his age, he set down to a chill brought on "ejus inobedientia et mulierum contumacia[1]."

The cooling regimen, as well as the danger of it, was familiar long before Sydenham's time. There could be no better proof of this than a bit of dialogue in Beaumont and Fletcher's 'Fair Maid of the Inn' (Act II. scene 2), a comedy which was licensed in January, 1626:

Host. And you have been in England? But they say ladies in England take a great deal of physic....They say ladies there take physic for fashion.
Clown. Yes, sir, and many times die to keep fashion.
Host. How! Die to keep fashion?
Clown. Yes: I have known a lady sick of the smallpox, only to keep her face from pit-holes, take cold, strike them in again, kick up the heels, and vanish.

Sydenham says that the heating regimen was the practice of empirics and sciolists. Per contra his distinguished colleague Morton says that every old woman and apothecary practised the cooling regimen, and he points the moral of its evil consequences in a good many of his sixty-six clinical cases[2]. He pronounces the results of the cooling regimen to have been disastrous; he had been told that Sydenham himself relaxed the rigour of his treatment in his later years. There was so

[1] "First of all," he says, "let the patient be kept with all care and diligence from cold air, especially in winter, so that the pores of the skin may be opened and the pocks assisted to come out. Therefore let him be kept in a room well closed, into which cold air is in no manner to enter, and let him be sedulously covered up in bed. . . . I desire the more to admonish my friends in this matter, for that Robert Cage, esquire, my dear sister's husband," etc.

[2] Besides cases to show the ill effects of blooding, vomits, purges and cooling medicines such as spirit of vitriol, he gives examples as if to refute Sydenham's favourite notion that salivation, diarrhoea and menstrual haemorrhage were relieving or salutary. Morton's chief object was to bring out the eruption, and to get it to maturate kindly; an eruption which languished, or did not rise and fill, was for him the most untoward of events. Sydenham, on the other hand, argued that the danger was in proportion to the number of pustules and to the total quantity of matter contained in them; and he sought, accordingly, to restrain cases which threatened to be confluent by an evacuant treatment or repressive regimen.

little smallpox for some fifteen years after the date of Morton's book (1694) that the controversies on its treatment appear to have dropped. But, on the revival of epidemics in 1710 and 1714, essays were written against blooding, vomits and purges in smallpox[1].

In 1718, Dr Woodward, the Gresham professor of physic and an eminent geologist, published some remarks on "the new practice of purging" in smallpox, which were directed against Mead and Freind. In 1719 Freind addressed a Latin letter to Mead on the subject (the purging was in the secondary fever of confluent smallpox), and a lively controversy arose in which Freind referred to Woodward anonymously as a well-known empiric. On the 10th of June, 1719, about eight in the evening, Woodward was entering the quadrangle of Gresham College when he was set upon by Mead. Woodward drew his sword and rested the point of it until Mead drew his, which he was long in doing. The passes then began and the combatants advanced step by step until they were in the middle of the quadrangle. Woodward declared (in a letter to the *Weekly Journal*) that he was getting the best of it, when his foot slipped and he fell. He found Mead quickly standing over him demanding that he should beg his life. This Woodward declined to do, and the combat degenerated to a strife of tongues[2]. Next year the controversy over the treatment of smallpox assumed a triangular form. The third side was represented by Dr Dover, who had been something of a buccaneer on the Spanish main and was now in practice as a physician. An old pupil of Sydenham's, he still adhered to blood-letting in smallpox; and in the spring of 1720, when the disease was exceedingly prevalent among persons of quality in London, he claimed to have rescued from death a lady whom Mead had given over, by pulling off the latter's blisters and ordering a pint of blood to be drawn. "He hath observed the same method with like success with several persons of quality this week, and is as yet in very great vogue... He declaims against his brethren of the faculty [especially Mead and Freind], with public and

---

[1] Walter Lynn, M.B., *A more easy and safe Method of Cure in the Smallpox founded upon Experiments, and a Review of Dr Sydenham's Works*, Lond. 1714; *Some Reflections upon the Modern Practice of Physic in Relation to the Smallpox*, Lond. 1715. F. Bellinger, *A Treatise concerning the Smallpox*, Lond. 1721.
[2] Letter from Woodward to the *Weekly Journal*, 20 June, 1719, in Nichols, *Lit. Anecd.* VI. 641.

great vehemence, and particularly against purging and blistering in the distemper, which he affirms to be the death of thousands[1]."

Huxham, another Sydenhamian, appears to have practised not only blooding in smallpox, but also blistering, purging and salivating[2]. But in that generation the practice was exceptional; so much so that when it revived in some hands about 1752 (including Fothergill's), it was thus referred to in a letter upon the general epidemic of smallpox in that year: "I have heard that bleeding is more commonly practised by some of the best physicians nowadays than it was formerly, even after the smallpox is come out[3]." In smallpox the lancet, like other methods, has been in fashion for a time, and then out of fashion; but the old teaching that smallpox did not call for blood-letting was ultimately restored. When Barker, in 1747, gave a discourse before the College of Physicians on the "Agreement betwixt Ancient and Modern Physicians," he did not venture to defend Sydenham's blooding in smallpox, although he would not admit that he was "a bloodthirsty man[4]."

Causes of Mild or Severe Smallpox.

Besides the errors of the heating or the cooling regimen respectively, there is another thing that may have had something to do with the greater fatality of smallpox, as remarked by many, about the middle of the 17th century. "How is it," asks Sydenham, "that so few of the common people die of this disease compared with the numbers that perish by it among the rich[5]?" Sydenham may not have known how much smallpox mortality there was in the poorer quarters of London. But the Restoration was certainly a great time of free living in the

---

[1] Rev. Dr Mangey to Dr Waller, 4 March, 1720, London. Nichols' *Lit. Anecd.* I. 135.

[2] Huxham, *Phil. Trans.* XXXII. (1725), 379.

[3] *Gent. Magaz.*, Sept. 1752.

[4] John Barker, M.D., *Agreement betwixt Ancient and Modern Physicians*, Lond. 1747. Also two French editions. It is on Van Helmont that Barker pours his scorn for "breaking down the two pillars of ancient medicine—bleeding and purging in acute diseases." That upsetting person forbore to bleed even in pleurisy; the only thing that he took from the ancient medicine was a thin diet in fevers; "and yet this scheme, as wild and absurd as it seems, had its admirers for a time."

[5] Lynn (u. s. 1714–15) agrees as to the matter of fact, namely, that the mortality from smallpox was greater among the richer classes, who were too much pampered and heated in their cure, than among the poorer, who had not the means to fee physicians and pay apothecaries' bills.

upper classes of society, and it is equally certain that smallpox was apt to prove a deadly disease to a broken constitution. Willis believed that excesses even predisposed people to take the infection: "I have known some to have fallen into this disease from a surfeit or immoderate exercise, when none besides in the whole country about hath been sick of it." There were, of course, families in which smallpox was for some unknown reason peculiarly fatal. Again, the origins of constitutional weakness are lost in ancestry, the poor stamina of children being often determined by the lives of their grandfathers or great-grandfathers. In the royal family of Stuart smallpox proved more than ordinarily fatal, but it was among the grand-children and great grand-children of James I. that those fatalities happened. Of the children of Charles I., the Duke of Gloucester and the Princess of Orange died of smallpox within a few months of each other in the year of the Restoration. The disease was not less fatal a generation after in the family of the Duke of York (James II.). Dr Willis fell into disgrace with that prince because he bluntly told him that the ailment of one of his sons was "mala stamina vitae." All his sons, says Burnet, died young and unhealthy, one of them by smallpox. Of his two daughters, Queen Mary died of haemorrhagic smallpox in 1694, and the Duke of Gloucester, only child of the other, Princess Anne of Denmark (afterwards Queen Anne), died at the age of eleven, of a malady which was called smallpox by some, and malignant sorethroat by others[1].

Among the medical writers of this period, who gave reasons why smallpox should be so severe or deadly in some while it was so slight in others, Morton was the most systematic. He made three degrees of smallpox—benign, medium and malignant: these did not answer quite to the discrete, confluent and haemorrhagic of other classifiers, for his malignant class included so many confluent cases that in one place he uses *malignae* as the equivalent of *confluentes seu cohaerentes*, while his middle class was made up of some confluent cases,—perhaps such medium cases as had confluent pocks on the face but not

[1] He was under the tutelage of John Churchill, duke of Marlborough, who does not give a name to the malady (Coxe's *Life of Marlborough*). Dr James Johnstone, junr., of Worcester, in his *Treatise on the Malignant Angina*, 1779, p. 78, claims the death of the Duke of Gloucester as from that cause, on the evidence of Bishop Kennet's account.

elsewhere,—and a certain proportion of discrete. The medium kind were the most common (*frequentissimae sunt et maxime vulgares variolae mediae*). Still, it was the benign type that he made the *norma* or standard of smallpox, from which the disease was "deflected" towards the medium type, or still farther deflected towards the malignant. He gives a list of fourteen things that may serve to deflect an attack of smallpox from the *norma* of mildness to the degrees of mean severity or malignity:

1. If the eruption come out too soon or too late.
2. If the patient be sprung from a stock in which smallpox is wont to prove fatal, as if by hereditary right.
3. If the attack fall in the flower of life, when the spirits are keener and more inclined to febrile heats.
4. If the patient be harassed by fever, or by sorrow, love or any other passion of the mind.
5. If the patient be given to spirituous liquors, vehement exercise or anything else of the kind that tends to irritate the spirits.
6. If the attack come upon women during certain states of health peculiar to them.
7. If cathartics, emetics and blooding had been used.
8. If the heating regimen had been carried to excess, or other ill-judged treatment followed.
9. If the patient had met a chill at the outset, checking the eruption.
10. If the attack happen in summer.
11. If the attack happen during a variolous epidemic constitution of the air.
12. If the patient be pregnant or newly married.
13. If the patient be consumptive or syphilitic.
14. If the patient be apprehensive as to the result.

Morton having made the benign type the norm, made the medium type the commonest; and that was really true of the first great epidemic in London in his experience, in the years 1667–68. Sydenham says of it that the cases were more than he ever remembered to have seen, before or after: "nevertheless, as the disease was regular and of a mild type, it cut off comparatively few among the immense number of those who took it." Pepys enters this epidemic under the date of 9 Feb. 1668: "It also hardly ever was remembered for such a season for the smallpox as these last two months have been, people being seen all up and down the streets newly come out after the smallpox." Let us pause here for a moment to ask what Pepys may have meant by recognising the people all up and down the streets newly come out after the smallpox. Did he mean that they were pock-marked? We may answer the question by the testimony of Dr Fothergill for a correspondingly mild and extensive prevalence of smallpox in London some three generations later, which I shall take out of its order because it bears upon the question of pitting. His report for December 1751 is:[1]

"Smallpox began to make their appearance more frequently than they had done of late, and became epidemic in this month. They were in general of a benign kind, tolerably distinct, though often very numerous. Many had them so favourably as to require very little medical assistance, and perhaps a greater number have got through them safely than has of late years been known." The January (1752) report is: "A distinct benign kind of smallpox continued to be the epidemic of this month; a few confluent cases, but rarely." In February he writes: "Children and young persons, unless the constitution is very unfavourable, get through it very well; and the height to which the weekly bills are swelled ought to be considered, in the present case, as an argument of the frequency, not the fatality, of this distemper." In June the type was still favourable: "Crowds of such whom we see daily in the streets without any other vestige than the remaining redness of a distinct pock."

This was an epidemic such as Sydenham alleges that of 1667–68 to have been; and the vestiges of smallpox by which Pepys recognized those who were newly come out of the disease were probably the same that Fothergill saw in 1752.

A practitioner at Chichester does indeed say as much of those treated by himself about the same date: "when the distemper did rage so much in and about Chichester, ten or a dozen years since [written in 1685], it was a great many that fell under my care, I believe sixty at the least, and yet I lost but one person of the disease. Nor was one of my patients marked with them to be seen but half a year after[2]." As these experiences must have been somewhat exceptional I shall give a section to the general case.

Pockmarked Faces in the 17th Century.

The smallpox of 1667–68 had among its numerous victims one of the king's mistresses, the beautiful Frances Stewart, duchess of Richmond, residing in Somerset House, who caught

---

[1] In the *Gentleman's Magazine*, under the dates.

[2] *A Direct Method of ordering and curing People of that Loathsome Disease the Smallpox, being the twenty years' practical experience of John Lamport alias Lampard,* London, 1685. The writer was probably an empiric, "Practitioner in Chyrurgery and Physick," dwelling at Havant, and attending the George at Chichester on Mondays, Wednesdays and Fridays, the Half Moon at Petersfield on Saturdays. He says: "One great cause of this disease being so mortal in the country is because the infection doth make many physicians backward to visit such patients, either for fear of taking the disease themselves or transferring the infection to others." He has another fling at the regular faculty: "Do not run madding to Dr Dunce or his assistance to be let bloud." Empirics, although they were commonly right about blood-letting, were under the suspicion of not speaking the truth about their cures.

Smallpox.

the disease in March 1668 and was "mighty full of it." Pepys, who records the fact, had seen her portrait taken shortly before: "It would make a man weep," he exclaims, "to see what she was then and what she is likely to be by people's discourse now." Happily the worst fears were not realized. Pepys saw her driving in the Park in August, and remarks, without a strict regard to grammar, that she was "of a noble person as ever I did see, but her face worse than it was considerably by the smallpox." The king, unlike the Lord Castlewood of romance, suffered no loss of ardour for his mistress, having visited her over the garden wall, as Mr Pepys relates, on the evening of Sunday, the 10th of May. It is rather the idea, and especially the historical idea, of these horrors that "would make a man weep," and it has moved a great and eloquent historian of our own time to deep pathos[1]. If there be anything that can counteract the effects of agreeable rhetoric it is perhaps statistics. The following numerical estimate of the proportion of pockmarked faces in London after the Restoration is accordingly offered with all deference. It applies mainly to the criminal and lower classes, who were as likely as any to bear the marks of smallpox.

In the *London Gazette*, the first advertisement of a person "wanted" appears in December, 1667; and thereafter until June, 1774, there are a hundred such advertisements of runaway apprentices, of footmen or other servants who had robbed their masters, of horse-stealers, of highwaymen, and the like. There is always a description more or less full; and in the consecutive hundred I have included only such persons as are so particularly described in feature that pock-pits would have been mentioned if they had existed. It is not until the ninth case that "pock-holes in his face" occurs in the description, the eleventh case following close, with the same mark of identity. Then comes a long interval until the twenty-fourth and twenty-fifth cases, both with pock-holes, two of a band of highwaymen concerned in an attempt to rob the Duke of Ormond's coach near London, one of them having emerged from Frying-pan Alley in Petticoat Lane. Fifteen cases follow, all described by distinctive features, without mention of pock-marks, until

---

[1] Macaulay, *History of England*, IV. 532. The moving passage on the former horrors of smallpox, *à propos* of the death of Queen Mary in 1694, is familiar to most, but it may be cited once more in the context of a professional history: "That disease, over which science has since achieved a succession of glorious and beneficent victories, was then the most terrible of all the ministers of death. The havoc of the plague had been far more rapid: but plague had visited our shores only once or twice within living memory; and the smallpox was always present, filling the churchyards with corpses, tormenting with constant fears all whom it had not yet stricken, leaving on those whose lives it spared the hideous traces of its power, turning the babe into a changeling at which the mother shuddered, and making the eyes and cheeks of the betrothed maiden objects of horror to the lover." It is not given to us all to write like this; but it is possible that the loss of picturesqueness may be balanced by a gain of accuracy and correctness.

we come to the fortieth, a boy of twelve or thirteen, who "hath lately had the smallpox." The next is the forty-ninth, a Yorkshireman, long-visaged, and "hath had the smallpox," and close upon him the fiftieth "marked with smallpox." Then come four in quick succession, the 56th, 59th, 61st and 63d; next the 71st; and then a long series with no marks of smallpox, until the 95th, 97th, 99th and 100th, three of these last four having been negroes.

The result is that sixteen in the hundred are marked more or less with smallpox, four of them being black men or boys. One had "lately had the smallpox," another had "newly recovered of the smallpox." One was a cherry-cheeked boy of twelve, "somewhat disfigured with smallpox," who had run away from Bradford school. Two are described as much disfigured, some as a little disfigured, several others as "full of pock-holes." The same mark of identity is occasionally mentioned in the advertisements beyond the hundred tabulated, but not more frequently than before, the usual term in the later period being "pock-broken." This proportion of pock-marked persons among the London populace, sixteen in the hundred, or about twelve in the hundred excluding negroes, does not err on the side of under-statement, if it errs at all. Some such small ratio is what we might have expected in the antecedent probabilities, arising out of the varying degrees of severity of smallpox and the various textures of the human skin. Pitting after smallpox has always been a special risk of a certain texture of the skin, namely, a sufficient thickness of the vascular layer to afford the pock a deep base. Such complexions are common enough even in our own latitudes; and those are the faces that have always borne the most obvious traces of small-pox. It was some of the confluent cases, or rather, of such of them as recovered, that became pock-marked: the babe that became a changeling was not likely to survive. Adults retained the marks more than children, so that there must always have been a good many pock-marked faces in a population where the incidence of the disease was largely upon grown persons, as in the 17th century and in our own time. When smallpox was something of a novelty at the end of the Elizabethan period, a poet addressed a pathetic lyric to his mistress's pock-marked face. A medical writer of the same period reproduces the old Arabian prescription against pitting, to open the pocks on the face with a golden pin, and adds: "I have heard of some, which, having not used anythinge at all, but suffering them to drie up and fall of themselves, without picking or scratching,

have done very well, and not any pits remained after it[1]."
Whitaker, in 1661, dismisses the risk of pitting very briefly,
remarking that the means of prevention was "commonly the complement of every experienced nurse[2]." Morton, in his sixty-six
clinical cases and in his commentary, makes but slight reference
to pitting. In his 14th case, a severe one, "no scars remained";
in his general remarks he treats pitting as a bugbear: "women
set the fairness of their faces above life itself," which may mean,
as in Beaumont and Fletcher's comedy, that they would chill
themselves at all risks by the cooling regimen so they might drive
the pocks in[3].

The Epidemiology continued to the end of the 17th century.

What little remains to be said of smallpox in England to
the end of the seventeenth century may be introduced by the
following table of the deaths in London.

Smallpox Deaths in London 1661 to 1700.

Year	Total deaths	Smallpox deaths	Year	Total deaths	Smallpox deaths
1661	16,665	1246	1681	23,951	2982
1662	13,664	768	1682	20,691	1408
1663	12,741	411	1683	20,587	2096
1664	15,453	1233	1684	23,202	1560
1665	97,306	655	1685	23,222	2496
1666	12,738	38	1686	22,609	1062
1667	15,842	1196	1687	21,460	1551
1668	17,278	1987	1688	22,921	1318
1669	19,432	951	1689	23,502	1389
1670	20,198	1465	1690	21,461	778
1671	15,729	696	1691	22,691	1241
1672	18,230	1116	1692	20,874	1592
1673	17,504	853	1693	20,959	1164
1674	21,201	2507	1694	24,100	1683
1675	17,244	997	1695	19,047	784
1676	18,732	359	1696	18,638	196
1677	19,067	1678	1697	20,972	634
1678	20,678	1798	1698	20,183	1813
1679	21,730	1967	1699	20,795	890
1680	21,053	689	1700	19,443	1031

[1] Kellwaye, u. s., 1593.

[2] Dr Richard Holland in 1730 (*A Short View of the Smallpox*, p. 75), says: "A
lady of distinction told me that she and her three sisters had their faces saved in a bad
smallpox by wearing light silk masks during the distemper."

[3] As I do not intend to come back to the subject of pockmarked faces, I shall add
here that I have found nothing in medical writings of the 18th century, nor in its fiction
or memoirs, to show that pockpitting was more than an occasional blemish of the
countenance. At that time most had smallpox in infancy or childhood, when the
chances of permanent marking would be less. The disappearance of pockpitted faces

Sydenham's remarks throw some light on the smallpox of the several years. While the epidemic of 1667–68 was of a regular and mild type, that of 1670–72, which has fewer deaths in the bills, was of the type of black smallpox complicated with flux. The year 1674 has the highest figures yet reached; the type of the disease was confluent, and so severe that it "almost equalled the plague"; while the smallpox of the year 1681, with a still higher total, was "confluent of the worst kind."

It is not easy to make out what the differences of "type" described by Sydenham depended on; but it may be hazarded that those who fell into smallpox in an otherwise unhealthy season would die in larger numbers, being weakened by antecedent disease, such as measles or epidemic diarrhoea, influenza or typhus fever. An epidemic of measles in the first six months of 1674 was most probably the reason of the great fatality of smallpox in the second half of that year (see the chapter on Measles). The high figures of smallpox mortality in 1681 followed two hot summers, unhealthy with infantile diarrhoea, and coincided with a third season unhealthy in the same way. The deaths by smallpox in the last week of August, 1681, reached the very high figure of 168, the next highest cause of death that week, and the highest the week after, being "griping in the guts," or infantile diarrhoea. The smallpox of 1685 was more uniformly distributed over the months of the year, which was one of malignant typhus, the worst week for fever having 114 deaths (ending 29 Sept.), and the worst week for smallpox 99 deaths (ending 18 Aug.).

The deaths by smallpox in the London bills are the only 17th century figures of the disease. According to later experience, a high mortality in London in a certain year meant an epidemic general in England in that or the following year; and the same appears to have held good for the period following the

was discovered long ago. The report of the National Vaccine Board for 1822 says: "We confidently appeal to all who frequent theatres and crowded assemblies to admit that they do not discover in the rising generation any longer that disfigurement of the human face which was obvious everywhere some years since." The members of this board were probably seniors who remembered the 18th century; and it is quite true that the first quarter of the 19th century was singularly free from smallpox in England except in the epidemic of 1817–19. But the above passage became stereotyped in the reports: exactly the same phrase, appealing to what they all remembered "some years since," was used in the report for 1825, a year which had more smallpox in London than any since the 18th century, and again in the report for 1837, the first year of an epidemic which caused forty thousand deaths in England and Wales. These stereotyped reminiscences are apt to be as lasting a blemish as the pockholes themselves.

Restoration. In the parish register of Taunton, a weaving town, the smallpox deaths are many in 1658 ("all the year," which was one of agues and influenza), in 1670, 1677, and 1684 ("very mortal," the year being noted for a very hot summer and for fevers and dysenteries[1]). The highest total of deaths in London to the end of the 17th century fell in 1681, which is known to have been a year of very fatal smallpox at Norwich[2] and at Halifax. Thoresby's friend Heywood lost three children by it at the latter town in the epidemic of 1681, which does not appear to have visited Leeds. In 1689 Thoresby himself lost his two children at Leeds within a few days. In 1699 the epidemic returned, and he again lost two of the four children that had been born to him in the interval[3]. Similar calamities befell country houses, of which the following from the correspondence of a titled family in Cumberland is an instance:

"17th April, 1688,—Captaine Kirkby came hither, and told me that Mrs Skelton, my god-daughter, of Braithwaite, dyed the last week, and her two children, of the smallpockes[4]."

Rumours of "smallpox and other infectious disease" at Cambridge in the summer of 1674[5], and at Bath in the summer of 1675[6], threatened to interfere with the studies of the one place and the gaieties of the other.

Smallpox in London in 1694: the death of the Queen.

The epidemic of smallpox in London in 1694 was made memorable by the death of the queen. On 22 November Evelyn notes, "a very sickly time, especially the smallpox, of which divers considerable persons died"; on 29 December:

---

[1] Collinson, *Hist. of Somerset*, III. 226, citing Aubrey's *Miscellanies*, 33.
[2] Blomefield, *Hist. of Norfolk*, III. 417.
[3] Thoresby, *Ducatus Leodiensis*, ed. Whitaker. App. p. 151.
[4] *Cal. Le Fleming MSS.* p. 408 (*Hist. MSS. Com.*). There are also many references to smallpox from 1676 onwards in the letters of the Duke of Rutland at Belvoir, lately calendared for the Historical MSS. Commission.
[5] In the *London Gazette* of 11–14 May, 1674, the Vice-Chancellor and two doctors of medicine of the University of Cambridge contradicted by advertisement a report that smallpox and other infections were prevalent in the university.
[6] Marquis of Worcester to the Marchioness, [London] 8 June, 1675 (Beaufort MSS. *Hist. MSS. Commis.* XII. App. 9, p. 85): "They will have it heere that the smallpox and purple feaver is at the Bath, and the Dutchesse of Portsmouth puts off her journey upon it. The king askt me about it as soon as I came to towne. Pray enquire, and lett me know the truth." The *London Gazette* of 17–21 June and 28 June–1 July, 1775, had advertisements "that it hath been certified under the hands of several persons of quality" that Bath and the country adjacent was wholly free of the plague or any other contagious distempers whatsoever.

"the smallpox increased exceedingly, and was very mortal," the queen having died of it the day before. Queen Mary came of a stock to which smallpox had been peculiarly fatal, a brother and sister of her father, James II., having died of it at Whitehall in 1660. Some of the particulars of her illness and death come from bishop Burnet[1], who saw her in the first days of the attack and was about the Court until the end of it; the authentic medical details are by Dr Walter Harris, one of the physicians in attendance, who published them, by leave of his superiors, in order to meet the censures passed on the doctors "by learned men at a great distance[2]."

The symptoms of illness on the first day did not prevent the queen from going abroad; but, as she was still out of sorts at bedtime, she took a large dose of Venice treacle, a powerful diaphoretic which her former physician, the famous physiologist Dr Lower, had recommended her to take as often as she found herself inclined to a fever[3]. Finding no sweat to appear as usual, she took next morning a double quantity of it, but again without inducing the usual effect of perspiration. Up to that time she had not asked advice of the physicians. To this severe dosing with one of the most powerful alexipharmac or heating medicines, the malignant type of the ensuing smallpox was mainly ascribed by Harris, who was a follower of Sydenham and a partizan of the cooling regimen. On the third day from the initial symptoms the eruption appeared, with a very troublesome cough; the eruption came out in such a manner that the physicians were very doubtful whether it would prove to be smallpox or measles. On the fourth day the smallpox showed itself in the face and the rest of the body "under its proper and distinct form." But on the sixth day, in the morning, the variolous pustules were changed all over her breast into the large red spots "of the measles"; and the erysipelas, or rose, swelled her whole face, the former pustules giving place to it. That evening many livid round petechiae appeared on the forehead above the eyebrows, and on the temples, which Harris says he had foretold in the morning. One physician said these were not petechiae, but sphacelated spots; but next morning a surgeon proved by his lancet that they contained blood. During the night following the sixth day, Dr Harris sat up with the patient, and observed that she had great difficulty of breathing, followed soon after by a copious spitting of blood. On the seventh day the spitting of blood was succeeded by blood in the urine. On the eighth day the pustules on the limbs, which had kept the normal variolous character longest, lost their fulness, and changed into round spots of deep red or scarlet colour, smooth and level with the skin, like the stigmata of the plague. Harris observed about the region of the heart one large pustule filled with matter, having a broad scarlet circle round it like a burning coal, under which a great deal of extravasated blood was found when the body was examined after death. Towards the end, the queen slumbered sometimes, but said she was not refreshed thereby. At last she lay silent for some hours; and some words that came from her shewed, says Burnet, that her thoughts had begun to break. She died on the 28th of December, at one in the morning, in the ninth day of her illness.

[1] Burnet, *History of his own Time,* IV. 240.
[2] Walter Harris, M.D., *De morbis acutis infantum.* Ed. of 1720, p. 161.
[3] John Cury, M.D., *An Essay on Ordinary Fever.* Lond. 1743, p. 40.

The case of Queen Mary was one of discrete smallpox turning
to the haemorrhagic form; and it had from first to last the most
striking resemblance to that of her uncle, the Duke of Gloucester,
in September, 1660[1]. The smallpox, says Burnet, came out,
but the pustules "sunk so that there was no hope of raising
them"; and in sinking they turned to livid spots or blotches.
It is quite possible that the repeated doses of Venice treacle at
the outset, which failed in their usual effect of inducing sweat,
may have had something to do with the result, as Dr Harris
certainly believed and afterwards publicly said with the leave of
his superiors.   But the queen, with eminent qualities of mind
and heart, was not physically of good constitution.   She was
one of those children of James II. whom Willis had brusquely
pronounced, some twenty-five years before, to be affected with
mala stamina vitae; and her father's brother, the Duke of
Gloucester, who was not treated in the same way, and, by one
account, not treated at all, died in exactly the same kind of
haemorrhagic smallpox[2].

[1] See p. 438.
[2] Macaulay hardly realized the anomalous character of the queen's attack of
smallpox.   "The physicians," he says, "contradicted each other and themselves in a
way which sufficiently indicates the state of medical science in that day.   The disease
was measles; it was scarlet fever; it was spotted fever; it was erysipelas...Radcliffe's
opinion proved to be right."   There had been some doubt on the first appearance of
the eruption whether it would turn to measles or smallpox.   Sydenham says that it was
often difficult to make the diagnosis at that stage, and in the queen's case the first
signs were anomalous as well.   Next day, however, the eruption all over the body
became "smallpox in its proper and distinct form."   But it did not long remain so;
the livid spots, into which the pustules subsided, again raised doubts in the minds of
some of the physicians whether it was not measles after all; and there was undoubtedly erysipelas of the face.   Harris took the middle course of diagnosing
"smallpox and measles mingled," a name by which the form that we now call
haemorrhagic smallpox had been known from the early part of the seventeenth
century.   It was at this late and ominous stage of the illness that Radcliffe was called
in; it is not correct to say, as the historian says, that he was the first to pronounce
"the more alarming name of smallpox."   The diagnosis was then a matter of little
moment, for the queen was dying.   He declared that "her majesty was a dead
woman, for it was impossible to do any good in her case when remedies had been
given that were so contrary to the nature of her distemper; yet he would endeavour
to do all that lay in his power to give her ease."   (Munk's *Roll of the College of
Physicians*, II. 458.)   For some unexplained reason Radcliffe was made to bear the
blame of the queen's death, an accusation which he deserved as little as he deserved
the credit given him by the historian of having been the only physician to make the
correct diagnosis.
     Macaulay is equally unfortunate in his remark that smallpox "was then the most
terrible of all the ministers of death," in his comparison of it to plague, and in his
rhetoric generally.   The haemorrhagic form, of which the queen died, was rare.
Dover adds it as a fourth variety, but admits that he had seen only five cases of it.
Ferguson, of Aberdeen, as late as 1808, in a paper on measles (*Med. and Phys.
Journal*, XXI. 359), described a haemorrhagic case of smallpox which he once saw,
without knowing that it was a recognized variety of smallpox at all.   However terrible
a minister of death smallpox may sometimes have been, it happened that there was

Circumstances of the great Epidemic in 1710.

For fifteen years after the year of Queen Mary's death by haemorrhagic smallpox, there was comparatively little of the disease in London. In seven of the years the deaths were counted by hundreds, while the average of the whole period from 1695 to 1710, which included the years of Marlborough's campaigns, was unaccountably low. There was a corresponding lull in the fever mortality in London; and as precisely the same kind of lull took place both in fever and smallpox during the next great war with France a century after, it may seem as if a state of war, instead of spreading infectious disease as it did in the countries where the war raged, had the effect in England of reducing it. The period of comparative immunity came to an end, both for fever and smallpox, with the great epidemic of each disease in 1710, in which year smallpox cut off 3138 in London and "great numbers in Norwich[1]." In 1714 there was another severe epidemic of smallpox in London, again in company with one of fever, and thereafter a high average for many years.

Smallpox deaths in London, 1701–1720.

Year	Deaths from smallpox	Deaths from all causes	Year	Deaths from smallpox	Deaths from all causes
1701	1099	20,471	1711	915	19,833
1702	311	19,481	1712	1943	21,198
1703	398	20,720	1713	1614	21,057
1704	1501	22,684	1714	2810	26,589
1705	1095	22,097	1715	1057	22,232
1706	721	19,847	1716	2427	24,436
1707	1078	21,600	1717	2211	23,446
1708	1687	21,291	1718	1884	26,523
1709	1024	21,800	1719	3229	28,347
1710	3138	24,620	1720	1442	25,454

The marked increase of smallpox deaths in 1710 and 1714, after an interval of low or moderate annual mortalities, caused

comparatively little of it in London during the period covered by Macaulay's history; and it certainly did not "fill the churchyards," as he might have found out by referring to that not altogether recondite source, the bills of mortality. From 1694 to 1700 fevers caused three and a half times more deaths than smallpox. In the year 1696, when "the distress of the common people was severe," the smallpox deaths in London were 196, or about one-hundredth part of the mortality from all causes.

[1] Blomefield, III. 432. The following are two cases from the London epidemic of 1710: June, 15.—"Lord Ashburnham's brother has the smallpox, and the first, concluding he had had it, went to him, and now himself very ill of them. Doctor Garth, who says none has them twice, examined the servants, and they tell him he was but six days ill then; so he concludes that was not the smallpox." *Cal. Belvoir MSS.*, II. 190.

the same cry to be raised as in the Restoration period, namely, that the medical treatment was to blame. Lynn, writing in 1714, says that many complaints were made of the destructiveness of smallpox in the epidemic four years before (1710), and of "the great want of better help, care or advice therein[1]." Woodward also ascribed the great increase of smallpox fatalities from 1710 onwards to erroneous treatment[2]. All the lives that might have been saved by better medical treatment or by more assiduous visiting of the sick would, in the then circumstances of the London populace, have made little difference to the bills of mortality. The causes that made fever so mortal in the same years were in great part the causes that made smallpox mortal, the former chiefly among those in the prime or maturity of life, the latter chiefly among the children. London had nearly reached its maximum of overcrowding; its population advanced but little for a good many years, and its mortality from all causes was so great that the numbers were only kept up by a constant recruit from the country. The necessity of doing something for the health of the poorer classes was felt, but nothing adequate was done or could be done[3]. So far as concerned the richer classes, they incurred constant danger of smallpox infection. In one of those fatal years, probably 1720, when there was smallpox among persons of quality in London, the Duchess of Argyll wrote to the Countess of Bute, to congratulate her on the birth of a daughter and on having two fine boys in her family already, "and he that has had the smallpox as good as two, so mortal as that distemper has been this year in town was never known[4]."

The domestics also of great houses frequently caught

---

[1] Lynn, u. s. He recalls a remark made by a writer in 1710 that the severity of that epidemic " was not due to a peculiar state of the air, but to a defect in some of our great physicians, who, being too fully employed, could not give due attendance to all or even to any of their patients through the multiplicity of them : for want of which, and the severity of their injunctions, which hindered others from applying anything in their absence, many persons were lost who might otherwise have been saved with due care."

[2] John Woodward, M.D., *The State of Physick and Diseases, with an inquiry into the causes of the late increase of them, but more particularly of the Smallpox; with some considerations on the new practice of purging in that disease.* London, 1718.

[3] See the account of the Dispensary of the College of Physicians in Warwick Lane, in Munk's *Roll of the Coll. of Phys.* II. 499, under the head of Sir Samuel Garth. The dispensary was started in 1687 and languished until 1724. The General Dispensary in Aldersgate Street was opened in 1770 with Dr Hulme as physician, and Dr Lettsom as additional physician in 1773.

[4] Letter of 27 March, year not given. *Hist. MSS. Com.* v. 618. See also the letter of 4 March, 1720, from Mangey to Waller, cited above, p. 450.

smallpox and spread it, a trouble which gave occasion at length, in 1746, to the first Smallpox Hospital for the admission of such of them as brought subscribers' letters. Before that it had been the practice of the rich to send their domestics to private houses kept by nurses[1].

It was in these circumstances, and for the benefit of the upper classes and their domestics, that a project of getting through smallpox on easy terms was brought to the notice of London society in 1721.

Inoculation brought into England.

The first that was heard in England of engrafting the smallpox was through a communication by Dr Timoni, a Greek of Constantinople, to Dr Woodward, Gresham professor of physic, who had the paper printed in the *Philosophical Transactions* of the Royal Society[2]. After a statement that "the Circassians, Georgians and other Asiatics" had brought the practice to Constantinople, and that it had been followed there for forty years by "the Turks and others" (statements never confirmed but on inquiry contradicted by those who knew), he proceeds to matters more within his own competence. During these eight years past "thousands" of subjects have been inoculated, and the value of the practice has now been put beyond all suspicion and doubt. The practice is to take fluid smallpox matter from the pustules of a discrete case of the natural disease, and convey it warm in a stopped phial to the scene of inoculation. A few punctures with a three-edged surgeon's needle are made in any of the fleshy parts (but preferably over the muscles of the arm or forearm) until the

---

[1] Dr Philip Rose, of Bedfordbury ("over against a baker, next door to the Old Black Horse, two doors from Chandos Street, St Martin's parish"), having been called by Lady Wyche to see her butler, pronounced him to be in the smallpox; whereupon the lady informed the physician that "she knew an eminent nurse who had managed above twenty of my Lord Cheyney's servants in the smallpox, and every one of them had recovered." Her butler was accordingly carried to this nurse's house in a by street near Swallow Street. *An Essay on the Smallpox.* By Philip Rose, M.D. Lond. 1724, p. 18.

[2] "An Account or History of the Procuring the Small Pox by Incision, or Inoculation; as it has for some time been practised at Constantinople." Being the Extract of a Letter from Emanuel Timonius, Oxon. et Patav. M.D., S.R.S., dated at Constantinople, December, 1713. Communicated to *Phil. Trans.* XXIX. (Jan.–March, 1714) 72, by Dr Woodward, Gresham Professor of Physic. Timoni had been in England in 1703, and had been incorporated a doctor of medicine at Oxford on his Padua degree: hence, perhaps, his correspondence.

blood comes; a drop of the fluid matter of smallpox is then to be mixed with the blood, and the inoculated part to be protected by a walnut shell bound over it. The symptoms that follow are very slight, some being scarce sensible that they are ill. The pocks that ensue are for the most part distinct, few, and scattered; commonly ten or twenty break out; now and then the patient may have only two or three; few have a hundred. The matter is hardly a thick pus, as in the common sort, but a thinner kind of *sanies*. There are some in whom no pustules appear except at the points of insertion, where purulent tubercles arise; yet these have never had the smallpox afterwards in their whole lives, though they have consorted with persons having it. On one occasion fifty were inoculated together, and of these four developed smallpox which was nearly confluent; but there was a suspicion that they must have been already infected by contagion. Timoni had never observed any mischievous accident from this incision hitherto; reports of such had sometimes spread abroad among the vulgar, "yet having gone on purpose to the houses whence such rumours have arisen I have found the whole to be absolutely false." But, to keep nothing back, he will mention two fatalities of children inoculated; both of them were cases of hereditary *lues* with marasmus, and it was about the fortieth day from their inoculation that death ensued. The rest of Timoni's paper is printed in the original Latin, being devoted to a theory of engrafting which afterwards passed current:—one attack of smallpox secures from a second, a mild attack serves as well as a severe, as also in the natural way, the reason being that smallpox, in whatever degree, causes a fermentation of the mass of the blood.

A year after this, in 1715, there was published in London *An Essay on External Remedies*, of which the 37th chapter was "Of the Variolae or Small Pox, the manner of ingrafting or giving them, and of their Cure." The author was Peter Kennedy, Chir. Med., a Scot of good but impoverished family, who had spent several years in various parts of Europe visiting the schools of medicine and surgery, and had found his way to Constantinople[2]. His account of the engrafting of smallpox,

[1] *An Essay on External Remedies*, Lond. 1715, p. 153. Kennedy settled in practice in London as an ophthalmic surgeon, and appears to have enjoyed the patronage of Arbuthnot. His other work, *Ophthalmographia, or Treatise of the Eye*

which he had seen or heard of there, differs somewhat from that of Timoni, whom he just refers to: "Dr Timoni, a Grecian who resides there, had taken or followed this same method with his two sisters a little before my arrival at Constantinople."

Kennedy says that engrafting the smallpox was practised in the Peloponnesus or Morea, "and at this present time is very much used both in Turkey and Persia, where they give it in order to prevent its more severe effects by the early knowledge of its coming; as also probably to prevent them being troubled with it a second time." In Persia, however, the smallpox was taken internally in a dose of dried powder. In Constantinople the matter was inserted at scarifications upon the forehead, wrists, and ankles. After eight or ten days the smallpox came forward in a kindly manner, and not nearly so numerous as if naturally taken. "The greatest objection commonly proposed is, whether or not it hinders the patient from being infected a second time. But, in answer to this, it is advanced that we do rarely or never find any to have been troubled with this distemper twice in the same manner or the same fulness of malignity"—i.e. we rarely find this in the natural way.

Kennedy's object was, not to recommend the engrafting of smallpox in England, but to show how easily distempers or contagions, "as well as medicines," may be communicated to the blood from the surface of the body: "and this is more confirmed by some of the country people in Italy, in the more remote parts from towns, so also in some parts of the highlands of Scotland, where they infect their children by rubbing them with a kindly pock, as they term it."

Meanwhile Timoni's essay in the *Philosophical Transactions* had stirred up Sir Hans Sloane to make farther inquiries[1]. He applied to the British consul at Smyrna, Dr Sherrard, who was fortunately able to get information at first hand from an old Smyrna colleague, Dr Pylarini, consul for Venice, who had practised inoculation at Constantinople in the first years of the century. Pylarini, who had retired to Venice, was induced to draw up an account of what he knew of the beginnings and

and its Diseases, with appendix on Diseases of the Ear, Lond. 1723, which is dedicated to Arbuthnot, shows a knowledge of optics and of the structure of the parts concerned in operations on the eye.

[1] Sloane, *Phil. Trans.* XLIX. (1756), p. 516, "An Account of Inoculation given to Mr Ranby to be published, anno 1736."

original methods of engrafting, which was printed at Venice, with a dedication to Sherrard, in 1715, and at once copied into the *Philosophical Transactions*[1]. This, the most trustworthy account of the Constantinople practice, ignores the earlier essay of Timoni altogether.

Pylarini carries the authentic history of the practice at Constantinople back to the year 1701. Its history before that was obscure; but it is most certain, he says, that it began in Greece, more particularly in Thessaly, and crept gradually from place to place until it reached Constantinople, where it attracted little notice for several years, being rarely practised and only among the lower class. A noble Greek having spoken of it to him in 1701, with a view to the protection of his children from the epidemic then raging, Pylarini had to confess his entire ignorance of it, but being at the Greek's house four days after he there met a Greek woman who expounded the practice clearly in detail and gave him many instances of persons who had gone through it safely. Pylarini inquired into some of these cases and found them to be genuine; but in that great city he could not search them all out. Soon after this interview, the woman came and operated on the four children of the rich Greek, of whom the three younger had a very mild disease, but the eldest a severe attack, which nearly cost her life. Many other rich Greek families followed suit, so that, says Pylarini in 1715, "every one wishes to have the advantage of transplantation." He adds, however, that "the Turks have hitherto neglected it." He confirms Timoni in saying that the pocks raised by transplantation were nearly always of the distinct kind and few in number—ten to twenty or thirty, rarely a hundred, very rarely two hundred,—although he does not reach Timoni's minimum of "two or three," or the pustules only at the punctured spots.

These accounts from Constantinople, printed in London in 1714, 1715 and 1716 were regarded, says Douglass, "as virtuoso amusements[2]" until the spring of 1721, when inoculation began to be tried tentatively in London, and in a bold and

---

[1] Jacobus Pylarinus, *Nova et Tuta Variolas excitandi per Transplantationem Methodus, nuper inventa et in usum tracta, qua rite peracta immunia in posterum praeservantur ab hujusmodi contagio corpora.* Venetiis, 1715. Privilege dated 10 Nov., 1715. Reprinted in *Phil. Trans.* XXIX. (Jan.–March, 1716), p. 393.

[2] *A Dissertation concerning Inoculation of Smallpox.* By W. D[ouglass], Boston, 1730.

confident way during the very same weeks at Boston, New England.

Dr Pitcairn, of Edinburgh, had received an account of inoculation from Bellini, an Italian physician, who had read Pylarini's essay. Douglass says that Pitcairn "was very fond of it, but could not persuade himself to venture it in practice[1]." Sometime in March, 1721, one à Castro had issued in London a pamphlet on inoculation, full of inaccuracies and of no moment[2]. In a lecture on the plague given at the College of Physicians on the 17th of April, 1721, Dr Walter Harris made a passing reference to the Constantinople practice of engrafting smallpox[3]; and shortly after that, or shortly before, the Lady Mary Wortley Montagu set about having her younger child inoculated in London, her elder child having been inoculated at Constantinople three or four years before. This lady had, in 1717, accompanied her husband as ambassador to the Porte, where the embassy remained about a year. During her residence at Pera she heard of the Greek practice of engrafting or transplanting the smallpox; the French ambassador had said in pleasantry to her: "They take the smallpox here by way of diversion, as they take the waters in other countries." According to her information, there was a set of old women who made it their business to perform the operation every autumn, in the month of September, when the great heat is abated. People send to one another to know if any of their family has a mind to have the smallpox; they make parties for this purpose, and when they are met (commonly fifteen or sixteen together) the old woman comes with a nut-shell full of matter. Every year thousands undergo the operation (but according to the information of the British embassy in 1755 not more than twenty in a year, which may perhaps mean that it had fallen into disuse[4]). There is no example of anyone that has died of it. She intended to have it performed upon her little son, and had patriotic visions of bringing "this useful invention" into fashion in England. Accordingly her boy, aged five, was inoculated in March, 17$\frac{1}{18}$, by a Greek woman, under the direction of Maitland, a Scots surgeon who attended the embassy. The child suffered very

---

[1] *loc. cit.*   [2] Published under the initials J. C., M.D.
[3] *De Peste dissertatio habita Apr.* 17, 1721, *cui accessit descriptio inoculationis Variolarum,* a Gualt. Harris, Lond. 1721.
[4] *Phil. Trans.* XLIX. 104.

little inconvenience and, according to Maitland, "had about an hundred pox all upon his body."

Lady Mary returned to London in 1718; but it was not until some three years after, in the spring of 1721, that she stirred the matter again. Whether it was that she herself was the cause of the talk about inoculation in London in April, 1721, or that she merely had the subject brought back to her mind by the essay of à Castro, the lecture by Harris, or by what others were saying, she sent sometime in April for Maitland, who had assisted at the inoculation of her elder child at Pera, with a view to having the operation done on the younger, who was now four or five years old. In a week or two Maitland found suitable smallpox matter and engrafted the child on both arms; on the tenth night she was a little feverish, but the smallpox began to appear next morning and in a few days she was perfectly recovered. Three physicians of the College visited the case, as well as several ladies and other persons of distinction. One of those physicians, Dr Keith, resolved to have a boy of his own, aged six, engrafted, which was done by Maitland on both arms on the 11th of May, 1721, five ounces of blood having been drawn before the operation.

Among Lady Mary's intimates was the Princess of Wales, who became interested in the project for the sake of her own children[1]. She proposed to the king (George I.) that he should remit the capital sentence of six Newgate felons on condition that they would submit to be inoculated. The king consulted Sir Hans Sloane, who applied to Dr Terry of Enfield, formerly in practice at Constantinople. Terry's report was that not more than one in eight hundred had died from the effects of inoculation in Turkey. The upshot was that the six Newgate convicts, three men and three women, were inoculated by Maitland on the 9th of August, 1721, in the presence of several eminent physicians, surgeons, Turkey merchants, and others. The matter was inserted on both arms and on the right leg of each, and the insertion was repeated on the arms of five of them three days after. Dr Mead, having heard that the Chinese procured smallpox by stuffing the matter up their noses, got a pardon for a seventh convict under sentence of death, a young woman, on condition that she would submit to a pledget of cotton dipped in smallpox matter being inserted in her nostril:

[1] Sloane, u.s., 1736.

it produced, besides a fair smallpox, much severe pain along the Schneiderian membrane and the frontal sinuses, and was not thought a satisfactory experiment. The trial upon the other six was reassuring; they all escaped with the slightest possible eruption; "the most that anyone had was sixty pustules."

The next step was on the part of the Princess of Wales, who procured the inoculation of six charity children of the parish of St James's. Four of them had smallpox "very favourably"; one did not have it at all, "having evidently had the smallpox before"; and the sixth had not only the prolonged effects of inoculation, but also an attack of the natural smallpox, of a favourable kind, eleven weeks after. This experiment was followed by the inoculation of five more hospital children, from eight to fourteen weeks old, of whom three had no effects, their bodies being "morbid." The Princess of Wales was at length resolved in April, 1722, to run the risk of the operation on her two daughters, the princess Amelia, aged eleven, and the princess Caroline, aged nine, being urged by the fact that another daughter, the princess Anne, afterwards princess royal of Orange, had just had the natural smallpox so dangerously that Sloane feared for her life. The inoculations were done on the 19th of April, by serjeant-surgeon Amyand under the direction of Sir Hans Sloane. What passed between that physician and the king shows at once the apprehension of danger from a novel operation and the temper in which it was undertaken:

"I told his Majesty," says Sloane, "that it was impossible to be certain but that, raising such a commotion in the blood, there might happen dangerous accidents not foreseen; but he replied that such might, and had happened, to persons who had lost their lives by bleeding in a pleurisy, and taking physic in any distemper, let never so much care be taken. I told his Majesty that I thought this to be the same case; and the matter was concluded upon, and succeeded as usual, without any danger during the operation, or the least ill symptom or disorder since."

The news of the successful inoculation of the two princesses had hardly time to create a vogue for the practice, when there came word, in the same month of April, of the death by inoculation of the Earl of Sunderland's son, aged two and a half, and of Lord Bathurst's footman, aged nineteen.

Meanwhile, in the autumn of 1721, Maitland had gone down to Hertford, where smallpox would seem to have been more rife than elsewhere, and had done several inoculations. In the family of a Quaker, near Hertford, an infant of two and a half years developed no more than twenty pustules, which lasted only three or four days; but six domestics of the house, four men and two maids, "who all in their turn were wont to hug and caress this child whilst under the operation and the pustules were out upon her" (Maitland), caught natural smallpox in varying degrees of severity, some of them having a narrow escape, while one of the maids died.

The question that people were really anxious about was the immediate risk to the inoculated; and as there were occasional fatalities, especially to the age of childhood, inoculation made little progress. In the first year of its trial in England it was done on the greatest scale by Dr Nettleton, of Halifax, whose practice remains for more particular notice. Apart from his cases, which numbered sixty-one, the following are all that were known in England from the month of April, 1721, to the end of 1722[1]:

By Mr Amyand, surgeon, London	17
„ Mr Maitland, surgeon, London and elsewhere	57
„ Dr Dover, London	4
„ Mr Weymish, London	3
„ Rev. Mr Johnson, London	3
„ Dr Brady, Portsmouth	4
„ Messrs Smith and Dymes, Chichester	13
„ Mr Waller, Gosport	3
„ A woman at Leicester	8
„ Dr Williams, Haverfordwest	6
„ Two others near Haverfordwest	2
„ Dr French, Bristol	1

The inoculations in all England in 1723 reached the considerable total of 292; but in 1724 they were no more than 40, being distributed among the various operators as follows:

Amyand, London	11
Maitland, London	4
Pemberton, London	3
Cheselden, London	1
Pawlett, London	1
Howman and Offley, Norwich	3
Beeston, Ipswich	3
Lake, Sevenoaks	3
Goodwin, Winchester	1
Mrs Ringe, Shaftesbury	2
Skinner, Ottery St Mary	6
Tolcher, Plymouth	2

[1] Jurin, *Account of the Success of Inoculating the Smallpox.* Annual reports from 1723 to 1726.

In the next two years, 1725–26, Amyand and Maitland had respectively 66 and 37 cases in London, the other known cases in London being 30. Maitland had also 16 cases in Scotland. Sir Thomas Lyttelton had 4 at Hagley. All the known cases in those two years, including Nettleton's at Halifax, came to 256, with four deaths of somewhat conspicuous persons. In 1727 the inoculations fell to 87, and in 1728 to 37. The total in eight years was 897, with 17 deaths. For the next ten or twelve years none were heard of in Britain. The check, however, was only temporary. The practice revived, extended among the rich, at length reached the common people in some counties, and gave rise to important developments of scientific doctrine. The greater these developments the more interesting the origins, which we shall now examine.

The popular Origins of Inoculation.

Six years before the Greek inoculation was tried in London, Kennedy, the travelled Scot, had compared the Constantinople practice with one that he knew of in his native country: "So also in some parts of the highlands of Scotland they infect their children by rubbing them with a kindly pock." This indigenous Scots practice was confirmed by Professor Monro, the first, of Edinburgh, in 1765:

"When the smallpox appears favourable in one child of a family, the parents generally allow commerce of their other children with the one in the disease ; nay, I am assured that in some of the remote highland parts of this country it has been an old practice of parents whose children have not had the smallpox to watch for an opportunity of some child having a good mild smallpox, that they may communicate the disease to their own children by making them bedfellows to those in it, and by tying worsted threads wet with the pocky matter round their wrists."

And, to make it clear that this was not the same as the method afterwards used of procuring the smallpox, he adds that the latter was not known in Scotland until Maitland introduced it, in 1726[1]. In Wales the curious practice of buying the smallpox was found to be indigenous[2]. One young woman in a village near Milford Haven testified in 1722 that, some eight or nine

[1] Alexander Monro, primus, *An Account of the Inoculation of the Smallpox in Scotland.* Edin. 1765 (Reply to circular of queries issued by the dean and delegates of the Faculty of Medicine of Paris).
[2] *Phil. Trans.* 1722: papers by Perrot Williams, M.D. (p. 262), and Richard Wright (p. 267).

years before, she had bought twenty pocky scabs of one in the smallpox, and had held them in her hand, with the result that she sickened with the infection in ten or twelve days and had upwards of thirty large pustules in her face and elsewhere—at least ten more than she had bargained for. A schoolboy of Oswestry, who had since become an attorney and must have known the nature of an affidavit, bought, as he positively affirmed, for three-pence of a certain lady twelve pustules of smallpox (at a farthing each), and rubbed the matter into his hand with the back of his pocket-knife ; a sore remained on the hand as well as pockpits in his face.

There was nothing remarkable in these methods of procuring smallpox except an occasional element of superstition or freak. It was not unusual in England for educated persons to let smallpox go through all their children after it had attacked one of them, just as it is regarded an economy by many to have done with the measles. On 15 September, 1685, Evelyn travelling to Portsmouth in the company of Pepys, stopped to make a call at Bagshot at the house of Mrs Graham, a former maid of honour to the queen. " Her eldest son was now sick of the smallpox, but in a likely way to recover, and others of her children ran about and among the infected, which she said she let them do on purpose that they might whilst young pass that fatal disease she fancied they were to undergo one time or other, and that this would be for the best." It would be for the best because children from five to ten or fifteen (the older writers said even infants) ran far less risk from the attack than at the higher ages, and seldom died of it.

Similar means of procuring smallpox for children were used in other countries. La Motraye, who rode through the Caucasus in 1712, was told that children, to give them the smallpox, were placed in the same bed with one who had it, the mothers sometimes carrying them a whole day's journey to any village where they heard of someone being attacked. He professes also to have seen a child of four inoculated with smallpox matter at five places (the region of the heart, the pit of the stomach, the navel, the right wrist and the left foot) by an old woman who used " three needles tied together[1]." The idea

---

[1] *Voyages du Sr. A. de la Motraye.* Tome II. La Haye, 1727, Chap. III. p. 98. He saw Timoni at Constantinople on his return from the Caucasus. Timoni used " a three-edged surgeon's needle," which is more intelligible than three needles

of barter was widely spread in those practices of procuring smallpox on favourable terms. We have seen that the Welsh had it. Bruce found it in his travels to the sources of the Nile[1]. African negroes are known also to have carried with them to the West Indies the practice of "buying the yaws," which is also a contagious and inoculable disease of the skin. The earliest medical notices of buying the smallpox come from Poland in 1671 and 1677. A case having been published in the *Miscellanea Curiosa* of the Imperial German Academy, in which a quartan ague was alleged to have been got rid of by transferring it to a brute animal, Dr Vollgnad, of Warsaw wrote: "There is a similar superstition not uncommon among our nurses, who instruct the children under their charge to buy for a few farthings a certain number of pocks from one infected with the smallpox, in the belief that those who purchase that disagreeable commodity will be affected with a more scanty eruption and will be the sooner freed from the disease and with the less risk[2]." Six years after, Dr Simon Schultz, of Thorn, physician

tied together. La Motraye's travellers' tales have not enjoyed the best credit. But this of the inoculation in Circassia has been made by Voltaire the sole basis of his spirited account of inoculation as the national practice of that country (*Lettres sur les Anglais*, Lettre XI. "Sur l'insertion de la petite-vérole," 1727, reprinted as the article "Inoculation" in his *Dict. Philosophique*, 1764). There has never been a grosser instance of a myth constructed in cold blood. The fable does not need refutation because it is mere assertion, in the manner of a *philosophe*. But the British ambassador at Constantinople made inquiries concerning the alleged Georgian or "Circassian" practice in 1755, at the instance of Maty, the foreign secretary of the Royal Society (*Phil. Trans.* XLIX. 104). A Capuchin friar, "a grave sober man" who had returned shortly before from a sixteen years' residence in Georgia and "gives an account of the virtues and vices, good and evil, of that country with plainness and candour," solemnly declared to Mr Porter that he never heard of inoculation "at Akalsike, Imiritte or Tiflis," and was persuaded that it had never been known in the Caucasus. It was impossible that either the public or private practice of inoculation could have been concealed from him, as he went in and out among the people practising physic. He had often attended them in the smallpox, which, he said, was unusually severe there. On the other hand La Motraye says: "I found the Circassians becoming more beautiful as we penetrated into the mountains. As I saw no one marked with the smallpox, it occurred to me to ask if they had any secret to protect them from the ravages which this enemy of beauty makes among all nations. They told me, Yes; and gave me to understand that it was inoculating, or communicating it to those whom they wished to preserve by taking the matter from one who had it and mixing the same with the blood at incisions which they made. On this I resolved to see the operation, if it were possible, and made inquiry in every village that we passed through if there was anyone about to have it done. I soon found an opportunity in a village named Degliad, where I heard that they were going to inoculate a young girl of four or five years old just as we were passing." This was published fifteen years after, Timoni's account being given in an Appendix.

[1] *Travels*, IV. 484. See also for Algiers, *Lond. Med. Journ.* XI. 141. In those cases there was no inoculation by puncture or otherwise.

[2] *Miscell. Curiosa s. Ephemer. Med.-Phys. Acad. Nat. Curios.* Decuria I., An. 2, Obs. CLXV. 1671. D. Thomae Bartholini, "Febris ex Imaginatione." Scholion by D. Henr. Vollgnad, Vratislaviae practicus.

to the king of Poland, wrote that the same practice of buying the smallpox obtained also in that part of Poland: "What I have first to remark," he says, "is that, in most cases if not in all, those infants that buy of the infected (whether in their proper persons or through others), while they may have few pocks, yet fall into a more serious illness than otherwise (*gravius reliquis decumbant*): which I remember to have happened to my younger brother Johannes, to say nothing of others[1]."

These early references to buying the smallpox were made *à propos* of the 17th century practice of sympathetic transference of disease from one to another, or from man to brute, or to plants, stones, holes in the ground, etc.[2], and were published as instances of "a similar superstition." The case of a transferred ague which called them forth had been sent to the *Curiosa* of the Academy by Thomas Bartholin, the celebrated anatomist of Copenhagen. Ten years before, he had written in the *Theatrum Sympatheticum Auctum*[3] (to which also Dr Sylvester Rattray, of Glasgow, and Sir Kenelm Digby contributed): "I disclose a great mystery of nature. The transplantation of diseases is a stupendous remedy, by means of which the ailments of this or that person are transferred to a brute animal, or to another person, or to some inanimate thing" —various methods being instanced. He returned to the subject in 1673 under the title of the Transplantation of Disease, the name by which Pylarini first described the engrafting of smallpox[4]. It was the transfusion of blood, a foible of the time, especially at the Royal Society in London, which set Bartholin to his second essay. He expected that health, in the one case, or disease in the other, might be transplanted to another's veins with the blood. It would be an incomparable addition to the amenities of life to be able to draw off in a syringe the diseased blood of a familiar friend and bring it to a better coction by one's own juices[5].

---

[1] *Miscell. Curiosa, l. c.* 1677.

[2] See Drage, *Pyretologia.* Lond. 1665.

[3] Nuremberg, 1662, p. 529.

[4] La Condamine cites Bartholin's essay on Transplantation as if it really contained the germ of inoculation, which it does not, the single reference in it to smallpox being in a passage where the contagion of that, as well as of plague, syphilis and dysentery, is said to be capable of being turned aside from one to another.

[5] Drage (*Pyretologia*) gives a case where an ague passed from one person to another in the fumes of blood drawn in phlebotomy. He says also (*Sicknesses and Diseases from Witchcraft*, 1665, p. 21) that a witch could be made to take back a disease by scratching her and drawing blood.

Bartholin discovered the germ of these scientific developments in the scape-goat of the Israelites and in the miracle of the swine of Gadara[1]. In his own doctrine of transplantation, others in turn have found the germ of inoculation, Pylarini having actually adopted the 17th century name, with the proviso that the transplantation of smallpox was not sympathetic but *res vera mera pura.* The older idea of transplanting smallpox was to get rid of it. "Some persons in the smallpox," says Slatholm, of Buntingford, in 1657, "keep a sheep or a wether beside them in the chamber, those animals being apt to receive the envenomed matter and to draw it to themselves[2]." The developments of folk-lore are erratic ; one thing leads to another, but not necessarily in a logical sequence. Transference had somehow become the inoculation which Pylarini first found in the practice of a woman from the Morea or from Bosnia, being still in its superstitious stage. The woman drew blood and rubbed the smallpox matter into the bleeding points ; but whether she did so with a physiological or a symbolical intent we shall probably never know. She told Dr Le Duc[3], who submitted to inoculation at her hands, that she had received the secret from the Virgin ; during the operation she muttered prayers to the Virgin, and, on finishing it, requested an oblation of two wax candles to be sent to the shrine of the Virgin her patroness in Thessaly. She pricked the skin of the face at the four points which are touched in making the sign of the Cross, and at the points of the hands and feet which are pierced by the nails in the Crucifix. Voltaire says that Lady Mary Wortley Montagu's chaplain objected to inoculation because it was an un-Christian practice. He must have been strangely ill-informed if he did so ; for at Constantinople it was practised by the Christians only and not at all by the Mussulmans, who, by Kennedy's account, were somewhat doubtful of its utility.

Pylarini and Timoni very properly dropped the symbolism of the Greek woman, and inserted the matter at any convenient spot, choosing usually the skin of the forearm. Therewith they

[1] *De Transplantatione Morborum.* Hafniae, 1673, p. 24.
[2] *De Febribus,* u. s. In the plague, a live cock applied to the botch was thought to draw the venom ; the cock was then to be buried. Also crusts of hot ryeloaf hung in the room where one had died of plague absorbed the venom. Gabelhover, *The Boock of Physicke,* Dort, 1599, p. 298. Bread was used for the same purpose in fevers as late as 1765. Muret, *Mém. par la Société Econom. de Berne,* 1766.
[3] *Dissertationes in Inoculationem Variolarum,* a J. à Castro, G. Harris, et A. le Duc. Lugd. Bat. 1722.

took the practice under scientific protection. At the same time Pylarini was careful to explain that this transference of disease, although he called it by Bartholin's old name of "transplantation," was a real thing, and in no way akin to the sympathetic or magnetic transference whose name it bore. A real thing it undoubtedly was: a visible effect did follow in most cases—some ten, or twenty or thirty watery pimples on the skin. The effect being thus real, Pylarini and Timoni laid down at the outset the doctrine that the smallpox matter inserted in minute quantity was a ferment, which produced an ebullition in the mass of the blood. The common people, who had been procuring the smallpox for their children in other ways than by puncture and insertion, also knew that the transplanting was a real thing : it was smallpox, and nothing else, that they designed to procure, peradventure it might be mild smallpox.

While Pylarini used the name of Transplantation, Timoni used the name of Inoculation. Both names were figures of speech taken from the gardener's art. Inoculation, or ineying, was a form of grafting, the taking of the "eye" or resting-bud of one kind of fruit-tree and fixing it upon the stock of another kind. The effect of a graft upon a fruit-tree is one of the most remarkable in nature : the incorporation of a bud from a nearly allied species at a particular part of the stock causes the whole tree to assume some characters of the other tree, the change being greatest in the fruit. An effect at once so real, so useful, and so familiar could not fail to take hold of the imagination. Accordingly we find the ineying or grafting of trees used in a correct figure, as in Hamlet's "for virtue cannot so inoculate our old stock but we shall relish of it." Between a fruit-tree modified as to its fruit by the permanent incorporation of a strange shoot, and an animal body infected of purpose with diseased matter, there is no very exact analogy. Figurative names, as well as metaphors, are apt to be mixed ideas. Correct science avoids the one vice, as correct style avoids the other. Transplantation had in any case too many fanciful associations to be retained as the name for the new practice in smallpox ; inoculation, on the other hand, was still unspoiled as a medical term, while its wonderful effects were obvious in the familiar art of the gardener.

In all the developments or modifications of this practice, the intention was still to procure the smallpox by art. The idea of antidote or counter-poison did not enter into it at all. Yet the idea of a counter-poison was quite familiar, as in the following passage from a medical writer of the time of James I.[1] :

" But here a great doubt and controversie may arise : whether, as sometimes we see one poyson to be the expeller of another poyson, so in like sort, whether one stinking savour, and graveolent or ill odour, and vapour of some pestilent breath or ayre, may bee the proper amulet or preservative against any such poyson, to bee hanged about the necke : for at this time let it bee granted (to please some) that tabacco is of no good smell or sent, and that it is a little poysonous.   For wee see some daily in the time of any generall or grievous infection of the plague, for avoidance thereof, and for preservation sake, will smell unto the stinking savour of some loathsome privie, or filthy camerine and sinke ; and this they make reckoning is one of the best counter-poysons that may be devised against any pestiferous infection : for their nature being inured to these, they will afterwards not seeme to passe for any pestilent malignitie of the ayre, and dare boldly adventure without any prejudice, or impeachment to their health, into any place or companie whatsoever.   And to perswade us the more easily to this, they object to us for example sake, those women that spend their dayes continually in hospitals for pilgrims, and for poore travellers, who are accustomed to every abominable savour of the sicke ; whereof we shall never see, or very seldome, any of them either to be taken or die with any pestiferous infection though never so dangerous."

While he admits these to be instances of counter-poisons having a prophylactic effect against epidemic sickness, he denies, what some had maintained, that "either the French Pockes or the quartan ague is a *Superseder* of the plague[2]."

Results of the first Inoculations; the Controversy in England.

Thus far we have traced the rise of inoculation as an idea. It was one way of procuring the smallpox, which had gradually arisen out of other fanciful or real modes of infection. The populace for long retained a preference for giving their children the smallpox by exposing them to the contagion of it ; in the last quarter of the 18th century, Haygarth found the common people of Chester still following the earlier practice of inviting the smallpox in the natural way[3]. It is even more remarkable

---

[1] Gardiner's *Triall of Tabacco*. London, 1610, fol. 38.

[2] *Ibid.* fol. 43.   *The City Remembrancer*, 1769, a work claiming to be Gideon Harvey's, says that in the Great Plague of London, 1665, some low persons contracted the French pox of purpose to keep off the infection of plague.

[3] *Inquiry how to prevent the Smallpox*, Chester, 1785 :—" No care was taken to prevent the spreading ; but on the contrary there seemed to be a general wish that all the children might have it."   Cited from Mr Edwards, surgeon, of Upton, near Chester.   Again (*Sketch of a Plan, &c.*, 1793, p. 491), "They neither feared it nor shunned it.   Much more frequently, by voluntary and intentional intercourse, they endeavoured to catch the infection."

that Huxham, the ablest epidemiologist in England during the first period of inoculation, preferred that children should take the disease naturally, believing that they might be so "prepared" to receive the seeds of it by the breath as to have always a sufficiently mild but effective dose of it.   Still, the insertion of smallpox matter at a puncture or wound of the arm appeared to many to have advantages over the natural way.   In London it was taken up by the Court, by the Court doctors, and by the Royal Society, the leading physicians in favour of it having been Sloane, Mead, Arbuthnot and Jurin.   It appears that Freind, a more learned physician than any of these, was adverse to it.   It was to him that Wagstaffe, physician to St Bartholomew's Hospital, dedicated a hostile essay on inoculation when it was new; and Freind himself brought into his *History of Physic*, published in 1725–26, the following sarcastic passage upon John of Gaddesden, whom he regarded as a high-placed charlatan :

"He had an infallible plaster and caustick for a rupture; could cure a cancer from an outward cause with red dock.   And if he had lived in our day, he would, I don't question, have been at the head of the Inoculators ; and in this case the position he lays down, contrary to the experience of the best physicians, that one may have the smallpox *twice*, might have served him in good stead for salvo's upon many occasions."

—which means that, in Freind's opinion, the inoculated smallpox was no security against a subsequent attack in the natural way[1].

Wagstaffe, in his printed letter to Freind, sums up the objections to inoculated smallpox as follows :

"Some have had the distemper not at all, others to a small degree, others the worst sort, and some have died of it.   I have given instances of those who have had it after inoculation in the common way; and consequently as it is hazardous, so 'twill neither answer the main design of preventing the distemper for the future.   I have considered what the effects may be of inoculating on an ill habit of body, and how destructive it may prove to spread a distemper that is contagious : and how widely at length the authors in this subject disagree among themselves, and how little they have seen of the

[1] *History of Physic*, Lond. 1725–26, II. 288.   This was written at a time when the novelty of inoculation had passed off, and may be taken as Freind's mature opinion.   Douglass, of Boston, writing in 1730, implies that Freind's objections had been overcome; which may mean no more than he says in general : "Yet from repeated tryals the Anti-Inoculators do now acknowledge that inoculation, generally speaking, is a more easy way of undergoing the smallpox."   Condamine, in his French essay of 1755, counts Freind among the original supporters of inoculation, and ridicules the opposition to it.   Munk, in citing the title of Wagstaffe's *Letter to Dr Freind showing the danger and uncertainty of Inoculating the Smallpox* (London, 1722), omits the words "to Dr Freind," at the same time describing the pamphlet as "specious." There seems no reason to doubt that Freind shared Wagstaffe's views.

practice :—all which seem to me to be just and necessary consequences of these new-fangled notions, as well as convincing reasons for the disuse of the practice[1]."

These objections were shared by several, including Blackmore, Clinch, and Massey, the apothecary to Christ's Hospital.

On the other hand Jurin, who took the lead in defending inoculation, reduced the issues to two[2]:

1. Whether the distemper given by inoculation be an effectual security to the patient against his having the smallpox afterwards in the natural way?

2. Whether the hazard of inoculation be considerably less than that of the natural smallpox?

These questions, thus put forward as of equal moment, did not receive equally full handling. Jurin dismissed the former question in a brief sentence: "Our experience, so far as it goes, has hitherto strongly favoured the affirmative side"—a conditional assent which became an absolute affirmative after a short time. Having thus disposed of the question which has all the scientific or pathological interest, he turned with his whole energy to give a precise arithmetical demonstration of what no one could doubt, namely, that inoculated smallpox was many times less fatal than smallpox in the natural way,—having got the idea of such a comparison from Nettleton as well as a large part of the statistics necessary for it. Jurin's statement of the questions at issue, and his manner of answering them, became the received mode, so much so that even towards the end of the eighteenth century one finds capable medical men contrasting the almost infinitesimal mortality from inoculation, as then practised, with the high mortality from the natural smallpox, as if that were the question at issue. The permanent impression in favour of inoculation made by Jurin's arithmetic was shown a generation later, when Dr George Baker pronounced an eulogy upon him in the Harveian Oration before the College of Physicians in 1761[3]. "It was his special glory," said the orator, to have "confirmed the practice of inoculation by his ex-

---

[1] Hecquet, of Paris, who is supposed to have been the original of Dr Sangrado in 'Gil Blas,' gave the following reasons against inoculation (*Raisons de doutes contre l'Inoculation*) : "Its antiquity is not sufficiently ascertained : the operation rests upon false facts : it is unjust, void of art, destitute of rules :......it doth not prevent the natural smallpox :......it bears no likeness to physic, and savours strongly of magic."

[2] James Jurin, M.D., *Account of the Success of Inoculation*, 1724, p. 3.

[3] G. Baker, M.D., *Oratio Harveiana*, 1761, p. 24.

periments and his authority." There was only one experiment, and it was a remarkable one. The Princess of Wales had begged George I. to pardon six Newgate criminals under sentence of death on condition that they would submit to be inoculated. It was assumed that those six had not had smallpox in infancy or childhood, and Sloane, relating the facts in a letter to Ranby some years after, does in fact call them "six condemned criminals who had not had the smallpox[1]." The concurrence of six persons belonging to the criminal classes and about to be hanged together in Newgate, of whom none had already gone through the common infantile trouble of London and other large towns, was singular. They were inoculated, and it was found that they had escaped the death penalty on very easy terms: John Alcock, aged twenty, had most smallpox, but even he had "not more than sixty pustules"; Richard Evans, aged nineteen, had none, but his antecedents were inquired into, and then it was found that he had had smallpox in gaol only six months before. One of the others, a woman named Elizabeth, was chosen for the grand crucial experiment. Sir Hans Sloane and Dr Steigerthal clubbed together to pay her expenses to Hertford where smallpox was then very prevalent; thither Elizabeth went and ministered among the sick; she lay in bed with one in the smallpox, or she lay in bed with various in the smallpox; at all events she exposed herself to contagion and did not catch it, according to certificates from the woman she lodged with and from another person, which certificates were published with much formality and lawyer-like precision[2]. This was the single experiment in which Jurin had any part. What were the chances of her having had smallpox in childhood? What were the chances of her knowing anything about it, or telling the truth about it if she knew? (One of her fellows in the experiment upon the pardoned convicts had smallpox only six months before, but the fact was not discovered until it was wanted.) What were the chances of her taking smallpox at Hertford, supposing that she had hitherto escaped it? These questions do not appear to have been debated[3].

---

[1] Sloane, *Phil. Trans.* XLIX. 516.

[2] They are given in Maitland's *Vindication*, 1722, and in one of Jurin's papers.

[3] In regard to the last of them, when Frewen in 1759 was controverting the fancy of Boerhaave and Cheyne that smallpox might be hindered from coming on in a person exposed to contagion by a timely use of the Aethiops mineral, he said there was a fallacy in the evidence, because many persons ordinarily escape smallpox "who had been supposed to be in the greatest danger of taking it." Huxham also pointed out

Such was the experiment by which Jurin "confirmed the practice of inoculation." As for his authority, it was doubtless considerable; but it was more as a follower of the Newtonian mathematics than as a pathologist or physician, and most of all as one of the secretaries of the Royal Society in the last years of Newton's presidency, that he spoke with authority[1]. His influence, such as it was, availed little. The practice of inoculation fell into total disuse in England after a few years' trial, so that in 1728 Jurin himself was prepared to see it "exploded."

The principal reason of inoculation having been tried upon decreasing numbers in England after the first year or two, and of its having been dropped absolutely for a time, was the death of some persons of good family, both adults and children—a sacrifice of life which could not but seem gratuitous. Those deaths were not from the fulness of the eruption but from anomalous effects. When inoculation began in London in 1721, it was according to the Greek method of inserting a minute quantity of matter at two or more places. In the case of the Newgate felons, Maitland had reason to do the inoculations over

that a person might be susceptible at one time but not at another, or insusceptible altogether; and the elder Heberden wrote: "Many instances have occurred to me which show that one who had never had the smallpox may safely associate, and even be in the same bed with a variolous patient for the first two or three days of the eruption without any danger of receiving the infection." William Heberden, sen., M.D., *Commentaries on Disease*, 1802, p. 437.

[1] Dr James Jurin was educated at Cambridge, and elected a fellow of Trinity College. He became a schoolmaster at Newcastle, where he also gave scientific lectures. Coming to London, with a Leyden medical degree, he devoted himself to the Newtonian mathematics and was made one of the secretaries of the Royal Society, Newton being the president. He was one of the original physicians of the new hospital founded in the Borough by Guy, the rich bookseller. He made a fortune by medical practice, and was elected president of the College of Physicians a few weeks before he died. In medicine his name is associated with the inoculation statistics, the idea of which, as well as most of the substance, he got from Nettleton, and with "Jurin's Lixivium Lithontripticum," or solvent for the stone, the idea of which belonged originally to Mrs Johanna Stevens, and was sold by her to the State for five thousand pounds on the 16th of June, 1739, the prescriptions having been made public in the *London Gazette* of 19th June. On the 15th of December, 1744, Jurin was called to see the Earl of Orford (Sir Robert Walpole), who was suffering from stone, either renal or vesical. He began administering his alkaline solvent, "four times stronger than the strongest capital soap-lye," and during the six weeks of his attendance had given his patient thirty-six ounces of it. Horace Walpole made him angry by arguing on the medicine: "It is of so great violence that it is to split a stone when it arrives at it, and yet it is to do no damage to all the tender intestines through which it must first pass. I told him I thought it was like an admiral going on a secret expedition of war with instructions which are not to be opened till he arrives in such a latitude." (*Letters of Horace Walpole*, Cunningham, I. 339.) His services were at length dispensed with, and the earl, whose case was probably hopeless before, died in a few weeks. A war of pamphlets followed, Ranby, the serjeant-surgeon, maintaining that the patient had "died of the lixivium." Mead, also, expressed himself strongly upon the attempt to use a modification of Mrs Stevens's solvent.

again after three days, being dissatisfied with the appearance of
the original punctures.   They are admitted to have had a slight
disease (the man who had most had only some sixty pustules on
his whole body), so that Dr Wagstaffe, who went to see them,
said in his letter to Dr Freind: "Upon the whole, Sir, in the
cases mentioned, there was nothing like the smallpox, either in
symptoms, appearances, advance of the pustules, or the course of
the distemper."   Many of the other early cases had likewise a
slight eruption ; when numbers are given, the pocks are "not
more than eleven to eighteen" (as in Maitland's case of Prince
Frederick at Hanover in 1724), or "not above twenty in all upon
her" (as in Maitland's case of a child near Hertford, in 1721).   Of
the first six charity children inoculated, one had no eruption; of the
next five, three had no smallpox from inoculation.   The cases that
died after inoculation during the first seven years of the practice
—seventeen in England and Scotland and two in Dublin, most
of them children—owed the fatal result for the most part to some
peculiar prostration or lowered vitality, in two cases actually to
pyaemia, the eruption being kept back altogether or but feebly
thrown out[1].   This was the danger of arbitrarily procuring the
smallpox which Dr Schultz remarked upon in 1677, with
reference to the Polish practice of "buying" the disease ; most,
if not all the cases known to him, although they may have had
few pocks, yet fell into more serious illness (*gravius reliquis
decumbant*).   The risk of arbitrarily forcing infection upon a
child at a time when it might not be ready for it, or in a position
to deal with it in its blood, was afterwards recognized, and was
provided against in the long and tedious preparation which the
subject for inoculation had to undergo.

While those in England who followed Maitland in inoculating after the Greek fashion produced for the most part an
infinitesimal number of pustules or watery pimples, there were
others at a distance from London who inoculated by a method
of their own and gave their patients a more real smallpox.   The
chief of these were Dr Thomas Nettleton of Halifax, and
Dr Zabdiel Boylston, of Boston, New England[2].   Nettleton
made a long incision through the whole thickness of the skin of

[1] The fatalities are given somewhat fully in Jurin's annual accounts of the *Success
of Inoculation*, 1723—27.
[2] John Wreden, body-surgeon to the Prince of Wales, author of *An Essay on the
Inoculation of the Smallpox* (Lond. 1779), may also be counted among those who
gave a more real smallpox. See especially his cases at Hanover.

one arm and of the opposite leg, and laid therein a small piece
of cotton soaked in smallpox matter, which he secured in the
wound with a plaister for twenty-four hours.   Boylston says:
"The Turkey way of scarifying and applying the nutshell &c.,
I soon left off, and made an incision through the true skin," the
rest also of his procedure being the same as Nettleton's.   And
just as those two inoculators devised for themselves a more real
method of giving the smallpox by insertion, taking means to
ensure the absorption of the matter into the blood, so they
procured in many cases, although not in all, an eruption of
pustules on the skin which came near to being the same as that
of natural smallpox of the average discrete type.

In the Boston practice, "the number of the pustules is not
alike in all; in some they are very few; in others they amount
to an hundred; yea in many they amount unto several hundreds,
frequently unto more than what the accounts from the Levant
say is usual there[1]."   Nettleton's account, which was printed in
the same number of the *Philosophical Transactions* as that from
New England, says of the pustules on the skin at large: "The
number was very different: in some not above ten or twenty,
most frequently from fifty to two hundred; and some have had
more than could well be numbered, but never of the confluent
sort....They commonly come out very round and florid, and
many times rose as large as any I have observed of the natural
sort, going off with a yellow crust or scab as usual[2]."

The smallpox procured by inoculation in these English and
American trials was thus a more real form of that disease than
at Constantinople; compared with the number of pustules
given by Timoni and Pylarini, the Boston and Halifax numbers
are multiplied ten times.

Nettleton thus expressed his belief that inoculated smallpox
saved from the natural disease, at the same time grounding that
belief on the reality or substantial nature of the artificial
disease:

"Some of those who have been inoculated, that are grown up, have
afterwards attended others in the smallpox, and it has often happen'd that in
families where some children have been inoculated, others have been afterwards seized in the natural way, and they have lain together in the same bed
all the time; but we have not yet found that ever any had the distemper

---

[1] H. Newman, "Way of Proceeding in the Smallpox Inoculation in New
England." *Phil. Trans.* XXXII. (1722), p. 33.
[2] Thomas Nettleton, Letter to Whitaker. *Ibid.* p. 39.

twice; neither is there any reason to suppose it possible, there being no difference that can be observed betwixt the natural and artificial sort, but only that in the latter the pustules are fewer in number, and all the rest of the symptoms are in the same proportion more favourable[1]."

Nettleton returned to the question of the reality of inoculated smallpox, which is the root of the whole matter, in his second letter, to Jurin[2]: "The question whether the distemper raised by inoculation is really the smallpox is not so much disputed now as it was at first....There is usually no manner of difference to be observed betwixt the one sort and the other, when the number of pustules is nearly the same; but in both there are almost infinite degrees of the distemper according to the difference of that number. All the variation that can be perceived of the ingrafted smallpox from the natural is, that in the former the pustules are commonly fewer in number, and all the rest of the symptoms are in the same proportion more favourable. They exactly resemble what we call the distinct sort....It will follow as a corollary, that those who have been inoculated are in no more danger of receiving the distemper again than those who have had it in the ordinary way. And this is also thus far confirmed by experience."

It does not appear that Nettleton based so much upon the subsequent experience as upon the antecedent probability. Thus he says of some cases :

"These had the eruptions so imperfect as to leave me a little in doubt, but two of these have since been sufficiently try'd by being constantly with those who had the smallpox, without receiving any infection; which makes me inclined to believe they will always be secure from any danger. As to all the rest, neither I nor anybody else who saw them did in the least question that they had the true smallpox."

Nettleton began his inoculations in and around Halifax during a considerable epidemic of smallpox in the winter of 1721–22, of which the following figures were collected by himself (as well as statistics for Leeds, Bradford, Rochdale and other places):

	Cases	Deaths
Halifax	276	43
Part of Halifax parish towards Bradford	297	59
Another part of Halifax parish	268	28

In the town of Halifax the smallpox was of a more favourable type than usual, whereas in Leeds at the same time (792 cases and 189 deaths) it was more than usually mortal. In the country round Halifax there was more smallpox than in the town ; but the epidemic in general ceased in the spring of 1722. As the people mostly disliked the idea of inoculation, Nettleton did not urge it upon them, but inoculated only the children of those who favoured it. Down to the 22nd of April, 1722, he had inoculated about forty, with one death ; at the date of 16

---

[1] *Phil. Trans. l. c.* p. 46. A remark follows which is not quite clear: "There is one observation which I have made, tho' I would not yet lay any great stress upon it, that in families where any have been inoculated, those who have been afterwards seized never had an ill sort of smallpox, but always recovered very well."

[2] *Phil. Trans.* 1722, p. 209. Dated from Halifax, 16 Dec. 1722.

June, he had done fifteen more, his total to the end of 1722 being 61.   In 1723 he did nineteen inoculations, in 1724 none, in 1725 and 1726 about forty (in an epidemic of 230 cases, and 28 deaths in Barstand Ripponden and another part of Halifax parish), and in writing to Hartley of Bury St Edmunds in 1730, he gave his total at that date as 119, from which it appears that he had ceased to inoculate after 1726.   His name does not appear again in the controversy, and it is probable that he acquiesced in the tacit verdict against inoculation which Jurin himself, in 1728, seemed to think was imminent.

Besides this centre of inoculation in Yorkshire in the midst of epidemic smallpox, the only other of importance in the first trials of the practice was at Boston, New England.   The smallpox epidemic there in 1721 was a very severe one.   There had been no smallpox in Boston since 1702, so that a large part of the population were susceptible of it.   The infection was brought by a ship from Barbados in the middle of April, 1721, and made slow progress at first, according to the following table of deaths from it[1] :

Deaths from Smallpox in Boston.

1721–1722

May	1	October	402
June	8	November	249
July	20	December	31
August	26	January	6
September	101		
		Total	844

In the course of the epidemic some 5989 persons were attacked, or more than half the population (10,565).   All the rest, save about 750, had been through the smallpox before.   Inoculation played a very subordinate part amidst these dreadful scenes of smallpox.   Its instigator was the Rev. Dr Cotton Mather, who had been shown by Dr Douglass the numbers of the *Philosophical Transactions* with Timoni's and Pylarini's papers in them.   The reverend doctor "surreptitiously" employed Douglass's rival, Dr Boylston, to begin inoculating, in July, 1721, or a few months after the first trials in London.   Boylston

---

[1] Dr William Douglass to Dr Cadwallader Colden, 28 July, 1721, and 1 May, 1722, in *Massachu. Hist. Soc. Collections*, Series 4, vol. II. pp. 166-9.   Also *A Dissertation concerning Inoculation of Smallpox*. By W. D[ouglass]. Boston, 1730; and *A Practical Essay concerning the Smallpox*. By William Douglass, M.D. Boston, 1730.

inoculated 244, whites and negroes, and admitted the deaths of six of them, probably by inhaled infection[1]. But Douglass says:

"The precise number of those who dyed by inoculation in Boston, I am afraid will never be known because of the crowd of the sick and dead whilst inoculation prevailed most, the inoculator and relations inviolably keeping the secret....Some porters who at that time were employed to carry the dead to their graves say that it was whispered, in sundry houses where the dead were carried from, that the person had been inoculated. I could name some who are suspected, but having only hearsay and conjectural evidence, I forbear to affront the surviving relations. I myself am certain of one more who died 'after inoculation' as they express it."

He then gives the case, which was clearly one of the natural contagion of smallpox acquired at the same time as the inoculation. In the Charleston inoculations of 1738, which were also done in the midst of an epidemic, there is little doubt that the fatalities were mostly from natural smallpox which the inoculated infection had failed to anticipate or prevent. The inoculators were often in that dilemma with their fatal cases: either the inoculation had killed the patient or it had been powerless to keep off the contagion ; sometimes they confess the former as an untoward accident, at other times they plead the latter, which appears to me to have been the more usual of the two in a time of epidemic smallpox[2].

Douglass, for all his bitterness against his rival Boylston, and his severity against the extravagant assertions and loose reasoning of the first inoculators, was far from denying the merits of inoculation, whether in theory or in practice. "We may confidently pronounce," he says, "that those who have had a genuine smallpox by inoculation never can have the smallpox again in a natural way, both by reason and experience ; but there are some who have had the usual feverish symptoms, a discharge by their incisions, with a few *imperfect* eruptions,

---

[1] Boylston, *Account of the Smallpox inoculated in New England.* London, 1726.

[2] This was admitted, in a manner, for the great Boston epidemic of 1752, by the Rev. T. Prince, *Gent. Magaz.* Sept. 1753, p. 414. The epidemic attacked 5545 (in a population of 15,684), and cut off 569. The numbers inoculated were 2124 (including 139 negroes), of which number 30 died and were included in the total of 569. Many of the inoculated, says Prince, were not careful to avoid catching the infection in the natural way ; "for I have known some, as soon as inoculated, receive visits from their friends, who had been with the sick of the same disease and 'tis likely carried infection with them ; it seems highly probable that the inoculated received the infection from them into their vitals." It may be supposed that the inoculated who were more careful formed a part of the 1843 who "moved out of town." More than a third of the population took natural smallpox in some four months (April to July) of 1752, more than a third had had it before, a severe epidemic having occurred in 1730 as well as in 1721.

that may be obnoxious to the smallpox,"—of which he gives instances. In like manner Nettleton, in Yorkshire, who took pains to make his smallpox a real thing, and succeeded in doing so as well as any inoculator ever did succeed, was persuaded that inoculated smallpox counted for a natural attack. He admitted only one failure, a case at Halifax which had been inoculated without an eruption ensuing and took smallpox by contagion a month after. Failures in England, in that sense, were fewer than the deaths directly from inoculation. The deaths were freely admitted, but any alleged failure of inoculation to ward off the natural smallpox was challenged, investigated, and denied, so that Mead, writing in 1747, declared that he knew of none. There were, however, a few cases recorded, which appear to be authentic. One of the six charity children inoculated at the instance of the Princess of Wales had taken natural smallpox twelve weeks after. The child of one Degrave, a surgeon, had a similar experience. Another familiar case was the son of a person of distinction, inoculated on 7 May, 1724, by the Rev. Mr Johnson.

On the 14th a rash came out, on the 15th there was fever, on the 16th, very little eruption to be seen and the fever gone, and on the 18th he was pronounced "secure." On that day (18th May), his sister was inoculated in the same place, both children remaining together at the inoculator's house until the 2nd of June, when the boy went home. For a day or two before the 8th of June the boy was ill, and on the 9th he began to have smallpox in the natural way, of a good sort, the disease keeping its natural course. He was supposed to have caught it from his sister, who was inoculated after his own protection was over, and was "very full of smallpox" until the 27th of May, her brother being with her[1].

Another case of failure, which must have been known to some at the time, was not published until some ten years after, when Deering brought it to light[2]:

"I was an eyewitness of the inoculation of a little boy, the child of Dr Craft, who is now a sugar-baker in the Savoy. He was inoculated by one Ahlers under the direction of Dr Steigerthal, the late king's physician in ordinary; and notwithstanding the great care there was taken in the choice of the pus, had the confluent kind severely; and twelve months after had them naturally, and though a favourable sort, yet was very full."

A boy aged three, the son of Mr Richards, M.P. for Bridport, was inoculated in 1743, and had fifty to sixty pocks which maturated and scabbed. About two years after ("one year ago") he had smallpox again, the pustules numbering from 200

<hr/>

[1] Clinch, *Rise and Progress of the Smallpox, with an Appendix to prove that Inoculation is no Security from the Natural Smallpox.* 2nd ed. 1725.
[2] C. Deering, M.D., *An Account of an Improved Method of treating the Smallpox.* Nottingham, 1736, p. 27. Woodville appears to accept this case as authentic.

to 300; when the eruption came out the fever declined and did not return. These facts are given in a letter to Dr Dod from Dr Brodrepp, grandfather of the child, who attended him on both occasions[1].

Such cases were not often heard of. As Mead said, "If such a thing happened once, why do we not see it come to pass oftener?" There was, however, little encouragement for anyone to come forward with adverse evidence; witness the case of an unfortunate Welshman, one Jones, of Oswestry, who had innocently mentioned, in writing to his son in London, that natural smallpox had followed an inoculation done by him, on 9th August, 1723, and was frightened out of his wits by the *apparatus criticus* which Jurin brought to bear upon him[2]. Another reason why so few failures could be discovered was that the inoculated were not kept long in sight. A child of Dr Timoni, the first writer on inoculation, was inoculated at Constantinople in December, 1717, at the age of six months, and had an average effect, namely ten small *boutons*. She died of smallpox in 1741, at the age of twenty-four. This failure came to light by the vigilance of the celebrated De Haën, of Vienna, an opponent of inoculation, who had been told of it by a Scots physician at Constantinople[3].

A good instance of the same thing came to light long after in the practice of the celebrated Dr Rush of Philadelphia. "I lately attended a man in the smallpox," he wrote to Lettsom, "whom I inoculated six-and-twenty years ago. He showed me a deep and extensive scar upon his arm made by the variolous matter"—without which evidence, and the man's own reminder, confirmed by his mother's recollection, Dr Rush would probably have had no reason to believe that this particular one of his inoculations had failed[4].

---

[1] Pierce Dod, M.D., F.R.S., *Several Cases in Physic.* London, 1746.

[2] Kirkpatrick, and after him Woodville, treat the alleged experience of Jones as pure fiction.

[3] La Condamine, of Paris, an amateur enthusiast for inoculation, did all he could to upset the case. He got his friend Dr Maty, foreign secretary of the Royal Society, to make inquiry through the British ambassador to the Porte. It happened that Angelo Timoni, son of the inoculator, was at that time an interpreter at the British Embassy; he applied to his mother, who re-affirmed the facts as to the inoculation of her child in infancy, and her death by the natural smallpox twenty-four years after. The only defence left was that the inoculation had not been done by Dr Timoni's own hand. La Condamine, *Mémoires pour servir à l'Histoire de l'Inoculation.* 2me Mémoire. Paris, 1768.

[4] Rush to Lettsom, Philadelphia, 17 June, 1808, in Pettigrew's *Memoirs of Lettsom,* III. 201.

In the nature of the case, such evidence of failure would seldom be opportune. It would have needed a more dramatic presentation of these cases, and many more of them, to discredit the practice of inoculation. It was, indeed, discredited, so much so that it was not practised at all in England from 1728 until about 1740; but that was owing to the disasters directly resulting from it. No amount of evidence as to the inoculated taking natural smallpox afterwards could have touched the popular imagination like the following paragraphs in the London newspapers in 1725:

> March 16, died Mrs Eyles, niece of Sir John Eyles, alderman of London, of the smallpox contracted by inoculation. June 17, died of the smallpox contracted by inoculation Arthur Hill, esquire, eldest son of Viscount Hilsborough. August 12, died of the smallpox by inoculation — Hurst, of Salisbury, esquire.

Inoculation seemed hardly worth having on these terms, granting all that was alleged of its protective power; so that it fell in England into total disuse[1]. It came on again after a time and had a long career, at first among the richer classes, and at length among the common people, who did not cease to use it for their children until it was made a felony by the Act of 1840. After its first brief success, it was revived about 1739–40, in consequence of highly favourable accounts from Charleston, South Carolina, and from Barbados and St Christopher. This second period of inoculation brings in certain modifications of the practice by which the casualties of the earlier period were avoided. The danger from blood-poisoning, pyaemia, or the like, was surmounted. At the same time the inoculated smallpox ceased to have anything of that reality, or approximation to the natural disease, which Nettleton succeeded for a time in giving to it.

Revival of Inoculation in 1740: a New Method.

As early as the Boston inoculations of 1721, the matter had now and again been taken, not from a case of the natural

---

[1] Fuller, in his *Exanthematalogia*, makes a somewhat late defence of it in 1729. But Richard Holland, who published in 1730 *A Short View of the Smallpox*, does not mention inoculation, and in the following passage he writes of smallpox as if the extravagant hopes of the preceding years had vanished: "This last season having afforded too many melancholy instances of the fatal effects of the distemper, though under the care and direction of the most eminent physicians, since the disease, notwithstanding the plainness of its symptoms, is become the *opprobrium medicinae*," &c. (p. 3).

smallpox, but from the pustules of a previous inoculation[1]. But at Charleston in 1738 there really began, doubtless in the way of empirical trial, a systematic attenuation of virus, which has had great scientific developments in our time and has come to be considered as of the essence of the inoculation principle. Describing the South Carolina practice, Kilpatrick says[2]:

"Some persons were of opinion that *the pock of the inoculated* would be too mild to convey the disease; or, at least, that it must become effete by a second or third transplantation. Experience manifested the contrary. I have inoculated from those who were infected by the matter taken from others of the inoculated, and found no defect. Mr Mowbray, who inoculated many more than any other practitioner, assured me he had infused matter in the fifth or sixth succession from the natural pock, and observed no difference....The smallest violation of the surface, if it was stained with blood, was a sufficient entrance for the matter, and the least matter was sufficient."

The last point was a return to the Greek practice, and an abandonment of the more severe method of Nettleton and Boylston.

The Charleston smallpox of 1738, imported by slave-ships from Africa, became extensively epidemic and mortal. It had been last in Charleston fourteen or fifteen years before, but only one or two died on that occasion, and hardly more than ten were attacked. But for that small outbreak, it had not been known in the South Carolina port for a generation previous to 1738. The number of victims in that year is not known precisely. As at Boston in 1721, the epidemic dragged through the spring months, and became very extensive and mortal in the hot weather of June and July. It was then that Mowbray began inoculating, most of the Charleston faculty being opposed to it. He was soon followed by Kilpatrick, who had lost one of his children in the epidemic, and was moved thereby to inoculate the other two. No exact account was kept of the inoculations, nor, we may be sure, of the protective effects; some said a thousand were inoculated, Kilpatrick says eight hundred, but the total of four hundred is also given. Eight died after

[1] *Phil. Trans.* Jan.-March, 1722: "The way of proceeding in the Small Pox inoculated in New England." Communicated by Henry Newman, Esq. of the Middle Temple, p. 33, § 3: "Yet we find the variolous matter fetched from those that have the inoculated smallpox altogether as agreeable and effectual as any other."

[2] *An Essay on Inoculation: occasioned by the Smallpox being brought into S. Carolina in the year* 1738. By J. Kilpatrick. London, 1743, p. 50. The essay had been "first printed in South Carolina," the London edition of 1743 having an Appendix dealing historically with the Charleston epidemic of 1738.

inoculation, six whites and two negresses. One child of ten months died in convulsions on the ninth day after inoculation, with few signs of smallpox; a minister, aged 40, sickened on the third or fourth day, which was too soon for the artificial disease, and was almost certainly the effects of the inhaled virus; two other adult whites died in such circumstances as to make it doubtful whether they died of inoculation or of coexistent natural smallpox; one negress died of confluent smallpox, having treated herself unwisely; while two other children and a negress died after inoculation, of whom no particulars are known.   Besides the fatal cases after inoculation, some "had an eruption that might be called a moderate confluence"; but in these cases also it is not clear that infection was not taken in the natural way: as regards one gentlewoman who had confluent smallpox, it was not certain in what manner she received the infection, whilst "Miss Mary Rhett's eruption did not appear until the 14th day, yet was supposed to be effected by art."   To meet such cases Kilpatrick adopted the doctrine that there was "no precise term for the artificial eruption." Among those "hardly dealt with" by the disease, supposed to have been given by art, were two ladies who had their eyes permanently injured. "With regard to a second infection of the inoculated *who took*, this was asserted by some who wished for it, but were as soon refuted."   Nineteen in twenty of the inoculated had an exceedingly slight eruption, so slight indeed that they thought the confinement indoors irksome and unnecessary. As to the negroes, who had all been born in Africa (and commonly have smallpox there or in the voyage across), it was not easy, he admits, to find out whether they had had smallpox before or not, the pits on their faces being less obvious than in whites, and the marks of other distempers easily mistaken for them. On the whole Kilpatrick was confident that inoculation in this epidemic had saved many lives; and it was the rumour of its success, together with corresponding reports from the plantations in the West Indies relating the valuable lives of negroes saved, that gave a fresh impulse to the practice in England. In 1743 Kilpatrick came to London, where he republished his Charleston essay, with an historical appendix, and soon got into the leading practice as an inoculator, having proceeded to the degree of M.D. and changed the spelling of his name to Kirkpatrick. Woodville says "he was esteemed the most scientific inoculator in London." During the eleven years from his setting up in practice there until the publication of his *Analysis of Inoculation* (1754), he had almost certainly been applying the arm-to-arm method which he learned from Mowbray in Charleston, having briefly indicated it in his first essay and avowed it more explicitly in his second. The establishment of Kirkpatrick in London, to practise the Charleston method of inoculation, corresponds, as nearly as one can trace it, with the revival of the practice in the south of England, to the extent of some two thousand cases in the counties of Kent, Surrey, Sussex, Hampshire and Dorset. We have a glimpse of that practice in the essay on inoculation published in 1749 by Dr Frewen, of Rye in Sussex[1], a physician of considerable learning (of the school of Boerhaave), whose theories of the effects of inoculation are reflected in Kirkpatrick's *Analysis* of 1754. In 350 cases, Frewen had only one fatality, the death of a child, aged four, from worm fever on the eighth day of a discrete eruption. He still used the incision on the arm, but less deep than Nettleton's, keeping the pledget of lint, moistened with matter, bound upon it for twenty-four hours ; also he encouraged the rendering from the incision for some weeks, giving the same reason as before, that "Nature by means of a continual drain is greatly aided in her attempts to throw off the matter of the disease." In his general account of the effects of inoculation, we seem to be reading of as real symptoms and as many pocks as Nettleton described—the eruption, always of the simple distinct kind, beginning on the 9th day, all out in three or four days after, the pocks filling and turning yellow for the next four or five days, then scabbing and falling, leaving temporary shallow marks. But it is clear that he had other results than these from trying new ways of procuring matter. "Experience," he says, "has convinced me that it is in reality of no consequence from what kind of smallpox it [the matter] is procured." If taken from the natural smallpox, it should be taken from ripe pustules : "yet I have sometimes applied it sooner, while only a limpid water." Oftentimes it happened that an inoculation produced too "slight" pustules to furnish matter for the succeeding operations. The question then arose whether the matter rendering from the incisions on the arms in these cases was

---

[1] Thomas Frewen, M.D., *The Practice and Theory of Inoculation.* London, 1749.

merely common pus or whether it had the property of "variolosity." This abstract quality, as it were the essence or quiddity of the pustular exanthem, was assumed to be present if the pus of the rendering incision could be made to raise a pustule on another arm, and if the person so infected could stand exposure to natural smallpox with impunity. One person so inoculated did have an attack of smallpox by contagion, so that Frewen concluded that the matter used for his protection had " run off all its variolosity." But others inoculated with the same, "in whom the symptoms were remarkably light, and in some few no pustules at all," were equally exposed to contagion without catching it, so that they were "judged to be secure from ever taking the smallpox again." Frewen's general conclusion, if it be not very logical, is at least modest:

"However, it may be worth the attention to reflect seriously whether it be not highly probable, from the success attending the numbers I have been concerned for, that inoculation has been often times a security against taking the most dangerous kinds of the natural smallpox."

Whether Frewen got the ideas of these novelties of method from Kirkpatrick's first account of the South Carolina practice, or struck them out for himself, it is clear that Kirkpatrick, in his next essay of 1754, has adopted variolosity as an abstract doctrine to surmount certain difficulties in the concrete reason. Many of his inoculated cases had only a few bastard pustules of smallpox, some had none. Was their disease smallpox? Did it warrant their future security?

"As many of the inoculated have very few pustules, and they are sometimes disposed to scab and wither away with very little suppuration, it might be of service to discover that the matter from the incisions would infect. But it would be certainly satisfactory to find it would where there was no eruption from inoculation, as its variolosity would greatly warrant the future security of the person it was taken from. That it is variolous is now evinced by the fact that it infected others to the like slight degree[1]."

The movement towards attenuating the virus used for inoculation was general in Europe. One of the mild methods, invented by Tronchin, of Amsterdam and afterwards of Paris, was to raise a small blister on the arm and to pass through the fluid a thread moistened with smallpox matter. This became one of the most common continental methods and was in use until the beginning of the 19th century. Kirkpatrick, who went

[1] J. Kirkpatrick, M.D., *Analysis of Inoculation, with a consideration of the most remarkable appearances in the Small Pocks.* Lond. 1754.

to see the practice of Tronchin, found the method by blister to produce as slight effects in the way of eruption as he describes for his own method :

"I attended and infected five poor children:—three, about seven years old, by incision; and two, about five years old, by vesication. Of the first three, one, a girl, had a pretty moderate but very kindly sprinkling ; the two boys very few. The two by blisters, a boy and a girl, had rather less,—the boy Dudin, a very fair delicate little child, not having above three or four, all which had not matter enough to infect one patient[1]."

Everywhere after the middle of the eighteenth century inoculation was coming into fashion again. In France it was lauded by the *philosophes*, while it was scouted by the medical faculty. La Condamine, a mathematician who had acquired fame by his journey to the Amazon to measure the three first degrees of the meridian, became interested in the subject by hearing from a credulous Carmelite missionary at Para how he had saved half of his Indian converts by inoculation after the other half had been destroyed by the natural smallpox. The mathematical philosopher on his return became an enthusiast for inoculation, and twice harangued the Académie des Sciences thereon. "The practice of inoculation," he said, "was improved during the time of its disgrace." What this improvement consisted in he also explained : "Neither the eruption is essential to the natural nor the pustules to the artificial smallpox: and perhaps art will one day come to effect what one hopes for and what Boerhaave and Lobb have even tried—I mean a change in the external form of this malady without any increase of its danger[2]."

[1] Kirkpatrick, *Analysis.*
[2] La Condamine, *Mémoires pour servir, &c.* (Deuxième Discours), 1768, p. 91. It matters little what Lobb may or may not have done. But it does not appear that Boerhaave ever tried to get rid of the eruption of smallpox by means of drugs. In the chapter of his *Aphorisms*, "De Variolis" (§ 1392) he says that he imagines a specific might be found, in the class of antidotes, to correct and destroy the variolous virus, indicating antimony and mercury as likely agents for the purpose owing to certain physical properties of the medicinal preparations of them. Ruston (*An Essay on Inoculation*, 3rd ed. 1768) says that Boerhaave, who died in 1738, "never practised it himself; nor seems to have understood the manner in which these medicines operate to produce their salutary effects." However they were known as the Boerhaavian antidotes to smallpox, and were used in Rhode Island, it is said with great success and as a secret. Ruston used them in England, and discovered by an analysis that Sutton's secret powders were the same. They seem also to have been used by Cheyne to prevent the development of smallpox in persons who had been exposed to contagion and had presumably taken the contagion. Frewen, in 1759, published a pamphlet to show the improbability of antimony and mercury having any such action, and the fallacy of the claims made for their success.

The Suttonian Inoculation.

Daniel Sutton, though an empiric, has given his name to the slight and safe method of inoculation which had been used in England for a good many years before his advent. So completely was his name joined to the practice of smallpox inoculation in its later period that in a Bill before Parliament in 1808 it is called " the Suttonian inoculation," to distinguish it from cowpox inoculation. The idea of attenuating the virus used for inoculation, and of making the effects minimal, was not his. It had been reached empirically years before by Mowbray, of Charleston, in 1738, who carried inoculation from arm to arm to the fifth remove, by Frewen, of Rye, in 1749, who was satisfied with an abstract " variolosity" of the incisions, in cases where there was no eruption at all or only a few pustules that did not fill, by Kirkpatrick, "the most scientific inoculator in London," who endorsed the doctrine of variolosity, by La Condamine, and most of all by Gatti of Paris.

Gatti used the unripe matter from a previous inoculation and inserted a most minute quantity of it at a very small puncture; and, to make sure that no general eruption should follow, he used the cooling regimen in various ways, including the prolonged immersion of the hands in cold water. Thus he promised his clients "the benefits of inoculation without its risks." But Gatti's career of prosperity was cut short by a series of conspicuous failures of his artificial smallpox to prevent the natural or real disease when it was epidemic. One of his patients, the Duchess de Boufflers, a great lady whose *salon* was frequented by the *philosophes* and *beaux esprits*, fell into the natural smallpox two years and a half after her inoculation[1].

[1] The Duchess gave the following account of her own case (*Gent. Magaz.* Nov. 1765, p. 495, sent by Gatti to a friend in London): "On the 12th of March, 1763, I was inoculated for the smallpox, and about four or five days afterwards a redness appeared round the orifice, which Mons. Gatti called an inflammation, and assured me was a sign that the smallpox had taken effect : these were the very terms he used. The redness or inflammation increased every day, and about the seventh or eighth day, the wound began to suppurate. There appeared also about the wound six small risings, or pimples, which successively suppurated and disappeared the next day. Mons. Gatti, upon their appearance, again assured me that the smallpox had taken effect. In the afternoon of the eleventh or twelfth day of my inoculation I felt a general uneasiness and emotion, a pain in my head and my back, and about my heart, in consequence of which I went to bed sooner than ordinary. I slept well, however, and rose without any disorder in the morning. These symptoms Mons. Gatti assured me were the forerunners of the eruption. The next day a pretty large rising

So many others in Paris had the same disappointment that a discussion arose in the Faculty of Medicine, the result of which was that the Parliament of Paris prohibited the practice of inoculation, for various reasons, within the limits of the capital.

Gatti's friend and correspondent in London was Dr Maty, who, "though born in Holland might be considered a Frenchman, but he was fixed in London by the practice of physic and an office in the British Museum[1]." Having conducted the foreign correspondence of the Royal Society, he became in 1765 its secretary in ordinary, and about the same time Principal Librarian of the British Museum. His interest in inoculation, which was shown by his translating La Condamine's first discourse on that subject in 1755, led him in 1765 to suggest to Gatti that he should write an essay for publication in England, "both to reclaim the thinking part of Paris, and to vindicate his own operations from the contemptuous treatment of his antagonists." The essay was written in due course, and Maty brought it out in English[2].

Gatti's own experiments and those which had previously been made in England by the most experienced inoculators had satisfied him of the truth of what he had long suspected, namely, that the operation could be made "still more harmless, though not less efficacious" (p. 29). There would be hardly any fever, certainly a very slight eruption and perhaps none at all (p. 68), It had, indeed, been questioned whether a patient who had but very few pustules, or only one, has had the smallpox as truly as

or pimple appeared in my forehead, turned white, and then died away, leaving a mark which continued many days.

"The wound in my arm continued to suppurate seven or eight days, and Mons. Gatti now assured me that I had nothing to fear from the smallpox; and upon this assurance I relied without the least doubt, and continued in perfect confidence of my security till the natural smallpox appeared. I continued very well during the whole time of my inoculation, except one day, as mentioned above, and I went out every day.   "Monmorency, D. de Boufflers."

[1] Gibbon's *Autobiography*. It was to Dr Maty that Gibbon, in 1759, submitted his French essay on the Study of Literature, having had a fair copy of it transcribed by one of the French prisoners at Petersfield. Of Maty he says: "His reputation was justly founded on the eighteen volumes of the *Journal Britannique*, which he had supported almost alone, with perseverance and success. This humble though useful labour, which had once been dignified by the genius of Bayle and the learning of Le Clerc, was not disgraced by the taste, the knowledge and the judgment of Maty."

[2] Angelo Gatti, M.D., *New Observations on Inoculation*. Translated from the French by M. Maty. Lond. 1768. The French edition was published at Brussels in 1767.

one who has been very full, and whether he is equally safe from catching it. He answers in the affirmative, according to the doctrine of variolosity: "No reason can be alleged, why we should have the smallpox but once, that will not equally hold good for one as for ten thousand pustules" (p. 69). Some, however, will not believe that one pustule is as good as ten thousand, "notwithstanding the obviousness of this truth." If one were absolutely bent upon giving a certain number of pustules, he would advise to inoculate according to his method (insertion with a needle) at twenty, thirty, or fifty places: "then you would be sure of one pustule at least at each puncture, and, probably, of many more in other parts." He would do this, however, only to humour prejudice, and with a feeling that he was doing the patient "more harm than was necessary." He was seriously satisfied of the "sufficiency of a single pustule," and believed that every wise man should run the venture of it and "embrace the method here laid down."

There was no theoretical objection to this method, but there was the practical one, that it might be *too* slight in its effects. Patients could hardly rest satisfied with so little to show for smallpox; and inoculators themselves found that they might have all their work to do over again. An eminent Irish physician wrote in 1765 to Dr Andrew, of Exeter, that crude matter from a previous inoculation was "less communicative of the disorder and more apt to disappoint us" than matter from a natural smallpox eruption taken "five or six days before the maturation of it[1]." It was also the experience of Salmade, of Paris, in 1798, that serous matter, taken from arm to arm through a long succession of cases, was apt to go off altogether, or to be "weakened to the point of nullity," whereby it disappointed the operator[2]. Reid, of Chelsea Hospital, was said to have carried the succession to thirty removes from the natural smallpox. Bromfeild knew for certain of matter being used at the sixteenth remove.

So long as the operation held at all, and had not to be repeated, Dr Andrew believed that effects which "no one would have taken for the smallpox," were "sufficient security against

---

[1] John Andrew, M.D., *The Practice of Inoculation impartially considered.* Dated 17 June, 1765, Exeter, p. 61.
[2] *La Pratique de l'Inoculation.* Paris, An. VII. (1798), p 51.

any future infection[1]." Heberden, indeed, has recorded a case
adverse to that view; but one case is not enough, even if it had
been in as eminent a person as Madame de Boufflers[2].

Daniel Sutton, who gave his name to the slighter kind of
smallpox inoculation, was not a regular practitioner. His
father, a doctor of medicine in Suffolk, was a specialist inoculator, as others of the regular profession here and there were
becoming, and had operated upon 2514 patients from 1757 to
1767. In 1763 Daniel began business on his own account at
Ingatestone in Essex, where patients from all parts were
boarded and subjected to his regimen, as at a water-cure. In
1764 he made 2000 guineas, and in 1765 £6300. In the three
years 1764–66 he inoculated 13,792 persons, and his assistants
some 6000 more—without a single death. Sutton kept his
method at first a secret, and for that reason was looked at
askance by eminent physicians. He used pills and powders,
which were found, by the analysis of Ruston, to be a preparation
of antimony and mercury, the drugs supposed to be antidotes
to natural smallpox, or the means of preventing its pustular
eruption. But the essence of his method was found to be, in
Chandler's words, "the taking of the infective humour in a crude
state [from a previous inoculation] before it has been, if I may
allow the expression, variolated by the succeeding fever[3]," or, in
Dimsdale's words, "inoculating with *recent* fluid matter," or in
Sir George Baker's words, "with the moisture taken from the
arm before the eruption of the smallpox, nay, within four days
after the operation has been performed[4]."

Sutton made it known that the effects of this method were
exceedingly mild—no keeping of bed, no trouble at all: "if any

[1] Andrew, u. s. p. 53.

[2] "I am sorry to have found that this operation has not always secured the
patient from having the smallpox afterwards, if the eruptions have been imperfect
without maturation. I attended one in a very full smallpox, which ran through all
its stages in the usual manner; yet this patient had been inoculated ten years before,
and, on the 5th day after inoculation, began to be feverish, with a headache, followed
by a slight eruption, which eruption soon went off without coming to suppuration;
the place of inoculation had inflamed and remained open ten days, leaving a deep
scar, which I saw." William Heberden, Senr., M.D., *Commentaries on Disease*
(p. 436). This was published in 1802, after the author's death; but as he was in the
height of his practice from 1760 onwards, the case, which is undated, may be taken
as illustrating Heberden's position in the Suttonian controversy.

[3] Benj. Chandler, M.D., *An Essay on the Present Method of Inoculation.* Lond.
1767.

[4] *Method of Inoculating the Smallpox.* Lond. 1766. Baker thought he was "an
enemy of improvement and no philosopher," who stood upon the antecedent
improbability of securing the patient by a minimal inoculation such as Sutton used.

patient has twenty or thirty pustules, he is said to have the smallpox very heavy." Being put on his trial at Chelmsford for spreading abroad the contagious particles of smallpox by the number of his inoculations, his defence was to have been (if the bill had not been thrown out by the grand jury), that he "never brought into Chelmsford a patient who was capable of infecting a bystander." The mildness of his artificial smallpox was acknowledged with satisfaction by some, with dissatisfaction by others. Dr Giles Watts, an inoculator in Kent, says it was "a most extraordinary improvement. The art of inoculation is enabled to reduce the distemper to almost as low a degree as we could wish... There is now an opportunity of seeing what a very small number of the multitude of persons of all ages, habits and constitutions, who have been inoculated in these parts, have been ill after it." Comparing it with the method which he had practised before, he says that he never knew ten or twelve inoculated together "in the old way" but one or more had the distemper in a pretty severe manner; on the other hand, he had inoculated four of his children in the new way and all of them together had not so many as eighty pustules. He adds that sometimes the inoculated had not even a single pustule (besides the one at the point of insertion) or at other times not more than two or three[1].

The Suttonian practice was objected to by Bromfeild in an essay dedicated to Queen Charlotte. Tracing it to Gatti, whose manifesto had been published in England two years before, he said that it was mere credulity "to have given credit to a man who should assert, that he would give them a disease which should not produce one single symptom that could characterize it from their usual state of health... Inoculation, though hitherto a great blessing to our island, will in a very short time be brought into disgrace," if it were assumed "that health and security from the disease can be equally obtained by reducing the patients so low as only to produce five to fifteen pimples[2]."

Bromfeild was not openly supported except by Dr Langton, of Salisbury, who contended that "the matter communicated is not the smallpox, because numbers have been inoculated a

[1] Giles Watts, M.D., *Vindication of the Method of Inoculating.* London, 1767.
[2] William Bromfeild, *Thoughts on the Method of treating Persons Inoculated for the Smallpox.* Lond. 1767. He was a Court surgeon and a man of some eminence. Morgagni dedicated one of the books of his *De Sedibus et Causis Morborum* to him as representing the Royal Society.

second, third and fourth time, that therefore it is no security against a future infection." He cites Gatti's case of the Duchess de Boufflers, and declares, as to the English inoculations, that not above one in ten have so many variolous symptoms as may be remarked in her case. "The old method of inoculating," he says, "was to take the infection from a good subject where the pustules were well maturated, whereby the operation was sure of succeeding; but the present practice is to take the matter from the incision the fourth day after the incision is made [this was Sutton's avowed practice]. By this means you have a contagious caustic water instead of laudable pus, and a slight ferment in the lymph is raised, producing a few watery blotches in the place of a perfect extrusion of the variolous matter[1]."

There was no difference of opinion as to the exact purport and upshot of the new method; it was to reduce the eruption to the lowest point or to a vanishing point. Nothing can be more emphatic than Gatti's profession of belief that a single pustule, at the place of insertion, was as effectual as ten thousand; and it is not only likely, on the face of it, that such a mitigation as Reid's to the thirtieth remove from natural smallpox, would produce merely the local pustule, but it is clear that Gatti saw no way of ensuring more by his method, supposing he were to gratify the prejudices of the laity in favour of more, than by puncturing the skin at twenty, thirty, or fifty separate points. It is not to be supposed, however, that the minimum result was obtained in all cases, or that all inoculators were equally adroit in procuring it; even Sutton had to admit that some of his thirteen thousand patients had more pustules on the skin than he desired.

Perhaps the most exact record of the number of pustules produced in a comparative trial of various methods is that of Sir William Watson at the Foundling Hospital in 1768[2]. Of 74 children inoculated in October and November, twelve had no eruption at all, but yet were held to have been protected by the operation. The remaining sixty-two had a very small average

[1] W. Langton, M.D., *Address to the Public on the present Method of Inoculation.* London and Salisbury, 1767. Dr Thomas Glass, of Exeter, replied in 1767 to Bromfeild and Langton, in *A Letter to Dr Baker on the Means of procuring a Distinct and Favourable Kind of Smallpox.* Lond. 1767, and in a *Second Letter to Dr Baker,* 1767.
[2] W. Watson, M.D., *An Account of a Series of Experiments instituted with a view of ascertaining the most successful Method of Inoculating the Smallpox.* London, 1768.

of pustules in addition to the local pustules, which average, small as it was, came mostly from two or three severer cases (e.g. one with 440 pustules, one with 260, and one with near 200), the most having three or four or a dozen or perhaps two dozen (e.g. three had only 7 pustules among them, or, in another batch of ten done with crude or ichorous matter, "the most that any boy had was 25, the least 4, the most that any girl had was 6, the least 3," or, in another batch of ten, also with crude lymph, two had no eruption, seven had 35 pustules among them, and one had 30). Of the amount of smallpox upon the whole sixty-two cases which had some eruption Watson says: "Physicians daily see in one limb only of an adult person labouring under the coherent, not to say confluent smallpox, a greater quantity of variolous matter than was found in all these persons put together."

Watson's sole measure of "success" in inoculating was the slightness of the effect produced ; and as he found that crude or watery matter from the punctured spot of a previous inoculation had the least effect, he decided to use that kind of matter always in future at the Foundling Hospital. On the other hand, Mudge, of Plymouth, raised a different issue and put it to the test of experiment on a large scale. Did crude matter infect the constitution ? Did it make the patient insusceptible of the effects of a second inoculation with purulent matter ? The experiment came out thus :

At Plympton, in Devonshire, in the year 1776, thirty persons were inoculated with crude or watery matter from the arm of a woman who had been inoculated five days before, and ten persons were at the same time inoculated with purulent matter from the pustules of a case of natural smallpox. The thirty done with crude matter had each "a large prominent pustule" at the place of puncture, "but not one of them had any eruptive fever or subsequent eruption on any part of the body." Matter taken from their local pustules produced exactly the same result in the next remove, namely, a local pustule, but no eruptive fever nor eruptive pustules. The thirty were inoculated again, this time with purulent matter (five from natural smallpox, twenty-five from inoculated smallpox), and all of them had, besides the local pustule, an eruptive fever and an eruption "in the usual way of inoculated patients." The ten who were originally inoculated with purulent matter had that result at first[1].

[1] John Mudge, Surgeon at Plymouth, *A Dissertation on the Inoculated Smallpox.*

In the subsequent history of inoculation it would appear that the method known by the name of Sutton, of using crude or watery matter from a previous inoculated case, was the one commonly preferred. But it was not always preferred. One of the medical neighbours of the afterwards celebrated Dr Jenner took matter from the pustules and kept it in a phial; his patients inoculated therewith had somewhat active effects, even "sometimes eruptions." But "many of them unfortunately fell victims to the contagion of smallpox, as if they had never been under the influence of this artificial disease," so that Jenner, who had probably not heard of Mudge's experiment, was confirmed in his preference for the crude matter (before the eruptive fever) from a previous inoculation. It was of great importance, he said, to attend to that point, as it would "prevent much subsequent mischief and confusion[1]." Of course there were many more chances of getting matter from natural smallpox than from inoculated; but it would appear that in the former also it was taken in the ichorous or unripe stage of the eruption, according to the practice of Sutton, and despite the experimental proof that Mudge gave of its merely superficial or formal effects.

Mudge's experiment was on a large scale, and designed to test a general or scientific issue. The testing experiment usually made was merely for the sake of the particular case; the patient was inoculated a second time, shortly after the first, with the same matter as before, or a third time, or even a fourth time. Whatever the significance of this for the doctrine of inoculation in general (as in the issue raised by Mudge), the individual was both reassured and fortified so far as concerned his own safety. The experiment of the former generation that was usually cited was that of the Hon. John Yorke. On his leaving the university at the age of one and twenty it was thought prudent that he should be inoculated for smallpox before entering on the great world. He was inoculated by serjeant surgeon Hawkins, and had the local suppuration, some fever, but little or no eruption. The inoculator was satisfied, but not so the youth:

London, 1777. A copy of this essay was found in the library of Dr Samuel Johnson. The Doctor was a friend of the author's father, the Rev. Archdeacon Mudge, whose published sermons he has characterized in one of his most amusing balanced sentences of praise qualified with blame. Johnson stood godfather to one of John Mudge's children. Notes on "Dr Johnson's Library," by A. W. Hutton.

[1] Edward Jenner, M.D., *Inquiry into the Causes and Effects of the Variolae Vaccinae, or Cowpox.* Lond. 1798, p. 56. See also his *Further Observations on the Cowpox.* 1799.

he insisted upon a second inoculation, which had no effect. This was considered a leading case. When the Suttonian method came in, and the absence of eruption (barring a few pimples or bastard pustules) became the usual thing, the occasions for a second inoculation became more common, owing to the prejudice, as Gatti said, of the laity in favour of something tangible although not excessive[1].

Dimsdale inoculated many of his patients a second time, and produced the local pustule again, as at first. Of the 74 foundlings in Watson's experiment of Oct.–Nov. 1767, there were twelve who had no eruption, of whom four were re-inoculated with no better result or with no result. Of the whole twelve he says: "Although they had no eruption, I consider them as having in all probability gone through the disease, as the punctures of almost all of them were inflamed and turgid many days." It was so unusual for a second inoculation, in a doubtful case, to produce more than the first, that Kite, of Gravesend, communicated to the Medical Society of London two cases where that had happened, as being "anomalous." He had never before been able to communicate the smallpox, on a second attempt, "to any patient whose arm had inflamed, and who had even a much less degree of fever" than Case 1, who had only the local pustule and "on the eighth day was quite well:" and he cites Dimsdale to the same effect[2].

Perhaps enough has been said to illustrate the subtle casuistry that had gradually arisen out of the old problem of procuring the smallpox by artifice. I make one more citation, from a Hampshire inoculator in 1786, to show how fine were the distinctions, depending, one might suppose, upon the subjective state of the practitioner, drawn between effective and non-effective inoculation :

"The incisions sometimes have a partial inflammation for a few days, which then vanishes without producing any illness ; in this case the patient

[1] Langton cites the following advertisement put out on 18 June, 1767, in his own district by Messrs Slatter and Duke, surgeons, of Ringwood, Hants: "The first objection I shall take notice of is that the disorder being in general so light, it is imagined there is danger of a second infection [i.e. a natural attack]. Whenever this has been supposed to have happened, I am certain the operation has failed, which not being discovered by the operator, proves to me that he was not experienced in the practice; for it may always be determined in four, five, or six days, sometimes sooner; and if there is the least reason to doubt, it is very easy to inoculate a second, third or fourth time, which may be done without the least inconvenience. I have inoculated several patients three or four times for their own satisfaction, having very little or perhaps no eruption."

[2] *Mem. Med. Soc. Lond.* IV. 114.

is certainly still liable to infection; but I believe it very rarely happens that there is any matter, or even ichor, in the present slight manner they are made, without producing the smallpox....I have constantly remarked that when the punctured part inflames properly, and is attended with an efflorescence, rather inclining to a crimson colour, for some distance round the same, about the eleventh or twelfth day from the inoculation, although the patient should have very little illness and no eruption, yet that he is secure from all future infection[1]."

Extent of Inoculation in Britain to the end of the 18th Century.

From 1721 to 1727 the inoculations in all England were known with considerable accuracy to have been 857; in 1728 they declined to 37; and for the next ten or twelve years they were of no account. The southern counties led the revival in the fifth decade of the century, so that before long some two thousand had been inoculated in Surrey, Kent, Sussex and Hampshire. Frewen, however, who could point to 350 cases done by himself in Sussex previous to 1749, says that it "gained but little credit among the common sort of people, who began to dispute about the lawfulness of propagating diseases, and whether or no the smallpox produced by inoculation would be a certain security against taking it by infection," etc.

In London, after the revival under Kirkpatrick's influence in 1743, inoculation became a lucrative branch of surgical practice, and was done by the heads of the profession—Ranby, Hawkins, Middleton and others, and almost exclusively among the well-to-do. In 1747 Ranby had inoculated 827 without losing one; in 1754 his total, still without a death, had reached 1200. In 1754 Middleton had done 800 inoculations, with one death. The operation was by no means so simple as it looked. It required the combined wits of a physician, a surgeon, and an apothecary; while the preparation of the patient to receive the matter was an affair of weeks and of much physicking and regimen. Thus inoculation was for a long time the privilege of those who could pay for it. As late as 1781, when a movement was started for giving the poor of Liverpool the benefits of inoculation, it was stated in the programme of the charity that, "as the matter now stands, inoculation in Liverpool is confined almost exclusively to the higher ranks," the wealthier

[1] John Covey, of Basingstoke, 8 May, 1786, in *London Medical Journal*, VII. p. 180.

inhabitants having generally availed themselves of it for many years[1].

The first project in London for gratuitous inoculation took shape, along with the plan of a smallpox hospital, at a meeting held in February, 1746, in the vestry-room of St Paul's, Covent Garden[2]. The original house of the charity, called the Middlesex County Hospital for Smallpox, was opened in July, 1746, in Windmill Street, Tottenham Court Road, but was shortly removed to Mortimer Street, and again, to Lower Street, Islington. The charity opened also a smallpox hospital in Bethnal Green, which eventually contained forty-four beds. The Inoculation Hospital proper, used for the tedious preparation of subjects, was a house in Old Street, St Luke's, with accommodation for fifteen persons. Besides the smallpox hospital at Islington, the charity had, in 1750, a neighbouring house in Frog Lane, for the reception of patients after they had been inoculated in the Old Street house. Down to the middle of 1750 there had been admitted 620 patients in the natural smallpox, while only 34 had gone through the process of inoculation. The latter involved a month's preparation, and about a fortnight's detention after the operation was done; so that a new batch of subjects was inoculated but once in seven weeks. In 1752 the governors of the charity purchased a large building in Coldbath Fields, which they fitted with one hundred and thirty beds, as a hospital both for cases of the natural smallpox and for preparing subjects to undergo inoculation (the Old Street house being still retained for the latter purpose). The next important change was in 1768, when a large new hospital was opened at St Pancras, to be solely a house of preparation, the old hospital in Coldbath Fields being now turned to the double purpose of receiving the patients from St Pancras after their inoculation and of receiving patients in the natural smallpox. Thus the inoculation business of the charity, which had begun with being subordinate to the treatment of those sick of the natural smallpox, gradually encroached upon the latter and became paramount. The inoculations, which had been only 112 in the year 1752, reached the total of

[1] *Address to the Inhabitants of Liverpool on the subject of a General Inoculation for the Smallpox.* 1 September, 1781.
[2] The account of the London charity is taken from the *History of Inoculation in Great Britain* (1796) by Woodville, who became physician to it in 1791.

1084 in the year 1768, while the admissions for smallpox "in the natural way" from 24 March, 1767, to 24 March, 1768, were 700.

In the year 1762–63, the admissions for natural smallpox had been 844, and for inoculations 439. One reason of the great increase of patients received for inoculation after that date was the rise of the Suttonian practice, which had vogue enough to attract numbers, and at the same time was so much simplified in the matter of preparation and in its results that many more could go through the hospitals in a given time. The inoculations by the Smallpox Charity were done in batches, men and boys at one time, women and girls at another, on some eight or twelve occasions in the year, of which public notice was given.

The following table is taken from the annual report of the Smallpox and Inoculation Hospitals for the year 1868.

Period	Inoculations	Period	Inoculations
Previous to Oct. 1749	17	1758 } 1759 }	446
Oct. 1749–Oct. 1750	29	1760	372
Oct. 1750–Oct. 1751	85	1761	429
1752	112	1762	496
1753	129	1763	439
1754	135	1764	383
1755	217	1765	394
1756	281	1766	633
1757	247	1767	653
		1768	1084

These charitable efforts to keep down smallpox in London hardly touched the mass of the people, and did not touch at all the infants and young children among whom nearly all the cases occurred. The charity admitted no subjects for inoculation under the age of seven years. It aimed at giving to a certain number of the working class, or of the domestics or other dependents of the rich, the same individual protection that their betters paid for. Meanwhile there were on an average about twelve thousand cases of smallpox in London from year to year, mostly in infants and young children. The first proposal to apply inoculation to these came in 1767, from Dr Maty, in a paper on "The Advantages of Early Inoculation." This physician, distinguished in letters and now become a librarian, sought to recommend inoculation for infants by glorifying the purity of their juices and the natural vigour of their constitutions, which was something of a paradox at a time when half the infants born in London were dying before the end of their third year. He saw as in a vision how smallpox would be extinguished by making inoculation universal :

"When once all the adults susceptible of the infection should either have received it or be dead without suffering from it, the very want of the variolous matter would put a stop to both the natural and artificial smallpox. Inoculation then would cease to be necessary, and therefore be laid aside[1]."

Eight years after, in 1775, Dr Lettsom seriously took up the project of inoculating infants in London[2]. He started a Society for Inoculation at the Homes of the People, which effected nothing besides some inoculations done by Lettsom himself during an epidemic " in confined streets and courts." In 1779 he launched another scheme for a " General Inoculation Dispensary for the benefit of the poor throughout London, Westminster and Southwark, without removing them from their own habitations[3]." That also was frustrated by the active opposition of Dimsdale[4]. The objection to it was that there was no prospect of making the practice universal, and that partial inoculations in the crowded quarters of London would merely serve to keep the contagion of smallpox more active than ever. Lettsom answered that the danger of contagion from inoculated smallpox was more theoretical than real, inasmuch as the amount of smallpox matter produced upon the inoculated was a mere trifle[5].

At Newcastle, Lettsom's design had at least a trial, under the influence of his friend Dr John Clark[6]. The Dispensary, founded in 1777, was designed from the outset to undertake gratuitous inoculations; but it was not until 13 April, 1786, that it got to work. The "liberality of the public" enabled the managers in that year to offer premiums to parents, to cover the expense of having their children sick from inoculation—five shillings for one child, seven shillings for two, nine shillings for

---

[1] *Med. Obs. and Inquiries*, III. (1767), p. 287. The passage quoted (p. 306, *note*) is almost exactly in the words of Hufeland long after, with reference to the probable extinction of smallpox by cowpox. See his *Journal*, x. pt. 2, p. 189.

[2] J. C. Lettsom, *A Letter to Sir Robert Barker, F.R.S. and G. Stacpoole, Esq. upon General Inoculation.* London, 1778.

[3] *A Plan of the General Inoculating Dispensary, &c.* Lond. (no date).

[4] T. Dimsdale, *Thoughts on General and Partial Inoculation.* Lond. 1776. *An Introduction to the Plan of the Inoculation Dispensary.* 1778. *Remarks on Dr Lettsom's letter to Barker and Stacpoole.* 1779.

[5] Lettsom, *Obs. on Baron Dimsdale's Remarks, &c.* 1779; and other pamphlets on both sides.

[6] Clark, *Report of the Newcastle Dispensary.* 1789.

three, and ten shillings for four or more of a family. On the first occasion, 208 children were inoculated, and all recovered. From 1786 to 1801, the cases numbered 3268. It was the aim of Dr Clark to get the operation done in infancy; accordingly in the space of four and a half years (1786–1790), of 1056 inoculations 460 were on infants under one year, 270 from one to two, 122 from two to three, 69 from three to four, 62 from four to five, 66 from five to ten, and 7 from ten to fifteen. This was perhaps the most systematic attempt at infant inoculation from year to year. The other dispensaries at which inoculation was steadily offered to the children of the poor were at White-haven (1079 inoculations from 1783 to 1796), at Bath, and at Chester.

Before the society was started at Chester for the purpose, the inoculations were some fifteen or twenty in a year, and these, we may suppose, in the richer families. The society got to work in 1779, but its operations were stopped in 1780 by a singular cause—the general diffusion of smallpox in the town by a regiment of soldiers. The whole inoculations of poor children from the spring of 1780 until September, 1782, were 213, besides which 203 were done in private practice. The year 1781 was tolerably free from epidemic smallpox (8 deaths), but in January, 1782, a very mortal kind prevailed in several parts of the town.

At Liverpool the first gratuitous general inoculation was in the autumn of 1781, to the number of about 517. "The affluent," says Currie, "being alarmed at the advertisement for this purpose, presented their children also in great numbers, and 161 passed through the disease." There was a second gratuitous inoculation in the spring of 1782 (to which some of the above numbers may have belonged), and it was intended to continue the same at regular intervals; but there is no record of more than those two[1].

Although Dimsdale opposed "general" inoculations in the large towns, for the reasons mentioned, he was in favour of inoculating together all the susceptible subjects in a smaller place or country district; and that kind of general inoculation was not unfrequently undertaken, sometimes hurriedly at the beginning of an epidemic, at other times after an epidemic had

---

[1] Currie to Haygarth, 28 Nov. 1791, in *Sketch of a Plan, etc.*, pp. 451, 207.

been running its course for months, and here or there, it would seem, during a free interval and by way of general precaution.

Dimsdale himself, with the help of Ingenhousz, carried out on one occasion, in Berkhamstead and three or four other villages of Hertfordshire, a general inoculation to the number, he guesses, of some six hundred persons of all ages, including some quite old persons. In 1765 or 1766 Daniel Sutton at Maldon, Essex, inoculated in one morning 417 of all ages, who were said to be all those in the town that had not had smallpox in the natural way. Some hundreds were also inoculated by him at one time in Maidstone.

In the small Gloucestershire town of Painswick in 1786, a very violent and fatal smallpox broke out during a time of typhus and intermittent fever. In consequence of the epidemic, one surgeon inoculated 738 persons from the 26th of May to the end of June[1]. In another Gloucestershire parish, Dursley, a single surgeon in the spring of 1797 inoculated 1475 persons of all ages, "from a fortnight to seventy years." But in certain villages near Leeds in 1786–7 a general inoculation, organised by a zealous clergyman and paid for by a nobleman, mustered only eighty. About the same time, during an epidemic of malignant smallpox at Luton, Bedfordshire, 1215 were inoculated, and thereafter about 700 more; the average number annually attacked by smallpox during a period of nine years had been about twenty-five[2].

Inoculation was tried first in Scotland in 1726 by Maitland, during a visit to his native Aberdeenshire, but was not persevered with owing to one or two fatalities among the half-dozen cases. About 1733 it was begun at Dumfries by Gilchrist, who practised it during the next thirty years upon 560 persons, most of them, doubtless, paying patients. The returns made to Professor Monro, of Edinburgh, showed in the chief medical practices 5554 inoculations down to 1765; of which 703 were in Edinburgh and Leith, 950 in Glasgow, 208 in Stirling, 260 in Irvine, 157 in Aberdeen, 310 in Banff, 243 in Thurso, and 560 in Dumfries as above[3]. Seventy-two deaths are put down to the

---

[1] J. C. Jenner, "An Account of a General Inoculation at Painswick." *Lond. Med. Journ.* VII. 163–8.
[2] *Gent. Magaz.* April, 1788, reported by the Hon. and Rev. Mr Stuart, who was a grandson of Lady Mary Wortley Montagu.
[3] Monro, *Account of Inoculation in Scotland*, 1765; in his *Works*. Edin. 1781, p. 693.

practice. When the Statistical Account of the 938 parishes was compiled in the last decade of the century, a few of the parish ministers made reference to inoculation.

Thus, in Applecross, Ross-shire, and three neighbouring parishes, an uneducated man is said to have inoculated 700 after a very fatal epidemic in 1789; it happened, however, that the pestilence reappeared, whereupon inoculation was "generally adopted[1]." Applecross may have been populous then; now there is not a smoke to be seen in it for miles. Again, the practice is said to have become "universal" in Skye from about 1780[2]. In Durness parish, which the tourist may now traverse for thirteen miles to Cape Wrath without seeing anyone but a shepherd, inoculation was rendered "general" about 1780 by the benevolence of a gentleman belonging to the parish[3]. From October, 1796, to July, 1797, a surgeon of Thurso inoculated 645 in that town and in country parishes of Caithness during a very severe epidemic[4]. In the parish of Jedburgh the cost of an inoculation was defrayed by the heritors, in that of Kirkwall by the kirk session, in another by the commissioners of annexed estates, in Earlstown, Berwickshire (on 70 children) by the chief proprietor. The ministers who mention it at all were mostly strong advocates of it, but they usually imply that the common people were (or had been) apathetic or prejudiced. It was sometimes recommended from the pulpit, and actually done by the ministers; it was even recommended that students of divinity should be instructed in the art. Statements that it had become "general" or "universal" are made for several parishes, mostly in the Highlands or Islands. The very full and trustworthy account of the parish of Banff says that "inoculation is by no means become general among the lower ranks[5];" which is perhaps about the truth for the country at large.

At the end of an epidemic at Leeds, in 1781, which had attacked 462 and killed 130 during six months, "in the next six months there were inoculated 385, of whom four died" (two by contagious smallpox). A second general inoculation was carried out in Leeds sometime previous to 1788. Lucas, writing in that year, says: "The result of two general inoculations in Leeds has been that the smallpox has since been less frequent and less fatal[6]." This will be a convenient opportunity of considering the gross effects of inoculation upon the prevalence of smallpox.

---

[1] *Statistical Account of Scotland.* 1791–99, III. 376.

[2] *Ibid.* IV. 130. It was about the year 1782 that the College of Physicians of Edinburgh appointed a committee to inquire into the mode of conducting the gratis inoculations of the poor, which had been tried at Chester, Leeds, Liverpool, &c. in 1781–82. Haygarth, u. s. 1784, p. 207.

[3] *Ibid.* III. 582.

[4] *Ibid.* XX. 502–7.

[5] *Ibid.* XX. 348. Account by Rev. Abercromby Gordon, who gives in a note (p. 349) the following instance of professional zeal: "A surgeon in the north, presuming that self-interest has a stronger hold on man than superstition, has lately opened a policy of insurance for the smallpox! If a subscriber gives him two guineas for inoculating his child, the surgeon in the event of the child's death pays ten guineas to the parent; for every guinea subscribed, four guineas, for half a guinea, two guineas, and for a crown one guinea."

[6] James Lucas, *Lond. Med. Journ.* X. 269.

The first and most obvious consideration is that it usually came too late. "Most born in London," said Lettsom quite correctly, "have smallpox before they are seven"—i.e. before the age for admission to the inoculation hospital. He might have added that, if they had run the gauntlet of smallpox in London until they were seven, they were little likely to take it at all. The inoculations in London were therefore done upon a very select class (they were, in fact, a very small number), who may be assumed to have escaped the perils of smallpox in London in their childhood, or to have come to London (as many did) from country places where smallpox broke out as an epidemic only at long intervals. In other large towns as well as the capital the inoculated must have been a residual class. At Leeds, with a population of 17,117, "the number of those who were still uninfected was found on a survey to be 700" at the end of an epidemic, of whom 385 were inoculated. If a general inoculation had been tried at Chester after the epidemic of 1774, there would have been only 1060, in a population of 14,713, to try it on. How many of these, above the age of childhood, were constitutionally proof against smallpox? The case of Ware, in Hertfordshire, after the epidemic in the summer of 1777, is so related by Lettsom as to bring out the ambiguity of much that was claimed for inoculation. "After about eighty had been carried off by it, a general inoculation was proposed, to prevent those who had not yet been attacked, and whose number was still considerable, from sharing the same fate. The alarm which had been excited induced most of the survivors to adopt this proposition, after which not one died, and the infection was wholly eradicated." Eighty deaths in one epidemic is a large mortality for such a place as Ware in any circumstances; the smallpox for once had done its worst. But, says Lettsom, there were a few families of those hitherto untouched by the epidemic who did not submit to inoculation. Not one of them caught the disease—from their inoculated neighbours (Lettsom is arguing that there was no danger in that way), nor, of course, from the epidemic contagion. It cannot but appear strange to us that the natural cessation or exhaustion of an epidemic should not have been thought of. Dr Currie, of Liverpool, records that in the first general inoculation there in 1781 there were 417 inoculated gratuitously and about 100 more in private practice, and that "about three or four thousand liable to the disease were scattered in the same manner [as the inoculated], not one of whom caught the infection." For a few weeks there was not a case of smallpox known in Liverpool, so that no matter could be got for inoculation. He adds, in the most ingenuous manner: "An important particular has been recalled to my mind by Mr Park; that previous to this first general inoculation, which extinguished the smallpox in so extraordinary a way, the disease raged in town with much violence and was very fatal[1]."

The general inoculations were often carried out in so haphazard a manner as to make them valueless for a scientific as well as for a practical purpose. A Bath surgeon of long experience wrote in 1800: "Whenever the inoculating rage once takes place whole parishes are doomed, without the least attention to age, sex, or temperament—no previous preparation, no after treatment or concern...Are not scores and hundreds seized upon at once, for the incisions, scratchings, puncturings and threadings, without even a possibility of their being properly attended to? and whether they may or may not receive the infection is just as little known or cared about[2]." It must have been equally little known or cared about whether they had had smallpox in the natural way before. What Dimsdale found to obtain at St Petersburg would have been the rule elsewhere: "The general method was to search for marks, and, if none were found, it was concluded the party had not had the disease[3]."

Thus in any attempt to estimate the gross advantages of inoculation in the 18th century we are met on every hand by sources of fallacy. Whatever its theoretical correctness, it does not follow that the inoculation of smallpox was a practical success to the extent of its trial; and even its theoretical correctness will be thought by some, and was so thought at the time, to have gone by the board when the artificial disease was brought down to a pustule at the point of puncture, with or without a few bastard pocks on the skin near. I have found two instances in the 18th century history in which there are data for a rough practical judgment, although not for a precise

[1] Currie to Haygarth, 28 Nov. 1791, in the latter's *Sketch of a Plan, &c.* p. 453.
[2] *A Conscious View of Circumstances and Proceedings respecting Vaccine Inoculation.* Bath, 1800. The author was probably James Nooth, senior surgeon to the Bath Hospital, who removed to London and practised in Queen Anne Street, holding the appointment of surgeon to the Duke of Kent. He wrote on cancer of the breast.
[3] *Tracts on Inoculation.* London, 1781.

statistical one. The first is the town of Blandford, in Dorset; the other is the Foundling Hospital in London.

During the smallpox year 1766, smallpox of a very malignant type broke out at Blandford in the first week of April[1]. It was estimated that 700 persons in the town (population 2110 in 1773) had not had the natural smallpox, and a general inoculation was resolved upon on the 13th April. "A perfect rage for inoculation," says Dr Pulteney[2], "seized the whole town," and in the week following the 16th April some 300 were inoculated, the total rising to 384 before the panic ceased; of these, 150 were paid for by the parish. There were thirteen deaths among the inoculated, but most of these confluent or haemorrhagic cases, seem to have been due to the epidemic contagious smallpox, which had been peculiarly fatal, with haemorrhagic symptoms, to the few that were seized before the inoculation began, and continued to be fatal to many. The mortality from smallpox for the year in the parish register was 44, and from all causes 104, or more than twice the normal[2]. The last epidemic of smallpox in Blandford had been in 1753, when 40 died of it, the deaths from all causes being 96. In that year also there had been a general inoculation to the number of 309. The parish register gives the deaths in an earlier epidemic, in 1741, which was a year of great distress and typhus fever all over England: 76 deaths are ascribed to smallpox (102 to all causes), which is a larger total from smallpox than in either of the subsequent occasions when general inoculations were tried. Comparing these three epidemics in a Table, with the associated circumstances, we get the following:

Statistics of Blandford in three Smallpox Years (Population in 1773, 2110).

Year of Epidemic	Deaths from all causes	Deaths from Smallpox	Inoculations	Annual Averages of eight previous years		
				Marriages	Births	Deaths
1741	102	76	—	24·87	63·37	49·25
1753	96	40	309	19·37	50·62	49·62
1766	104	44	384	20·62	54·12	49·12

It will be seen that the higher mortality from smallpox in 1741 was associated with other things besides the absence of inoculation. The annual average of deaths for eight years preceding each of the three epidemics is almost the same. But the marriages and births for eight years preceding 1741 were much in excess of those in the periods preceding the other two epidemic years. In the former there was a much larger susceptible population of children, upon which the smallpox mainly fell; and that alone would account for more deaths from smallpox in the epidemic of 1741. But the year 1741 was peculiar in another way; it was the worst year of typhus fever and general distress in the whole of the 18th century, and in the circumstances the deaths from smallpox would have been unusually numerous for the cases. Another epidemic of smallpox without inoculation, in 1731, showed how mild smallpox could be. At a time when sixty families had the disease

---

[1] R. Pulteney, M.D., in a letter of 21 June, 1766, to Dr G. Baker, given in his *Inquiry into the Merits of a Method of Inoculating the Smallpox.* Lond. 1766.
[2] Pulteney, "Births, Deaths and Marriages of Blandford Forum, 1733–1772." *Phil. Trans.* LXVIII. 615.

C. II. 33

among them, a fire broke out on 4 June, and burned down the town. It is said that 150 ill of smallpox were removed to gardens, hedgerows and the arches of bridges, and that only one of the whole number died[1]. This is usually cited to show the benefits of fresh air; but if it be true, it shows more than that.

The Foundling Hospital may seem to offer all the conditions for a fair trial of the question. It had been a standing rule of the Governors, since the opening of the charity in 1749, that all children received into it should be inoculated. Sir William Watson, who states the fact, adds that he himself was "in a situation of superintending every year the inoculation of some hundreds." Still, the rule may not have been uniformly carried out; and even in this community of children, it was not always possible to learn on their admission whether they had had smallpox before in the natural way[2].

The lists of the inoculated are longer in the later periods than in the earlier: thus, from March, 1759 to May, 1766, the annual average is something under a hundred, the inmates having been 312 in 1763; but from May, 1766 to July, 1769, the annual average is some two hundred and fifty, the inmates in 1768 having been 438. Sir William Watson, in his essay upon the inoculations at the Foundling, breathes no hint that such a thing as natural smallpox ever happened there[3]; but in another context he does casually mention that there was an epidemic of sixty cases, with four deaths, in the end of 1762, and another epidemic in the following summer, of "many" cases, nineteen of which, with eleven fatalities, occurred in children who had lately been through the measles and were weakened in consequence[4]. Another epidemic, as I find by the apothecary's book of weekly admissions to the infirmary, happened in the winter of 1765–66, twenty-six names being entered as admitted for "natural smallpox." After that date all the great epidemics appear to have been of measles, whooping-cough, influenza or scarlatina; but almost every year smaller groups of "natural smallpox" occur, of which the following have been collected from the available records:

Foundling Hospital, London.

Year	Natural Smallpox	Year	Natural Smallpox
1766	8	1774	4
1767	2	1775	3
1768	8	1783	1
1769	7	1784	0
1770	1	1785	8 (or 16?)
1771	2	1786	0
1772	3	1787	5
1773	1	1788	4

[1] Pulteney to Baker, App. to *Inquiry into the method of Inoculating.* 1766; Hutchins, *Dorsetshire*, I. 217.

[2] On 23 July, 1785, the apothecary makes a note in his book: "Some inspectors are not sufficiently careful to send information to the Hospital when children have had the smallpox." MS. Records.

[3] *Experiments, &c.* 1768.

[4] Sir W. Watson, M.D., F.R.S., "On the Putrid Measles of London, 1763 and 1768." *Med. Obs. and Inquiries*, IV. 153.

The occurrence of one or more cases seems to have been the signal for a general inoculation; or, again, it may be that the few cases of natural smallpox in the infirmary at one time had followed a general inoculation. Thus, in June–July, 1767, one case is entered on the second day from the inoculation (of a large number), and another on the fourth day. Again, in Nov.–Dec., 1768, one of the four cases of natural smallpox is marked "soon after his inoculation."

The received cases in which inoculation failed to save individuals from the natural smallpox are few. Besides those already given for the first period of the practice, and the case from Heberden, there are six fully detailed by Kite of Gravesend, in two groups of three each, all in the spring of 1790[1]. Apart from exact records, there are various testimonies more or less trustworthy. The Marquis of Hertford is said to have told Dr Jenner that his father, having been inoculated by Caesar Hawkins, the serjeant surgeon, and thereafter attended by him during a tour abroad, caught smallpox at Rheims and died[2]. Bromfeild, surgeon to Queen Charlotte, is said to have "abandoned the practice of inoculation in consequence of its failure[3]." Jenner and his friends made a collection of cases in which inoculation had failed, to the number of "more than one thousand, and fortunately seventeen of them in families of the nobility[4]." A Bath surgeon said he had heard of "innumerable" cases of attacks of natural smallpox long after inoculation, and had himself professionally seen "not a few[5]." A surgeon of Frampton on Severn knew of four cases, out of five inoculated together in 1784, that took smallpox afterwards in the natural way, of whom one died[6]. In an epidemic of smallpox at Enmore Green, a suburb of Shaftesbury, in 1808, a surgeon from Shaston found that "nearly twenty" of the victims had been inoculated "by the late Mr John White" about ten years before, and were supposed to have had it "very fine[7]." Dr John Forbes learned that some nineteen cases of natural smallpox in and around

---

[1] Charles Kite, surgeon, Gravesend, "An Account of some anomalous Appearances consequent to Inoculation of Smallpox." *Memoirs Med. Soc. Lond.* IV. (1794), p. 114.

[2] Fosbroke, *Lond. Med. Repository.* June, 1819, p. 466.

[3] Jenner to James Moore, in Baron's *Life of Jenner*, II. 401 : "Is not that a precious anecdote for your new work?" See also *Court and Private Life of Queen Charlotte* (Journals of Mrs Papendiek). Lond. 1887, I. 41, 70, 270.

[4] In Baron, u. s.

[5] *A Conscious View, &c.* u. s.

[6] Earle, in Jenner's *Further Observations.* 1799.

[7] T. Adams to Richard Pew, M.D., of Sherborne. *Lond. Med. and Phys. Journ.* April, 1829.

Chichester in 1821–22 were of inoculated persons[1]. It would be incorrect to say that such cases could be multiplied indefinitely; on the contrary, they are hard to find. Whether that shows that inoculation was on the whole a success, to the extent that it was tried, or that its failures are in part unrecorded, I am not competent to decide. But it cannot be doubted that the usual estimates of the saving of life by inoculation were extravagant and fallacious. La Condamine, a mathematician, counted up the saving to the slave-owner in an ideal plantation of three hundred negroes[2]. Watson, with the epidemics in the Foundling fresh in his memory, estimated that inoculation might have saved 23,000 out of the 23,308 who had died of smallpox in London in ten years, 1758–68[3]. Haygarth[4] reckoned that 351 might have been saved by inoculation of the 378 children who died of smallpox at Chester from 1772 to 1777. Woodville, who wrote the history of inoculation down to the advent of Sutton, declared in 1796 that the art of inoculation, originally a fortuitous discovery, "is capable of saving more lives than the whole *materia medica*[5]." Arnot, the historian of Edinburgh (1779), asserted inoculation to be "a remedy so compleat that we hesitate not in the least to pronounce those parents, who will not inoculate their children for the smallpox, accessory to their death[6]." The College of Physicians, in a formal minute of 1754, pronounced it "highly salutary to the human race."

Despite all those academic pronouncements, inoculation was somehow not a practical success. It cannot be maintained that it failed because the people were averse to it; for it continued to be in popular request far into the 19th century, until it was at length suppressed by statute. For the present we may return to the proper subject of epidemic smallpox, premising, on the ground of what has been said, that inoculation made but little difference to the epidemiological history.

---

[1] John Forbes, M.D., "Some Account of the Smallpox lately prevalent in Chichester and its vicinity." *Lond. Med. Reposit.* Sept. 1822, p. 218.

[2] *Discourse on Inoculation.* Eng. Transl. 1755.

[3] *A Series of Experiments, &c.* 1768.

[4] John Haygarth, M.B., *Inquiry how to prevent the Smallpox.* Chester, 1784, p. 154.

[5] *History of Inoculation in Britain.* Vol. I. London, 1796, p. 33.

[6] *History of Edinburgh.* Edin. 1779, p. 260.

The Epidemiology continued from 1721.

The ordinary course of smallpox in Britain was little touched by inoculation. The inoculators were like the fly upon the wheel, with the important difference that they did indeed raise the dust. The writers who kept up the old Hippocratic or Sydenhamian habit of recording the prevalent maladies of successive seasons, such as Huxham, Hillary[1], and Barker, of Coleshill, while they dealt with epidemics impartially and comprehensively, were as if by a common instinct adverse to the fuss made about inoculation. Says Barker, in an essay against inoculation during the Suttonian enthusiasm, "It is undoubtedly a great error that the smallpox is now considered the only bugbear in the whole list of diseases, which, if people can get but over, they think they are safe." This hits fairly enough the disproportionate share given to inoculation in the medical writings of the time, while it is made more pointed by the author's suggestions for a scientific study of the conditions of smallpox itself[2]. It is still possible, with much trouble, to bring together the data for a scientific handling of the disease in the 18th century, thanks most of all to the exact school of observers or statisticians which began with Percival, of Manchester, and was continued to the end of the century by Haygarth, Heysham, Ferriar, Aikin and others. The best of the original English inoculators, Nettleton of Halifax, has also left a large number of interesting statistics relating to epidemics in Yorkshire and other northern counties in the years 1721–23; also, upon his suggestion, the figures were procured from many more smallpox epidemics in other parts of England down to 1727. It will be convenient to resume the history with these, as they come next in order after the London epidemic of 1720, at which point the interlude of inoculation came in. The following is a complete table of the figures collected from various sources: it will be observed that most parts of England are represented, the fullest representation being of the northern counties.

---

[1] W. Hillary, *Rational and mechanical Essay on the Smallpox.* Lond. 1735.

[2] J. Barker, *The Nature of Inoculation explained and its Merits stated.* London, 1769, p. 33. He taught that a depraved habit, by ill diet, &c., "serves for a nidus wherein the variolous matter rests." If the variolous matter to be expelled is small, "by reason of natural health, temperance, or the power of preparation," the disease is of the distinct kind; when large, of the confluent. "And wise indeed must he be who can find out any laws respecting the reception and expulsion of diseases superior on the whole to those which are original." p. 9.

Censuses of Smallpox Epidemics in England, 1721–30.

Locality of the Epidemic	Period	Authority	Cases	Deaths	Percentage of Fatalities
[1] Halifax	winter of 1721 to April 1722	Nettleton, *Phil. Trans.* XXXII. 51	276	43	15·9
[2] Rochdale	,,	,,	177	38	21·4
[3] Leeds	,,	,,	792	189	23·8
Halifax parish towards Bradford	1722	*Ibid.* p. 221	297	59	19·9
Halifax parish, another part	,,	,,	268	28	10·4
Bradford	,,	,,	129	36	27·9
Wakefield	,,	,,	418	57	13·6
[4] Ashton under Lyne	,,	,,	279	56	20·0
Macclesfield	,,	,,	302	37	12·2
Stockport	,,	,,	287	73	25·4
Hatherfield	,,	,,	180	20	11·1
[5] Chichester	1722 (to 15 Oct.)	Whitaker, *Ibid.* p. 223	994	168	16·9
Haverfordwest	1722	Perrot Williams, *Ibid.*	227	52	22·9
Barstand, Ripponden, Sorby, and part of Halifax parish 4 miles from the town	,,	Nettleton, in Jurin's *Acct.* for 1723, p. 7	230	38	16·5
Bolton	1723?	Jurin's *Acct.* for 1723, p. 8	406	89	21·6
Ware	,,	,,	612	72	11·7
Salisbury	,,	,,	1244	165	13·2
Rumsey, Hants	,,	,,	913	143	15·6
Havant	,,	,,	264	61	23·1
Bedford	,,	,,	786	147	18·4
Shaftesbury	1724?	*Ibid.* for 1724, p. 12	660	100	15·1
Dedham, near Colchester	,,	,,	339	106	31·3
Plymouth	,,	,,	188	32	17·2
Aynho, near Banbury	27 Sept. 1723 to 29 Dec. 1724	Rev. Mr Wasse, rector, *Ibid.* for 1725, p. 55	133	25	18·8
Stratford on Avon	,,	Dr Letherland, *Ibid.*	562	89	15·8
Bolton le Moors	,,	Dr Dixon, *Ibid.*	341	64	18·8
Cobham	,,	Sir Hans Sloane, *Ibid.*	105	20	19·0

[1] "I have taken an account in this town [Halifax], and some parts of the country, and have procured the same from several other towns hereabouts, where the smallpox has been epidemical this last year, with as much exactness as was possible." *Phil. Trans.* XXXII. 211.

[2] "A small neighbouring market town."

[3] "More than usually mortal."

[4] "A small market town in Lancashire, including two neighbouring villages."

[5] Account taken "by a person of credit" and sent to Dr Whitaker. Jurin says, more generally: "Taken in several places by a careful enquiry from house to house." *Account, &c.* 1724, p. 7.

Locality of the Epidemic	Period	Authority	Cases	Deaths	Percentage of Fatalities
Dover	29 Sept. 1725 to 25 Dec. 1726	Dr Lynch of Canterbury, in Jurin's *Acct.* for 1726, p. 17	503	61	12·1
Deal	25 Dec. 1725 to 29 Nov. 1726	„	362	33	9·1
Kemsey, near Worcester	„	Dr Beard, in Jurin, *Ibid.*	73	15	20·5
[1] Uxbridge	1727	Dr Thorold, in Scheuchzer's *Acct.* for 1727 and 1728	140	51	36·4
Hastings	1729–30	Dr Frewen, *Phil. Trans.* XXXVII. 108	705	97	13·7

The years 1722 and 1723, to which most of these epidemics belong, were one of the greater smallpox periods in England. In Short's abstracts of the parish registers those years stand out very prominently by reason of the excess of deaths over births in a large proportion of country parishes (see above, p. 66); and, according to Wintringham's annals, it was not fever that made them fatal years, but smallpox, along with autumnal dysenteries and diarrhoeas. Of one epidemic centre in the winter of 1721–22, which is not in the table, the district of Hertford, we obtain a glimpse from Maitland, who repaired thither from London to practise inoculation.

" I own that it seem'd probable that the six persons in Mr Batt's family might have catched the smallpox of the girl that was inoculated; but it is well-known that the smallpox were rife, not only at Hertford but in several villages round it, many months before any person was inoculated there: witness Mr Dobb's house in Christ's Hospital buildings, where he himself died of the worst sort with purples, and his children had it; some other families there, and particularly Mr Moss's, (where the above-named Elizabeth Harrison, inoculated in Newgate, attended several persons under it to prove whether she would catch the distemper by infection); both Latin boarding-schools, Mr Stout's and Mr Lloyd's families, Mr John Dimsdale's coachman and his wife, and Mr Santoon's maid-servant, who was brought to the same house and died of the confluent kind of the smallpox[2]."

Here we have the same indication of adults attacked as well as children, which we find in Dover's practice in London in 1720 and in all the 17th century and early 18th century references to smallpox. The most detailed account is that

1 " At Uxbridge and in the neighbourhood, the smallpox having been exceedingly fatal all thereabouts."
2 *Mr Maitland's Account of Inoculating the Smallpox vindicated.* 2nd ed. Lond. 1722.

given for the epidemic of 1724–25 at Plymouth by Huxham, who was not an inoculator but purely an epidemiologist and practitioner in the old manner.

The epidemic was a very severe one and of an anomalous type. Adults, according to his particular references and his general statement, must have been freely attacked. The major part of the adult cases, he says, proved fatal, including one of an old gentlewoman of 72,—"a very uncommon exit for a person of her years"! When the disease raged most severely, some children had it very favourably and required no other physic than to be purged at the end of the attack. The pustules were apt to be small and to remain unfilled. In some there were miliary vesicles, dark red or filled with limpid serum, in the interstices between the smallpox pustules. Some had abundance of purple petechiae among the pocks, the latter also being livid. Only one person survived of all who had that haemorrhagic type. Swelling of the face and throat was also seldom recovered from; in such cases that did well, the maxillary and parotid glands would remain swollen for some time. "It was a remarkable instance of the extraordinary virulence of these smallpox that the women (tho' they had had the smallpox before and some very severely too) who constantly attended those ill of the confluent kind, whether children or grown persons, had generally several pustules broke out on their face, hands and breast....I knew one woman that had more than forty on one side of her face and breast, the child she attended frequently leaning on those parts on that side."

Huxham appears to have adopted the whole Sydenhamian practice of blooding, blistering, purging, and salivating. For the last he used calomel: "Two adults and some children in the confluent sort never salivated. Some very young children drivelled exceedingly through the course of the distemper. A diarrhoea very seldom happened to children[1]."

Corresponding very nearly in time to Huxham's malignant and anomalous constitution of smallpox at Plymouth, and agreeing exactly with his generalities as to children and adults, there is an interesting table of the ages and fatalities of those who were attacked at Aynho, in Northamptonshire, six miles from Banbury. It was then a small market town, and its smallpox for some fifteen months of 1723–24, as recorded by the rector of the parish, may be taken as a fair instance of what happened at intervals (usually long ones) in the rural districts in the earlier years of the 18th century[2]:

Ages	0–1	–2	–3	–4	–5	–10	–15	–20	–25	–30	–40	–50	–60	–70	above 70	Total
Cases	0	0	3	4	6	15	33	14	16	9	12	10	4	4	2	132
Deaths	0	0	2	1	0	1	3	1	3	3	3	4	1	2	1	25

The small fatality of the disease between the ages of five years and twenty is according to the experience of all times.

[1] *Phil. Trans.* XXXIII. 379. "A short account of the Anomalous Epidemic Smallpox beginning at Plymouth in August, 1724, and continuing to the month of June, 1725, By the learned and ingenious Dr Huxham, physician at Plymouth."

[2] The totals are given in Jurin's *Account* for 1725. The ages are in the original communication of the Rev. Mr Wasse, among the MS. papers which Jurin had deposited with the Royal Society.

But the considerable proportion of attacks at the higher ages would hardly have been found anywhere in England, not even in a country parish, a generation or two later, although it is consistent with all that is known of smallpox in the 17th century and in the first years of the 18th[1].

Another glimpse of a prolonged smallpox epidemic of the same period in a town is given in Frewen's census of Hastings, with a population of 1636 (males 782, females 854). The disease was prevalent for about a year and a half, and had ceased previous to 28 January, 1732[2]. The table accounts for the whole population:

The number of those that recovered of the smallpox (including four that were inoculated)	608
Died of it	97
Escaped it	206
Died of other diseases since the smallpox raged there	50
The whole number of inhabitants in that town are	1636

Leaving out the fifty who died of other diseases as persons who may or may not have had smallpox, it appears that 725 of the inhabitants of Hastings had been through the smallpox in previous epidemics, that 705 were attacked in this epidemic, and that 206 had hitherto escaped, some of them to be attacked, doubtless, in the future. The proportion of attacks above the age of childhood in the epidemic of 1730–31 would have depended on the length of time since the last great epidemic; the interval was probably a long one, by the large number of susceptible persons in the town, just as at Boston, Massachusetts, in 1721 and 1752, and at Charleston, Carolina, in 1738[3]; and, as the fact is known for these places, so it is probable that the epidemic at Hastings had included many adolescents and adults.

On the other hand, where smallpox came in epidemics at short intervals, or where it was always present, the incidence,

---

[1] The most singular thing in the Aynho experience is that there should have been no cases in infants under two years. It was observed, however, some two generations after this, that smallpox attacked children at the earliest ages in the great towns (Haygarth, *Sketch of a Plan, &c.*, 1793, p. 31), and even in the worst conditions of infancy it has attacked relatively few in the first three months of life. Again, it is nearly as remarkable that there should have been only three cases at Aynho in the third year of life and only four in the fourth. However, the fewness of cases in the five first years of life must be taken as exceptional, even for a village epidemic. If Nettleton, who made the first of these censuses of smallpox epidemics and suggested to Jurin that they should be carried out elsewhere, had given the ages, he would certainly have included some in infancy, for he mentions, in the course of his inoculation experiences, particular cases at nine months, eighteen months, etc.

[2] Frewen, *Phil. Trans.* XXXVII. 108.

[3] See above, pp. 485–6 and 490–1.

even in the first half of the 18th century, was much more exclusively upon childhood. Thus at Nottingham there was always some smallpox, with a great outburst perhaps once in five years. The year 1736 was one of those fatal periods of smallpox, the victims being "mostly children." From the end of May to the beginning of September, great numbers were swept away; the burials in St Mary's churchyard were 104 in May; the burials from all causes for the whole year exceeded the baptisms by 380; there had been no such mortality since thirty years. Such excessive incidence of smallpox upon the earliest years of life happened in places where the infant mortality was high from all causes. Nottingham was one of those places. Leaving out the great smallpox year, 1736, the other seven years of the period 1732–39 had a total of 2590 baptisms to 2226 burials, of which burials no fewer than 1072 were of "infants," meaning probably children under five years, although the work of Harris on the Acute Diseases of Infants, which was current at that time, defines the infantine age as under four years[1].

The years of distress and typhus fever in England, Scotland, and Ireland from 1740 to 1742 were another great period of smallpox epidemics throughout the country. The mortality from that cause is known to have been excessive in Norwich, Blandford, Edinburgh and Kilmarnock, which may be taken as samples of a larger number of epidemics in the same years. The association of much smallpox of a fatal type with much typhus fever, which can be traced in the London bills from an early period, is at length seen to be the rule for the country at large. After 1740–42, the next instances of it were in 1756 and 1766: it is most definitely indicated again in 1798–1800, very clearly in 1817–19, and in 1837–39. In all the later instances smallpox was the peculiar scourge of the infants and children in times of distress, while the contagious fever was as distinctively fatal to the higher ages. There is some reason to think that the law of incidence was the same in populous cities in 1740–42.

Thus at Edinburgh there died in the two worst years of the distress (population in 1732 estimated at 32,000)[2]:

---

[1] Deering, *Nottingham vetus et nova.* 1751, pp. 78, 82. He says, in an essay on smallpox (*Improved Method of treating Smallpox.* Nottingham, 1737) that he treated fifty-one cases in the epidemic of 1736, of which only three proved fatal.

[2] *Gent. Magaz.* 1741, p. 704.

Edinburgh Mortalities.

	1740	1741
Under two years	439	562
From two to five	198	269
From five to ten	53	93
Above ten	547	687
	1237	1611
Fever	161	304
Flux	3	36
Consumption	278	349
Aged	102	156
Suddenly	56	62
Smallpox	274	206
Measles	100	112
Chincough	26	101
Convulsions	22	16
Teething	111	141
Stillborn	29	50
Other diseases	77	78

More than half the deaths were under five years, and among those deaths it will be necessary to include most of the smallpox mortality. That disease in the two exceptional years made 17 per cent. of all deaths, or one in six. But in its somewhat steady prevalence among children in Edinburgh from year to year, smallpox accounted for one death in about ten, as in the following[1]:

Deaths by Smallpox and all causes in Edinburgh, including St Cuthbert's parish, 1744–63.

Year	All Burials	Dead of Smallpox	Year	All Burials	Dead of Smallpox
1744	1345	167	1754	1215	104 .
1745	1463	141	1755	1187	89
1746	1712	128	1756	1316	126
1747	1200	71	1757	1267	113
1748	1286	167	1758	1001	52
1749	1132	192	1759	1136	232
1750	1038	64	1760	1123	66
1751	1241	109	1761	903	6
1752	1187	147	1762	1305	274
1753	1105	70	1763	1160	123
	12709	1256 or 1 in 9·6		11613	1185 or 1 in 9·8

As in other epidemics, it was not until its second year that the smallpox reached Norwich. The mortality had been enormous

[1] Alex. Monro, primus, in his Report to the Dean of the Faculty of Medicine of Paris on Inoculation in Scotland, 1765. Reprinted in his *Works*. Edin. 1781, p. 485. He does not give ages, but an inspection of the burial registers is said to show that they were nearly all under five.

in 1741, owing to the distress and the fever, 1456 burials to 851 baptisms; but in 1742 the burials were 1953 (to 825 baptisms), the excess over the previous year being ascribed, in general terms, to the smallpox[1]. It is probable that the enormous excess of burials over baptisms at Newcastle in 1741 was due in great part to the same disease among the children; but the statistics do not show it.

Northampton is an instance of a town with very moderate mortality for the 18th century; for that and other reasons its bills were used by Price as the basis of a table of the expectation of life. It had certainly shared in the fever epidemic of 1741 and 1742, for in the latter of those years the annual bill shows the very high fever-mortality of 37 in 130 deaths from all causes in All Saints' parish, which had fully one-half of the population. But in that year there are no smallpox deaths recorded, and only nine in the next four years. The great periodic outburst of smallpox came in 1747[2] :

Smallpox in Northampton, 1747.

Parish	Cases	Deaths	Percentage of Fatalities
All Saints	485	76	15·6
St Sepulchre	175	21	12·0
St Giles	131	23	17·5
St Peter	30	6	20·0
	821	126	15·3 or 1 in 6·5

Of the 76 deaths in All Saints' parish only 58 were buried there. The deaths from all causes in that parish were 189, of which 103, or 54 per cent., were under five years of age, and 10 between five and ten years. Next year, when things had improved much, although the mortality was still high, All Saints' parish had 119 burials, of which 47, or 40 per cent., were under five years, and 4 from five to ten, only three of the deaths being from smallpox. Only a few smallpox deaths appear in the bills of All Saints' parish until 1756 and 1757, when an epidemic occurred, part of it in each year, which produced in that greatest of the four parishes 85 burials, or half as many again as

---

[1] *Gent. Magaz.* 1742, p. 704. Blomefield gives 1710 and 1731 as great smallpox years in Norwich.

[2] *Ibid.* 1747, p. 623. The population of Northampton in 1746 was 5136. Price, *Revers. Payments.* 4th ed. I. 353.

in the epidemic of ten years before. It is singular that the deaths under and over five are in a very different ratio in the two successive years of the epidemic:

All Saints' Parish, Northampton.

	1756	1757
All deaths	140	135
Smallpox deaths	31	54
All deaths under 2	54	24
„ „ 2—5	12	18
„ „ 5—10	7	21
„ „ 10—20	5	6
„ „ 20—30	13	18
„ „ 30—40 .	7	12
„ „ 40—50	4	5
„ „ above 50	38	31

This looks as if a good many more had died of smallpox at the higher ages in the second year of its prevalence than in the first; but the great difference between the deaths under two in 1756 and 1757 is explained chiefly by the article "convulsions," which is 28 in the former year and only 10 in the latter.

In Boston, Lincolnshire, a town almost as healthy as Northampton, the intervals between epidemics of smallpox were almost as long, and the effect in raising the mortality for the year nearly the same. The population in the last year but one of the table was 3470. The deaths averaged 104 in a year, the smallpox deaths 9·45, or one in eleven[1].

Smallpox in Boston, Lincolnshire, 1749–68.

Year	Baptised	Buried	Died by Smallpox	Year	Baptised	Buried	Died by Smallpox
1749	68	120	48	1759	102	91	—
1750	80	93	—	1760	106	84	2
1751	55	59	—	1761	80	94	—
1752	88	85	—	1762	95	134	3
1753	79	73	—	1763	92	206	69
1754	88	111	1	1764	130	102	5
1755	74	102	19	1765	112	113	—
1756	66	110	34	1766	144	117	—
1757	93	86	4	1767	129	95	—
1758	83	88	4	1768	131	117	—

[1] Part of the account extracted from the parish registers by the Rev. Samuel Partridge, F.S.A., vicar of Boston, and sent to Dr George Pearson, who published it in the *Report of the Vaccine Pock Institution for* 1800–1802. London, 1803, p. 100.

This was a favourable instance of urban smallpox in the 18th century, Boston having "no circumstances of narrow streets, crowded houses, manufactories or want of medical assistance." We may compare with it an industrial town only a little larger, the weaving town of Kilmarnock, Ayrshire, the smallpox epidemics of which came as follows[1]:

Smallpox in Kilmarnock, 1728–63.

Year	Baptised	Buried	Died by Smallpox	Year	Baptised	Buried	Died by Smallpox
1728	111	162	66	1746	—	—	8
1729	—	—	—	1747	—	—	—
1730	—	—	—	1748	—	—	2
1731	—	—	—	1749	134	149	79
1732	—	—	—	1750	—	—	5
1733	—	—	45	1751	—	—	1
1734	—	—	—	1752	—	—	—
1735	—	—	—	1753	—	—	1
1736	135	147	66	1754	146	203	95
1737	—	—	—	1755	—	—	—
1738	—	—	—	1756	—	—	—
1739	—	—	—	1757	125	132	37
1740	95	164	66	1758	—	—	9
1741	—	—	—	1759	—	—	—
1742	—	—	—	1760	—	—	—
1743	—	—	—	1761	—	—	—
1744	—	—	—	1762	132	173	66
1745	116	102	74	1763	—	—	2

Although Kilmarnock had an average annual excess of baptisms over burials (134 to 107), which was more than that of Boston, its smallpox mortality was higher than that of the Lincolnshire market town. On an annual average, one death in eleven from all causes was by smallpox at Boston, one in six at Kilmarnock. In the former the epidemics came at intervals of about five years, in the latter at intervals of three or four. The oftener the epidemic came, the earlier in life it attacked children; and in all subsequent experience it has been found that smallpox is far more mortal to the ages below five than to the ages from five to ten or fifteen. More generally, the conditions were worse for young children in a weaving town than in a market town of nearly the same size. In the populous

---

[1] J. C. M'Vail, M.D. in *Proc. Philos. Soc. Glasgow*, XIII. 1882, p. 381, from a MS. register kept by the session clerk of Kilmarnock, now in the General Register House, Edinburgh. The baptisms and burials have not been extended from the MS. for more years than the table shows.

weaving parish of Dunse, 130 children are said to have died of smallpox in 1733, during a space of three months[1].

The ages at which deaths from smallpox occurred in Kilmarnock from 1728 to 1763 are strikingly different from those already given for the small market town or village of Aynho, near Banbury, in 1723–24; at the latter the greater part of the fatalities, although not of the attacks, happened to persons between twenty and fifty; at the former nine-tenths of the deaths were of infants and young children, as in the following:

Ages at Death from Smallpox, Kilmarnock, 1728–63.

Deaths at all ages	Under One	One to Two	Two to Three	Three to Four	Four to Five	Five to Six	Above Six	Age not stated
622	118	146	136	101	62	23	27	9

This almost exclusive incidence of fatal smallpox upon infants and young children in a weaving town during the middle third of the 18th century we shall find abundantly confirmed for English manufacturing and other populous towns in the last third of the 18th century, and thereafter until the middle of the 19th century. On the other hand, the less populous towns and the country districts continued in the 18th century to furnish a fair share of adult cases, for the reason that epidemics came to them at longer intervals, wherein many had passed from infancy to childhood, and even from childhood to youth or maturity, without once encountering the risk of epidemic contagion.

Of such less populous places we have an instance in Blandford, Dorset. Particulars of its smallpox have been given in connexion with general inoculations; here let us note that in this typical market town of 2110 inhabitants (in 1773), the known epidemics were in 1731, 1741, 1753 and 1766—at intervals of ten or a dozen years. In the villages the intervals were longer. Haygarth gives the instance of three parishes in Kent with only ten deaths from smallpox in twenty years, and of Seaford, in Sussex, with one death "eleven years ago[2]." An authentic instance is the parish of Ackworth, Yorkshire, whose register of burials contains only one smallpox death in the ten years 1747–57, while there are thirteen such deaths in it in the next ten-

---

[1] *Statist. Acct. of Scotland.*
[2] *Sketch of a Plan, &c.* 1793, pp. 33–34.

years period, clearly the effects of an epidemic, perhaps in 1766[1]. This parish, judged by the excess of births, was not so healthy as many[2], while its mortality by "fevers" was considerable. The following somewhat general statements are made for the parish of Kirkmaiden, Wigtonshire[3]:

1717. "Nearly thirty-seven died of the smallpox."
1721. Forty-eight died, "mostly of fevers."
1725. Forty-three died, "mostly of the smallpox."

By means of this law of periodic return, at short intervals in the populous industrial towns, at longer intervals in the market towns, and at very long intervals in the villages, we may realize in a measure what smallpox was at its worst. It was the great infective scourge of infancy and childhood, admitting but few or feeble rivals or competitors, as we shall see in the historical accounts of measles, whooping-cough and scarlatina. The table of epidemics from 1721 to 1727, given at p. 518, is of a kind that might have been furnished by any series of years in the 18th century; they were so much of a commonplace that hardly anyone thought of chronicling them unless for a special statistical purpose, such as the inoculation controversy. Thus, the Salisbury epidemic of 1723, with 1244 cases and 165 deaths, must have been only one of a series at intervals, which may or

---

[1] The following is the Ackworth bill given by Price, *Phil. Trans.* LXV. 443.

	1747–57	1757–67
Christened	127	212
Buried	107	156
Consumption	23	38
Dropsy	5	3
Fevers	35	23
Infancy	13	13
Old age	24	30
Smallpox	1	13
Chincough	—	2
Convulsions	—	6
Dysentery	—	2
Measles	—	2
Sundries	6	24
Total deaths in ten years	107	156

[2] The following are some examples of rural fecundity and health : Middleton, near Manchester, 1763–72, births 1560, deaths 993, average of 4·75 children to a marriage. Tattenhall, near Chester, 1764–73, births 280, deaths 130; Waverton, same county and years, births 193, deaths 84. Stoke Damerel (now the dockyard near Plymouth), in 1733 (in part an influenza-year), births 122. deaths 62, population 3361. Landward townships of Manchester in 1772, births 401, deaths 246. Darwen, in 1774–80, births 508, deaths 233, population 1850. From Papers in *Phil. Trans.* by Percival and others.

[3] *Statist. Acct. of Scot.* I. 155.

may not have become more frequent, or of different age-incidence, or of more fatal type, as the century proceeded. We have a glimpse of one of them in 1752–3. Lord Folkestone having given a hundred pounds to the poor of Salisbury, it was ordered on 15 December, 1752, "that five shillings be given to every inhabitant who hath had the smallpox in the natural way since 1 September, or that shall have it hereafter." The epidemic went on for months; it was not until the end of 1753 that the mayor advertised the city free of smallpox. In September of that year ten guineas were voted to Mr Hall, the apothecary, for his trouble during the smallpox, and a like sum to Mr Dennis, the surgeon[1].

The year 1753 was also the time of one of the periodical Blandford outbreaks. For a year or two before there had been much smallpox at Plymouth, the account of which by Huxham will serve as a sample of his numerous references to the disease there from the beginning of his annals in 1728.

In May, 1751, smallpox was brought in by Conway's regiment; it spread in July and August, becoming worse in type in the autumn as it became more common. In January 1752 it was still prevalent, the pustules often crude, crystalline, undigested to the end; sometimes very confluent, small and sessile; sometimes black and bloody, attended now and then with petechiae. In March the type grew more mild; in April the malady was still up and down, some cases being of a bad sort. It became more frequent again in June, and was epidemic all the summer, the eruption often confluent, small, sometimes black, with haemorrhages from the nose, especially in children. In August it was epidemic everywhere, and more fatal, becoming milder in September and October. In December, "the crusts of the black confluent kind many times remained for at least thirty days after the eruption." It declined from January, 1753, and entirely ceased in May, having had a prevalence of two years[2].

Smallpox in London in the middle of the 18th century.

There is hardly any epidemic malady in London of which so few particular records remain as of smallpox, except in the bills of mortality. The monthly notes in the *Gentleman's Magazine* from 1751 to 1755 by Dr Fothergill, who practised at that time in White Hart Court, Lombard Street (having afterwards removed westward to Harpur Street, Red Lion Square), contain the following references to it:

[1] Hoare's *Wiltshire*, VI. 521. There had been a general inoculation to the number of 422, from 13 August, 1751, to February, 1752, just before the epidemic. Brown to Watson, in *Phil. Trans.* XLVII. 570.
[2] Huxham, *Ulcerous Sore-throat*, 1757.

1751, May. Smallpox uncommonly mild in general, few dying of it in comparison of what happens in most years.

1751, December. Smallpox began to make their appearance more frequently than they had done of late, and became epidemical in this month. They were in general of a benign kind, tolerably distinct, though often very numerous. Many had them so favourably as to require very little medical assistance, and perhaps a greater number have got through them safely than has of late years been known.

1752, January. A distinct benign kind of smallpox continued to be the epidemic of this month....A few confluent cases, but rarely. February— Children and young persons, unless the constitution is very unfavourable, get through it very well, and the height to which the weekly bills are swelled ought to be considered in the present case as an argument of the frequency, not fatality, of this distemper.

1752, April. Smallpox continued to be the principal epidemic, as in the preceding months; during which time it attacked most of those who had not hitherto had the distemper, and it is now spread into the suburbs and the neighbouring villages, but still in a favourable way in general. Some have the confluent, a few the bleeding kind, but these are not very common.

1752, June. Smallpox still continues, not many escaping who have not had it before.

1752, July. Smallpox inclined to become malignant, but the constitution on the whole remarkably mild. Children from one to three years old have, I believe, suffered more from the distemper during this constitution than those of any other ages; at least it has so fallen out under the writer's observation.

1753, December. Smallpox of a bad type.

1754, August. Smallpox frequent in many parts of the City, and eastern suburbs especially. In general the kind was mild, distinct and favourable. Out of sixteen who had the disease in a certain district, of different ages, one only died. In some it was very virulent, with livid petechiae.

1754, December. Smallpox not unfrequent. Many had the worst kind seen for years.

1755, January. Smallpox more favourable.

Fothergill, who pointed out the defects of the London bills of mortality and made a serious attempt to get them reformed[1], was disposed to take their figures of smallpox deaths as on the whole trustworthy: " The smallpox, of all diseases mentioned in the weekly bills, is perhaps the only one of which we have any tolerably exact account, it being a disease which the most ignorant cannot easily mistake for another." Reserving this opinion for some critical remarks in the sequel, we may now resume the London statistics from the year last given.

---

[1] *Gent. Magaz.* 1751, Supplement, p. 577. See also June, 1751, p. 244, and letter of "Devoniensis," *ibid.* 1752, p. 159. The subject had been raised by Corbyn Morris in his *Observations on the past growth and present state of London,* and was discussed, from an actuary's point of view, by Dodson in *Phil. Trans.* XLVII. (Jan. 1752), p. 333.

Smallpox Mortality in London, 1721-60.

Year	Deaths from smallpox	Deaths from all causes
1721	2,375	26,142
1722	2,167	25,750
1723	3,271	29,197
1724	1,227	25,952
1725	3,188	25,523
1726	1,569	29,647
1727	2,379	28,418
1728	2,105	27,810
1729	2,849	29,722
1730	1,914	26,761
1731	2,640	25,262
1732	1,197	23,358
1733	1,370	29,233
1734	2,688	26,062
1735	1,594	23,538
1736	3,014	27,581
1737	2,084	27,823
1738	1,590	25,825
1739	1,690	25,432
1740	2,725	30,811
1741	1,977	32,169
1742	1,429	27,483
1743	2,029	25,200
1744	1,633	20,606
1745	1,206	21,296
1746	3,236	28,157
1747	1,380	25,494
1748	1,789	23,069
1749	2,625	25,516
1750	1,229	23,727
1751	998	21,028
1752	3,538	20,485
1753	774	19,276
1754	2,359	22,696
1755	1,988	21,917
1756	1,608	20,872
1757	3,296	21,313
1758	1,273	17,576
1759	2,596	19,604
1760	2,181	19,830

The year 1752, to which Fothergill refers most fully in the notes cited, had the highest total of deaths from smallpox in the period 1721-60, namely, 3538, and was exceeded by only two years in the latter part of the century, 1772, with 3992 deaths and 1796 with 3548. Fothergill says twice that the disease in 1752 was on the whole mild, but so universal that not many escaped it who had not had it before; and that children from one to three years suffered most from it. As the year was not

34—2

an unhealthy one in general, this epidemic of smallpox may be chosen to show its effect upon the weekly mortalities, of children in particular.

London Weekly Mortalities: Smallpox Epidemic of 1752.

Week ending		All deaths	Under two years	Two to five	Five to ten	Smallpox deaths	Convulsions deaths
March	3	438	162	54	19	64	113
	10	441	165	40	16	63	116
	17	477	177	56	15	76	110
	24	456	161	61	19	87	111
	31	471	169	62	8	96	117
April	7	500	185	58	14	87	129
	14	431	144	52	27	76	99
	21	397	145	37	18	77	106
	28	458	161	47	25	94	98
May	5	421	133	52	17	81	85
	12	414	140	62	24	93	101
	19	461	235	52	20	119	104
	26	456	157	66	24	120	92
June	2	452	159	65	28	125	98
	9	415	172	51	17	113	87
	16	421	165	56	20	120	98
	23	380	160	57	15	102	82
	30	353	127	52	19	92	74
July	7	390	142	68	19	107	87
	14	339	142	44	12	79	98
	21	351	144	38	23	73	97
	28	368	168	53	14	92	93
Aug.	4	316	141	37	13	72	90
	11	350	155	44	13	58	99
	18	297	145	26	9	43	98
	25	371	168	46	12	57	109

The weeks with highest smallpox mortalities have not always the highest deaths from all causes; but they correspond to a marked rise of the deaths from two to five years. If the table were continued to the end of the year, to show the decline of smallpox to a fourth or fifth of its highest weekly figures, the decline in the deaths from two to five, as well as from five to ten, would be seen to correspond more strikingly[1]. The other notable suggestion of the figures is that the article "convulsions," which included at that time nearly the whole of infantile diarrhoea, is not so high as usual when the article smallpox rises most. The highest weekly deaths from convulsions are in the first months of the year, when the smallpox epidemic was beginning, and in September and October, the season of

[1] The weekly average deaths for eight weeks of September and October is 30·5 from two to five years and 11·1 from five to ten, which are about half the average at each age period during the maximum prevalence of smallpox.

infantile diarrhoea, when the smallpox epidemic was nearly spent.

The ages at which persons died in the several diseases were not given in the Bills, although they were recorded in the books of Parish Clerks' Hall; so that the incidence of smallpox mortality upon infants and young children cannot be proved for the capital as it can for other great towns in the 18th century. Not only can it not be proved, but it was not the fact that the disease was so exclusively an affair of childhood as it was in the populous provincial centres. The London population was peculiar in receiving a constant recruit direct from the country. Many of them came from parishes where, as Lettsom says, "the smallpox seldom appears"; they must often have passed their childhood without meeting with it, to encounter the risk when they came to London[1]. Many of the class of domestic servants were in that position; and it was especially for them that the London Smallpox Hospital existed, the admission to it being by subscribers' letters, as in the voluntarily supported hospitals at present.

Its small accommodation was given up to some extent also to persons in exceptionally distressed circumstances[2]. From its opening on 26 September, 1746, to 24 March, 1759, it had admitted 3946 cases, of which 1030 had died; these are stated in the annual reports to have been "mostly adults, in many cases admitted after great irregularities and when there was little hope of a cure"; so that the practice of this hospital alone may be taken as evidence of several hundreds of adult cases of smallpox in the year in London (the whole annual cases averaging perhaps twelve thousand).

The exact statistics which we shall come to in a later period of the century, for Manchester, Chester, Warrington and Carlisle, show that nearly all the deaths by smallpox were under five

---

[1] W. Black, M.D. (*Observations Medical and Political on the Smallpox, etc.* London, 1781, p. 100) says : "I am induced by various considerations to believe that whatever share of smallpox mortality takes place in London amongst persons turned of twenty years of age, is almost solely confined to the new annual settlers or recruits, who are necessary to repair the waste of London, and the majority of whom arrive in the capital from twenty to forty years of age."

[2] Maddox, bishop of Worcester, preaching a sermon in 1752 for the Smallpox and Inoculation Charity, enforced his pleading by relating the recent case of "a poor man sick of this distemper, of which his wife lay dead in the same room, with four children around her catching the dreadful infection, but destitute of all relief, till they found *some* in that too narrow building which now importunately begs your compassionate bounty to enlarge its dimensions."

years; and it can hardly be doubted that the bulk of them in
London also, with all its influx of country people, were at the
same age-period. "Most born in London," said Lettsom, "have
smallpox before they are seven." It is singular, therefore, that
smallpox should have caused a much smaller proportion of the
deaths from all causes in London than in the populous provincial
cities. The annual average for London was one smallpox death
to about ten or twelve other deaths; in other large towns it was
one in about six or seven. Lettsom held that the proportion in
London would have come out nearly the same if the classification
of deaths in the London bills had been correct, the generic
article "convulsions" having swallowed up, in his opinion, a
large number of the smallpox deaths of infants. An assertion
such as that is more easily made than refuted. Everyone
agreed that there was no difficulty in recognising smallpox[1].
Whoever had seen confluent smallpox all over an infant's body
was not likely to have set down its death under any other
name, for there is hardly anything more distinctive or more
loathsome. It is possible, however, that many infants with mild
smallpox had died of complications, such as autumnal diarrhoea.
Sydenham, indeed, says as much under the year 1667, blaming
the nurses for killing the infants by trying to check the
diarrhoea. The truly incredible sacrifice of infant life in
London in the 17th and 18th centuries by summer diarrhoea, as
shown in another chapter, may have caused a certain number of
deaths of infants to be classed under "griping in the guts" in
the earlier period, and under "convulsions" in the later, which
were primarily cases of smallpox. But the true probability of
the matter—and it is wholly for us a question of probability—is
that London's smaller ratio of smallpox deaths and greater
ratio of infantile deaths from other causes, was not artificially
made by transferring deaths from the one to the other, but was
actual, owing to a really greater liability of the London infants
to die of other more or less nondescript maladies before smallpox could catch them[2].

[1] The *Gent. Magaz.* Sept. 1752, p. 402, contains a long letter to refute the very
prevailing notion among many people that there is very little occasion for doctors and
apothecaries in smallpox, but that a good nurse is all the assistance that is usually
wanted. "Whence this notion took its rise I cannot conceive, unless it was from the
disease being visible, so that every one who has been at all used to it knows it when
they see it."

[2] This was an argument used in the first writings on Inoculation, so as to prove
the real hazard of dying by the natural smallpox. Thus, Maitland in his *Vindication*

The Epidemiology continued to the end of the 18th century.

The London bills, which are the only continuous series of figures, show the following annual mortalities by smallpox from 1761 to the end of the century:

Smallpox Mortality in London, 1761–1800.

Year	Smallpox deaths	All deaths	Year	Smallpox deaths	All deaths
1761	1,525	21,063	1781	3,500	20,709
1762	2,743	26,326	1782	636	17,918
1763	3,582	26,148	1783	1,550	19,029
1764	2,382	23,202	1784	1,759	17,828
1765	2,498	23,230	1785	1,999	18,919
1766	2,334	23,911	1786	1,210	20,454
1767	2,188	22,612	1787	2,418	19,349
1768	3,028	23,639	1788	1,101	19,697
1769	1,968	21,847	1789	2,077	20,749
1770	1,986	22,434	1790	1,617	18,038
1771	1,660	21,780	1791	1,747	18,760
1772	3,992	26,053	1792	1,568	20,213
1773	1,039	21,656	1793	2,382	21,749
1774	2,479	20,884	1794	1,913	19,241
1775	2,669	20,514	1795	1,040	21,179
1776	1,728	19,048	1796	3,548	19,288
1777	2,567	23,334	1797	522	17,014
1778	1,425	20,399	1798	2,237	18,155
1779	2,493	20,420	1799	1,111	18,134
1780	871	20,517	1800	2,409	23,068

The last twenty years of the century show a decrease in the annual averages of smallpox deaths, along with a decrease of deaths from all causes. The health of the capital had undoubtedly improved since the reign of George II., especially in the saving of infant life. But it is not worth while instituting a statistical comparison, for the reason that some large parishes, containing poor and unwholesome quarters, had become populous in the latter part of the century, but were not included in the

of 1722, which Arbuthnot is said to have had a hand in, deducts a quarter of the annual London deaths before he begins to estimate the ratio of smallpox among them, for the reason that eight out of nine infants who die in their first year are "nonentities" *quâ* smallpox, other causes of death having had the priority (p. 19). Jurin used the same argument for the same purpose in his *Letter to Caleb Cotesworth, M.D.*, 1723, p. 11: "It is notorious that great numbers, especially of young children, die of other diseases without ever having the smallpox"; and again, "very young children, or at most not above one or two years of age," including the stillborn, abortives and overlaid, chrisoms and infants, and those dead of convulsions. "It is true, indeed, that in all probability some small part of these must have gone through the smallpox, and therefore ought not to be deducted out of the account"; but he does deduct 386 in every 1000 London deaths before he estimates the ratio of smallpox deaths, which so comes out 2 in 17.

bills, while some of the old parishes, including those of the City, were probably become less populous owing to the conversion of dwelling-houses into business premises of various kinds. The decrease of fever-deaths in the bills is closely parallel with the decrease of smallpox, and it is probable that both were real ; but as there is an element of uncertainty in the data it would be unprofitable to abstract statistical ratios from them, or to aim at demonstrating numerically what can only be in a measure probable. Perhaps the safest generality from these London figures is that smallpox once more fluctuates a good deal from year to year, seldom, indeed, falling below a thousand deaths, but showing a considerable drop for several years after some greater epidemic, as in the earlier history. This becomes most obvious by exhibiting the mortality in a graphic tracing.

Manchester, which was a healthier place than the capital, having an excess of births over deaths, had a smallpox mortality for six successive years, 1769–1774, as follows, the population, exclusive of Salford, having been 22,481 by a careful survey in 1773[1]:

Smallpox Deaths in Manchester.

Year	All deaths	Smallpox deaths
1769	549	74
1770	689	41
1771	678	182
1772	608	66
1773	648	139
1774	635	87
	3,807	589

Between a seventh and a sixth part of all the deaths in Manchester (15·3 per cent.) were from smallpox. All but one were under the age of ten years :

All deaths by smallpox	Under One year	One to Two	Two to Three	Three to Five	Five to Ten	Ten to Twenty
589	140	216	110	93	29	1

Manchester was one of the towns that had smallpox continuously from year to year at this period. It had a rapidly growing population, and an excess of births over deaths which was in great part due to the very large number of new families settling in it. It was probably this rapid increase of children that

---

[1] Percival, *Med. Obs. and Inquiries,* v. 1776, p. 287 ; population in *Phil. Trans.* LXIV. 54.

explained the great height of the smallpox mortality in 1781, namely, 344, rising from three deaths in January and falling to thirteen in December, the maximum being in the third quarter of the year[1].

Liverpool, like Manchester, had smallpox among its infants and children steadily from year to year, and a higher rate of fatality from that cause than Manchester. With a population half as great again as that of Manchester, namely, 34,407 in 1773, it had the following deaths from smallpox, according to the figures taken from the registers by Dobson and supplied to Haygarth[2]:

Smallpox Deaths in Liverpool.

Year	Baptisms	Burials	Dead of smallpox
1772	1160	1085	219
1773	1192	1129	200
1774	1207	1420	243

The smallpox deaths were 1 in $5\frac{1}{2}$ of all deaths. The figures also mean that nearly all the infants born in Liverpool, who survived the first months, must have gone through the smallpox.

Warrington, with a population (about 9000) one-fourth that of Liverpool, had a great periodic outbreak of smallpox in 1773, which caused about the same number of deaths that Liverpool had steadily in three successive years. The deaths were 207, with an incidence upon infants as remarkable as at Manchester. I reserve the figures for another section. Whether Warrington had much or any smallpox in the years between, it is known to have had fifty deaths in 1781, most of them in the first half of the year. Chester, in 1774, with a population half as great again as Warrington, namely, 14,713, had 1385 cases of smallpox, with 202 deaths, or 1 in 6·85, all the deaths being of children under five except 22, and those of children from five to ten. At the end of the epidemic a census showed that there were only 1060 persons in Chester who had not had smallpox. It was one of the healthier towns, which had a great smallpox mortality only in certain years; in 1772 it had 16 deaths, in 1773, only one death; the next great mortality after 1774 falling in 1777, when the deaths were 136, of which only 7 were in children above the age of seven years. In 1781 it had 7 deaths.

---

[1] Haygarth, *Inquiry how to prevent the Smallpox*, 1784.
[2] Haygarth, *Sketch of a plan to exterminate the Natural Smallpox.* Lond. 1793, p. 139.

In the year 1781, when smallpox was so fatal to Manchester, Leeds also had an epidemic, 462 cases, with no fewer than 130 deaths, the population (in 1775) being 17,111, of whom only some seven hundred (or eleven hundred) at the end of the epidemic had not been through the natural smallpox.

At Carlisle, where the conditions of a greatly increased population (4158 in 1763 increased to 6299 in 1780) and weaving industries were the same as at Leeds, the smallpox deaths in a series of years were as follows[1]:

Deaths by Smallpox at Carlisle, 1779–87.

	Total	Under Five years	Over Five years			Total	Under Five years	Over Five years
1779	90				1784	10	9	1
1780	4	} 136	7		1785	38	39	0
1781	19				1786	—	—	—
1782	30				1787	30	28	2
1783	19	17	2			—	—	—
						241	229	12

The smallpox deaths were 13·37 per cent. of the deaths from all causes. The deaths from all causes under five years were 44·13 per cent.

Whitehaven, which had, like Liverpool, a large part of its labouring population housed in cellars, suffered severely from smallpox in 1783: "incredible numbers," says Heysham, of Carlisle, were attacked, of whom " scarcely one in three survived." The annual reports of its dispensary, which begin from that year, show a small number of calls to smallpox cases in most years; but it must have happened there, as Clark found it in Newcastle, that medical aid was not often sought for the children of the poor in smallpox unless they were dying. Smallpox was perhaps not peculiar among infantile troubles in that respect; but it is remarkable that it should have fallen so little under the notice of practitioners considering how important its aggregate effects were on the death-rate. In 1753 the readers of the *Gentleman's Magazine* took some interest in the question whether smallpox required the aid of a physician or an apothecary, or whether a nurse were not sufficient: instances were adduced in support of the latter view, while the serious claims of smallpox to regular medical attendance were elabo-

---

[1] John Heysham, M.D. " An Abridgement of Observations on the Bills of Mortality in Carlisle, 1779–1787," in Hutchinson's *History of Cumberland.* 2 vols. Carlisle, 1794, and separate reprint, Carlisle, 1797; also reprinted in Appendix to Joshua Milne's *Treatise on the Valuation of Annuities.* London, 1815, pp. 733–752.

rately urged in a letter several columns long. At Newcastle, at all events, the prevalence and fatality of smallpox were actually unknown to Dr Clark, for all his zeal and statistical accuracy. Assuming from the experience of some other populous industrial towns, that it made a sixth part of the deaths from all causes, he estimated its annual mortality at 130.

Smallpox in Glasgow towards the end of the 18th century appears to have been more mortal to children than anywhere else in Britain. The figures are not known previous to 1783, from which year the laborious researches of Dr Robert Watt in the burial registers begin; but it is probable that the conditions were as favourable to smallpox at an earlier period[1]. In the year 1755 its mortality is given thus: "buried, men 273, women 206, children 584, total 963[2]."

The following table shows the Glasgow deaths from small-pox, and from all causes at all ages and at three age-periods under ten:

Glasgow Mortality by Smallpox and all causes, 1783–1800.

Year	All deaths	Smallpox deaths	All deaths under Two	All deaths 2—5	All deaths 5—10
1783	1413	155	479	174	66
1784	1623	425	671	161	45
1785	1552	218	576	126	42
1786	1622	348	706	179	56
1787	1802	410	746	205	65
1788	1982	399	770	221	68
1789	1753	366	794	188	76
1790	1866	336	903	247	86
1791	2146	607	984	320	63
1792	1848	202	664	184	54
1793	2045	389	807	239	80
1794	1445	235	553	144	62
1795	1901	402	761	225	62
1796	1369	177	562	181	54
1797	1662	354	586	241	57
1798	1603	309	642	181	41
1799	1906	370	783	244	78
1800	1550	257	545	148	53

Dividing the period into three of six years each, and abstracting the ratios, Watt got the following result[3], by which it appears

[1] See Loveday's *Diary of a Tour,* 1732, p. 120.
[2] *Gent. Magaz.* 1755, p. 595. In a parish near Glasgow, Eaglesham, eighty children are said to have died of smallpox in 1713. Chambers, *Domest. Annals,* III. 387.
[3] Robert Watt, M.D., *Treatise on the History, Nature and Treatment of Chin-cough...to which is subjoined an Inquiry into the relative mortality of the Principal Diseases of Children, and the Numbers who have died under ten years of age in Glasgow during the last thirty years.* Glasgow, 1813.

that smallpox made between a fifth and a sixth of the whole mortality, and presumably a full third of all the deaths under five years:

Six-years period	All deaths	Ratio of fevers	Ratio of smallpox	Ratio under five years, all deaths
1783 to 1788	9994	12·65	19·55	50·06
1789 to 1794	11103	8·43	18·22	53·28
1795 to 1800	9991	8·24	18·70	51·03

The Glasgow figures bear out the rule that the greater the mortality of children from all causes, the greater the mortality from smallpox. The ratio of infantile deaths (under two) was actually higher in Glasgow in the end of the 18th century than in London during the very worst period of its history, the time of excessive drunkenness in the second quarter of the 18th century: the London deaths under two years were 38·6, and from two to five 11·37 per cent. of the annual average deaths from 1728 to 1737, while the Glasgow maxima were 42·38 and 11·90.

The examples last given are all of crowded industrial towns, the sanitary condition of which has been referred to in the chapter on Typhus. The market towns and the villages doubtless had the same relatively favourable experiences of smallpox which have been shown for them in the first half of the 18th century. It happens that the figures for Boston, Lincolnshire, of which a twenty-years series has been given already, are complete to the end of the century.

Smallpox Deaths in Boston, Lincolnshire, 1769–1800.

Year	Births	All deaths	Smallpox deaths	Year	Births	All deaths	Smallpox deaths
1769	159	120	3	1785	168	124	4
1770	140	166	78	1786	152	114	—
1771	150	133	2	1787	168	130	—
1772	138	130	6	1788	181	145	—
1773	157	143	27	1789	184	185	27
1774	160	112	—	1790	204	126	—
1775	162	186	55	1791	218	93	2
1776	165	176	7	1792	219	152	—
1777	165	131	6	1793	195	141	1
1778	166	174	18	1794	197	148	—
1779	173	195	3	1795	217	161	1
1780	137	247[1]	—	1796	214	205	64
1781	136	193	19	1797	240	166	—
1782	133	177	—	1798	227	112	—
1783	162	149	—	1799	229	133	—
1784	147	202	58	1800[2]	225	147	1

[1] This high mortality was probably caused by the epidemic agues of 1780, which specially affected Lincolnshire.

[2] In 1802 the smallpox epidemic recurred, with 33 deaths. In 1801 there was one death.

The second division of the table covers the same years as the Glasgow table, but tells a very different tale.   It shows a great excess of births over deaths, and smallpox coming at the same long and regular intervals as in the twenty-years period before 1769, but now causing only a fifteenth part of the whole annual average deaths, or about one-third as many of them as in Glasgow.   Whether the other market towns and villages of England had improved equally cannot be proved, owing to the almost total absence of smallpox statistics from the country south of the Trent.   It was partly an accident that the best statistics of smallpox all came from the northern half of the country, where population and industries were growing most; but it was in part also because there was more epidemic disease there than elsewhere in England.

Some particulars or generalities were recorded for the parishes of Scotland in the last ten years of the 18th century by parish ministers writing for the *Statistical Account*:

Some of the Highland parishes suffered greatly from time to time by epidemics of contagious fever and by smallpox.   Kiltearn, in Eastern Ross, a parish in which "the greatest number of cottages are built of earth, and are usually razed to the ground once in five or seven years, when they are added to the dunghill," was visited at intervals by infectious fever which spread from cottage to cottage, and by smallpox so disastrously in two successive years, 1777 and 1778, that above thirty children died in the first and no fewer than forty-seven in the second, owing, the minister thought, in part to improper management (*Statistical Account of Scotland*, I. 262). Something similar, although the numbers are not given, had happened in 1789 in the Western Ross parish of Applecross, which is now one vast deer-forest with two or three poor fishing hamlets.   Of Kilmuir, in the extreme north-west of Skye, it is said, "In former times the smallpox prevailed to a very great extent, and sometimes almost depopulated the country."

In the parish of Holywood, Dumfriesshire, the yearly average marriages were 5, the baptisms 16, and the burials 11 ; but in 1782, the burials rose to 20, "owing to an infectious fever in the west part of the parish" (said elsewhere to be "chiefly owing to poor living and bad accommodation during the winter season ") ; and in 1786 "the large number of deaths "— namely fourteen all told—" was owing to the ravages of the natural small-pox " (I. 22).

In Galston parish, Ayrshire, "smallpox makes frequent ravages."   In Eaglesham parish, near Glasgow, most of the infectious deaths are by fever, but smallpox also carries off great numbers (II. 118).

In the parish of Largs, Ayrshire, the number of deaths varied in different years "according as the smallpox or any species of dangerous fever prevailed " ; in such cases the number of deaths were above forty, but in ordinary years between twenty and thirty, the mean annual average of births being about thirty.   (II. 362.)   But in Dunoon " we have commonly no sickness or fatal distemper except from old age and the complaints peculiar to children ; and even these last are not in general fatal." (II. 390.)   In Forbes and Kearn, Aberdeenshire, "some children are lost by the smallpox, measles, and hooping-cough. But as the people in a great measure have got over their prejudices against inoculation, very few now die of the smallpox," (IX. 193).

In Monquhitter, in the same county: "the chincough, measles and smallpox return periodically ; but the virulence of these disorders is now greatly lessened by judicious management" (VI. 122). In Grange, Banffshire, "of late neither the smallpox nor any inflammatory disorders have been very prevalent or mortal ; the complaints are principally nervous " (IX. 563). In Fyvie, Aberdeenshire, "there has been no prevalent distemper for some time except the putrid sore-throat " (IX. 461). But, in Dron, Perthshire, smallpox owing to the prejudice against inoculation, continues to carry off a great number of children ; the hot regimen, and the keeping of the patients too long in their foul linen and clothes, are bad for the disease (IX. 468). In Fordyce, the ravages of the smallpox are very much abated by the practice of inoculation ; the most prevalent distemper is fever (III. 48). In the sea-board parish of Rathen, smallpox occurred among the fishers (VI. 16). The fullest account is under the head of Thurso (XX. 502), supplied by John Williamson, surgeon : In December, 1796, the confluent smallpox became highly epidemic and fatal in the county of Caithness. In Thurso, more particularly, the epidemic was almost general, "and by my calculation one in four fell a victim." The mortality became so general that a general inoculation was proposed, and more or less carried out in most parishes except Latheron.

The most exact record is for the parish of Torthorwald Dumfriesshire ; in two ten-year periods and one of seven years the mortality was as follows (II. 12):

	All deaths	Smallpox	Measles	Chin-cough	Fevers	Infants under one, cause unknown
1764—73	100	2	1	1	10	9
1774—83	100	5	0	3	7	14
1784—90	80	7	0	0	8	6

Ages at deaths from all diseases.

	All deaths	Under One	One to Two	Two to Five	Five to Ten	Ten to Forty	Forty to Seventy	Above Seventy
1764—73	100	9	2	1	2	19	28	39
1774—83	100	16	7	2	2	8	34	31
1784—90	80	8	2	1	4	12	23	30

Twelve of the fourteen smallpox deaths occurred after the introduction of inoculation in 1776, and were ascribed by the parish minister to that source. Again, in the parish of Whittinghame, among the Lammermuir hills, "it is not remembered that this parish has ever been visited with any epidemical distemper"—its vital statistics for ten years, 1781–90, being (II. 352):

Marriages	Baptisms	Burials
54	189	81

On the other hand another Berwickshire parish, Dunse, much more populous and occupied with weaving, had an epidemic of smallpox in 1781, which brought the annual deaths up to 85, the births for the year being 54.

Authentic accounts of smallpox in Ireland in the 18th century are not easy to find, but it is clear from such notices of it as do exist that it could be widely prevalent and malignant in type. Rogers gives it a bad name in Cork in the first third of the century. During the great famine and fever of 1740–41 the deaths by smallpox are said to have been twice or thrice as many in Dublin as the deaths by fever[1]. The smallpox mortality, being chiefly of infants and children, attracted no special notice, just as the smallpox deaths in the famine of 1817–18, although more than those by fever, are all but unmentioned in the various accounts for those years. Rutty, of Dublin, under the year 1745, says: "The smallpox was brought to us by a conflux of beggars from the north, occasioned by the late scarcity there; whose children, full of the smallpox, were frequently exposed in our streets." His next mention of smallpox is in the winter of 1757–58, when the disease "kept pace in malignity," with the prevalent spotted or typhus fever. Amidst numerous entries of fevers of all kinds (typhus, agues, miliary fevers), as well as scarlatina and angina, these are the only two references to smallpox in Rutty's Dublin annals from 1726 to 1766. The annals kept by Sims of Tyrone overlap those of Rutty by a few years; and his first reference to smallpox is under the year 1766, which was a year of almost universal smallpox in England. Towards the close of 1766 and in the spring of 1767 the smallpox caused unheard-of havoc, scarcely one-half of all that were attacked escaping death. The disease had appeared the year before along the eastern coast, and proceeded slowly westward with so even a pace that a curious person might with ease have computed the rate of its progress. It had not visited the country for some years, and was not seen again until 1770, when it was less severe than in 1766–7[2].

Little is heard of smallpox in the army and navy in the 18th century. Pringle says, "We have never known it of any consequence in the field." On board ships of war it is mentioned occasionally, but very rarely in comparison with fever. Lind says that it prevailed in 1758 in the 'Royal George,' among a ship's company of 880 men: "it destroyed four or five persons

---

[1] Barker and Cheyne, u. s.
[2] James Sims, M.D., *Observations on Epidemic Disorders.* London, 1773.

and left nearly a hundred unattacked[1]." Trotter has an occasional reference to it in his naval annals from 1794 to 1797[2]. One reason, and doubtless the chief reason, for its rarity in the services was that comparatively few escaped having it in childhood. The surgeon to the Cheshire Militia told Haygarth in 1781 that he found the whole regiment of six hundred to have had smallpox, except thirty[3]. It does not appear that so great a ratio of sailors or marines were protected by a previous attack; for Trotter counted 70 in a 74-gun ship of war who had not had it, and based a calculation thereon that there were about 6000 men in the navy in the like case. It was comparatively rare, also, in the gaols, doubtless for the same reason that has been suggested for the army and navy. Howard mentions it in only three of the prisons visited by him[4].

The range of severity in Smallpox, and its circumstances.

It has been abundantly shown in the foregoing, by the figures of Nettleton and others for Yorkshire and many other parts of England in 1722–27, of Frewen for Hastings in 1731, by the figures for each of the four parishes of Northampton in 1747, and by Haygarth's census of each of the nine (or ten) parishes of Chester in 1774, that the average fatality of smallpox was one death in six or seven attacks[5]. Any average of the

---

[1] *Two papers on Fever and Infection*, 1763, p. 112.
[2] *Medicina Nautica.*
[3] Haygarth, *Sketch of a Plan, &c.*, 1793, p. 32.
[4] Gaol at Bury St Edmunds: In the winter of 1773, five died of the smallpox. No apothecary then. Leicester County Gaol: In 1774 three debtors and one felon died of the smallpox. "Of that disease, I was informed, few ever recover in this gaol." Oxford Castle: In 1773 eleven died of the smallpox. In 1774 that distemper still in the gaol. In 1775 one debtor died of it in May, three debtors and a petty offender in June; three recovered. No infirmary, no straw to lie on. *State of the Prisons.*
[5] I append Haygarth's full table of the Chester smallpox epidemic, 1774:

	Parish	Families	Persons	Recovd. from smallpox	Died of smallpox	Not had smallpox
Suburbs	St Oswald	924	4027	321	40	350
	St John	774	3187	284	52	218
	St Mary	583	2392	240	45	205
	Trinity	330	1605	127	24	97
Old parishes	St Peter	193	920	52	6	39
	St Bridget	154	623	52	6	35
	St Martin	154	611	47	18	35
	St Michael	135	575	15	2	31
	St Olave	134	536	42	8	43
	Cathedral	47	237	3	1	7
		3428	14713	1183	202	1060

kind represents a very wide range, as indeed the table of epidemics on p. 518 sufficiently shows ; and as it is a matter of scientific interest to ascertain, if possible for smallpox as for other epidemic infections, the circumstances of its greater or lesser fatality, I shall endeavour to illustrate still farther the fact of its wide range from an extremely mild to an extremely severe disease, and to inquire into the circumstances or conditions of the same.

In the first place, selected ages were below or above the average. Isaac Massey, apothecary to Christ's Hospital school, having boys to deal with at the most favourable of all ages for smallpox, found that not one had died of the 32 children "who are all that have had the smallpox, in the last two years, in that family"; and that "upon a strict review of thirty years business, and more, I have reason to think not 1 in 40 smallpox patients of the younger life have died, that is, above five and under eighteen[1]." On the other hand the London Smallpox Hospital, whose patients, as the stereotyped phrase in the reports said, were "most of them adults, often admitted after great irregularities and when there are hardly any hopes of a cure," had to acknowledge about one death in four or five cases on an average, which average, again, included such an unfavourable year as 1762, with 224 deaths in 844 cases.

Small groups of cases might perchance incline to mildness or to severity. Those of the former kind in the practice of one person were the more likely to be recorded. Thus Deering says that, in London about the year 1731, his method answered so well that "out of one hundred smallpox patients who were under my care within the course of two years, I lost but one. However, sincerity obliges me to own that the smallpocks were not during that whole time generally malignant, for some had them favourable, and the matter in others who had the confluent kind came in most by the eighth day to a good suppuration[2]." This might be matched with an experience from the seventeenth

---

[1] Isaac Massey, *Remarks on Dr Jurin's last yearly Account of the Success of Inoculation.* Lond. 1727, p. 6. Huxham held that children might be "prepared" for the natural smallpox, as it was then the custom to prepare them for the inoculated disease, so that few of them need have it severely: "I am persuaded, if persons regularly prepared were to receive the variolous contagion in a natural way, far the greater part would have them in a mild manner." *On Fevers.* 2nd ed. 1750, p. 133.
[2] C. Deering, M.D., *Account of an improved Method of treating the Smallpocks.* Nottingham, 1737.

century already given on the doubtful authority of an empiric[1]. At Nottingham, in 1737, Deering claimed to have treated fifty-one cases with three deaths. Dr Robertson, physician to the fleet, says of his practice ashore: "When I arrived at Hythe in the beginning of April, 1783, the smallpox was pretty general...My patients, about fifty in number, all did well[2]."

The hold of a slave-ship may not seem a very good place to have smallpox in; and yet, in the voyage of the 'Hannibal,' 450 tons, 36 guns, from Guinea to Barbados in 1694, with 700 slaves on board, of whom 320 died on the passage from dysentery and white flux, the fatality of smallpox was so slight that "not above a dozen" were lost by it, "though we had a hundred sick of it at a time, and that it went through the ship[3]." This gives some colour to that remarkable experience in the treatment of smallpox which occupied so much of the attention of Bishop Berkeley and of his friend Prior about the years 1746–7. The captain of a slave-ship on his return home made affidavit before the mayor of Liverpool, "in the presence of several principal persons of that town," that smallpox attacked the slaves on board, when on the Guinea Coast, to the number of 170, that 169 of them who were induced to partake of tar-water recovered, and that the one negro who proved recalcitrant against the bishop of Cloyne's panacea died of the disease[4]. The somewhat low fatality of the Boston epidemic of 1752 (569 deaths in 5545 attacks not including the attacks among inoculated persons) was thought possibly due to the use of tar-water by many[5].

Sometimes a run of highly favourable cases was followed by a succession of fatalities, or *vice versa*. Dr Mapletoft, to whom

[1] John Lamport alias Lampard, u. s.
[2] *Obs. on Ship Fever, &c.* New ed. Lond. 1789, p. 448.
[3] Thomas Phillips, "Journal of a Voyage," &c. in Churchill's *Collection of Voyages*, VI. 173.
[4] Berkeley's claim for tar-water in smallpox was a double one, as a preventive or modifier, and as a cure. Of the former he says: "Another reason which recommends tar-water, particularly to infants and children, is the great security it brings against the smallpox to those that drink it, who are observed, either never to take that distemper, or to have it in the gentlest manner." *Further Thoughts on Tar-water*, 1752. In his *Second Letter to Thomas Prior, Esq.* 1746 (in *Works*. 4 vols. Oxford, 1871, III. 476) he gives the famous case of curing by it:—"the wonderful fact attested by a solemn affidavit of Captain Drape at Liverpool, whereby it appears that of 170 negroes seized at once by the smallpox on the coast of Guinea one only died, who refused to drink tar-water; and the remaining 169 all recovered, by drinking it, without any other medicine, notwithstanding the heat of the climate and the incommodities of the vessel. A fact so well vouched must, with all unbiassed men, outweigh, &c."
[5] Prince, *Gent. Magaz.* Sept. 1753, p. 414.

Sydenham dedicated a book, was originally in good physician's practice and Gresham professor of physic; but he gave up these emoluments to enter the Church, and it is related by one who conversed with him in his extreme old age that he gave a singular reason for changing his profession, namely that, having treated smallpox cases for years without losing one (his treatment being to do nothing at all), he thereafter found that two or three died under his hands[1].

Fothergill's sixteen cases, in a certain locality of London in 1752, with only one death, are an instance of a run of mild cases. At the Whitehaven Dispensary in 1796 there was a good instance of how an average is made up; of the first seven cases attended from the dispensary three died, and then followed a run of thirty-four cases with only two of them fatal. Again, a high or low degree of fatality might seem to pertain to a particular spot. Bateman gives an instance in 1807 of 28 deaths within a month in a single court off Shoe Lane; also in 1812, "in one small court in Shoe Lane, seventeen individuals have lately been cut off by this variolous plague[2]." One can understand that of the old Shoe Lane; but why should Nantwich have been reputed never to have its smallpox mortal? Worse things are told of country smallpox in Scotland than in England. In 1758, it is said, 8 died out of 28 near Cupar Fife, and in some parts of Teviotdale "three or four died for one that recovered[3]." Similar unparalleled mortalities are reported by some parish ministers in the 'Statistical Account.'

Cleghorn stationed with British troops in Minorca had a good opportunity of comparing two epidemics of smallpox, one in 1742 and the other in 1746. There had been no smallpox since 1725, so that when it did come in March, 1742, it found many susceptible of it: "every house was a hospital"; but "in proportion to the numbers, not many died; and what mortality there was happened chiefly among children at the breast and the common soldiers. About the end of July the disease suddenly disappeared, most of those who were susceptible of it having by that time undergone it." Four and a half years after, in December, 1745, the infection was brought in by one of H. M. ships from Constantinople, and produced in many cases attacks of

---

[1] Walter Lynn, u. s. 1715, *ad init.*
[2] *Reports, &c.* 1819.
[3] Whytt, *Med. Obs. and Inquiries*, II. (1762), p. 187.

a bad type; which leads Cleghorn to remark that "it is a matter of chance whether the best or the worst kind is got in the natural way[1]." Barbados had its epidemic maladies noted from season to season for several years by Hillary, who enters smallpox once: "May, 1752, smallpox epidemic: in general of the distinct kind; and in those few who had the confluent sort, they were generally of a good kind[2]." Foreign observers were sometimes struck by the same mildness of a whole epidemic[3].

The often cited remark of Wagstaffe in 1722, that there were cases which a physician could not save and cases which a nurse could not lose, had many illustrations. The cases of Queen Mary, in 1694, with the best physicians at her bed-side, and of the Duke of Gloucester in 1660, show the one event; the following from the *Gentleman's Magazine*, shows the other:

In the parish of Whittington, Derbyshire, seventeen patients in all had the smallpox in the year 1752; the first was seized June 7, and the last August 12. They were all children, of various ages, and all did well. An apothecary was called to one only of them[4].

A note added says:

"William Cave, a tradesman of Rugby, had twelve children, who, with three nephews, were seized with the smallpox; some of them had it severely, but all did well through the care of their mothers, without the intervention of an apothecary."

Or there might be the average fatality in village epidemics left to domestic treatment only. At Kelsall and Ashton, two small Cheshire villages, sixty-nine persons had smallpox during seven months of 1773, of whom twelve died. "No medical practitioner visited any of the patients during the whole disease[5]."

To find a single principle of cleavage through the smallpox of the 18th century, dividing it into good and bad, is impossible. The determining things were manifold, and they are to us obscure. Things proper to the individual constitution or temperament, hidden in what has been called "the abysmal deeps of personality," cover a good deal in our reactions towards smallpox as in more important relationships. Generalizing such facts to the utmost, we do not get beyond the notion that the

[1] Cleghorn, *Diseases of Minorca*. London (under the years).
[2] Hillary, *Changes of the Air, and Epidemical Diseases of Barbados*.
[3] Muret, *Mém. par la Société Économique de Berne*, 1766. "Population dans le pays de Vaud": p. 102, "J'ai vu à Veney, la petite vérole être générale dans toute la ville, des centaines d'enfans attaqués de cette maladie, et qu'à peine il en mouroit sept ou huit."
[4] *Gent. Magaz.* 1753, p. 114. Letter from Sam. Pegge, rector, 17 Feb. 1753.
[5] Haygarth, *Phil. Trans.* LXV. 87.

greater or lesser degree of proclivity runs in families. Morton
could recall no case of smallpox fatal in his own family, nor,
curiously enough, among his wife's relations. On the other
hand he introduces a case, his 53rd, as if to illustrate the
contrary—a fair and elegant young lady, sprung of a distinguished stock, but one to which this disease was wont to
prove calamitous as if by hereditary right[1]. The royal family
of Stuart had a peculiar fatality in smallpox; and so, it appears,
had the family of the earl of Huntingdon, who wrote to Thomas
Coke on 18 June, 1701: "I am informed Lord Kilmorey
[married to his sister] is ill of a fever, and that some think it
may prove the smallpox. For the love of God, send for my
sister to your house. She never has had them and they have
proved fatal in our family[2]." A similar fatality in the family of
John Evelyn can be traced in the pages of his diary.

Next to the individual constitution, we may take the
epidemic constitution, in the Hippocratic sense. No one
keeping before him the strange diversities of type in whole
epidemics of scarlatina and measles will say that the Hippocratic
doctrine of varying constitutions is not requisite to cover a
certain element of mystery. But we should rationalize it
wherever we can; and there are some obvious considerations
that may be used to explain why smallpox, throughout a whole
epidemic, had so high an average fatality in some years or in
some localities. Rutty, who noted the fevers and other
prevalent maladies in Dublin and elsewhere in Ireland from
year to year, and the associations of the same with famine or
the like, says that some had dysentery in 1757, "promoted
perhaps by the badness of their bread, as it was a time of great
scarcity," that a low, putrid, petechial fever followed in the
winter, fatal to not a few of the young and strong both in
Dublin and in the country, and that as the cases of petechial
fever increased much beyond the usual number in January,
1758, "it was observable that the smallpox kept pace in

[1] Morton, *Pyreologia*, II. 338: "Et quidem omnes haereditario quasi jure benignis
istis variolis tentabantur, quae (Deo favente) eventum secundum habuerunt; nunquam
enim quemquam meâ vel conjugis meae stirpe ortum hoc morbo periisse memini."
The case of hereditary tendency to fatal smallpox is No. 53, p. 470: "Domina
Theodosia Tytherleigh, virgo elegans ac formosa, stirpe celeberrima (sed cui hic
morbus jure quasi haereditario funestus esse solebat)" &c. She died in a late stage
of the disease.
[2] *Cal. Coke MSS.* (Hist. MSS. Commis.) II. 429.

malignity with the fevers[1]." That was the same year, 1758, for which Whytt records, along with the fatal smallpox of Fifeshire and Teviotdale, a dysentery and pestilential fever a month or two before, disastrous in Argyllshire, less mortal in Haddington and Newcastle, as well as an influenza all over Scotland[2]. Again, in the country town and parish of Painswick, Gloucestershire, there was an epidemic of smallpox in the summer of 1785 so fatal that nearly one in three of the infected died. "This fatality," says J. C. Jenner, "may in some measure perhaps be attributed to a contagious fever and epidemic ague which prevailed at the same time, and to the heat of the atmosphere" —many being dropsical from the agues that had afflicted them for months, and many reduced by the typhus fever[3]. A striking instance of the fatality of smallpox among children in a poor state of health owing to previous disease is given by Sir William Watson :

At the Foundling Hospital of London, containing upwards of 300 children, there were 60 cases of smallpox during the last six months of the year 1762, of which only 4 died, or 1 in 15. In April and May of next year (1763) measles of a bad type broke out among the 312 inmates, attacking 180, of whom 19 died (over 1 in 10), while many who recovered were greatly weakened, having ulcerations of the lips and mouth for some time after. In May and June, when the children were recovering from measles, the smallpox attacked many in the hospital, including 18 who had lately gone through the measles. No fewer than 11 of those 18 died of smallpox. A corresponding fatality of smallpox was observed shortly before among children at the Foundling who were recovering from or had lately passed through the dysentery or "dysenteric fever[4]."

It happens that we can compare a mild or average smallpox with an unusually fatal one, and the conditions on which they respectively depended, in the two neighbouring towns of

---

[1] Rutty, *Chronological History of the Weather and Seasons, and prevailing Diseases in Dublin during forty years.* London, 1770, under the dates.

[2] Short (*Comparative History of the Increase and Decrease of Mankind in England, &c.* Lond. 1767) has found somewhere a statement that in 1717 there was "a most fatal continual fever in the West of Scotland, in January and February, and not less fatal confluent smallpox in March and April."

[3] *Lond. Med. Journ.* VII. 163.

[4] W. Watson, in *Medical Observations and Inquiries by a Society of Physicians in London,* IV. (1771), p. 153. Whether the epidemic that preceded the smallpox was measles or scarlatina is a question that was raised by Willan, and is referred to in the chapter on "Scarlatina and Diphtheria."

Warrington and Chester in the two successive years 1773 and 1774. Chester in 1774 had the average kind of epidemic—1385 cases with 202 deaths (1 in 6·85), all in children. The Chester populace, as described by Haygarth, lived for the most part in poor houses of the newer suburbs; they were filthy in their persons and their houses were often visited by typhus fever (supra, p. 41). But the occupations of the men were not unhealthy, and the women would seem to have been left to their domestic duties in the usual way. At Warrington the circumstances were different. A seat of the sailcloth weaving from the Elizabethan period (as early as 1586 the "poledavies" of Warrington are mentioned), it had retained its repute and extended its industry as sailcloth came more into demand[1]. The American War, and the earlier war with the French in Canada, caused an immense number of ships to be commissioned for the royal navy, and the Warrington looms are said to have furnished half of all the sailcloth that the fleets needed[2]. Its manufacturers made their fortunes, new looms were added, population was drawn to the town from the country, marriages multiplied and were unusually prolific, and the swarms of children were hardly into their teens before they were set to earn wages along with their fathers and their mothers. We have vital statistics from the parish register by Aikin[3], and an account of the industries by Arthur Young, as he saw them in 1769[4]. During the twenty years from 1702 to 1722, each marriage, according to the register, produced only 2·9 children; from 1752 to 1772, the marriages averaged 73 in a year, and the baptisms 237, being 3·25 children to each marriage[5]. But in the last three years of that period, 1770–72, the marriages had risen rapidly to an annual average of 95, and the baptisms to 331, being about 3·5 children to each marriage. From 1773 to 1781 the marriages averaged 85 and the fecundity reached 4·5 children to each. Arthur Young found the whole of this

[1] *Annals of the Lords of Warrington and Bewsey from* 1587. By W. Beamont. Manchester, 1873, p. xix.
[2] John Aikin, M.D., *Descriptions of the Country from thirty to forty Miles around Manchester.* London, 1795, p. 302.
[3] Taken out of the register by Aikin at the request of Dr Richard Price, and published by the latter in the 4th ed. of his *Obs. on Reversionary Payments.* Lond. 1783, II. 5, 100.
[4] Arthur Young, *Six Months Tour through the North of England.* 4 vols. London, 1770–71, III. 163.
[5] Percival, *Phil. Trans.* LXV. 328.

community, men, women, and children, engaged in sailcloth or sacking manufacture, boot-making, and pin-making.

"At Warrington the manufactures of sailcloth and sacking are very considerable. The first is spun by women and girls, who earn about 2*d.* a day. It is then bleached, which is done by men, who earn 10*s.* a week; after bleaching, it is wound by women, whose earnings are 2*s.* 6*d.* a week; next it is warped by men, who earn 7*s.* a week; and then starched, the earnings 10*s.* 6*d.* a week. The last operation is the weaving in which the men earn 9*s.*, the women 5*s.*, the boys 3*s.* 6*d.* a week. The spinners (women) in the sacking branch earn 6*s.* a week. Then it is wound on bobbins by women and children, whose earnings are 4*d.* a day....The sailcloth employs about 300 weavers, and the sacking 150; and they reckon 20 spinners and 2 or 3 other hands to every weaver."

On that basis of reckoning, Young estimated that the Warrington manufactures employed about eleven thousand hands; but as Aikin, in 1781, counted the whole inhabitants of the borough and three adjoining hamlets at 9501, it is clear that a good many spinners of the flax and hemp who lived in the country near Warrington must be allowed for in the eleven thousand. At all events Warrington was an early and an extreme instance of that hurry and scramble of wage-earning, by fathers, mothers and children, which the growth of manufactures in the latter part of the 18th century gave rise to, and of which many particulars came to light long after during the discussions that preceded the passing of the Factory Act. The mothers were workers, and all the while breeders at a somewhat high rate. It is difficult to imagine how the household duties were got through, and the infants reared, in such an industrial hive. Nor was there much attention given, during those great days of the sailcloth industry, to the scavenging and lighting of the town, and probably little to the overcrowded state of its old-fashioned streets and lanes. It was in January and February, 1775, fully a year after the great smallpox epidemic had ceased, that Mr Blackburne, who had become lord of the manor in 1764, "promoted the design of establishing a court of requests at Warrington, cleansing and lighting the town, and removing the butchers' stalls." These proposals, we are told, gave rise to a paper war[1].

Ferriar has described what was apt to happen when country people migrated to manufacturing towns, got married, and had children born to them:

---

[1] Beamont, u. s. p. 116–17.

"A young couple live very happily, till the woman is confined by her first lying-in. The cessation of her employment then produces a deficiency in their income, at a time when expenses unavoidably increase. She therefore wants many comforts, and even the indulgences necessary to her situation : she becomes sickly, droops, and at last is laid up by a fever or a pneumonic complaint ; the child dwindles, and frequently dies ; the husband, unable to hire a nurse, gives up most of his time to attendance on his wife and child ; his wages are reduced to a trifle ; vexation and want render him diseased, and the whole family sometimes perishes, from the want of a small timely supply which their future industry would have amply repaid to the public[1]."

What Ferriar saw so often some years after at Manchester must have been a not uncommon case at Warrington during the bustling time that Arthur Young describes. Its infantile mortality was certainly excessive, according to the following comparison with that of Chester, from the figures supplied to Price by Aikin from the Warrington burial registers of nine years, 1773–81, and by Haygarth from the Chester bills for ten years, 1772–81[2]. The deaths are reduced to annual averages, and those of Warrington are raised, in the third column, to the ratio of the population of Chester by making them half as much again.

Annual average of deaths from all causes under five years.

Ages at death	Warrington. Pop. 9,501 in 1781	Chester. Pop. 14,173 in 1774	Warrington raised to the ratio of Chester
Under one year	72·7	80·6	109·0
One to two	43·5	36·1	65·2
Two to three	20·1	23·4	30·1
Three to four	11·5	14·4	17·2
Four to five	7·0	8·7	10·5

It was among infants and young children born and brought up with such comparatively poor chances of surviving, that smallpox broke out at Warrington in January, 1773, reaching its climax in May and ending about October, with a mortality of 209 or 211. Aikin says :

"Its victims were chiefly young children, whom it attacked with such instant fury that the best-directed means for relief were of little avail. In general the sick were kept sufficiently cool, and were properly supplied with diluting and acidulous drinks ; yet where they recovered, it seemed rather owing to a less degree of malignity in the disease or greater strength to struggle with it, than any peculiar management. When it ended fatally, it was usually before the pustules came to maturation ; and, indeed, in many they showed no disposition to advance after the complete eruption, but remained quite flat and pale"—a sure sign of poor *stamina vitae*. "In one neighbourhood I found that out of 29 who had the disease, 12 died, or about 2 in 5 ; in others the mortality was still greater, and I have reason to believe it was not less on the whole."

[1] Ferriar, *Med. Obs. and Reflections.*
[2] Price, *Reversionary Payments.* 4th ed. II.

The monthly progress of the mortality at Warrington and Chester respectively was as follows[1]:

	Deaths. Warrington, 1773	Deaths. Chester, 1774			Deaths. Warrington, 1773	Deaths. Chester, 1774
Jan.	4	0		July	33	11
Feb.	4	1		Aug.	11	26
March	13	0		Sept.	7	28
April	23	0		Oct.	3	46
May	63	3		Nov.	0	44
June	49	3		Dec.	1	40[2]
					211	202

The following are the ages at which the children died of smallpox, and of all causes, in each town during the epidemic year[3]:

Ages	Warrington (pop. in 1781, 9501)		Chester (pop. in 1774, 14,713)	
	Smallpox	Other deaths	Smallpox	Other deaths
Under one month	0	18	0	17
One to three months	4	9	3	19
Three to six months	4	9	4	10
Six to twelve months	39	15	44	8
One to two years	84	24	38	14
Two to three years	33	5	42	3
Three to five years	33	14	49	13
Five to ten years	12	15	22	8
Above ten years	0	—	0	—
	209	—	202	—

Comparing the ages at death in the two epidemics, we see at a glance that the second year was most fatal to children at Warrington, whereas at Chester the deaths fell more at the higher ages, although in ratio of its population it was only on a par with Warrington even at these ages.

If the great smallpox year at each town be left out, 1773 at Warrington, 1774 at Chester, the mortality of infants in their second year from all causes is found to be one-third more at Warrington than at Chester on an annual average of eight (or nine) years. Some such difference Haygarth says was well

---

[1] Aikin, *Phil. Trans.* LXIV. (1774), p. 438; Haygarth, *ibid.* LXVIII. 131.
[2] "Almost ended at the winter solstice, only 19 remaining ill in January, 1775."
[3] Percival, for Warrington, *Med. Obs. and Inquiries,* V. (1776), p. 272 (information from Arkin); Haygarth, for Chester, *Phil. Trans.* LXVIII. 150. Haygarth (*Sketch of a Plan, &c.* p. 141) gives the following table of the smallpox deaths and the deaths from all causes at several ages of children up to ten years at Chester from 1772 to 1777 inclusive:

	Under one	1—2	2—3	3—5	5—10	Total
Smallpox deaths	91	75	83	86	34	369
All other deaths	392	155	68	68	53	736

known between the smallpox of great and small towns, namely, that it "attacks children at an earlier age, and consequently is fatal to a larger proportion of people, in great than in small towns[1]." Although Warrington was the smaller town, infants died earlier there than at Chester (from smallpox and from all causes), or the probability of life was less ;—a statistical fact which Price made out, but was unable to explain. The explanation is the poor stamina of the Warrington children, which was due most of all to the circumstance that the married women were at once wage-earners and prolific breeders.

In the smallpox year at Warrington, the deaths from all causes under five years of age were 62·5 of the whole mortality, (in infants under two years they were 43·5 per cent. of all deaths) smallpox having caused them in the ratio of 199 to 291. Although Aikin's estimate of two deaths in five cases is improbable for the whole epidemic, we may admit a rate of one death in four, which would give Warrington in 1773 about as many cases in proportion to its numbers as Chester had in 1774— 844 in a population of some 9000, as compared with 1385 in a population of 14,713.

The epidemics of smallpox at Carlisle in 1779 and Leeds in 1781 were unusually mortal, for reasons analogous to those assigned in the case of Warrington. Both towns had increased fast in numbers, owing to the growth of the weaving and spinning industries, both were overcrowded, ill ventilated, and filthy, and both had high mortalities from typhus fever among the adults, as described in another chapter. At Carlisle, the great epidemic of smallpox, which was the children's special scourge, came in 1779, two years before the typhus fever reached a height. The smallpox caused 90 deaths, while "a species of scarlet fever" at the same time caused 39 deaths. Heysham estimated somewhat vaguely that these 90 deaths occurred in 300 cases, or one case fatal in 3·3, which is double the average[2]. Lucas gives the proportion at Leeds more exactly—462 cases, in six months, with 130 fatalities, or 1 in 3·5. The epidemic at Leeds in 1721–22, which Nettleton described as "more than usually mortal," caused 189 deaths in 792 attacks, or 1 in 4·2. There were fewer attacks in the much larger population (17,117) of

---

[1] *Sketch of a plan, &c.* p. 31.
[2] Heysham, *Obs. on Bills of Mortality in Carlisle,* 1779–1787. Carlisle, 1797. Reprinted from App. Vol. II. of Hutchinson's *Cumberland.*

1781, perhaps because there were fewer persons who had not had the disease already, and these almost exclusively the infants born and the young children who had grown up since the last epidemic[1]. In those circumstances it is hardly surprising that the Leeds smallpox of 1781 should have been a degree more mortal than that of 1721–22, which was itself "more than usually mortal."

A complete survey of smallpox in its great period, the eighteenth century, in all places and continuously from year to year, is impossible even if it were to be desired. Had it not been for the exact diligence of a few, especially in the North of England, we should have been left in doubt on some of the main epidemiological generalities. A system of registration such as was applied for the first time in the epidemic of 1837–39 would have saved much research and would have made it possible to bring the facts within a smaller compass. By comparison and classification of many scattered particulars we may still acquire a tolerably clear notion of what smallpox was in the 18th century. It was chiefly a disease of infancy and early childhood. It was always present in one part or another of the capital and of the larger towns, rising at intervals to the height of a great and general epidemic[2]. At its worst, as in Glasgow, it took about a third part of the lives under the age of five, and perhaps a sixth part of the lives at all ages. It came in epidemics at somewhat regular intervals in the smaller towns, and at longer intervals in the country parishes. The village epidemics were apt to be very searching when they did come. Haygarth gives the instance of Christleton, a small village two miles from Chester, in 1778: "The distemper began in March and continued till October. At the commencement of the epidemic, 107 poor children had never been exposed to the variolous infection; of these 100 had the distemper, probably all who were capable of receiving the smallpox." In all places, with the possible exception of London where the risks from

---

[1] Lucas, *Lond. Med. Journ.* x. 260: "The number of those who were still uninfected was found on a survey to be 700."

[2] Dr Henry, of Manchester, to Haygarth, 20 March, 1789, in the latter's *Sketch of a Plan, &c.* p. 369: "In large and populous places such as Manchester, the smallpox almost always exists in some parts of the town. I have known it strongly epidemic in one part without any appearance of it in others... At present it is prevalent and fatal in the outskirts, but very rarely occurs in the interior parts of the town."

infantile diarrhoea and " convulsions " were peculiar, it cut off the infants and young children more than any other single disease, infectious or other; and indeed it had few rivals among infectious diseases until towards the close of the century, being for a time the grand epidemic scourge of the first years of life just as the plague was once the unique scourge of youth and mature age. It was more mortal in some seasons than in others, and at certain places. Towards the end of the 18th century, much more is heard of it in the northern industrial towns than in England south of the Trent. If the statistics of Boston, Lincolnshire, are at all representative, smallpox certainly declined much in market towns in the last twenty years of the century. It appears to have declined also in the capital during the same period. In the parishes of Scotland, by the almost unanimous testimony of the articles which refer to it in the 'Statistical Account,' it had become much less frequent and less dangerous for some years previous to the publication of that work (1792–98). In Glasgow, with the worst statistics of children's deaths in the whole kingdom, the maximum had been reached, and passed, in the period between the close of the American war and the first years of the great war with France. As the French war proceeded, and vast sums of public money were poured out (the bill being left to Prince Posterity to pay), the effects of this abundance were seen in the remarkable decline, and almost total disappearance, of fevers all over England, Scotland and Ireland. Corresponding with the lull in fevers there was a lull in smallpox, not so marked as the former, but very significantly covering the same period and lasting until the great depression of trade in 1816 which followed the Peace. This will appear in continuing the chronology of epidemics; but before we come to that, it remains to make clear the scientific or pathological nature of a new kind of inoculation which became at this juncture the rival of the old. The extent to which each of the rival methods was practised will become a subject of inquiry after the epidemic of 1817–19 has been dealt with.

Cowpox.

Much has been said, in previous sections of this chapter, as to the efforts of inoculators to reduce the effects of inoculated virus "to as low a degree as we could wish." What kind of matter do you use? one inoculator would ask of another. The comparative trials of Watson had shown that serous or watery matter from an unripe pustule of smallpox, preferably from the unripe pustule of a previous inoculation on the arm, was most "successful," the success being measured by the slightness of the effect produced at the time. The comparative trials of Mudge had confirmed that, but had gone a little farther in showing that these slight effects of crude or unripe matter left the constitution still open to the same effects by the same means, or to more severe effects by more severe means. What kind of matter to use was, accordingly, still an open question, which offered some scope for originality and ingenuity. Among other sources of crude or watery matter with bland properties was the glassy or watery variety of eruption called swinepox, which, like its congener chickenpox, was peculiar to man; and among those who tried that source of non-purulent matter for inoculation was Jenner, of Berkeley. It was in 1789 that he inoculated his child, aged eighteen months, with matter from the so-called swinepox of man. There was still another pox bearing the name of a brute animal, which was, however, a true affection of brutes—the cowpox or pap-pox. A farmer at Yetminster, Dorset, named Benjamin Jesty, had used matter from that source for the inoculation of his wife and two young children in 1774, with the result that the arm of the former was much inflamed and had to be treated by a surgeon. There seemed to be no good reason for preferring matter of such dangerous tendency, and the experiment was not repeated. A few years after, an apothecary of Lyme, in Dorset, is said to have heard of another case of the domestic use of cowpox matter for inoculation by the mistress of a farm house, and to have pressed this fact upon the attention of Sir George Baker; who, although a supporter of the mild or Suttonian inoculations with crude lymph, and by his own avowal a friend of experiments, did not favour the trial of matter from the pap-pox of cows, probably for the reason that he should have been departing from the ground-principle of inoculating for the smallpox if he were to go outside the class of variolous disease for his matter. The true virtuoso, however, has no antecedent objection to experimenting with anything. Sometime after Jenner had used the swinepox matter, he began to talk among his medical neighbours of using cowpox matter. But it was known that cowpox matter had properties and effects of its own, and that it would be a radical innovation to use it, a departure *toto coelo* from every modification hitherto tried in the inoculation procedure. Although it was also a pox by name, and although cowpox to the apprehension of a man of words or notions might seem to be in the same class as swinepox, glasspox, hornpox, waterpox or chickenpox, yet those who had ever seen it on the chapped hands of milkers would hardly admit that matter from such a source could serve for inoculation purposes unless upon wholly independent and original proof of efficacy. Jenner's colleagues are reported to have denied that cowpoxed milkers escaped natural smallpox any more than their fellows[1]. About the year 1794 Jenner began to press the subject upon the attention of his friends. His clerical neighbour, Worthington, mentioned it in one of his letters to Haygarth, of Chester, who replied, on 15 April, 1794:

" Your account of the cowpox is indeed very marvellous, being so strange a history, and so contradictory to all past observations on this subject, very clear and full evidence will be required to render it credible. You say that this whole rare phenomenon is soon to be published, but do not mention whether by yourself or some other medical friend. In either case I trust that no reliance will be placed upon vulgar stories. The author should admit nothing but what he has proved by his own personal observation, both in the brute and human species. It would be useless to specify the doubts that must be satisfied upon this subject before rational belief can be obtained. If a physician should adopt such a doctrine, and much more if he should publish it upon inadequate evidence, his character would materially suffer in the public opinion of his knowledge and discernment[2]."

It is clear that Haygarth, who was well acquainted with epidemic smallpox and with inoculation, saw in this Gloucester-shire idea something quite new as well as antecedently im-probable. What the real novelty was will appear from the next historical reference to cowpox in an original work upon Morbid Poisons by Joseph Adams, a writer of the Hunterian school. All that Adams knew of the nature of cowpox previous to March, 1795, came from Cline, surgeon to St Thomas's Hospital, who had been a fellow student of Jenner's five and twenty years before, and kept up some correspondence with him. Adams is writing on the peculiar danger of ulceration and sloughing, or phagedaena, from transferring animal matters from one body to another, his last illustration having been the notorious

[1] "Most of them [Jenner's colleagues] had met with cases in which those who were supposed to have had cowpox had subsequently been affected with smallpox." Baron, *Life of Jenner*, I. 48.
[2] Haygarth to Worthington, 15 April, 1794, in Bacon's *Life of Jenner*, I. 134.

phagedaenic ulceration of the gums, with rashes of the skin and constitutional effects so severe as to be fatal, which followed the transplantation of fresh teeth from one person to another in a number of cases about the year 1790 and led to the speedy abandonment of that unnatural practice[1]. He proceeds to say, "Thus far we have only traced the poisonous effects of matter applied from one animal to another of the same class," and then he brings in the illustration of cowpox to finish the chapter:

"The cowpox is a disease well known to the dairy-farmers in Gloucestershire. The only appearance on the animal is a phagedaenic ulcer on the teat, with apparent inflammation. When communicated to the human subject, it produces, besides ulceration on the hand, a considerable tumour of the arm, with symptomatic fever, both which gradually subside. What is still more extraordinary, as far as facts have been hitherto ascertained, the person who has been infected is rendered insensible to the variolous poison[2]."

Jenner's own essay on the cowpox, when it appeared at length in 1798, confirmed these statements as to the phagedaenic or corroding ulcerous character of the milkers' sores, in his brief accounts of several cases, of which it will suffice to mention these two: William Stinchcomb, farm servant, had his left hand severely affected with several corroding ulcers, and a tumour of considerable size appeared in the axilla of that side; his right hand had only one small sore. A poor girl, unnamed, "produced an ulceration on her lip by frequently holding her finger to her mouth to cool the raging of a cowpox sore by blowing upon it[3]." Inquiries made by Dr George Pearson in various other dairy counties of England brought out the same character of cowpox in milkers: the painful sores might be as large as a sixpenny piece, and might last a month or two, causing the milker to give up his work[4].

As to the pap-pox itself, or cowpox in the cow, the most circumstantial account was obtained, a few months after Jenner's first essay, by interrogating a veterinary surgeon or cow-doctor, one Clayton, who attended at most of the farms within ten miles of Gloucester:

---

[1] See the cases and remarks by John Hunter, Sir W. Watson, Lettsom and others.

[2] Joseph Adams, *Observations on Morbid Poisons, Phagedaena and Cancer.* 1st ed. Lond. 1795. Preface, 31 March.

[3] I have collected all the scattered references in Jenner's writings to cowpox in the cow or in infected milkers in my *Natural History of Cowpox and Vaccinal Syphilis.* London, 1887, pp. 53–57.

[4] G. Pearson, *Inquiry concerning the History of Cowpox.* Lond. 1798.

"That the chief diseases of the cow are the lough, swellings of the udder, and cowpox; that the two former are the most common, the latter being rarely seen except in spring and summer.

That cowpox begins with white specks upon the cow's teats, which, in process of time, ulcerate; and, if not stopped, extend over the whole surface of the teats, giving the cow excruciating pain.

That, if this disease is suffered to continue for some time, it degenerates into ulcers, exuding a malignant and highly corrosive matter; but this generally arises from neglect in the incipient stage of the disease, or from some other cause he cannot explain.

That this disease may arise from any cause irritating or excoriating the teats; but that the teats are often chapped without the cowpox succeeding. In chaps of the teats, they generally swell; but in the cowpox, the teats seldom swell at all, but are gradually destroyed by ulceration.

That this disease first breaks out upon one cow, and is communicated by the milker to the whole herd; but if one person was confined to strip the cow having this disease, it would go no farther.

That the cowpox is a local disease, and is invariably cured by local remedies.

That he never knew this disease extend itself in the highest degree to the udder, unless mortification had ensued; and that he can at all times cure the cowpox in eight or nine days[1]."

No account of cowpox in the cow has ever been given which differs materially from that of this experienced Gloucester cow-doctor in 1798[2]. Cowpox is not only a local disease, but it is peculiar to certain individuals of the species, namely cows in milk; in them it occurs on the teats, so that it was correctly known in Norfolk by the name of pap-pox. The common observation has been that one cow starts it, and that an infection is rubbed into the teats of others by the fingers of the milkers. The cow which develops this ulceration of the paps is usually either a heifer in her first milk, from which the calf has been taken away, or a cow in milk which has been bought in a market, with the udder "overstocked" or left distended for appearance sake, but as yet with no blemish of the paps. The cause of cowpox is the rough handling of a highly sensitive part, which was originally adapted only for the lips and tongue of the calf. Ceely, a correct observer in the Vale of Aylesbury, uses no exaggerated phrase when he speaks of "the merciless

[1] Beddoes' *Contributions to Physical and Medical Knowledge.* Bristol, 1799, p. 387.
[2] See my *Natural History of Cowpox, &c.* u. s. 1887. The most systematic descriptions, both for cows and milkers, are by Ceely, in *Trans. Provinc. Med. and Surg. Assocn.* VIII. (1840) and X. (1842). Professor E. M. Crookshank has reproduced these valuable memoirs, with the coloured plates, in his *History and Pathology of Vaccination.* 2 vols. London, 1889. The plates are in vol. I., the memoirs in vol. II. Crookshank's volumes, which are a convenient repertory of the more important earlier writings on cowpox, contain also the author's original observations (with plates), of cowpox in Wiltshire in 1887–88.

manipulations of the milkers." Men milkers are well known to
lack the delicate tact of women ; and cowpox has been most
common in the great dairying districts where men-milkers are
employed. But in some animals cowpox may be produced even
under gentler handling or with slighter provocation, of which I
give a recent case from my notebook, taken during a visit to the
country :

27 April, 1891. Case of cowpox. A maid in the service of Mr J. R.
has on the ulnar side of the fore finger of the right hand, over the joint of the
first and second phalanges, a collapsed bleb the size of a sixpenny piece,
pearly white round the margin, bluish towards the centre, which is brown.
The forefinger, as well as the wrist and hand generally, bears traces of recent
inflammation, and was said to have been greatly swollen and painful, the
pain extending up the arm. There is a symmetrical rash of bright red
papules on both arms as high as the elbows, more copious and bright on the
right arm but abundant on the left also. The papules are elevated and
pointed, with a small zone of bright redness of the skin round the base
of each. The history is as follows : A cow was bought four or five weeks
ago to supplement the supply of milk from the three ordinarily kept. The
new comer proved "tough" to milk, so that the maid was obliged, contrary
to usual practice, to take the paps in the cleft of the fore and middle fingers ;
under this mode of "stripping," the animal would hardly stand quiet to be
milked. After a time it was found that one of the paps had a black crust
upon it, which might have covered originally a chap of the skin. The crust
would have been displaced in the milking, and would have grown again ; the
sore beneath soon healed. Only one pap was affected. None of the other
cows was infected. The "tough" cow was at length sold as an unsatisfactory
milker, and had been sent to a distance on the morning of the day on which
these notes were made. The maid's finger began to be affected after two or
three weeks of milking the cow, the beginning of the large and tumid bluish-
white vaccine vesicle having been like a small wart.

Jenner's opinion that cowpox was a specific disease "coeval
with the brute creation," and that it had been the parent of
the great historical smallpox of mankind, is not now received as
correct. His other opinion, that cowpox was derived from the
hocks of horses affected with "grease," which held a central
place in his original essay, especially in connexion with his
doctrine of "true" and "spurious" cowpox, was rejected by
most of his contemporaries, and is perhaps unsupported by
anyone at the present time[1].

[1] In my essay of 1887 (u. s.) I maintained, as an original opinion, that the true
affinity of cowpox was to the great pox of man, and that the occasional cases of
so-called vaccinal syphilis were not due to the contamination of cowpox with
venereal virus but to inherent (although mostly latent) properties of the cowpox virus
itself. This opinion was at first received with incredulity, but is now looked upon
with more favour. See Hutchinson, *Archives of Surgery*, Oct. 1889, and Jan. 1891,
p. 215. The concessions hitherto made are only for cases that have arisen since my
book was published, such as the case at the Leeds Infirmary in 1889. I believe that
my explanation of vaccinal "syphilis" will at length be accepted for all cases, past or
future.

In the title-page of his first essay, Dr Jenner called this singular malady of the cow's paps by a new name—*variolae vaccinae*, or smallpox of the cow. Pearson, the earliest and most ardent of Jenner's original supporters, and for several years thereafter a convinced vaccinist, at once took exception to the name *variolae vaccinae* " for the sake of precision of language and justness in thinking." It is a palpable catachresis, says he, to designate what is called the cowpox by the denomination *variolae vaccinae*, because the cowpox is a specifically different distemper from the smallpox in essential particulars, namely, in the nature of its morbific poison and in its symptoms[1].

That the term *variolae vaccinae* in Jenner's title-page is used tropically can hardly be doubted ; but it is not so easy to say which of the great classical tropes it is. It may be objected that "catachresis" is too general for the misuse of a word when that word is a scientific one and occurs in the leading title of a scientific book. Here we have the somewhat specific and purposeful use of a word in an unwonted sense, which, if it fall under any of the scholastic figures of speech, ought to be a figure more specifically defined than mere catachresis. In a matter so important as this one should find the exact figure if possible ; but at the outset a difficulty arises, namely whether we should look for it in the usage of the rhetors, as Isocrates teaches, or in the usage of the logicians, as Aristotle lays down the definitions of tropes. If among the former class, the nearest is perhaps the hypocorisma, or attractive, agreeable name for something that is not so nice in itself. If among the latter, we shall hardly find a better than the metalepsis, which is a change more of mood than of meaning, namely the transition without proof from a supposition to an assertion. But in truth no single figure of the ancient teachers suits this modern instance. We require at least two. Metalepsis carries us so far, but synecdoche must supplement it. The term *variolae vaccinae* is a synecdoche in that it names the cause from the effect ; it is a metalepsis in that it passes abruptly from the hypothetical mood to the categorical; and in respect that it does both at a stroke it is probably unique, and without precedent among the examples known to the ancients. Or again, leaving the graver figures, and translating the Latin name of Jenner's title-page, one may try the figurative conversion of cowpox into smallpox by the standard of pure and legitimate

[1] *An Inquiry, &c.* 1798. " Remarks on the term Variolae Vaccinae."

paronomasia, of which there is a familiar English example in the conversion of a plant into an animal by the verbal play of horse-chestnut and chestnut horse in the minor premiss.

Some in more recent times, mistaking the figurative or rhetorical intention of Jenner, have understood his Latin name of cowpox as if there really were a smallpox of the cow (although not of the bull, nor of the steer, the maiden heifer or the calf of either sex). Not being able to find a smallpox of the cow in the natural way, they have thought to satisfy the legitimate requirements of proof by manufacturing it. Certain Germans of the Lower Rhine, where the cows ordinarily wear blankets, have wrapped the blankets taken from smallpox beds round the bodies of cows, after clipping the hair close ; nothing was found to ensue in these interesting experiments except an occasional pimple which had probably been caused by the shears in the preliminary clipping. Others in England, France, America and India, have succeeded in raising a smallpox pustule at the point of puncture in the epidermis of the cow or in the more delicate transitional epithelium, the matter from which has produced smallpox in its turn[1]. But these are academic exercises. The natural cowpox of the cow has been likened by none to the natural smallpox of man in a sustained comparison of all the anatomical and epidemiological particulars of each; nor, I am persuaded, will anyone ever attempt to draw out such a comparison. *Variolae vaccinae* as a name for cowpox was a figure of speech, and it is to misunderstand its original use to treat it as anything else.

The proof that cowpox had some power over smallpox consisted in trying to inoculate with the latter those who had been previously inoculated with the former. The accepted mode of testing the power of inoculated smallpox itself was to inoculate it again ; at first the test for cowpox was to inoculate with smallpox, but after a few years the testing inoculation was done with cowpox itself. The effects of Suttonian inoculation with smallpox, as we have seen, were nearly always slight, and sometimes invisible (as in Watson's practice at the Foundling

---

[1] That Dr Jenner foresaw this line of proof, and dismissed it as irrelevant, is made clear by G. C. Jenner, *Monthly Magazine*, 1799, p. 671, in reply to Dr Turton, of Swansea : "It is possible that variolous virus inserted into the nipples of a cow, might produce inflammation and suppuration, and that matter from such a source might produce some local affection on the human subject by inoculation. But all this tends only to show, what was well known before, that virus taken from one ulcer is capable of producing another by its being inserted into any other part of the body."

Hospital). A previous inoculation with cowpox made them slighter still; but even with cowpox in the system, the pustules of smallpox rose where the matter had been inserted on the arm. It may be thought that there were only fine shades of difference between the effects of inoculation after cowpoxing and the effects of the same in a virgin soil; but some difference must have been perceived, for it was upon that, and upon nothing else, that the authority in favour of cowpox as a substitute for smallpox in inoculation was promptly established. The relationship between cowpox and smallpox was admitted by all to be in the nature of things "extraordinary," as Jenner said, or a mystery, as others said; but as an empirical fact many believed it to be true, because the cowpoxed had less to show for the effects of inoculation with smallpox than if they had not been cowpoxed. Jenner himself is known to have made only two variolous tests. He used crude or watery matter from the local pustule of inoculated smallpox, and advised all his readers to do the same. In one of his two trials, a child Mary James had nearly the same effects from inoculation after cowpox that her mother and another child had from it without having been cowpoxed, namely the pustule or confluent group of pustules at the place of puncture, and the eruptive fever at the ninth day[1].

In the earliest tests made independently of Jenner, five at Stonehouse[2], near Stroud, and five at Stroud[3], in the first months of 1799, the cowpoxed received smallpox afterwards by inoculation "in the usual slight manner." In the practice at the Smallpox and Inoculation Hospital, London, in the spring and summer of 1799, many of the cowpoxed took smallpox by contagion from the atmosphere of the hospital, so that Woodville, after a period of perplexity, at length concluded that cowpox, while it was still active upon the arm, did not shut out the action of the smallpox virus in the constitution[4].

[1] Jenner, *Further Observations on the Variolae Vaccinae*, 1799.
[2] Thornton, in Beddoes' *Contributions to Physical and Medical Knowledge.* Bristol, 1799.
[3] Hughes, *Med. and Phys. Journ.* I. (1799), p. 318. Many other tests, English and foreign, are detailed in my book, *Jenner and Vaccination.* London, 1889, for which see the Index under "test."
[4] Woodville tabulated 511 cases of applicants for inoculation at the hospital in whom cowpox matter was used, giving "the number of pustules" opposite the name of each; 90 had from a thousand to a hundred pustules, 215 had less than one hundred. William Woodville, M.D., *Reports of a Series of Inoculations for the Variolae Vaccinae or Cowpox; with remarks on this disease considered as a substitute for the Smallpox.* London, 1799. In a subsequent letter (*Med. Phys. Journ.* V.,

The antecedent objections to cowpox, arising out of its non-variolous nature, were met by appealing to the results of experiments. The authority in favour of cowpox was speedily established on that ground, and has been continuous to the present time. The experimenters had to decide very nice points both in the way of observation and of reasoning. They had to appraise the margin of difference between the effects of Suttonian inoculation where cowpox had preceded and where it had not preceded. They had to allow for the first virus causing a swelling in the absorbent glands, which would obstruct the entrance of the second testing virus into the blood. They had to average the varying effects of Suttonian inoculation for its own sake, and the equally varying effects of it as the variolous test, and to find a broad difference between the two averages. Having decided that preceding cowpox infection did make a real and appreciable difference to the number of pustules resulting, at the spot or elsewhere, from the insertion of inoculated smallpox matter, or to the amount of fever, they had next to consider whether that degree of resistance by a cowpoxed person to inoculation were a good measure of his power to resist contagion reaching his vitals in the natural way. Their diligence and acumen may or may not have been equal to these things—it was a slack tide in medical science. Also they received little or no help from Dr Jenner himself, whose inventive genius was of the kind that is apt to leave the practical value, and even the theoretical probability, of the project to be tried by others. The inventor made interest with great personages—with the king, the duke of York, and the aristocracy of his county. His priority, and the merits of his project, were referred in 1802 to a

Dec. 1800), he thus explained the occurrence of smallpox among those recently inoculated with cowpox : "If a person who has been exposed to the contagion of smallpox for four or five days be then inoculated for this disease, the inoculation prevents the effects of the contagion, and the *inoculated* smallpox is produced. But if the vaccine inoculation be employed in a case thus circumstanced, the smallpox is not prevented, although the tumour produced by the cowpox inoculation advance to maturation. It was not before the commencement of the present year [1800], that I ascertained that the cowpox had not the power of superseding the smallpox. For, though from the first trials that I made of the new inoculation it appeared that these diseases, as produced in the same subject from inoculation, did not interrupt the progress of each other; yet as the casual does not act in the same manner as the inoculated smallpox, and may be anticipated by the latter, I thought it still probable that the cowpock infection might have a similar effect. Numerous facts have, however, proved this opinion to be unfounded, and that the variolous effluvia, even after the vaccine inoculation has made a considerable progress, have in several instances occasioned an eruption resembling that of smallpox."

Committee of the House of Commons, with Admiral Berkeley as chairman, which entered on its labours with a strong recommendation from the king, endorsed by Addington, the prime minister. They decided in favour of Dr Jenner's claim for remuneration on all the issues, and on 2 June, 1802, the Committee of the whole House unanimously voted: "That it is the opinion of the Committee that a sum not exceeding £10,000 be granted to his Majesty to be paid as a remuneration to Dr Edward Jenner for promulgating the discovery of the Vaccine Inoculation, by which mode that dreadful malady the smallpox was prevented[1]." On 29 July, 1807, a farther sum of £20,000 was voted to him; and on 8 June, 1808, a National Vaccine Establishment was appointed, at an annual cost of about £5,000.

Chronology of epidemics resumed from 1801.

In resuming the history of smallpox from the beginning of the present century, we come first to the deaths in the London Bills of Mortality, which are the only continuous figures. The bills of Parish Clerks' Hall had failed, before they ceased, to include more than two-thirds, perhaps not much more than a half, of all the deaths in the capital. The great parishes of St Pancras and St Marylebone, which returned a somewhat excessive share of the deaths both from smallpox and from fever in the first two or three years of the Registration Act (1837–39), as well as the parishes of Chelsea and Kensington, were never included within the Bills; also much of the suburban extension on the other sides of London was never taken in. Meanwhile the area of the old Bills had actually become less populous owing to the displacement of dwelling houses by warehouses, workshops, counting houses, and the like, in the City, the Liberties and in certain out-parishes such as those bordering the Thames at the east end.

Still, the bills of mortality may be taken as showing on the whole fairly the proportion of smallpox deaths to other deaths, and the years of its greater outbursts.

---

[1] *European Magazine*, XLIII. 137.

Smallpox in the London Bills of Mortality, 1801–37.

	Smallpox deaths	All deaths		Smallpox deaths	All causes
1801	1461	19,374	1820	722	19,348
1802	1579	19,379	1821	508	18,451
1803	1202	19,582	1822	604	18,865
1804	622	17,034	1823	774	20,587
1805	1685	17,565	1824	725	20,237
1806	1158	17,938	1825	1299	21,026
1807	1297	18,334	1826	503	20,758
1808	1169	19,954	1827	616	22,292
1809	1163	16,680	1828	598	21,709
1810	1198	19,983	1829	736	23,524
1811	751	17,043	1830	627	21,645
1812	1287	18,295	1831	563	25,337
1813	898	17,322	1832	771	28,606
1814	638	19,283	1833	574	26,577
1815	725	19,560	1834	334	21,679
1816	653	20,316	1835	863	21,415
1817	1051	19,968	1836	536	18,229
1818	421	19,705	1837	217	21,063
1819	712	19,928			

The 18th century had ended with a severe epidemic of small-pox (2409 deaths) in the year 1800; and excepting in the year 1804, the deaths kept at a somewhat high level for ten years longer. The rise at the end of the last century corresponded to a time of distress and a severe epidemic of typhus fever. The fever declined after 1803, and remained for a dozen years at so low a level that Bateman, in his quarterly reports on the practice of the Carey Street Dispensary, expresses surprise that there should have been so little of it. The same writer, however, has occasion to remark upon the fatality of smallpox; twice he mentions large mortalities from it in courts adjoining Shoe Lane[1]. According to the figures, also, smallpox declined less than fever. This means that, in the same circumstances, adult lives fared better than infancy and childhood. But, on the whole, smallpox shared with fever the advantageous conditions for health which obtained in all parts of the kingdom (in Ireland as well as in Britain) from the decline of the epidemics of 1799–1803 until the rise of the next epidemics in 1816–19. This period of comparative freedom from smallpox and fever

---

[1] Bateman, u. s. 1819, Aug.–Nov. 1807: "In a court adjoining Shoe Lane, in the course of one month, twenty-eight persons had died of smallpox." Autumn, 1812: "In one small court in Shoe Lane, seventeen have lately been cut off by this variolous plague." Also in the summer of 1812, "perhaps universally through the metropolis."

corresponded to the second period of the great French War from its resumption after the failure of the Peace of Amiens until its termination with the Peace of Paris. It may seem surprising that this should have been a time of comparatively good public health in Great Britain and Ireland, inasmuch as it was a time of dear food and heavy taxes. The amount of typhus or relapsing fever is the best test; and those diseases, by all accounts, were at a lower level in all parts of the United Kingdom from 1804 to 1817 than they had been for many years before or than they were for many years after. Again, if precedents count for anything, the same kind of lull in smallpox and fever together is shown in the London bills during the war of the Allies against Louis XIV., and during the Seven Years War.

In Glasgow the decline of smallpox deaths for a few years in the 19th century was perhaps more marked than elsewhere because it was a decline from an excessively high level in the end of the 18th century.

Glasgow Mortalities, 1801–12.

Year	Smallpox deaths	Measles deaths	All deaths	Year	Smallpox deaths	Measles deaths	All deaths
1801	245	8	1434	1807	97	16	1806
1802	156	168	1770	1808	51	787	2623
1803	194	45	1860	1809	159	44	2124
1804	213	52	1670	1810	28	19	2111
1805	56	90	1671	1811	109	267	2342
1806	28	56	1629	1812	78	304	2348

Here it is not until 1805 that a marked fall in the smallpox deaths takes place. In Norwich there was a clear interval from the last severe period in the end of the 18th century, until the year 1805, when smallpox, "after being for a time almost extinct," became prevalent again. At the Whitehaven Dispensary, the contrast between the last years of the 18th century and first years of the 19th is not striking[1]:

Smallpox at Whitehaven Dispensary.

	Cases	Deaths		Cases	Deaths
1795	8	0	1800	120	11
1796	41	5	1801	9	3
1797	(no table)		1802	(no table)	
1798	51	3	1803	67	16
1799	7	1	1804	1	0

[1] Extracted from the Annual Reports of the Dispensary.

Carlisle, which used to share in smallpox as much as Whitehaven, seems to have been almost wholly free from it in the first twelve years of the century: at least Dr Heysham, who was no longer statistical, "had reason to believe" that no person died there of smallpox from the autumn of 1800 (when cowpox inoculation was introduced) until November, 1812[1].

The Newcastle Dispensary, like that of Whitehaven, treated a small fraction of all the cases of smallpox in the town; but it continued to have a fair average of cases and deaths after the century was turned:

Smallpox cases attended from Newcastle Dispensary.

	Cases	Deaths			Cases	Deaths
1795	7	1		1801	14	4
1796	19	3		1802	—	–
1797	12	0		1803	7	4
1798	15	3		1804	0	0
1799	—	–		1805	7	0
1800	—	–		1806	16	6

Most places continued to have their periodical epidemics of smallpox as before, although both measles and scarlatina were becoming more and more its rivals. Boston, Lincolnshire, had its sexennial epidemic in 1802 with thirty-three deaths. Besides the year 1805, there were two periods in which smallpox was somewhat general, 1807–9 and 1811–13. At Norwich from 1807 to the end of 1809 the bills of mortality showed 203 deaths from smallpox[2]. In 1808 we happen to hear of it also at Sherborne, in Dorset, at Ringwood, in Hampshire, at Cheltenham, at Cambridge and at Edinburgh, although the great epidemic malady of children in that year was measles[3]. Lettsom wrote on 25 January, 1808: "The smallpox (infanticides) and measles have been prevalent and fatal. The coffins for the parish poor in England for the smallpox deaths alone have cost £10,000[4]."

In 1811 it began to be somewhat general again, and rose in London to a considerable epidemic in 1812, the deaths in

[1] Heysham to Joshua Milne, in the latter's *Treatise on the Valuation of Annuities.* London, 1815. App. p. 755.
[2] Cross, 1819, u. i. p. 2.
[3] Most of these were brought to light by inquiries upon the alleged failures of cowpox to avert the epidemic. The serial numbers of the *Medical Observer* contain frequent references to them.
[4] Letter to Joshua Dixon, in *Memoirs*, III. 368.

summer rising to sixty in a week[1]. A village epidemic of 46 cases and 7 deaths is reported from North Queensferry, near Edinburgh, from 14 December, 1811 to 7 March, 1812[2]. At Norwich from 10 February to 3 September, 1813, there were 65 deaths[3]. The rise from 1811 to 1813 coincided with an increase of fever, the winter of 1811–12 having been a time of dearth and depressed trade, especially in the manufacturing districts. After that came a notable lull both in fever and smallpox, which was at length broken by the epidemics of each in 1817 in Ireland, Scotland and England, coincidently with the depression of trade and dislocation of commerce that began everywhere as soon as the great war was over.

The Smallpox Epidemic of 1817–19.

The same things that favoured the prevalence of typhus and relapsing fever in times of distress, favoured also the rise of smallpox to the height of an epidemic. Hence the greater epidemics of smallpox in the first half of the 19th century coincided somewhat closely with epidemics of relapsing or typhus fever,—in 1817–19, in 1825–27, in 1837–40, and in 1847–49. That which fever was to the adolescents and adults in times of distress, the same was smallpox to the infants and young children. The young children of a family did, indeed, take fever sometimes as well as the parents or the young persons in it; but the children seldom died of it. They died of smallpox (or of measles or whooping cough or the like), perhaps all the more readily that they would have been weakened by the fever, and by the want of food and comforts which attended it. Thus, while fever and smallpox went somewhat closely hand in hand during times of distress, it was the adolescents and adults that died of fever, the infants and young children that died of smallpox. The following table, compiled from the reports of the Whitehaven Dispensary from 1783 to 1800, will show how many children survived attacks of continued fever in comparison with their elders[4]:

[1] Bateman, *Edin. Med. Surg. Journ.* VIII. 515.
[2] C. Stuart, *ibid.* VIII. 380.
[3] Rigby, *ibid.* X. 120.
[4] Joshua Dixon, *The Literary Life of William Brownrigg, M.D.* Whitehaven, 1801, pp. 238–9.

Continued Fever at Whitehaven Dispensary, 1783—1800.

	Total	Under 2 years	2—5	—10	—15	—20	—30	—40	—50	—60	—70	—80
Cases	1712	40	142	240	223	150	240	236	202	92	47	15
Deaths	85	0	0	5	2	6	14	20	19	12	7	0

The deaths from smallpox are found nearly always to be high when the deaths from fever are high. The correspondence, however, is not always exact to months or quarters, or half-years; for it is not unusual in the London weekly bills to find a run of weeks with high deaths from smallpox just before or after a run of weeks with high deaths from fever. The domestic circumstances which spread the contagion of fever were such as might be expected to spread the contagion of smallpox, namely, the pawning of clothes, bedding and the like, on a vast scale in times of scarcity, the crowding of many in single rooms or in one bed, the wandering of men and women, attended by their children, in search of work, the exposure of children in the smallpox so as to extort alms. All these things were common in Ireland, Scotland and England during the long periods of depressed trade, alternating with periods of speculation and expansion, for which the generation following the Peace of Paris was remarkable. We hear far more of the fever than of the smallpox, because the former touched the lives of breadwinners, while the latter was often regarded as a matter of course[1]. Thus, in the Irish famine of 1817–18, it is possible to estimate the prevalence of dysentery, relapsing fever and typhus fever by the aid of various records, including two treatises and the reports of a Parliamentary Committee. There are also two or three brief references to smallpox; but no one would have supposed that smallpox caused actually more deaths than fever itself, as in the following returns of burials in the Cathedral churchyard of Armagh, from 1st May to 25th December, 1818[2]:

Smallpox deaths	180
Fever deaths	165
All other deaths	118

—the total of 463 being twice or thrice the numbers for the corresponding months of non-epidemic years. Whether there was as much smallpox in other provinces of Ireland as in

---

[1] Haygarth says: "With us in Chester, smallpox is seldom heard of except in the bills of mortality. *There* its devastation appears dreadful indeed." *Sketch of a Plan, &c.* 1793, p. 491.

[2] Barker and Cheyne, *Account of the Fever, &c.* 2 vols. 1821. I. 92.

Ulster, does not appear; but the following relating to Strabane and Londonderry will serve to prove that Armagh was not exceptional in the north of Ireland. In and around Strabane, smallpox began to spread in May, 1817, having been hardly known in the neighbourhood for years before; it was often confluent and was "fatal to hundreds" of children[1]. The same severity of the epidemic is reported also from the county of Derry in 1817: "Cases of smallpox appeared in greater numbers than I had ever before witnessed, even previous to the valuable discovery of Jenner[2]."

The vagrancy of the Irish peasants, not only cottiers but also many small farmers, began in Ulster in the end of the year 1816, after a wet autumn which ruined the crops; and it is probable that the contagion of smallpox began to be spread among their children about the same time. Whether a migration set in to England and Scotland at that time is not clear. It appears, indeed, that the first of the epidemic in England, in Whitehaven, Ulverston, and other places which were in direct communication with the North of Ireland, was at least as early as, and perhaps earlier than, the outbreak of the malady in that country. The whole of the United Kingdom was suffering in 1816 from depression of trade, and many of the labouring class were tramping from place to place in search of work. The following is the account of smallpox being brought to Ulverston[3]:

"The smallpox were brought to Ulverston from Wigan, by the wife of a nailer, who, with her child had slept in a house where the family had just recovered from them, in the latter end of January, 1816, or beginning of

---

[1] Francis Rogan, M.D., *Obs. on the Condition of the Middle and Lower Classes in the North of Ireland*. Lond. 1819, p. 17. He proceeds to say:—"The numerous cases, which came to my knowledge, of children in the neighbouring towns who had taken smallpox, after having been vaccinated by medical practitioners of high respectability, led me to pay particular attention to those whom I myself inoculated [with cowpox]; and, although they were numerous both in private practice and at the Dispensary, not one instance occurred among them." It comes out however that he did not keep them long in sight; he saw them on the 7th day after vaccination, and again on the 11th; and as they were meanwhile almost daily exposed to contagion, without catching it, he concluded that his own cases never would do so.

[2] W. L. Kidd. "A concise Account of the Typhus Fever at present prevalent in Ireland, as it presented itself to the Author in one of the towns in the North of that country." *Edin. Med. and Surg. Journ.* XIV. (1817), 144. He goes on: "A great number of those attacked were *reported* to have been formerly vaccinated. At Londonderry, in particular, great numbers who were *said* to have undergone vaccination were the subjects of smallpox; and, whether justly or not, vaccination has in that part of the country lost much of its credit as a preservative against smallpox."

[3] Redhead (dated Ulverston, 3 July, 1816) in *Med. and Phys. Journ.* Jan. 1817, p. 3.

February. She immediately returned to Ulverston and the eruption appeared on the child about ten days afterwards, when it was carried about by the mother and much exposed in different parts of the town. They soon removed from this place; and I believe the child died between this place and Kendal."

A young woman of Ulverston who was much in the company of the nailer's wife from Wigan, caught smallpox from her child, and died on 22 February; her sister sickened soon after, and had the disease favourably. An epidemic followed in the town, of which some particulars are known down to October, 1816; the disease was very fatal also in Whitehaven at the same time. Two things gave a particular interest to the Ulverston smallpox of 1816, two things which were found to characterize the epidemic everywhere in England and Scotland as it spread in 1817, 1818 and 1819. These were, first the numerous cases of smallpox among those who had been inoculated with cowpox, a sequel now obvious on a large scale for the first time; and secondly, the admixture of a good many cases of "crystalline" or "hornpox" eruptions among the usual pustular cases. There was nothing new in such crystalline eruptions in smallpox; for example Huxham mentions them at Plymouth in 1752. But they were always curious, and it was always a matter of wonder that they should happen in one epidemic and not in another. Of thirty-five cases tabulated from the Ulverston epidemic of 1816, twelve had the "horny pox," or the "small horny kind," all the rest having the ordinary pustules of smallpox, sometimes discrete, sometimes confluent, four being scarred, and one covered by "a complete cake of incrustation." All those thirty-five cases were above five years of age, except one child of three, and they seem to have nearly all recovered. Nothing is said of the infants and children under the age of five, who then contributed three-fourths of the mortality in every epidemic of smallpox. The crystalline eruption was not chickenpox; for the three first cases of it had all gone through chickenpox before.

Almost identical in tenour with this account from Ulverston is the narrative of an epidemic at Newton Stewart, in Wigton, just across the Solway from Cumberland, which began in the autumn of 1816, but did not extend until the following summer[1]. The first case was one of "hornpox" in a girl from London;

---

[1] James Black, "On Anomalous Smallpox." *Ed. Med. and Surg. Journ.* Jan. 1819, p. 39.

the second case was in a companion of the former, in the same family, her disease being ordinary pustular smallpox; both had been vaccinated. One hundred cases in the epidemic were thus assorted :

	Cases	Deaths
Smallpox	43	13
Modified hornpox, &c.	47	0
Varicella	10	0

That is to say, the mortality of the whole was thirteen per cent., an ordinary mortality for a country town. There were all extremes, from confluent smallpox to discrete, many of the discrete having no proper pustules "but hard vesicles of more or less tubercular appearance... These were termed by the people *nerles* or *hornpox*, and have long been noticed by very aged matrons, who pretend to no little skill in the diagnostics of smallpox, and who have distinct varieties by name, beyond the enumeration of any nosologist." Their diagnostic skill was natural enough, for the practice in smallpox had been almost entirely in their hands.

A certain proportion of hornpox cases was so characteristic of this epidemic (1816–19) as to have been remarked everywhere —in England as well as in Scotland. The epidemic was not well reported as a whole at any one place. Sometimes, as at Ulverston, only the vaccinated cases were given ; at other times, as at Cupar Fife and Edinburgh, only the "hornpox" cases were given; again, in the account of the Norwich epidemic, which is the fullest, the large number of cases with crystalline or horny eruption were not counted in as smallpox cases at all. Dewar's table of the Cupar Fife epidemic, in the spring of 1817, included 70 cases, all of crystalline or hornpox[1]. The latter variety was part of the epidemic at St Andrews[2].

The Edinburgh cases which Thomson heard of to the end of the epidemic numbered 556, assorted as follows[3] :

310 had been vaccinated.
41 had had smallpox (doubtless by inoculation).
205 had neither been vaccinated nor had smallpox.

[1] Henry Dewar, M.D., *Account of an Epidemic of Smallpox which occurred in Cupar in Fife in the Spring of* 1817. Lond. 1818.
[2] P. Mudie, M.D. to Thomson, 18 Oct. 1818: "Many of the cases occurring after vaccination so much resembled smallpox that, if my mind had not been prejudiced against the possibility of such an occurrence, I should have pronounced the eruption to have been of a variolous nature"—which, of course, it was.
[3] Thomson, *Account of the Varioloid Epidemic in Scotland, &c.* Edin. 1820.

A large proportion had the crystalline eruption, while some of the deaths are put down to "malignant crystalline water-pock." At Lanark and New Lanark the epidemic was also taken notice of[1]. At the latter were situated the cotton mills managed under Robert Owen's co-operative system; and it appears that vaccination had been somewhat generally carried out in this socialist community. The following was the incidence of smallpox upon 322 persons:

251 had been vaccinated.
3 were under vaccination at the time.
11 had been inoculated with smallpox, or had gone through the natural smallpox.
57 had neither been vaccinated nor variolated.

It is clear that this was the first severe and general epidemic in Scotland since the beginning of the century, although we have seen that the disease had never been out of Glasgow. Thomson saw well enough how that epidemiological fact told: "It is to the severity of this epidemic, I am convinced, that we ought to attribute the greatness of the number of the vaccinated who have been attacked by it, and not to any deterioration in the qualities of cowpox virus, or to any defects in the manner in which it has been employed. [Dewar said the same for Cupar Fife.] Had a variolous constitution of the atmosphere, similar to that which we have lately experienced, existed at the time Dr Jenner brought forward his discovery, it may be doubted whether it ever could have obtained the confidence of the public." Thomson himself, professor of military surgery in Edinburgh and a person of high character, drew the most astonishing inferences from the tolerably simple facts of the epidemic in 1817–19. The crystalline was mixed with the ordinary pustular smallpox in this epidemic, as it had been in some 18th century epidemics; it was common to those who had been vaccinated and to those who had not been so; it occurred in those who had previously gone through the chickenpox. Yet the professor concluded that crystalline or hornpox was smallpox "modified" by vaccination, that it should be called "varioloid," and that "modified" smallpox and chickenpox were the same disease.

Several cases of smallpox had occurred in the spring of 1816 at Quarndon, two miles from Derby, one or two of the nine cases proving fatal. Several of the Derby doctors went to see them,

[1] In Thomson, u. s.

some calling them "aggravated chickenpox," and others "mild smallpox after vaccination." In the spring following (1817), most of the children and young people in the villages of Breadsall, Smalling, Spondon, Heaver, and others near Derby, were afflicted with the epidemic, which declined in autumn. It came back in the spring of 1818, when it spread more generally than before, and was still prevalent at the end of that year, in Nottinghamshire and Staffordshire as well as in Derbyshire. In Herefordshire, also, in February, 1818, "typhus, measles and smallpox were at once raging." The disease proved fatal in many instances among the lower orders in Derbyshire, who still followed the heating regimen, giving the children saffron to drink, and holding them in blankets before a strong fire, to bring the eruption out ; but it was fatal also to some who were treated more rationally. In this part of England, as in Lancashire, Wigtonshire, Fifeshire, Edinburgh, and elsewhere, a large proportion of the cases had the crystalline eruption of smallpox, horny or glassy pimples or hard vesicles, which dried about the sixth day. But, said Dr Bent, the peculiar form "is the same in those persons who have never had the cowpox and in those who have passed through that disease satisfactorily." His two drawings of the characteristic hornpox were made from unvaccinated children. On the very day of his writing he had seen two children in the same family, both with the crystalline eruption, the one vaccinated and the other not. In his practice at the Derby Infirmary, one in-patient and one out-patient had died of smallpox after vaccination, and one out-patient had died of it who had not been vaccinated. He was greatly astonished, after all that had been said of the certainty of cowpox protection[1].

The epidemic of 1817–19 was longest in reaching the Eastern Counties, just as that of 1741–42 had been, and that of 1837–39

---

[1] Thomas Bent, M.D., "Observations on an Epidemic Varioloid Disease lately witnessed in the County of Derby." *Med. and Phys. Journal*, Dec. 1818, p. 457. One Jennerian, Dr Pew, of Sherborne, adopted an arrogant tone towards Bent (*Ibid.* April, 1819, and farther correspondence). Jenner employed Fosbroke, of Berkeley, son of his friend and neighbour the antiquary Fosbroke, to traverse the whole case of the epidemic of 1817–19, in a long paper in the *Medical Repository* for June, 1819. The object of the paper appears to be to confuse the issues with a view to a verdict of *non liquet.* The *Edinburgh Review* thought Thomson's book on the epidemic of 1817–19 important enough for an article, which has been attributed to Jeffrey. The article pronounced vaccination to be a very great blessing to mankind, but not a complete protection. This was not enough for Jenner, who wrote of the article : " It will do incalculable mischief: I put it down at 100,000 deaths at least."

was to be. It was also towards the close of 1818 and beginning of 1819 that the disease became frequent in Canterbury. When it did reach Norwich, Lynn and many other places in Norfolk and Suffolk it became unusually destructive. The history of smallpox in Norwich from the beginning of the century was a history of the usual periodic epidemics, such as the city had been visited by in former times, according to the records in Blomefield's *History* or other sources. The first epidemic was in the year 1805, when smallpox was unusually common in London also. The next, with 203 deaths, lasted from 1807 to 1809. In 1813, the bills again showed many deaths by it from 10 February to 3 September. For fully four years after that there was not a death from smallpox reported in Norwich. In June, 1818, by which time the epidemic had reached large dimensions in Ireland, Scotland, and part of England, it was brought to Norwich by a girl who had come with her parents from York; it spread little at the time, the deaths to the end of the year being only two. Meanwhile measles was a very frequent and fatal disease among the children in Norwich throughout the year 1818. The small-pox began to rage in April, 1819, after which the measles was hardly met with, and only a few cases of scarlatina. The following table shows the enormous rapidity with which smallpox went through the infants and children of the Norwich populace when it had once fairly begun[1]:

1819	Deaths from smallpox	Deaths from other diseases	Total
January	3	61	64
February	0	71	71
March	2	68	70
April	15	61	76
May	73	63	136
June	156	70	226
July	142	61	203
August	84	63	147
September	42	96	138
October	10	63	73
November	2	62	64
December	1	83	84
	530	822	1352

In one week of June, there were forty-three burials from smallpox. Half the deaths were of infants under two years; nearly all the rest were of children under ten:

[1] John Green Cross, *A History of the Variolous Epidemic which occurred in Norwich in the year* 1819. Lond. 1820.

Total	0—2	—4	—6	—8	—10	—15	—20	—30	—40
530	260	132	85	26	17	5	2	2	1

If the deaths were at the rate of one in about six cases, there would have been some three thousand children attacked in a population of 50,000 of all ages. Two hundred cases which Cross kept notes of were classified by him thus:

Mild	75		Confluent	42
Severe	78		Petechial	5

Forty-six of these died, a rather high rate of 23 per cent., which is due perhaps to the crystalline or hornpox cases being excluded from the definition of smallpox altogether; all the petechial or haemorrhagic cases died, and most of the confluent. Sloughing of the face, lips or labia, occurred in three children, and bloody stools in many of the worst cases. Those 200 cases occurred in 112 families, comprising 603 individuals, of whom nearly one-half (297) "had smallpox formerly" (including the inoculated form of it, doubtless).

This was a great epidemic for Norwich in the 19th century. The public health there, as elsewhere, had improved greatly since the 18th century. In 1742 the deaths had been increased 502 by smallpox; but in that year, a year of severe typhus, the deaths from all causes were 1953, against 1352 in 1819. One reason of the enormous smallpox mortality from May to September, 1819, was the number of susceptible children, all the greater that there had been hardly any smallpox for five years, whereas in towns such as Norwich in the 18th century it appears to have been perennial: all the greater, also, because "the removal of families from the country to Norwich, during a flourishing and improving state of our manufactures for two or three preceding years, gave a sudden increase to the number of those liable to the disease." Norwich may have been better off than many other towns; but the winter of 1816–17, when the smallpox epidemic began, was a time of depressed trade, many families being on the move in search of work; and it does not appear that all those who crowded to Norwich had found employment. The epidemic was "confined almost exclusively to the very lowest orders of the people;" the contagion was spread abroad among them by the shifts they were reduced to in their indigence—"the public exposure of hideous objects just recovering, loaded with scabs, at the street corners." Yet this deplorable state of want and beggary does not seem to have been accompanied with much typhus fever among the adult population, as it certainly was in 1742. Cross describes a petechial fever, in May, June and July, 1819, which was fatal in all the cases that he was called to; but he speaks of it only among children. Whenever the population increases rapidly, as it had been doing in the second decade of the 19th century, it is upon the young lives that epidemic mortality falls most. The smallpox epidemic at Norwich in 1819 caused rather more deaths than in 1742, when the public health was very much worse; but it would hardly have caused so many had it not been aided by the state of population.

The epidemic of 1819 spread all over East Anglia[1]. At Lynn there had been a good deal of the disease three years before; in 1819 there were so many deaths from it that in June the clergy ordered the smallpox burials to be specially marked in the register, from which date until the end of August they numbered forty. At Yarmouth the epidemic was still raging at the end of 1819. Of ninety-one surgeons in Norfolk and Suffolk who replied to a circular issued by Cross, all but eleven saw cases of smallpox in 1819, three had had cases in 1818, two had seen the disease in 1817, and one in 1816. Generally speaking, the disease had been in abeyance in those counties for seven years; a surgeon of Prudham, whose practice covered eleven parishes, had seen no case of smallpox for twelve years before. The largest number of deaths in the practice of any one surgeon was twelve. Twenty-eight surgeons together had 598 smallpox patients, with 97 deaths; but in their districts there had been 180 deaths besides from the same disease, in families unvisited by them.

The accounts of this epidemic in London are most meagre. In the bills of mortality, now become quite inadequate to the whole capital, the deaths rose to 1051 in 1817, fell next year to 421, and in 1819 were 712. But it was in the year 1819 that the admissions to the smallpox hospital were most numerous, namely, 193, the highest number since the epidemic of 1805, when they were 280 in the year. The horny or crystalline kind of smallpox was found in London, as elsewhere[2].

---

[1] Cross, u. s. Appendix.

[2] W. Shearman, M.D., "Cases illustrating the Nature of Variolous Contagion and the Modifying Influence of Vaccine Inoculation." *Lond. Med. Repos.* Dec. 1822.

In the spring of 1818, "smallpox *post vaccinationem*" was frequent among the boys of 'Christ's Hospital[1]. None of the cases proved fatal that year, but there was a death in the school from smallpox in 1820, probably the last fatality from that cause in the history of the school[2].

A few casual notices of smallpox in England in the years following the epidemic of 1817–19 lead one to suppose that the disease did not again fall to that apparent extinction which it had reached before the last epidemic began.   It is heard of in and around Chichester in 1821 ; nineteen surgeons who supplied Dr John Forbes with information had seen about 130 to 140 cases, with 20 deaths ; about 80 of the cases were in persons previously inoculated with cowpox, 19 cases (or the most of 19) were in persons previously inoculated with smallpox[3]. This was doubtless the experience of paying patients only ; according to the East Anglian precedent of 1819 there would have been twice as much smallpox in families who received no professional treatment.   Canterbury is another town from which a rapidly spreading epidemic of smallpox is reported—in the winter of 1823–4.   It continued into the winter and spring of 1824–25, among the poor, fatal cases being by no means rare.   Dr Carter frequently saw children exposed in the streets of Canterbury with smallpox upon them ; he appealed to the mayor to have some check imposed on the spread of contagion, but nothing was done, and smallpox was still prevalent at the date of his writing in the autumn of 1824[4].   The same year there was a

Case of a mother, with good vaccine marks, attacked with smallpox, which became dry and horny about the fifth day; case of her child, in which the eruption ran the full course of pustules, but also a mild case.

[1] *Lond. Med. and Phys. Journ.* May, 1818, p. 488 : "By Mr Field's report of Christ's Hospital smallpox in a mild form has been frequent *post vaccinationem.*"

[2] Thomas Stone, F.R.C.S. "Table of Deaths from Smallpox in Christ's Hospital, 1750 to 1850, with remarks," in Appendix to *Papers on the History and Practice of Vaccination : Parl. Papers,* 1857. In 1761 there were four deaths from smallpox. For ten years, 1775 to 1784, there were none. In some other years of the latter half of the 18th century there were one or two deaths from that cause.   There must have been some special reason for the four deaths in 1761. According to Massey (*supra,* p. 545), the apothecary in the beginning of the 18th century, not one death happened in forty attacks, the ages from five to eighteen being the most favourable of all for smallpox to fall in.   In the present century scarlatina has displaced smallpox as an infectious cause of death in that school as in others.   The deaths from scarlatina at Christ's Hospital during the six years 1851–56 were nine.

[3] John Forbes, M.D., "Some Account of the Smallpox lately prevalent in Chichester and its Vicinity." *Lond. Med. Repos.* Sept. 1822, p. 208.

[4] H. W. Carter, M.D., in *Lond. Med. Repos.* Oct. 1824, p. 267 : "The cases which came to light of smallpox after vaccination were unfortunately numerous ; some, it must be confessed, were exceedingly severe ; others were exaggerated."

severe epidemic at Oxford. These were probably only samples of epidemics filling the interval from 1819 to 1825, when smallpox again became general.

Extent of Inoculation with Cowpox or Smallpox, 1801–1825.

Twenty-five years had now passed since cowpox became the rival or substitute of the old matter of inoculation. The history at this point requires some notice of the extent to which each of those methods was practised. Professional opinion, or that part of it which found expression, was for the most part in favour of cowpox. The Smallpox and Inoculation Hospital of London took the lead, under Woodville, in substituting cowpox for smallpox, and other public institutions, such as the Newcastle and Whitehaven Dispensaries, quickly followed. The new mode was practised upon larger numbers than the old. At the Newcastle Dispensary the inoculations of smallpox from 1786 to 1801 had been 3268; the inoculations of cowpox from 1801 to 1825 were 20,264. At the Whitehaven Dispensary 173 children were inoculated with smallpox in 1796, the total inoculations before that having been 906. To the end of 1803 the total vaccinations were 490, of which many were done during the severe outbreak of smallpox in 1803.

In Glasgow, where the old inoculation was either little practised or of little use, the Jennerian mode was received with favour, and was offered to the children of the working classes gratuitously at the Hall of the Faculty of Physicians and Surgeons. From the 15th of May, 1801, to the 31st of December, 1811, these public vaccinations numbered 14,500, an average of about 1400 in the year. In the next seven years they declined as follows:

1812	950	1816	980
1813	1162	1817	820
1814	875	1818	650
1815	926		

On the revival of smallpox the Glasgow Cowpock Institution was opened on 28 August, 1818, and vaccinated 146 to the 1st of January, 1819. The smaller demand for even gratuitous vaccination of infants after 1812 was owing to the very small amount of smallpox in Glasgow in those years; in the six years, 1813–19, there were said (by Cleland) to have been only 236 deaths from smallpox in a total of 22,060 deaths from all causes, or 1·07 per cent. of all deaths[1]. Not more than a fourth part of all the infants born in Glasgow had been vaccinated in the years 1812 to 1818, and that was the time when smallpox was at its lowest point among the infantile causes of death. In some of those years when smallpox was in abeyance measles was most destructive. It was currently said in Glasgow that vaccination, if it discouraged smallpox, predisposed to measles, an opinion of the populace which Malthus shared from the *à priori* point of view. But in a survey of the individual cases in their practice the Glasgow doctors did not find that those were the relevant circumstances, whatever the truly relevant things may have been. Thus, Dr Robert Watt, a good observer and cautious reasoner, who became president of the Glasgow faculty, wrote: "The only family within my knowledge where three died of the measles in 1808 was one where none of the children had been either vaccinated or had had the smallpox. I met with another family where two died in the same circumstances"—that is to say, five children, in two families, escaped smallpox to die of measles, no artificial interference having been attempted[2].

Manchester was another populous district where vaccination had been freely offered to the poorer classes. Roberton, writing in 1827, says that it had been on the decline for several years, and gives the following figures for the earlier period, May, 1815, to May, 1823[3]: At the Manchester Lying-in Charity the annual average of deliveries was 2667, while the number of infants brought back for vaccination averaged 1392 in a year. During the same eight years public vaccinations at the Manchester Infirmary averaged 1700 annually. Great numbers of infants were said, also, to have been vaccinated gratuitously by druggists. The decline in the number of vaccinations, which had perhaps begun some time before (as at Glasgow), was shown conclusively by the returns for the two years May, 1824—May, 1826. The births at the Lying-in Charity averaged 3285 per annum; but the vaccinations in the infants brought back to the charity,

[1] The vaccinations are given in Cleland's *Rise and Progress of the City of Glasgow.* Glasgow, 1820. The smallpox deaths from 1813 to 1819 are given, on Cleland's authority, in the *Edin. Med. and Surg. Journal*, XXVI. p. 177.
[2] R. Watt, M.D., Appendix to *Treatise on Chincough.*
[3] John Roberton, *Obs. on the Mortality, &c. of Children.* Lond. 1827, p. 59, *note.*

together with those brought to the Manchester Infirmary, averaged only 1309 per annum.

Newcastle, Glasgow and Manchester were probably favourable instances of the extent of public vaccinations in the first quarter of the century. In London the proportion of vaccinations to births is known to have been smaller, although there was more money going and at one time four public charities—the Vaccine Pock Institution, the Royal Jennerian Society, Walker's offshoot from the latter, and the Inoculation Hospital. The following were the vaccinations at the Inoculation Hospital in four periods of five years each from 1806[1]:

1806—10	7,004
1811—15	9,339
1816—20	13,348
1821—25	16,666
	46,357

Annual average 2317.

At Norwich, Dr Rigby succeeded in 1812 in persuading the Board of Guardians to offer half-a-crown premium to parents for each child brought to be vaccinated. The premiums paid were as follows:

1812		1815	11
(12 Aug.—31 Dec.)	1066	1816	348
1813	511	1817	49
1814	47	1818	64

—the annual births being from a thousand to twelve hundred[2].

At the Canterbury Hospital the applications for free vaccinations fluctuated as follows:

1818	52	1822	35
1819	249	1823	50
1820	263	1824	
1821	47	(Jan.—July)	588

The sudden rise in 1819–20 and again in 1824 was owing to smallpox being epidemic in the city. During the severe epidemic of 1824 there were 250 vaccinations at the Dispensary, besides the 588 at the hospital[3]. At Kendal the following is the Dispensary record of vaccinations for three years, the annual average of births being 390[4]:

---

[1] Gregory, *Report of the London Smallpox Hospital for the year* 1825. Cited in the *Med. and Phys. Journ.* Feb. 1826, p. 176.
[2] Cross, u. s.
[3] Carter, u. s.
[4] T. Proudfoot, M.D., *Ed. Med. and Surg. Journ.* July, 1822.

1819	221
1820	102
1821	73

These are examples of the spasmodic demand for vaccination in the towns. The following is an instance of general vaccination in a village during an epidemic:

The village of North Queensferry, near Edinburgh, had a population of 390. There was an epidemic of smallpox from 14 December, 1811, to 7 March, 1812, during which time 46 children, from one to fifteen years, were attacked, and seven died, the same number that had died in the last epidemic, in 1797. When the epidemic was over there were only nine persons in the village, most of them aged, who had neither had smallpox nor cowpox. Those who had been vaccinated numbered 132; while of those "formerly vaccinated" only two were included among the 46 children who caught smallpox in 1811–12. The adult population must have nearly all gone through smallpox in former epidemics[1]. These general vaccinations during or towards the end of an epidemic were exactly comparable to the general inoculations by the old method. At Norwich, where a premium of half-a-crown was given to parents for each vaccination, the epidemic of smallpox in 1819 stimulated the practice somewhat, the increase in July and August having followed a public meeting of the inhabitants and a combined effort of the doctors:

	Progress of the mortality	Progress of premium vaccinations		Progress of the mortality	Progress of premium vaccinations
January	3	26	July	142	301
February	0	51	August	84	359
March	2	101	September	42	14
April	15	226	October	10	4
May	73	226	November	2	2
June	156	92	December	1	0

Cross estimated that a fifth part of the population of Norwich (50,000) were vaccinated—8000 before the epidemic of 1819, and 2000 during the epidemic. Many of the adults had been through the smallpox in the ordinary way in former epidemics. The state of vaccination throughout Norfolk and Suffolk was indicated in the answers made by ninety-one practitioners to the circular of queries sent out by Cross. Twenty-six had done 13,313 vaccinations during the epidemic of

---

[1] C. Stuart, u. s.

1819. The whole number in the practice of those ninety-one from first to last had been 120,000, two of the practitioners having vaccinated none.

To sum up, as well as the records enable us to do, the extent of the new practice in the first quarter of the century, it was systematically carried out from year to year among the infants of large towns, such as Glasgow, Newcastle, Manchester and London, and in these the maximum of gratuitous vaccinations in proportion to the births may have been one-half. In smaller towns and in country parishes the inoculations of cowpox, like those of smallpox, appear to have been irregular or by fits and starts, the alarm of smallpox being the occasion for them. But after the epidemic of 1817–19, which was the most general since cowpox had been tried, it was not mere negligence or procrastination that kept parents back, it was distrust of the new practice and preference for the old.

The original mode of inoculation, with the matter of smallpox itself, was far from being supplanted by its rival. In Jenner's first essay the latter was put forward tentatively, not indeed because of any want of confidence in asserting its protective powers, but because it was only in certain circumstances that a substitute was desired for the old inoculation. Some of those who took up the new matter soon discontinued the old altogether, as at the Newcastle and Whitehaven Dispensaries. At the London Inoculation Hospital the old practice was given up for out-patients after 1807, and for in-patients about 1821. In private practice, tastes or preferences differed. While ordinary people left it to the discretion of their medical advisers, commissioning them to inoculate their children "with either kind of pock," the upper classes "judge for themselves, and those among them who are philanthropists and converts to the new faith inoculate their own children and those of the poor together[1]." Moseley, in 1808, said that the "mere operative practice" in cowpox, by which phrase he meant to contrast the academic countenance of it by eminent physicians and surgeons, had been "chiefly carried on by lady-doctors, wrong-headed clergymen, and disorderly men-midwives," Dr Pearson being named as the only man of letters or pretensions to science who had been practically concerned in it of late[2].

---

[1] Dr Stokes, of Chesterfield, *Med. and Phys. Journ.* v. 17.
[2] Benjamin Moseley, M.D., *A Review of the Report of the Royal College of*

There was really little to choose between the new method and the old so far as concerned facility of operating; if anything, the inoculation of smallpox was the more difficult of the two, although that also was largely practised by amateurs[1]. Again, as regards remunerativeness, inoculation with smallpox no longer required the combined services of a physician, a surgeon and an apothecary; it had become a matter of simple routine, just as ill paid (or as well paid, according to circumstances) as inoculation with the matter from the cow. It was not on such grounds, but on grounds of scientific principle or of sentimental interest, that an active propaganda was kept up in favour of the old inoculation. The leading defenders of the latter, such as Moseley, physician to Chelsea Hospital, and Birch, surgeon to St Thomas's Hospital, maintained that cowpox was alien in nature to smallpox and could not be received as its equivalent. The foreign protagonists, such as Dr Müller, of Frankfort, and Dr Verdier, of Paris, emphasized still more the radical unlikeness of cowpox to smallpox. Said Verdier: "The vaccinists appeal to experience, setting aside all objections based upon the unlikeness of cowpox to smallpox. We are to be made invulnerable by vaccine as Achilles was made invulnerable by being dipped in the waters of the Styx. Protection by cowpox contradicts the received principle of inoculation. It is in vain to appeal to experience against established principles: for true principles are the result of the experience of all ages, and become the touchstone of each successive empirical innovation."

The English inoculators by the old method gave all sorts of reasons for their preference, and were doubtless actuated by the usual mixture of motives. There were medical families, such as the Lipscombs, who had an hereditary interest and pride in inoculation. It was a Lipscomb who had recited in the Sheldonian Theatre during the Oxford commemoration of 1772,

Physicians on Vaccination. 1808, p. 11. Jenner writing to James Moore, 18 Nov. 1812 (in Baron, II. 383), enumerates his various grievances against Pearson, "and finally, finding all tricking useless, his insinuations that vaccination is good for nothing."

[1] The equality of the two methods in this respect comes out incidentally in two reports of the Whitehaven Dispensary. In the report for 1796, when smallpox matter was in use, it is said that "173 were inoculated, all of whom, soliciting little medical assistance, recovered." In 1801, when cowpox matter had been substituted in every case, the same phrase is used: "We seldom find any medical assistance required in this disease."

a poem, " On the Beneficial Effects of Inoculation." Inoculators
to the third generation, it was not surprising that the Lipscomb
family should have caused to be printed in 1807, as if to shame
the changing fashion of the day, the prize poem of five-and-
thirty years before, which contained such spirited lines as these :

> "When, pierced with grief at sad Britannia's woes,
> Her country's guardian Montagu arose :
> Pure patriot zeal her ev'ry thought inspir'd,
> Glow'd on her cheek, and all her bosom fir'd.
> She saw the Tyrant rage without controul,
> While just revenge inflam'd her gen'rous soul.
> Full well she knew, when beauty's charms decay'd,
> Britannia's drooping laurels soon would fade :
> Pierc'd with deep anguish at the afflictive thought
> And whelm'd with shame, a heav'n-taught Nymph she sought,
> Whose potent arm, with wondrous power endued,
> Had oft on Turkey's plains the fiend subdued.
> Obedient to her prayer the willing Maid
> In pity came to sad Britannia's aid.
> 'Henceforth, fall'n Tyrant!' cries the Nymph, 'no more
> Hope that just Heav'n will thy lost pow'r restore :
> Let now no more thy touch profane defile
> The sacred beauties of Britannia's isle.
> By me protected shall they now deride
> Thy baffled fury and thy vanquish'd pride[1].'"

[1] *The Beneficial Effects of Inoculation.* Oxford University Prize Poem. Oxford,
1807. It seems probable that this was the "Oxford copy of verses on the two
Suttons" that Coleridge (*Biographia Literaria* (1817), Pickering's ed. II. 89)
professed to quote from in the following passage ; at least it would be remarkable if
there had been printed another Oxford poem on the same subject and in the same
manner : " As little difficulty do we find in excluding from the honours of unaffected
warmth and elevation the madness prepense of pseudopoesy, or the startling hysteric
of weakness over-exerting itself, which bursts on the unprepared reader in sundry odes
and apostrophes to abstract terms. Such are the Odes to Jealousy, to Hope, to
Oblivion, and the like, in Dodsley's collection and the magazines of the day, which
seldom fail to remind me of an Oxford copy of verses on the two Suttons, commencing
with

> ' Inoculation, heavenly maid ! descend !'"

It appears that Coleridge himself contemplated a poem on Cowpox Inoculation,
which was to have exemplified what poetry should be, just as the 18th century Oxford
poem on Smallpox Inoculation exemplified what poetry should not be. It was
clearly more than the difference 'twixt tweedle-dum and tweedle-dee. Writing
to Dr Jenner on 27 Sept. 1811, from 7, Portland-place, Hammersmith, he said :
" Dear Sir, I take the liberty of intruding on your time, first, to ask you where and
in what publication I shall find the best and fullest history of the vaccine matter as
the preventive of the smallpox. I mean the year in which the thought first suggested
itself to you (and surely no honest heart would suspect me of the baseness of flattery
if I had said, inspired into you by the All-preserver, as a counterpoise to the crushing
weight of this unexampled war), and the progress of its realization to the present day.
My motives are twofold : first and principally, the time is now come when the
'Courier'...is open and prepared for a series of essays on this subject ; and the
only painful thought that will mingle with the pleasure with which I shall write
them is, that it should be at this day, and in this the native country of the discoverer
and the discovery, be even *expedient* to write at all on the subject. My second
motive is more selfish. I have planned a poem on this theme, which after long

Still it was just among those classes to whom the *argumentum ad nitorem* came home most forcibly that the fashion had changed. Before the end of the 18th century, the danger to beauty from an attack of smallpox had become a matter chiefly of historical interest, carrying the mind back to the Restoration or the early Georgian era. The richer classes, while they seem to have countenanced cowpox inoculation as a good thing in general, were probably apathetic on their own account. Lord Mulgrave said in the House of Lords on 8 July, 1814 ; "If their lordships recollected how many persons of the higher order were reluctant to introduce vaccination into their families, it really must appear to them a harsh and arbitrary measure to lay the poor under the necessity of adopting the practice." The working class had been manifesting a devotion to the old practice which, indeed, they had never shown so long as it was unchallenged. Perhaps one reason to account for the undoubted preference of the poorer classes for the old inoculation was that they had only lately taken to it. Another was that a good deal of inoculation was done by amateurs of their own class— blacksmiths, farriers, tradesmen and women. A third reason was that the poorer classes, among whom smallpox prevailed most, saw their children take smallpox all the same, and cared little for the scientific explanation that a false or spurious kind of cowpox matter had been used. In October, 1805, a correspondent wrote from London to an Edinburgh journal: "The many late failures of supposed cowpock to prevent the smallpox have excited in some parts so much clamour among the lower orders of people that they insist upon being inoculated for the smallpox at some of the public institutions[1]." A report on vaccination made to Parliament by the College of Physicians in 1807, deplores "the inconsiderate manner in which great numbers of persons ever since the introduction of vaccination are still every year inoculated with the smallpox." When, in consequence of the same report, a vote was brought forward in Parliament to give Dr Jenner a national reward of twenty thousand pounds in addition to the ten thousand that he had

deliberation, I have convinced myself is capable in the highest degree of being poetically treated, according to our divine bard's [Milton's] own definition of poetry, as '*simple, sensuous*, (i.e. appealing to the senses by imagery, sweetness of sound, &c.) and *impassioned, &c.*'" *The Life of Edward Jenner, M.D.* By John Baron, M.D. 2 vols. II. 175.

[1] *Edin. Med. and Surg. Journ.* I. 507.

got five years before, the populace were so angry that one of their leaders, John Gale Jones, himself a medical man, sent a message to Jenner at his lodgings in Bedford Place to advise him "immediately to quit London, for there was no knowing what an enraged populace might do[1]."

Few particulars remain of the old inoculation at this time. One fact significant of the impression that the criticisms of cowpox had made is that Dr John Walker, director of the Royal Jennerian Society, who pushed "vaccination" among the poorer classes more than anyone in London, was all the while an inoculator in the old manner. He wrote to Lettsom, " I have from the first introduction of vaccination entertained an opinion respecting its nature different from those who suppose it a *substitute* only for smallpox....I have, from an early part of my practice, been in the habit of *diluting* smallpox virus with water previous to its introduction into the system ;" and this he had been doing in the name of Jenner, under the influence of a belief that, if cowpox were not smallpox, it ought to be, that it was a pity the disease had ever been called cowpox, and that the name (which was a very old one) " has only served to debase it in the eyes of the common people, and prevent its general adoption[2]." The very director of the Jennerian institute was among the prophets of the old inoculation.

With the revival of smallpox in general epidemic diffusion in 1816–19 we begin to hear more of the old inoculation. The account already cited of the outbreak at Ulverston contains a table of fourteen previously cowpoxed children whom it was thought desirable during the epidemic to inoculate with smallpox, all of them receiving the infection in one degree or another. A practitioner at Dunse, Berwickshire, not only returned to the old inoculation (thereby incurring "much odium," as he believed), but actually took his matter from the natural smallpox of his cowpox failures[3].

---

[1] Jenner to James Moore, 26 Feb. 1810, in Baron, II. 367.
[2] Walker to Lettsom, 1 Sept. 1813, in Pettigrew's *Memoirs of Lettsom.* Lond. 1817, III. 350.
[3] Dr Smith to Dr Monro, Dunse, 2 June, 1818, in Monro's *Obs. on the different kinds of Smallpox*, 1818. There appears to have been some reluctance to face the facts. "Though I have seen," says Smith, "a multitude of cases in which smallpox has in every possible shape taken place after vaccination, I feel myself placed in the painful situation [why painful ?] of bringing forward many facts to which gentlemen of the first eminence in the profession will probably give little or no credit."

When the epidemic reached the Eastern Counties, there were demands for the old kind of inoculation, not in Norwich only, but in numerous country parishes. Of ninety-one surgeons in Norfolk and Suffolk, who answered the queries of Cross, thirty-eight had practised the inoculation of smallpox in the epidemic of 1819; five of them, after having refused many private applications for inoculation in the old way, had at length yielded to the desire of the Overseers of the Poor, and had inoculated whole parishes. Cross's correspondents also testified that there was much inoculation going on at that time in the Eastern Counties by the hands of farriers, blacksmiths, tailors, shoemakers and women.

Dr John Forbes, who then practised at Chichester, brought to light an exactly similar state of public feeling in Sussex in 1821–22[1]. In the parish of Bosham there lived a farmer named Pearce who had an inherited skill in inoculating, his father having inserted smallpox into ten thousand persons in his day, without killing one of them. Pearce offered to wager with Forbes a considerable sum that he would inoculate any number of persons and that none of them should have more than twenty pustules. He believed that the smallpox matter became "as weak as water" by an uninterrupted transmission from one body to another.

In November, 1821, the Overseers of the Poor employed him to inoculate the pauper children, and his skill was soon in request for others, so that from two to three hundred in the parish were inoculated by him within a short time. He charged half-a-crown or a crown for each. From other parishes the people flocked to him in such numbers that he inoculated upwards of a thousand in the winter and spring of 1821–22. Before long he had three itinerant rivals, a knifegrinder, a tinsmith and a fishmonger, who claimed to have inoculated together a thousand persons, including four hundred previously cowpoxed. The surgeons of Emsworthy and Havant at length joined in the business, and in the space of six or eight weeks inoculated from twelve to thirteen hundred persons, who had not been previously vaccinated. Forbes also received from his medical friends in and around Chichester "an account of 680 cases of previously vaccinated individuals subjected by them to variolous inoculation." In the great majority of these the

---

[1] *Lond. Med. Repository.* Sept. 1822.

constitutional symptoms were so slight as to be only just observable, the eruption consisting of only a few pustules, which were all that the Pearces, of Bosham, father and son, ever expected to get with inoculated smallpox where no infection of cowpox had preceded. Disappointments with the new inoculation had led to a great revival of the old also at Canterbury, the operators being mostly women.

The same thing happened in Cambridgeshire and in Bucks. In a parish within eleven miles of Cambridge several hundred persons were inoculated with smallpox in 1824, and in April, 1825, a medical practitioner inoculated a number in a village near[1]. During a severe epidemic in the parish of Great Missenden, Bucks, which followed a general vaccination, and caused a prejudice against the latter, the old inoculation was generally resorted to[2]. It looked for a brief period, about the time of the epidemic of 1824–26, as if the old inoculation were to return to favour even with the profession itself. Dr John Forbes wrote of the two kinds of inoculation in a studiously impartial manner. Dr Robert Ferguson, who was also destined to make a name, addressed in 1825 a letter to Sir Henry Halford in which he advocated a singular compromise, namely, two inoculations, one with cowpox, the other with smallpox, the cowpox to neutralize the contagiousness of the smallpox for the occasion, while the latter was to be the prophylactic against itself for the future[3]. This reaction, if it deserves that name, corresponds in time to the great decline in the number of gratuitous vaccinations at Manchester, a decline which had been equally remarkable at Glasgow for some years before. There was at least an apathetic spirit towards cowpox inoculation during the epidemic of 1817–19, and for a good many years after

---

[1] J. J. Cribb, *Smallpox and Cowpox.* Cambridge, 1825.

[2] *Ibid.* Letter of Rev. R. Marks, of Great Missenden, 6 May, 1824 : "The summer I came here the smallpox was introduced, and as the weather was very hot, and the confluent sort was what appeared, the people began to die almost as fast as they took the plague. Great prejudice prevailed against vaccination, in consequence of the parish having some years ago been vaccinated by a gentleman who knew nothing of the matter, and contaminated the people with decomposed virus, when it was good for nothing but to make ulcers and produced very wretched arms, and left them all liable to smallpox, which they were all inoculated for the same year." This clergyman subsequently vaccinated 500 cases, and the parish surgeon 300 : " and here," says the former, " I had the happiness of seeing the plague and destruction of a most horrid smallpox completely stopped."

[3] Robert Ferguson, M.D. *A Letter to Sir Henry Halford, proposing a method of Inoculating the Smallpox, which deprives it of all its Danger, but preserves all its Power of Preventing a Second Attack.* London, 1825.

it, while there was something like toleration, even among medical men, for the old inoculation.

The Smallpox Epidemic of 1825-26.

Compared with the epidemic of 1837-40, which was the first in England to be recorded under the new system of registration of the causes of death, the smallpox of 1825-26 makes a poor figure in the records. Yet there is reason to believe that it was an epidemic of the same general kind, if not of the same duration or fatality. At the Newcastle Dispensary far more children in the smallpox were visited in 1825 than in any year since its opening in 1777, namely, 113 cases, with 28 deaths, which would have been a small fraction of all the cases in Newcastle. At the Rusholme Road Cemetery, Manchester, which received about a fourth part of the burials, 112 children, all under seven years, were buried from smallpox in the six months, 18 June to 18 December, 1826[1]. At Bury St Edmunds smallpox began to be epidemic about the end of 1824, when the guardians ordered a general vaccination, and reached its worst in July, 1825, the type being confluent in many of the cases[2]. It was in Cambridgeshire villages the same year, and is casually heard of in Bucks[3]. It had been severe at Oxford and Canterbury in 1824. At Glasgow the prevalence of fever is known for the corresponding years, but the smallpox deaths have not been taken out of the burial registers. The evidence from London is perhaps the best indication that the smallpox of 1825 was one of the more severe periodic visitations.

The extensive prevalence of smallpox was heard of in Paris before the epidemic attracted much notice in London; the news of persons of distinction dying by smallpox in the French capital reads like the old notices of it in 17th century letters. In the same year it was very severe also in Sweden after a long period of quiescence. As to London, Dr George Gregory, physician to the Smallpox Hospital, said[4]: "It may be inferred

[1] John Roberton, *Observations on the Mortality and Physical Management of Children.* London, 1827, p. 59, *note.*
[2] J. Dalton, "Smallpox as it prevailed at Bury St Edmunds in 1825." *Lond. Med. and Phys. Journ.* May, 1827, p. 406.
[3] Cribb, u. s.
[4] "Observation on Smallpox as it has occurred in London in 1825." *Med. and Phys. Journ.* Feb. 1826, p. 117.

that smallpox has been nearly as general in 1825 as in any of
the three great epidemics of the preceding century"—the demand
for admission to the Hospital being, in his opinion, a fair index;
while private information confirmed the estimate of its truly
epidemic prevalence, and of its incidence chiefly upon the lower
classes[1].   In the years of the 18th century to which he referred,
and in four maximum years of the 19th century, the cases and
deaths at the Smallpox Hospital had been as follows[2]:

London Smallpox Hospital.

Year	Cases	Deaths		Year	Cases	Deaths
1777	497	125		1819	193	61
1781	646	257		1822	194	57
1796	447	148		1825	419	120
1805	280	97				

While the demands upon the beds of the hospital pointed, as
Gregory supposed, to the existence of a great epidemic in London,
comparable to those of 1777, 1781 or 1796, in which years
the smallpox deaths were returned by the parish clerks at 2567,
3500 and 3548 respectively, yet in 1825 the bills showed only
1299 deaths from smallpox.   Gregory accepted without demur
the figures of the parish clerks' bills in 1825, although it is well
known that they had become more and more defective, even for
the original parishes, since the end of the 18th century[3].   "But
for the general prevalence of vaccination," he said, the smallpox
deaths in 1825 would have been 4000 in the same number of
attacks, the difference being in the rate of fatality.   His conclusion for all London was based upon the experience of the
Smallpox Hospital.   The patients received by that charity were
of the same class as formerly, most of them being adults, among
whom the proportion of fatalities was greater than at all ages.
Taking the three epidemics of the 18th century with which he
compared the epidemic of 1825 in respect of extent or number
of attacks, we find that 25 per cent. of the cases admitted died in

---

[1] *Med. and Phys. Journ.* 1826, p. 122.   "The general voice of the public satisfactorily showed that the upper ranks of society suffered during the past year from
smallpox much less than the lower."
[2] Gregory, *Report on the Smallpox Hospital,* 4 Dec. 1825.
[3] Farr, in the First Report of the Registrar-General (1839, p. 100), said: "It may
be safely asserted that the parish clerks registered little more than half the deaths
that occurred within the limits of the London bills of mortality."   Outside the limits
of the bills there were large parishes, such as St Pancras, Marylebone, Kensington
and Chelsea, which had large mortalities from smallpox in the first years of registration.

1777, 39 per cent. in 1781 (the seasons were unwholesome by epidemic agues, dysenteries, and typhus), and 33 per cent. in 1796. The average of fatalities at the hospital from its opening in 1746 to the end of the century was about 29 per cent., and that was exactly the ratio of deaths among the 419 patients in 1825. The rate of fatality was a little higher than in the epidemic of 1777, and a little lower than in each of the epidemics of 1781 and 1796. Gregory in 1825 was enabled to separate the sheep from the goats by the dividing line of cowpox, the former dying at the rate of 8 per cent., the latter at the rate of 41 per cent. There are various ways of apportioning a general average. The presence or absence of cowpox scars is one principle, which could not have been used to break up the 25 per cent of 1777, or the 39 per cent. of 1781, or the 33 per cent. of 1796, into two component parts. One thing common to all times is the different rate of fatality at different ages. All the deaths in the 8 per cent. division of 1825 were between the ages of eighteen and twenty-seven; the ages of the 41 per cent. division are written in the books of the hospital. In portioning out the general rate of fatality from typhus fever at the London Fever Hospital, it is found that the dividing line of age is nearly the same as the dividing line of social position; in one table the high ratio of deaths to attacks is among persons in the second half of life, and the low ratio among persons in the flower of their age; in another table the many deaths to cases are among paupers, and the few fatalities among paying patients[1]. However manifold the cutting up of a general average, some divisions would be identical, corresponding to natural lines of cleavage.

Having indicated the chief points in the vaccination controversy by the instance of Gregory's arguments sixty years since, (to which might have been added the question of efficient or inefficient vaccination according to the appearance of the scars in after life[2]), I shall for the rest depart from the usual practice of interlocking the history of smallpox epidemics with the history of vaccination. I shall treat the latter as *ex hypothesi*

---

[1] Tables in Murchison's *Continued Fevers of Great Britain.*
[2] *Med. Chir. Trans.* XXIV. 15. His other papers are: "Cursory Remarks on Smallpox as it occurs subsequent to Vaccination," *ibid.* XII. 324; and "Notices of the Occurrences at the Smallpox Hospital during the year 1838," *ibid.* XXII. 95. He contributed the treatise on Smallpox to Tweedie's *Library of Medicine*, I. 1840, and indicated his final opinions (which are interesting) in his *Lectures on the Eruptive Fevers*, 1843.

irrelevant, leaving it to each reader to incorporate, as matter of his own familiar knowledge or belief, whatever effects of cowpox upon smallpox, whether temporary effects or permanent, modifying effects or absolutely prophylactic, may suit his particular creed. I am led to take this course for several reasons. It leaves me free to look at the epidemics of smallpox from the same point of view as the other epidemics treated of in this work. It avoids a controversy which, unlike that of inoculation, is still actual, and unsuited to a historical treatise. It enables me to omit the excuses for failure, which are apt to be interminable and to usurp the whole space available for the epidemiology proper. Lastly, the irrelevancy which I here conveniently assume happens to be my real belief,—as elsewhere set forth in an examination of the antecedent probability arising out of the pathological nature and affinities of cowpox, and in a study of the grounds on which the authority of the profession was originally given to Dr Jenner's teaching.

The interval between the epidemic of 1825 and that of 1837–39 was occupied by a good deal of smallpox steadily from year to year in London, the deaths from which, in the following table from the bills of mortality, are to be understood as only a part of the whole, according to the explanation already given:

Year	Smallpox deaths	Year	Smallpox deaths	Year	Smallpox deaths
1826	503	1830	627	1834	334
1827	616	1831	563	1835	863
1828	598	1832	771	1836	536
1829	736	1833	574	1837	217

The inadequacy of these returns will appear from the fact that the 217 deaths in 1837 rose, under the new system of registration, from 1 July to 31 December, to 762, or to fully three times as many for the last six months as the parish clerks returned for the whole year. Their bills had become most defective when they were about to be, or had been superseded; but even on the special occasion of the cholera in 1832 they returned only some three-fifths of the known deaths. Besides these London figures there is little to show the extent of smallpox in England between the epidemic of 1825 and that of 1837–39. This was the time when many complaints were made of the so-called loss of power or strength in the current cowpox matter for inoculation. These complaints appear to have arisen from the greater frequency of smallpox among the cowpoxed, corresponding to the increasing numbers of the whole population who had received that kind of inoculation. "Secondary smallpox," says a report from Worcestershire in 1833, "has been very prevalent of late years[1]," the term "secondary" reflecting the teaching of Baron, chairman of the Smallpox Committee of the Medical Association, that cowpox itself was the primary smallpox. The increasing number of the vaccinated who took smallpox was clearly shown in the returns from the Smallpox Hospital of London, and was believed to be in proportion to the increasing number of the rising generation who had been vaccinated[2].

A generation of Smallpox in Glasgow.

Glasgow had afforded the most striking instance in Britain of the decline of smallpox after the beginning of the 19th century. The decline was observed everywhere, but it was most noticeable in Glasgow, partly because the smallpox mortality of infants at the end of the 18th century had been excessive there, partly because Dr Watt took the trouble to prove it statistically from the burial registers. In the last six years of the 18th century, 1795–1800, smallpox had contributed 18·7 per cent. of the deaths from all causes; from 1801 to 1806, it contributed 8·9 per cent., and from 1807 to 1812 only 3·9 per cent. In the next six years, 1813–19, if Cleland's search of the registers has been as laborious as Watt's, the share of smallpox was only 1·07 per cent. of the deaths from all causes, which would mean that Glasgow was hardly at all touched by the epidemic of 1817–19, reported from many other parts of Scotland[3]. But the lull in

[1] Kenrick Watson, "Medical Topography of Stourport and Kidderminster." *Trans. Prov. Med. and Surg. Assoc.* II. 195.

[2] John Roberton, "On the Increasing Prevalence of Smallpox after Vaccination." *Lond. Med. Gaz.* 9 Feb. 1839, p. 711. Roberton had been a warm supporter of the Jennerian method from as early a date as 1808, when he was resident in Edinburgh, and again in his book on *The Mortality of Children*, in 1827. The above cited paper is somewhat satirical, the disappointing facts of it being referred to the Island of Barataria. His conclusions are (p. 713): (1) "It is not fact, but conjecture, that the protective power of cowpox gradually ceases in the human system. (2) It is not fact, but conjecture, that a person successfully re-vaccinated is less liable to smallpox than he was before. (3) To affirm that, when re-vaccination fails in individuals, they are thereby proven to be secure from smallpox, is conjecture."

[3] Cowan, "On the Mortality of Children in Glasgow," *Glas. Med. Journ.* v. (1831), p. 358, does not give Cleland's figures, but says: "No bills of mortality except those for the Royalty in the *Glasgow Courier* are in existence for the period from 1812 to 1821"; and again: "Finding that the suburbs were excluded, and the Calton being the burying-place in which the greatest number of children are interred,

smallpox, which corresponded on the whole to the still greater
lull in fevers during the prosperous times of the second half of
the French war, was broken in Glasgow, if not in 1817, yet
before long. Unfortunately there is a break in the statistics
also. From 1821 the magistrates caused annual bills of mortality to be published, which did not, however, specify the
causes of death until 1835[1]. But we have some intermediate
glimpses of the state of the poorer classes and of the prevalence
of smallpox in particular. Writing in 1827, Dr Mac Farlane
one of the poor's surgeons, remarks upon the feeble stamina,
sallow complexions, and the like, of all but a few children in the
more crowded parts, adding that smallpox both in the virulent
and " modified " forms had been more prevalent during the last
three or four years than formerly[2]. Three years after, Drs
Andrew Buchanan and Weir gave an account of the state of the
poor in Glasgow, which shows that it had actually deteriorated
with the growth of the city. The poorer classes had been in
some part displaced from their old dwellings in the heart of the
town owing to the building of warehouses or the like, and had
been provided with no new habitations as good as the old.
"Apartments originally intended for cellars, and occupied as
such until lately, are now inhabited by large families, and the
only opening for light and air is the door, which when shut
encloses the poor creatures in a tainted atmosphere and in total
darkness. This is well exemplified in the cellars belonging to
the houses on the south side of St Andrew's Street." Not only
the notorious region of the Wynds, containing part of the three
parishes of the Tron, St Enoch's and St James's, but also the
Saltmarket and Gallowgate, were crowded with a destitute,
vagrant and often vicious class of people. Many of the houses
in the Wynds, with their network of alleys, were only one or
two storeys high, in the old Scotch fashion; here were the night
lodging-houses, with several beds in one room, two or three
persons in a bed, twelve to eighteen people in as many square

I thought it needless to insert any tabular view of the deaths by measles since the
date of Dr Watt's tables." Watt could have made no tables if he had not gone
direct to the sixteen MS. volumes of burial registers, including those of the Calton.

[1] J. C. Steele, *Glas. Med. Journ.* N. S. I. 60 : "From 1812 to 1835 it is much to
be regretted that no record of the deaths from smallpox has been kept for even a
limited period."

[2] *Glas. Med. Journ.* I. 105 : "There exists at present among the poorer classes an
increasing carelessness and aversion to vaccination, from a belief that it does not afford
adequate protection from the varioloid disease."

feet : " the extreme misery of these poor people is utterly inconceivable but to those who have actually witnessed it ; it has
certainly been carried to the very utmost point at which the
existence of human beings is capable of being maintained.
Some of them are lodged in places where no man of ordinary
humanity would put a cow or a horse, and where those animals
would not long remain with impunity." Buchanan found sometimes a horse, sometimes an ass, sometimes pigs, in the same
dungeon with one or more families[1]. Such was the region in
which Chalmers ministered from 1815 to 1822, first in the Tron
parish, afterwards in the poor and crowded parish of St John's.
Things got no better, certainly, after he left worn out by his
exertions, to become professor at St Andrews. Buchanan
thought the best index of the degradation of the people in 1830
to be that not one in ten ever entered a church (if they had, he
explains, the respectable congregation would have fled from
their filth and rags). " The people are starving," he exclaims,
" and there is a law against the importation of food[2]." It took
sixteen years longer to secure the benefits of free trade, and
meanwhile the public health of Glasgow got worse rather than
better. The infantile part of it attracted far less notice than
that which touched adults, so that we hear little of smallpox,
while the records of fever and cholera are fairly complete. When
the curtain is lifted in 1835 by the publication of statistics, the
mortality of infants and children by infectious diseases is found
to be proceeding as follows :

Glasgow Mortalities, 1835–39.

Year	Deaths from all causes	Deaths from smallpox	Deaths from measles	Deaths from scarlatina
1835	7198	473	426	273
1836	8441	577	518	355
1837	10270	351	350	79
1838	6932	388	405	87
1839	7525	406	783	262

According to the following table of the ages at death from
smallpox, it will appear that a higher ratio of infants died of it

[1] Andrew Buchanan, M.D. " Present Condition of the Poor in Glasgow." *Glasg. Med. Journ.* III. (1830), 437.
[2] Chalmers had been urging the repeal of the Corn Law since 1819. In a letter to Wilberforce, Glasgow, 15 Dec. 1819, he says : '' From my extensive mingling with the people, I am quite confident in affirming the power of another expedient to be such that it would operate with all the quickness and effect of a charm in lulling their agitated spirits—I mean the repeal of the Corn Bill." Hanna's *Memoirs of Dr Chalmers,* 1850, II. 250.

in their first year at Glasgow than was the rule elsewhere, whether in the 18th or in the 19th century. It was only in the year 1837, when typhus was at its worst and smallpox had somewhat declined, that the deaths by the latter of infants under one year were fewer than those of infants in their second year:

Glasgow : Table of Deaths from Smallpox 1835 to 1839.

	Under 1	1—2	2—5	5—10	10—20	20—30	30—40	Above 40	Total
1835	204	154	75	17	14	8	1	0	473
1836	202	174	144	23	6	24	2	2	577
1837	93	116	94	24	10	11	4	0	352
1838	111	99	119	28	11	14	4	2	388
1839	137	98	113	19	15	17	5	2	406
Totals of five years	747	641	545	111	56	74	16	6	2196
Percentages	34%	29%	25%	5%		7%			

Cowan, who published these figures in 1840, had written eight years before, " I fear that if the list of infantile diseases were still published in the mortality bills many deaths from smallpox would annually be found." We do, indeed, hear of epidemics of smallpox not far from Glasgow. At Stranraer, in Sept.–Nov. 1829, " measles and smallpox attacked with scarcely an exception" all the children in the place who had not acquired immunity either by previous attacks or by the influence of vaccination ; " and even these powerful protectives were, in many instances, of no avail." The subjects of " unmodified " smallpox were nearly all infants of the poorer class. In St John's Street, occupied by decent Scots labouring people, ten children had " unmodified " smallpox and all recovered ; in Little Dublin Street, so called from its Irish tenants, fourteen children had smallpox, of whom six died[1]. At Ayr, about the same time, there was an epidemic, which came to a height in 1830, causing a considerable mortality[2]. At Edinburgh in the winter of 1830–31, it was unusually prevalent and fatal, the epidemic dying out in May, 1831[3].

For three or four years, 1843–46, there was another lull in the prevalence of smallpox in Glasgow ; but the mortality rose again, reaching in the two years 1851 and 1852 the total of

[1] J. Orgill, "Obs. on the Measles and Smallpox that prevailed epidemically in Stranraer, in the autumn of 1829." *Glasg. Med. Journ.* IV. 351.
[2] Mc Derment, *ibid.* IV. 201.
[3] Howison, *ibid.* V. 256–7.

1202, in a population of 360,138, which contrasted with the 2212 deaths in London in the same two years, and with the Paris mortality of 706 in the two years 1850 and 1851, in a population of about one million, the deaths being still almost wholly infantile in Glasgow while they were in great part of adults in Paris[1].

Glasgow Smallpox.

Year	Smallpox deaths	Year	Smallpox deaths
1840	455	1847	592
1841 (pop. 282, 134)	347	1848	300
1842	334	1849	366
1843	151	1850	456
1844	99	1851 (pop. 360, 138)	618
1845	195	1852	584
1846	not recorded		

Registration of the causes of death began in Scotland in 1855. In the first decennial period, to 1864, the smallpox deaths were 10,548, falling upon infancy and other age-periods as in the following table[2]:

Age-periods	Smallpox deaths
Under three months	774
Three to six months	668
Six to twelve months	1543
One to two years	1765
Two to three years	1132
Three to four years	798
Four to five years	514
Total under five years	7194
Above five years	3354
	10,548

Smallpox in Ireland, 1830–40.

Before coming to the epidemic in England let us glance at the prevalence of smallpox at this period in Ireland. Dr Cowan, of Glasgow, was struck by the fact that among ninety patients in the Infirmary with smallpox, all adults, only four

---

[1] J. C. Steele, *Glasg. Med. Journ.* N. S. I. 59.

[2] *Eleventh detailed Report of the Regr.-Genl. for Scotland,* 1865, p. xxxix. The Report says that vaccination was general during the above period, although there was no Vaccination Act for Scotland (until 1864). This was familiar knowledge in Scotland, so much so that the necessity for a compulsory law, on the English model, was not quite obvious in the medical circles of Edinburgh. See Christison's address to the Social Science Association at Edinburgh in 1863 (p. 106). In my own recollection of Aberdeenshire, the vaccination of infants was as little neglected as their baptism; the law made no real difference.

were from the considerable Irish population of the city, the larger number being natives of the Highlands of Scotland. This leads him to say: "The immunity of the Irish from small-pox is owing to the general practice of vaccination among the lower classes by the surgeons of the county and other dispensaries" (another Glasgow writer ascribes the prevalence of small-pox to the Irish negligence in the same matter). It happens that we can bring one part of this statement to a statistical test. The same volume of the *Journal of the Statistical Society* which contained the paper on the vital statistics of Glasgow contained also a statistical account of the public health of Limerick, by Dr Daniel Griffin, physician to the Dispensary[1]. Dr Griffin's figures were of the only kind that could then be got for an Irish town, and were representative rather than exhaustive. Struck by the seemingly enormous death-rate of infants in the poorest quarters of Limerick, he sought to bring out the facts with numerical precision. He provided a register-book at the Dispensary, in which he entered the results of his observations and retrospective inquiries among eight hundred families of the poorest class during "a good many years" down to 1840. The city of Limerick, and especially the parish of St Mary, was full of the misery and destitution that characterized Ireland in the years of its greatest over-population. The ejected cottiers and broken small farmers of the neighbouring county flocked to it, living in beggary in wretched lodging-houses with swarms of infants and children, the breadwinners finding only an occasional day's work as labourers. Among 800 such families during the years of his inquiries the chief causes of death among the infants and children were as follows:

Limerick Dispensary Deaths.

	Under Five years	Five to Ten	Above Ten	Total
Convulsions	569	18	7	594
Smallpox	333	55	5	393
Measles	187	32	7	226
Diarrhoea and Dysentery	108	19	24	151
Whooping cough	84	10	1	95
Croup	85	9	1	95
Scarlatina	8	2	0	10
Fever	70	33	66	169

[1] "An Enquiry into the Mortality among the Poor in the City of Limerick." *Journ. Statist. Soc.* Jan. 1841, III. 316.

The more exact ages at death from smallpox in male and female children were:

	Under One	One and Two	Three and Four	Five to Nine	Above Nine
Males	33	72	37	29	2
Females	52	92	47	26	3
	85	164	84	55	5

As compared with Glasgow, measles at Limerick has a much lower place than smallpox in the infantile mortality, while scarlatina hardly counts at all. Again, only 1·27 per cent. of the smallpox deaths are above the age of nine, whereas at Glasgow 7 per cent. are above the age of ten. Griffin's data for reckoning the probability of life were incomplete, as he was well aware; so that the following comparison of the poor attending Limerick Dispensary with all England and Wales probably errs in making the Irish town somewhat more fatal to infants of the poor than it really was:

	England and Wales in 1000 deaths	Limerick Dispensary in 1000 deaths
Under one year	214·54	327·71
One and under three	128·00	287·67
Three and under five	48·51	128·20
Five and under ten	46·07	97·29
Ten and under fifteen	25·91	24·93
Fifteen and under twenty	34·16	20·37

In a thousand deaths at all ages, 391·05 occurred before the age of five years in England and Wales, but 743·58 before the age of five years among a certain section of the poor of Limerick; and in the latter enormous sacrifice of infant life smallpox was the greatest single means next to convulsions. Perhaps that was the reason why so few of the Irish in Glasgow were attacked by smallpox in adult age. The experience of Limerick was not exceptional in Ireland. In the ten years 1831–40, for which the causes of death were ascertained by means of queries in the census returns of 1841, the total of deaths by smallpox was 58,006, nearly double the mortality by measles (30,735) and seven times that of scarlatina (7,886). It was almost wholly a malady of infants and children, the first and second years of life being its most fatal period. Only 129 of these deaths were returned from hospitals. The bulk of the decennial smallpox deaths fell in the two years 1837 and 1838, corresponding with the high epidemic mortality in England[1].

The Epidemic of 1837–40 in England.

The smallpox epidemic of 1837–40 was already in full force at Liverpool, Bath and Exeter when the mortality returns began to be made on 1st July, 1837, under the new Registration Act. Whether or not the contagion travelled from Ireland or the west of Scotland, the epidemic in England began in the west and south-west, and reached the Eastern counties last. The following table shows its rise and progress at selected places in the several quarters, beginning with the third quarter (July—September) of 1837[2]:

	1837		1838				1839			
	3rd qr	4th qr	1st qr	2nd qr	3rd qr	4th qr	1st qr	2nd qr	3rd qr	4th qr
Liverpool	375	132	32	24	18	36	11	29	75	138
Bath	154	18	15	1	1	2	1	25	17	30
Exeter	88	131	6	—	2	—	—	—	—	—
Bristol	21	74	72	44	4	7	6	—	—	—
Clifton	16	32	49	27	7	—	—	—	1	7
London	257	506	753	1145	1061	858	364	117	65	60
Manchester	23	98	127	120	111	180	94	40	33	53
Birmingham	34	55	85	86	66	47	26	12	7	10
Sheffield	14	14	27	36	22	12	9	3	4	—
Leeds	4	11	29	69	134	197	74	55	30	15
Newcastle	16	17	66	11	—	23	54	24	39	25
Abergavenny and Pontypool	13	85	102	50	22	21	22	30	26	10
Merthyr Tydvil	9	54	160	91	10	3	18	16	12	—
Weymouth, Bridport, and Beaminster	4	19	92	31	8	4	10	9	2	—
Plymouth	10	15	11	14	37	48	9	8	1	—
Taunton	—	7	66	40	4	3	—	—	—	—
Leicester	43	5	3	2	3	3	9	21	5	15
Norwich	1	—	—	—	—	17	180	204	10	7
Lynn etc.	—	1	2	10	7	4	127	81	6	—
Ipswich	—	—	2	6	38	95	23	—	1	—
Bury St Edmunds etc.	1	3	30	24	2	3	—	—	—	—
Woodbridge etc.	4	9	27	16	5	11	10	2	—	4

The epidemic having begun in the west and south-west in the summer of 1837, spread in the winter of 1837–38, all through the hills and valleys of Wales, causing high mortalities around

---

[1] *The Census of Ireland*, 1841. Parl. Papers, 1843. Report on the Tables of Deaths, by W. R. Wilde.

[2] From the Second Report of the Registrar-General, Lond. 1840, p. 180.

Abergavenny, Pontypool, Merthyr Tydvil and other towns in the first quarter of 1838, as well as in the rural parishes. It was not until the end of 1838 that the contagion spread widely over the Eastern counties. The epidemic in Norwich was again short and sharp, like that of 1819, most of the 418 deaths falling within six months of winter and spring, just as most of the 530 deaths in 1819 fell within six months of summer and autumn. The population in 1821 was 50,288, and in 1841, 62,344; the increase was only 1228 between 1831 and 1841, so that the smallpox of 1839 fell upon a stationary population, whereas that of 1819 had fallen upon a rapidly increasing one. In the autumn of 1839 and throughout 1840, a second outburst of smallpox took place in the towns where the epidemic had started two years before, namely, Liverpool, Bath, Bristol, Clifton, etc[1].

But the smallpox of 1840, which produced more deaths than that of 1839, was mostly centred in the Lancashire manufacturing towns, where also the mortality from scarlet fever was enormous. The circumstances of the working class in Lancashire at this time have been described in the chapter on fevers. The following shows the large proportion of smallpox deaths that fell in 1840 to the North-Western or Lancashire registration division.

Smallpox Deaths, 1840.

	1st qr	2nd qr	3rd qr	4th qr
England and Wales	2071	2476	2274	3613
Of which in the N.-W. Division (Lancashire)	1046	986	533	590

The epidemic continued in the manufacturing towns into 1841; in the more rural registration divisions of England it had almost ceased in 1839. From the 1st July, 1837 (beginning of registration) until the 31st December, 1840, the epidemic smallpox in England and Wales caused 41,644 deaths. In 1838 it eclipsed both measles and scarlatina as a cause of death among children; but in 1840 scarlatina gained the leading place and kept it.

1840.

	1st qr.	2nd qr.	3rd qr.	4th qr.
[1] Liverpool	172	184	90	85
Bath	25	42	22	8
Exeter	—	—	1	1
Bristol	6	54	49	76
Clifton	11	28	22	42

Legislation for Smallpox after the Epidemic of 1837–40.

The epidemic of smallpox in 1837–40, which was fatal chiefly to infants and young children, was one of the greatest, like the corresponding epidemic of typhus among adults, in the whole history of England. The troubles of the working class had been more or less chronic ever since the booming times of the Peninsular War had come to an end ; the climax was reached in the thirties ; the enormous sums spent upon railway construction gave a relief in the forties ; and the permanent cheapening of food by Free Trade made an entirely new era, which became visible in the public health after the contagion of the Irish famine had ceased in 1848. The great and hitherto permanent decrease of typhus was brought about by social and economic causes. There, at least, *laissez faire* was all powerful : " Let us be saved," said Burke, " from too much wisdom of our own, and we shall do tolerably well." But there has been at no time since the 18th century the same passiveness towards smallpox ; that is a disease against which we must always be doing something direct and pointed. The legislation against smallpox began in England (nothing was done for Ireland and Scotland until long after) with the Act of 1840.

It is a singular instance of the changes in medical opinion and of the vicissitudes of things that the first statute against smallpox should have been instigated by a desire to suppress the old inoculation. Parliament was first moved to action by the Medical Society of London through a petition presented by Lord Lansdowne ; but things had been moving that way for some time before in the councils of the British (then the Provincial) Medical Association, under the influence of Dr Baron, the executor and biographer of Dr Edward Jenner. The Bill of 1840 was brought into the House of Lords by the second Lord Ellenborough, and conducted through the Commons by Sir James Graham, who was not then in office. It purposed to enable the poorer classes to get their children vaccinated, if they so desired, at the cost of the ratepayers, and to prohibit under penalties the practice of the old inoculation by amateurs or empirics. Blomfield, bishop of London, said in the Lords' debate that many of the ignorant poor, in agricultural districts, were strongly prejudiced against inoculation with cowpox, and that they paid much greater attention to empirics, meaning inoculators by the old method, than to the advice of the clergy.   In the Commons, Mr Wakley, who was a Radical and the proprietor of one of the weekly medical journals, declared that " no one could be ignorant that the working classes entertained great prejudices against vaccination," although he did not explain why they were prejudiced.   According to this medical authority, whom the House took seriously on that subject if on no other, the epidemic of smallpox which the country had just passed through had been in effect due to the contagiousness of the smallpox matter used in inoculating; and he succeeded in carrying an amendment to put down the old practice, not only in the hands of amateurs but also in those of medical men.   The eighth clause of the Act decreed that any person convicted before two justices in Quarter Sessions of having wilfully procured the smallpox by inoculation shall be liable to a penalty of imprisonment for a term not exceeding one calendar month.   The penal clause against the original inoculation was an indirect compliment to its vitality.   Lord Lansdowne also paid it a compliment by recognizing the correctness of its principle; the rival inoculation-matter of cowpox, he said, was " perfectly identical" with smallpox, "although the symptoms were different."   This will be a convenient point in the history at which to review the rise and progress of the idea that the inoculation of smallpox was a wilful spreading of contagion and therefore a public nuisance.

The risk of spreading the contagion of smallpox by inoculating the disease was one of the objections to the practice raised by Wagstaffe in his letter to Dr Freind in 1722 : "I have considered," he says, "how destructive it may prove to spread a distemper that is contagious."   Still more explicit was Dr Douglass of Boston, New England, writing on 1 May, 1722 : "I oppose this novel and dubious practice...in that I reckon it a sin against society to propagate infection by this means, and bring on my neighbour a distemper which might prove fatal, and which, perhaps, he might escape (as many have done) in the ordinary way. ...However, many of our clergy have got into it, and they scorn to retract[1]."   Within a few months there was a striking instance of the alleged danger in one of Maitland's inoculations at Hertford, an inoculated child, with only twenty pustules, having been supposed the probable source of the natural smallpox in five domestics, of whom one died.   The death of the Duchess of Bedford by the natural smallpox in 1724 happened " after two of her children were recovered of that distemper, which they both had by inoculation[2]."   That risk, however, was little made of in the controversy, although it may have been one of the

[1] Douglass to Colden, 1 May, 1722, in *Massach. Hist. Soc. Collect.* Series 4, vol. II. p. 169.
[2] Philip Rose, M.D., *Essays on the Smallpox.* London, 1724, p. 76.

tacit reasons that led to the total abandonment of inoculation during the ten or twelve years after 1728. On the revival of the practice after 1740, when the serjeant-surgeons, the physicians and the apothecaries were all making it a considerable part of their business among the richer classes, the danger from contagion was either non-existent or it was not realized. In 1754 the College of Physicians of London, by a formal minute, recommended inoculation as "highly salutary to the human race," without one word of warning on the risk of contagiousness. That objection was raised again when Sutton's practice in 1765—67 was drawing large crowds to be inoculated. He was put on his trial at the Chelmsford Summer Assizes in 1766 on a charge of spreading the contagion of smallpox, which was epidemic in the town; but the grand jury, charged by Lord Mansfield, threw out the bill. Sutton's defence was to have been that he never brought into Chelmsford a patient capable of spreading the smallpox, that is to say, an inoculated person with smallpox enough on him to spread contagion[1]. Shortly after came the controversy between Lettsom and Dimsdale as to inoculation of infants at their homes, which turned upon the risk of increasing the natural smallpox by a constant succession of artificial cases. Lettsom's position was the same as Sutton's, that the quantity of smallpox matter (he might have said the quality also) produced by inoculation was not sufficient to create an appreciable risk. As to the matter of fact, the quantity was indeed small: Sir William Watson declared that a single limb of an adult person in a moderate attack of the natural smallpox had as many pustules on it as all the seventy-four children, in one of his inoculations at the Foundling Hospital, had on their whole bodies. In the theory of contagion, an infinitesimal quantity is sufficient; but in reality it appears that contagion must be in excess to be effective, just as, in the nearest physiological analogy, fertilization seems to depend upon the copiousness of the pollen or seminal particles[2].

The opposition to Lettsom's project of general inoculations among the infants of the working classes in cities shows that the risk of contagion was made to serve at least an argumentative purpose. As to experience, Lettsom in 1778 declared that he knew no instance of contagion from that source during two years of inoculations among the poor of London[3]. One writer of the time (1781) appealed boldly to the experience of sixty years : "Upon the first introduction of inoculation, physicians, divines, and innumerable other writers [who were they?] cried out that the infection would be spread, and the community suffer a greater loss ; but after sixty years' experience, we should expect those arguments, as well as the writers, had all died away, and that at this day the same stale dregs of ignorance and obstinacy would not be again retailed[4]." The risk, however, was not altogether imaginary. Some cases of smallpox caught from the inoculated were known. In Vienna

---

[1] Rev. R. Houlton, App. to *A Sermon in Defence of Inoculation*, Chelmsford, 1767, p. 59 : "For, had the indictment been found, he would have assuredly nonsuited his enemies, and have proved beyond a possibility of doubt that he never brought into Chelmsford a patient who was capable of infecting a bystander, notwithstanding such person would convey infection by inoculation. However paradoxical this may seem, it is truth, and would have been proved to a demonstration."

[2] Darwin, *Animals and Plants under Domestication*, II. 356 : "From these facts we clearly see that the quantity of the peculiar formative matter which is contained within the spermatozoa and pollen-grains is an all-important element in the act of fertilization, not only for the full development of the seed, but for the vigour of the plant produced from such seed."

[3] J. C. Lettsom, M.D., *A Letter to Sir Robert Barker, F.R.S. and G. Stackpoole, Esq. upon General Inoculation.* London, 1778, p. 8.

[4] W. Black, M.D., *Observations Medical and Political on the Smallpox, etc.* London, 1781, p. 103.

at that time the rule was to allow no inoculations except on groups of subjects isolated for the purpose. When Jenner, in 1798, enumerated the advantages of cowpox over smallpox for inoculation, in certain specified circumstances, one of his points was its non-contagiousness[1].

The favourable reception of his project seems to have been determined more upon that point than upon any other. The theoretical risk of contagion from inoculated smallpox became at once an actual danger to the community when it was perceived that they had in "smallpox of the cow" a non-contagious variety. Jenner was not slow to use that growing sentiment so as to discredit the old practice. As early as 1802 he began to urge privately the statutory prohibition of smallpox for inoculation, and Wilberforce, among others, took the matter up publicly. The College of Physicians, having been asked by Parliament in 1807 to inquire into the causes that hindered the progress of Jenner's inoculation, inserted the following paragraph in their report:

"Till vaccination becomes general, it will be impossible to prevent the constant recurrence of the natural smallpox by means of those who are inoculated, except it should appear proper to the Legislature to adopt, in its wisdom, some measure by which those who still, from terror or prejudice, prefer the smallpox to the vaccine disease, may in thus consulting the gratification of their own feelings, be prevented from doing mischief to their neighbours[2]." The same year, in the court of King's Bench, a medical practitioner was sentenced to fine and imprisonment for having neglected to prevent an inoculated person from communicating with others[3].

Next year, 1808, a bill was brought into the House of Commons by Mr Fuller, with the following preamble: "Whereas the inoculation of persons for the disorder called the Smallpox, according to the old or Suttonian method, cannot be practised without the utmost danger of communicating and diffusing the infection, and thereby endangering, in a great degree, the lives of his Majesty's subjects."...This bill, which had clauses also for notification and compulsory isolation of smallpox cases, the churchwardens to be the authority, was not persevered with. The inoculators by the old method opposed it, and they were joined by Joseph Adams, who had been the first English writer to mention cowpox, in 1795, and had been a staunch vaccinist subsequently[4]. In 1813 another attempt was made to restrict the practice of inoculating the smallpox on the ground of danger from its contagion, and to get cowpox substituted for it among the poorer classes. The Vaccine Board were the promoters, Lord Boringdon (afterwards Earl of Morley) having charge of the bill in the House of Lords. It was successfully opposed by the Lord Chancellor (Eldon) and by the Lord Chief Justice (Ellenborough), the latter contending that the common law was a better remedy than a statute against the nuisance of contagion from inoculated smallpox. Next year, 1814, Lord Boringdon brought in a new bill, which did not directly harass the inoculation interest, but made the rival method of cowpox obligatory upon the poor. Its provisions were ridiculed by Lord Stanhope, who got help from Lords Mulgrave and Redesdale to throw it out. Therewith ceased for many years

[1] "But, in the cowpox, no pustules appear, nor does it seem possible for the contagious matter to produce the disease from effluvia, or by any other means than contact, and that probably not simply between the virus and the cuticle; so that a single individual in a family might at any time receive it without the risk of infecting the rest, or of spreading a distemper that fills a country with terror."

[2] *Parliamentary Papers*, 1807, 8th July.

[3] Bateman, *Reports etc.* 1819, p. 102. The principle of the Common Law on which the judgment rested was, "Sic utere tuo ut alienum non laedas."

[4] Joseph Adams, *An Inquiry into the Laws of Epidemics, with Remarks on the Plans lately proposed for Exterminating the Smallpox.* London, 1809. The *Edin. Med. and Surg. Journal* (VI. 231), in a long review of this essay, declared that Adams was inconsistent in reaffirming his old faith in cowpox and at the same time demanding liberty for the inoculators.

the talk about the contagiousness of inoculated smallpox, together with the attempts in Parliament to enforce the rival inoculation. The next attempt, in 1840, was successful in making variolation a felony, and in throwing on the rates the cost of vaccinating the infants of the poorer classes. The danger of contagion from inoculated smallpox in 1840 was no greater than it had ever been, and it had never been appreciable among the things favouring an epidemic.

The common-law maxim, "sic utere tuo ut alienum non laedas," which gained statutory force as against inoculation by the Act of 1840, was farther extended and specifically applied in the Act of 1853, which enforced the inoculation of cowpox upon all infants before they were three months old. Legislation, as we know, broadens down from precedent to precedent. Parliament in 1853 did not debate the preamble of the Bill, but accepted the principle established by the Act of 1840,—in the constructive sense that to leave infants without the inoculation of cowpox was, in effect, "to expose them so as to be infectious," because they were sure to take smallpox, and so to become nuisances to others "unprotected" as well as (less obviously) to their cowpoxed neighbours.

Other effects of the epidemic of 1837–40 on medical opinion.

A second inoculation, except as a mere test of the first and within a few weeks thereof, was no part of the original 18th century teaching and practice. The theory of inoculation being based upon the familiar experience that we seldom have the same infectious disease twice in a lifetime, it was held that inoculation, if it were effective, was the giving of smallpox once for all, and that it could not really be given a second time unless the first inoculation had been ineffective. As soon as cowpox was recommended, it was remarked as a strange thing that this disease, according to current accounts of it, was actually acquired by milkers time after time. That fact in its natural history, said the *Medical and Physical Journal* of January, 1799, was "received with general scepticism merely on account of its improbability." Dr Pearson was so troubled by the apparent inconsistency that he wrote to Dr Jenner in 1798 to ask whether it were really so; and although the latter confirmed the matter of fact, Pearson went on denying it, and did actually deny it as late as the Report of the Vaccine Pock Institution for 1803. Again, the report of the Whitehaven Dispensary for 1801, while it admitted the matter of fact, adverted to the anomaly in these words: "As we know from experience that the cowpock can be repeatedly introduced by inoculation, it appears remarkable that it can act as a preventive of a similar equally specific but more malignant disease." Those were theoretical difficulties, which the practical minds of the profession did not stand upon. When we next hear of the possibility of having cowpox more than once, it is no longer an intellectual stumbling-block but is turned to account in the way of re-vaccination. *Lapidem quem reprobaverunt aedificantes, hic factus est in caput anguli.*

The practice of re-vaccination was usual on the Continent long before the English took to it. The reason of this was that a second inoculation of cowpox was not resorted to for the greater security of infants and young children, who were then the principal victims of smallpox in this country, but for the protection of adults, who made a great part of the subjects of the epidemics in other countries. There were so many adult deaths in the great Paris epidemic of 1825 that the news of it reads like the English references to smallpox in the time of the Stuarts. We obtain exact statistics of the ages in the 3323 fatal cases of smallpox in Paris from 1842 to 1851. Reduced to percentages they were as follows:

All ages	0—5	5—10	10—20	20—30	30—40	Over 40
100	33·8	5·9	13·25	32·95	10·95	3·15

Two-thirds of the deaths were above the age of five years, an age-incidence that was not reached in London until a whole generation after. The contrast with British experience comes out in concrete form in the following table of the age-incidence of 342 fatal attacks of smallpox in 1850 and 364 in 1851, in Paris (pop. 1,000,000), and of 584 fatal attacks in Glasgow in the single year 1852 (pop. 370,000)[1]:

Age-incidence of fatal Smallpox in Paris and in Glasgow

	Paris, 1850–51 (706 deaths)	Glasgow, 1852 (584 deaths)
Under one year	126	188
One to two	32	150
Two to five	94	189
Five to ten	31	20
Ten to fifteen	20	4
Fifteen to twenty	51	2
Twenty to twenty-five	109	19
Twenty-five to thirty	89	2
Thirty to forty	128	8
Forty to fifty	22	1
Over fifty	4	1

[1] J. C. Steele, M.D., "Increase of Smallpox in Glasgow." *Glas. Med. Journ.* N. s. I. 59. The Paris figures are cited from the *Annuaire pour l'an* 1852–53.

In other parts of the Continent of Europe the frequency of smallpox in adults was not less remarked than in France in the second quarter of the 19th century. English writers had been able at one time to point to foreign countries for the success of infantile vaccination. Sweden and Denmark were for a long time classical illustrations; then it was Germany's turn. "In Berlin during 1821 and 1822," said Roberton, "only one died of smallpox in each year. In the German States, vaccination has become universal, and in them as well as in various other countries the smallpox is almost unknown." When we next find German experience appealed to, it is to enforce the need of re-vaccination: "In 1829," said Gregory, "the principal Governments of Germany took alarm at the rapid increase of smallpox, and resorted to re-vaccination as a means of checking it. In Prussia, 300,000 had been re-vaccinated, and the same number in Würtemberg. In Berlin nearly all the inhabitants had undergone re-vaccination[1]." It was about the same time that a second vaccination became obligatory in the armies of Prussia, Würtemberg, Baden and other German States, and among the pupils of schools when they reached the age of twelve years. Dr Gregory, in his speech at the Medical and Chirurgical Society of London in December, 1838, urged the need of re-vaccination not only by the example of Germany, but also by the experience of Copenhagen, where a thousand cases of smallpox had been received into the hospital (it was nearly always adults that were taken to the general hospitals) in twenty-one months of 1833–34, nine hundred of them being of vaccinated persons[2]. Gregory was in advance of his age in advocating re-vaccination for England. His own cases at the Smallpox Hospital of London were, it is true, nearly all adults, according to the rules of the charity. But they were not representative even of the smallpox of the capital; and in England at large smallpox in 1839 was still distinctively a malady of the first years of life. It was not until youths and adults began to have smallpox in large numbers in the epidemic of 1871–72 that the doctrine of re-vaccination was generally apprehended in England. Medical truth, like every other kind of truth except that of geometry, is conditioned by time and place. What was a truth to the Germans in 1829 was not a

[1] I do not, of course, answer for the correctness of Gregory's statements.
[2] *Lancet*, 12 Dec. 1838.

truth to us until some forty years after. Dr Gregory, Sir Henry Holland and others advised re-vaccination after the epidemic of 1837–40; but as late as 1851 the National Vaccine Establishment denounced it as incorrect in theory and uncalled-for in practice.

After the great epidemic of 1837–40, there was an interval of a whole generation until smallpox broke out again on anything like the same scale, in 1871 and 1872. But it had risen to a considerable height at shorter intervals—in 1844–45, which were the years when vast numbers of navvies were employed making railroads all over England, in 1847 and successive years to 1852, which was the period of the great Irish migration after the potato-famine, in 1858, for which I find no explanation, and in the period from 1863 to 1865, which was again a time of somewhat high typhus mortality, not only in the Lancashire cotton-districts but also in London. The great epidemic of 1871 and 1872 finds no better explanation than our neighbourhood to Germany and Belgium, where the mortality from smallpox was far greater than in Britain, and was doubtless favoured by the state of war in 1870–71. The following tables for London, and for England and Wales in comparison with measles, scarlatina and diphtheria, show the progress of smallpox from the epidemic of 1837–40 to the present time:

Smallpox Deaths in London from the beginning of Registration.

Year	Deaths	Year	Deaths	Year	Deaths
1837 (6 mo.)	763	1856	531	1875	46
1838	3817	1857	156	1876	736
1839	634	1858	242	1877	2551
1840	1235	1859	1158	1878	1417
1841	1053	1860	898	1879	450
1842	360	1861	217	1880	471
1843	438	1862	366	1881	2367
1844	1804	1863	1996	1882	430
1845	909	1864	547	1883	146
1846	257	1865	640	1884	898
1847	255	1866	1391	1885	914
1848	1620	1867	1345	1886	5
1849	521	1868	597	1887	7
1850	499	1869	275	1888	5
1851	1062	1870	973	1889	0
1852	1150	1871	7912	1890	3
1853	211	1872	1786	1891	1
1854	694	1873	113	1892	11
1855	1039	1874	57	1893	206

England and Wales: Deaths by Smallpox, Measles, Scarlatina and Diphtheria from the beginning of Registration.

	Smallpox	Measles	Scarlet Fever	Diphtheria
1837 ($\frac{1}{2}$)	5811	4732	2550	—
1838	16268	6514	5862	—
1839	9131	10937	10325	—
1840	10434	9326	19816	—
1841	6368	6894	14161	—
1842	2715	8742	12807	—
1847	4227	8690	14697	—
1848	6903	6867	20501	—
1849	4644	5458	13123	—
1850	4665	7082	13371	—
1851	6997	9370	13634	—
1852	7320	5846	18887	—
1853	3151	4895	15699	—
1854	2868	9277	18528	—
1855	2523	7354	16929	385
1856	2277	7124	13557	603
1857	3236	5969	12646	1583
1858	6460	9271	23711	6606
1859	3848	9548	19310	10184
1860	2749	9557	9681	5212
1861	1320	9055	9077	4517
1862	1638	9860	14834	4903
1863	5964	11340	30473	6507
1864	7684	8322	29700	5464
1865	6411	8562	17700	4145
1866	3029	10940	11683	3000
1867	2513	6588	12380	2600
1868	2052	11630	21912	3013
1869	1565	10309	27641	2606
1870	2620	7543	32543	2699
1871	23062	9293	18567	2525
1872	19022	8530	11922	2152
1873	2308	7403	13144	2531
1874	2084	12235	24922	3560
1875	849	6173	20469	3415
1876	2468	9971	16893	3151
1877	4278	9045	14456	2731
1878	1856	9765	18842	3498
1879	536	9185	17613	3053
1880	648	12328	17404	2810
1881	3698	7300	14275	3153
1882	1317	12711	13732	3992
1883	957	9329	12645	4218
1884	2216	11324	11143	5020
1885	2827	14495	6355	4471
1886	275	12013	5986	4098
1887	506	16765	7859	4443
1888	10261[1]	9784	6378	4815
1889	23	14732	6698	5368
1890	16	12614	6974	5150
1891	49	12673	4959	5036
1892	431	13553	5618	6552
1893	1455	10764	6869	8918

[1] 409 of these in Sheffield.

The great epidemic of 1837–40 was the last in England which showed smallpox in its old colours. The disease returned once more as a great epidemic in 1871–72, after an interval of a whole generation (in which there had been, of course, a good deal of smallpox) ; but the epidemic of 1871–72 was different in several important respects from that of 1837–40. It was a more sudden explosion, destroying about the same number in two years (in a population increased between a third and a half) that the epidemic a generation earlier did in four years. It was an epidemic of the towns and the industrial counties, more than of the villages and the agricultural counties ; it was an epidemic of London more than of the provinces ; and it was an epidemic of young persons and adults more than of infants and children. The great epidemic of 1871–72 brought out clearly for the first time all those changes in the incidence of smallpox ; but things had been moving slowly that way in the whole generation between 1840 and 1871. Experience subsequent to 1871–72 has shown the same tendency at work.

To begin with the changed incidence upon rural and urban populations, a glance down the following Table, will show that the counties marked *, with a smaller share in 1871–72, in a total

Incidence of the Smallpox Epidemics of 1837–40 (*four years*) *and* 1871–72 (*two years*) *respectively upon the Counties of England and Wales.*

England and Wales	1837–40 41,253	1871–72 42,084	England and Wales	1837–40 41,253	1871–72 42,084
Metropolis	6421	9698	*Gloucestershire	1072	323
*Surrey (extra-metr.)	383	231	*Herefordshire	191	34
*Kent (extra-metr.)	817	537	*Shropshire	345	161
*Sussex	161	126	*Worcestershire	1002	529
Hampshire	348	1103	Staffordshire	1328	3050
*Berkshire	450	46	*Warwickshire	957	785
*Middlesex (extra-metr.)	418	306	Leicestershire	528	622
*Hertfordshire	260	157	Rutlandshire	8	7
*Buckinghamshire	268	53	Lincolnshire	482	498
*Oxfordshire	199	109	Nottinghamshire	562	983
Northamptonshire	399	563	*Derbyshire	329	297
*Huntingdonshire	65	14	*Cheshire	1141	310
Bedfordshire	125	128	†Lancashire	7105	4151
*Cambridgeshire	400	175	†Yorkshire W. Riding	2858	2609
*Essex	773	583	„ E. Riding	480	452
*Suffolk	506	348	„ N. Riding	236	405
*Norfolk	1038	895	Durham	798	4767
*Wiltshire	548	85	Northumberland	569	1512
*Dorsetshire	329	163	*Cumberland	549	366
*Devonshire	1097	838	*Westmoreland	98	41
*Cornwall	767	531	Monmouthshire	672	904
*Somersetshire	1466	412	*Wales	2699	2314

of deaths in all England and Wales which was nearly the same as in the great epidemic a generation before, are nearly all those with a population more purely rural[1]:

The counties which were most lightly visited in 1871–72, as compared with 1837–40, were the agricultural and pastoral. In the outbreaks subsequent to 1871–72, smallpox has almost ceased to be a rural infection in Scotland and Ireland as well as in England. The great change that has come over it in that respect is shown in the following table, in which the annual death-rates from smallpox per 100,000 living are contrasted, for children under five, in each of several agricultural counties, with the mean of all England and of London, 1871-80, and with the corresponding scarlatinal death-rates in the right-hand column:

Annual Death-rates of Children under five, per 100,000 living, 1871–80.

	Smallpox	Scarlatina
All England	53	349
London	113	307
Sussex	9	100
Berkshire	4	141
Bucks	4	160
Oxfordshire	9	167
Huntingdonshire	3	205
Bedfordshire	11	242
Cambridgeshire	18	112
Suffolk	12	136
Wiltshire	5	210
Dorsetshire	15	152
Herefordshire	5	166
Shropshire	12	247

But the history of smallpox since the great epidemic of 1871–72 has brought out still another tendency in the same direction, namely, the increasing share of London in the whole smallpox of England. In the epidemic of 1837–40, which reached to almost every parish of England and Wales, London had 6449 deaths in a total of 41,644, or between a sixth and a seventh part, having rather less than an eighth part of the population. In the epidemic of 1871–72, London had between a fourth and a fifth part of the deaths (9698 in a total of 42,084),

[1] There are two notable exceptions, marked †, Lancashire and Yorkshire; but, in regard to their higher mortality from smallpox in 1837-40, it should be kept in mind that they were the chief scenes of the great distress among the working class in those years, the same causes which produced an enormous mortality from typhus fever in adults having tended to increase the fatality of smallpox among the children.

having then about a seventh part of the population. In 1877, more than half of all the smallpox deaths were in London, and in the year after as many as 1417 in a total of 1856. In 1881, London had about two-thirds of the deaths from smallpox in all England and Wales; but in the epidemic of 1884–85, it had only over a third part (1812 in a total of 5043). This excess of London's share over that of the provinces is expressed in the following table, showing the respective rates of smallpox mortality per million of the population:

Smallpox Deaths in London and the Provinces, per million of population.

	1847–9	1850–4	1855–9	1860–4	1865–9	1870–4	1875–9	1880–4
London	460	300	237	281	276	654	292	244
Provinces	274	271	192	175	172	339	48	34

If the table were continued to the very latest date, it would show the provinces recovering their share, but upon a slight prevalence of the epidemic as a whole, the deaths in London having been mere units from 1886 to 1892, while in 1888 there was a severe epidemic in Sheffield and in 1892–93 a good deal of the disease in a few manufacturing towns of the North-western and Midland divisions. It would be a not incorrect summary of the incidence of smallpox in Britain to say, that it first left the richer classes, then it left the villages, then it left the provincial towns to centre itself in the capital; at the same time it was leaving the age of infancy and childhood. Of course it did none of these things absolutely; but the movement in any one of those directions has been as obvious as in any other. Measles and scarlatina have not shown the same tendency to change or limit their incidence. Smallpox may have surprises in store for us; but, as it is an exotic infection, its peculiar behaviour may not unreasonably be taken to mean that it is dying out,—dying, as in the death of some individuals, gradually from the extremities to the heart.

With all those changes, the fatality of smallpox, or the proportion of deaths to attacks, came out in the great epidemic of 1871–72 curiously near that of the 18th century epidemics, namely, one death in about six cases. This rate comes from the hospitals of the Metropolitan Asylums Board according to the following table:

Admissions for Smallpox, with the Deaths, at the hospitals of the Metropolitan Asylums Board, from the opening of the several hospitals to 30 April, 1872.

Age-periods	Males			Females			Both Sexes		
	Adm.	Died	Percentage of deaths	Adm.	Died	Percentage of deaths	Adm.	Died	Percentage of deaths
Under 5	434	235	54·15	469	236	50·32	903	471	52·15
5—10	851	236	27·73	821	196	23·87	1672	432	25·83
10—20	2827	265	9·37	2513	237	9·43	5340	502	9·40
20—30	2561	465	18·15	1922	285	14·82	4483	750	16·72
30—40	939	244	26·00	665	136	20·45	1604	380	23·69
40—50	316	100	31·64	242	64	26·45	558	164	29·39
50—60	85	18	21·17	88	31	35·22	173	49	28·32
Above 60	40	8	20·00	35	7	20·00	75	15	20·00
	8053	1571	19.49	6755	1192	17·64	14,803	2763	18·65

These admissions to hospitals included attacks of every degree of severity, the intention of the hospitals being to isolate all cases, mild and severe alike ; so that, although these are technically hospital cases, they are not comparable to the select class admitted to the old Smallpox Hospital of London, but to the cases of smallpox in former times in the community at large. Although the general average of deaths in 14,808 cases, namely, 18·65 per cent., is nearly the same as (being slightly higher than) that of the equally comprehensive totals of 18th century cases given at p. 518, yet the average is made up in a different way. In some of the 18th century epidemics, such as that of Chester in 1774, all the deaths were under ten years of age, and yet the average rate of fatality was only 14 or 15 per cent. The much higher rate of fatality from birth to five years and from five years to ten in the London epidemic of 1871–72 (which is confirmed in part by the Berlin statistics of the same years), must have had some special reasons. One reason, doubtless, was that the attack of smallpox in recent times has fallen upon comparatively few children, whereas in former times it fell upon nearly the whole; and it may be inferred that the infants who have been in recent times subject to the attack of smallpox have also been of the class that are most likely to die of it. The high rates of fatality at the ages above thirty in the table agree with the experience of all times.

The percentages of fatalities from smallpox in the hospitals of the Metropolitan Asylums Board have varied as follows from their opening to the present time :

	Cases	Percentage of deaths			Cases	Percentage of deaths
1 Dec. 1870—				1881	8671	16·61
3 Feb. 1871	582	20·81		1882	1854	12·96
4 Feb. 1871—				1883	626	16·06
31 Jan. 1872	13,145	18·95		1884	6567	15·98
1872–3	2362	17·84		1885	6344	15·8
1873–4	191 ⎫			1886	132 ⎫	
1874 (11 mo.)	120 ⎬	17·02		1887	59 ⎪	
1875	111 ⎭			1888	67 ⎬	14·28
1876	2150	21·64		1889	5 ⎪	
1877	6620	17·92		1890	27 ⎪	
1878	4654	17·99		1891	64 ⎭	
1879	1688	15·69		1892	348	11·29
1880	2032	15·95		1893	2376	7·75

The decline in average fatality in the last two years is remarkable, and is to be explained chiefly by the mild type of smallpox which has been prevalent; a very small fraction of the patients attacked between the ages of ten and twenty-five have died; and these are some two-fifths of the whole. This is shown in the following age-table of 2374 cases admitted to the Metropolitan Board Hospitals in 1893:

Smallpox in London, 1893.

Age-period	Cases	Deaths	%	Age-period	Cases	Deaths	%
0—5	168	53	31·5	30—35	250	14	5·6
5—10	191	16	8·3	35—40	182	13	7·1
10—15	230	7	3·0	40—50	199	18	9·0
15—20	340	7	2·0	50—60	79	9	11·4
20—25	393	13	3·3	60—70	35	6	17·1
25—30	298	23	7·7	70—80	9	1	11·1

The low rate of fatality during the slight epidemic revival of smallpox in 1892–93 has been found to obtain wherever the disease has occurred:

Smallpox in the Provinces, 1892-93.

	Cases	Deaths	Fatalities per cent.
Birmingham	1203	96	8
Warrington	598	60	10
Halifax	513	44	8·5
Manchester	406	27	6·7
Glasgow	279	23	8·2
Liverpool	194	15	7·7
Brighouse	134	15	11·2
Aston Manor	113	6	5·3
Leicester	362	21	5·8
St Albans	58	6	10·4
	3860	313	8·10

The ages under ten years had only 290 in 3644 of these cases; but those 290 cases had 70 in 302 of the deaths.

In the comparative table for Ireland, of deaths by smallpox, measles, scarlatina and diphtheria, measles in a decreasing population has changed little, while scarlatina has declined greatly, and smallpox has fallen during the last ten years almost to extinction.

Ireland: Deaths by Smallpox, Measles, Scarlatina and Diphtheria from the beginning of Registration.

	Smallpox	Measles	Scarlatina	Diphtheria
1864	854	630	2605	661
1865	461	1036	3683	480
1866	194	851	3501	317
1867	21	1292	2145	189
1868	23	1251	2696	202
1869	20	948	2670	243
1870	32	954	2978	188
1871	665	547	2707	226
1872	3248	1380	2459	257
1873	504	1303	2092	326
1874	569	667	4034	565
1875	535	898	3845	443
1876	24	664	2112	368
1877	71	1562	1117	288
1878	873	2212	1079	296
1879	672	860	1688	320
1880	389	1025	1344	314
1881	72	402	1230	323
1882	129	1518	2443	385
1883	16	801	1765	239
1884	1	559	1377	354
1885	4	1323	1147	296
1886	2	284	850	336
1887	14	1307	973	381
1888	3	1935	849	447
1889	0	574	457	358
1890	0	726	319	346
1891	7	240	308	281
1892	0	1183	419	286

In the great Irish famine of 1846–49, comparatively little is heard of smallpox. It would appear to have been less diffused through the country than in former famines, such as that of 1817–18, or those of the first part of the 18th century, just in proportion as the vagrancy of famine-times was checked by the establishment of workhouses. In the workhouses and auxiliary workhouses during the ten years 1841–51, smallpox is credited with 5016 deaths, while measles has 8943, fever 34,644, dysentery

50,019, diarrhoea 20,507, and Asiatic cholera 6716. Registration began in Ireland in 1864, and showed little smallpox for the first few years. The next great epidemic, of 1871–72, showed the incidence upon the large towns, and the comparative immunity of the country population, even more strikingly than in England. In a total mortality of 3913 during the two years of 1871 and 1872, the three counties of Dublin, Cork and Antrim had the following enormous share, which fell mostly to the three cities of Dublin, Cork and Belfast:

Dublin Co.	1825
Cork Co.	1070
Antrim	510

3405 deaths in 3913 for all Ireland.

In that epidemic the whole province of Connaught had only 25 deaths from smallpox; but a subsequent visitation, a few years after, fell mainly upon Connaught.

The epidemic which began in Scotland in 1871 was distributed over a somewhat longer period than the corresponding outbreak in England; but the bulk of it fell in the two years 1871 and 1872. The total of 3890 deaths in those two years was distributed as follows:

Eight largest towns	2441
Next largest towns	259
Small town districts	574
Mainland rural districts	586
Insular rural districts	30

3890

Glasgow had a considerably smaller relative share than Edinburgh, and altogether a much lighter incidence of the disease than in the years 1835–52, for which the figures have been given above (pp. 600–1). In the following table of the annual deaths in Scotland from the beginning of registration, the four other infective diseases of childhood included along with smallpox show by comparison the remarkable decline of smallpox since 1874, scarlatina being the only other infection of childhood which has become greatly less common or less fatal.

*Scotland.   Deaths by Smallpox, Measles, Scarlatina, Diphtheria and
Whooping-Cough, from the beginning of Registration.*

	Smallpox	Measles	Scarlatina	Diphtheria	Whooping-Cough
1855	1209	1180	2138	—	1903
1856	1306	1033	3011	—	2331
1857	845	1028	2235	76	1539
1858	332	1538	2671	294	1963
1859	682	975	3614	415	2660
1860	1495	1587	2927	480	1812
1861	766	971	1764	681	2204
1862	426	1404	1281	997	2799
1863	1646	2212	3413	1745	1649
1864	1741	1102	3411	1740	1993
1865	383	1195	2244	995	2318
1866	200	1038	2706	685	1860
1867	100	1341	2253	610	1728
1868	15	1149	3141	749	2490
1869	64	1670	4680	663	2461
1870	114	834	4356	630	1783
1871	1442	2057	2586	880	1504
1872	2448	925	2101	1045	2850
1873	1126	1450	2227	1203	1598
1874	1246	1103	6321	1163	1690
1875	76	1022	4720	867	2431
1876	39	1241	2364	861	2250
1877	38	1019	1374	956	1571
1878	4	1372	1870	1033	2788
1879	8	769	1592	862	2483
1880	10	1427	2165	838	2641
1881	19	1012	1573	816	1620
1882	3	1289	1583	961	2108
1883	11	1629	1336	747	2968
1884	14	1440	1266	830	2511
1885	39	1426	944	688	2157
1886	24	681	1058	583	1882
1887	17	1598	1179	805	3212
1888	3	1406	732	872	1722
1889	8	1948	701	968	2268
1890	0	2509	739	1018	3039
1891	0	1775	736	830	2437

The age–incidence of Smallpox in various periods of history.

Among the various changes of incidence that have attended
the recent decline of smallpox in England, Ireland and Scotland,
there is one that calls for more extended notice, namely, the fact
that the malady has in great part ceased to be an infection of
infancy and childhood and has become more distinctively an
infection of adolescence and mature age.   In no period of its
history has smallpox been so purely an infantile complaint

as measles[1], nor so purely a malady of childhood and early youth as scarlatina or diphtheria[2]. When it first rose to prominence in England, from the reign of James I. onwards, it attacked adults in a large proportion; of which fact the evidence, although not statistical, is sufficient. But, as the disease became nearly universal and ubiquitous, it was so commonly passed in infancy or childhood, that few grew to maturity without having had it. The number of adult cases diminished in proportion as the disease became more nearly universal. In the great period of smallpox in the 18th century, about nine-tenths of the deaths occurred under the age of five, and nearly all the remaining fraction between five and ten years, at Manchester, Chester, Warrington, Carlisle and Kilmarnock. But in London there were always a good many adult deaths, the reason commonly given being that there was a steady influx to the capital of domestic servants and others from country parishes where the epidemics came at sufficiently long intervals to let many children grow up without incurring the risk of it. Also at Geneva and the Hague, in the 18th century, there were many more deaths above the age of five than in the English provincial towns at the same time.

Ages at Death from Smallpox at Geneva (including Measles) and at the Hague (Duvillard).

	All ages	0–1	–2	–3	–4	–5	–6	–7	–8	–9	–10	–15	–20	–25	–30	–35	–40	–45
Geneva (1700–83)	3328	555	608	588	426	346	232	185	99	67	44	84	36	26	21	0	0	0
The Hague (15 years of 18th cent.)	1455	172	170	179	224	160	148	114	78	58	23	47	17	24	14	10	8	3

Twenty-four per cent. of the smallpox deaths in the 18th century at Geneva were above the age of five years, and at the Hague thirty-seven per cent., while in the former the ratio would probably have been higher but for the inclusion of measles. But, with this comparatively high ratio of deaths above the age of five, smallpox was a much less important cause of mortality at Geneva and the Hague than at Manchester, Glasgow, Chester, and most other provincial cities of this country, making about a fifteenth part of the deaths from all causes in the former, and as high as a sixth part in the latter.

[1] In the first universal and very fatal epidemic of measles, that of 1808, a good many adults, who had not had measles before, were attacked. See the chapter on Measles.

[2] The accounts by Fothergill, Wall and others, of the malignant sore-throat with scarlet rash about 1740 give prominence to cases in early manhood or womanhood.

The infantile character of smallpox was as marked as ever in the epidemic of 1817–19; of which the Norwich statistics are sufficient proof. As late as the epidemic of 1837–40, smallpox was still distinctively a malady of infants and young children in Britain, although that was by no means the case on the continent of Europe at the same time. The following was the age-incidence of fatal smallpox at Liverpool and Bath in the last six months of 1837.

		At all ages	Under 1	1–2	2–3	3–4	4–5	5–6	6–10	Above 10
Liverpool	Deaths	495	143	127	77	64	24	19	20	25
Liverpool	Ratios per cent.	100	28·65	25·45	15·43	17·63		7·81		5·01
Bath	Deaths	151	33	31	33	17	17	6	6	10
Bath	Ratios per cent.	100	21·56	20·26	21·56	22·2		7·84		6·53

In the third year of the epidemic, 1839, the ratio of deaths above the age of five was still less at Manchester, Liverpool and Birmingham, being only four and a half per cent. (26 in a total of 522). At Glasgow, from 1835 to 1839, twelve per cent. of the smallpox deaths were above the age of five (see p. 600). These are the rates of provincial cities; but in a total of 8714 deaths in the year 1839, added together from London and the provinces, about twenty-five per cent. were over five, and of these a moiety were over ten years:

All ages	Under five	Five to ten	Above ten
8714	6453	1122	1139

A good deal of that mortality above the age of five must have come from London, according to the probability of the following table, which is of six years' later date, but the nearest that can be got for London alone:

London, 1845. Ages at Death from Smallpox, Measles and Scarlatina.

	Smallpox	Measles	Scarlatina
Total at all ages	909	2318	1085
Under One year	209	353	88
One to Two	133	832	167
Two to Three	91	511	181
Three to Four	81	272	183
Four to Five	63	153	115
Five to Ten	136	168	254
Ten to Fifteen	33	18	46
Fifteen to Twenty	34	3	14
Twenty to Twenty-five	54	1	8
Twenty-five to Thirty	38	2	6
Above Thirty	37	5	23

The ratio of smallpox deaths above five was 37·5 per cent., of measles deaths 8·4 per cent., and of scarlatina deaths 32·3 per cent. Measles and scarlatina have kept these ratios somewhat uniformly to the present time, but the ratio of smallpox deaths above the age of five has increased according to the following table for England and Wales from 1851 to 1890:

Period	Percentage of smallpox deaths above five years	Percentage of measles deaths above five years	Percentage of scarlatina deaths above five years
1851–60	38	10	36
1861–70	46	8	36
1871–80	70	8	34
1881–90	77	8	36

The progressive raising of the age of fatal smallpox is shown in another way by taking the ratio of the deaths per million living at all ages and at each of eleven age-periods[1]:

Smallpox Deaths per million living at each age-period.

Period	All ages	0–	5–	10–	15–	20–	25–	–35	–45	–55	–65	75 and over
1851-60	221	1034	257	73	93	130	92	53	38	24	18	14
1861-70	163	654	145	56	86	136	102	73	49	36	26	22
1871-80	236	527	284	137	197	300	239	168	111	71	46	35

It was the great epidemic of 1871–72 that brought out the change of age-incidence most concretely, just as it brought out, in contrast to the last great epidemic in 1837–40, the decline in the rural and the increase in the industrial centres. In the three years before the outburst of 1871 the deaths under five and over five were approaching an equality; in the epidemic itself the old ratios were suddenly reversed:

Year	Smallpox deaths under five	Smallpox deaths over five
1868	1234	818
1869	892	673
1870	1245	1375
1871	7770	15356
1872	5758	13336

In the whole generation between 1840 and 1871, in which there was no great and general epidemic of smallpox, many had passed from childhood to adolescence and maturity without encountering the risk of it. When the epidemic of 1871 began, it found many in youth or mature years who had not been through the smallpox, and it attacked a certain proportion of

[1] *Supplement (Decennial) to the 45th Report of the Regr.-Genl.* 1885, p. cxii.

C. II.

40

them accordingly. The proportion above the age of five so attacked in 1871–72 was greater than it had been in this country since the beginning of the 18th century; indeed, as the information is not in statistical form for the earlier period, it may be asserted, and it may happen to be true, that it was greater than it had ever been in this country at any time. The reason for the large proportion of adult cases was the same in the rise of smallpox as in its decline, namely, that in the respective circumstances an epidemic found many who had not been through the disease in infancy or childhood. The same happened in those parts of the world where the epidemics of smallpox came at long intervals, during which many had passed from childhood to youth or mature age without once encountering the risk of smallpox.

Such were the epidemics at Boston, New England, and Charleston, South Carolina, in the 18th century. Not only do the accounts of them speak of the disease as if it were mainly one of the higher ages, but it follows from the ratio of attacks to population, known in the case of Boston, that adolescence and adult age must have had a full share, considering that these age-periods included all who were protected by a previous attack. The years of epidemic smallpox at Boston were 1702, 1721, 1730 and 1752: of these four the two worst were 1721 and 1752, the one epidemic following a clear interval of nineteen years, the other a more or less clear interval of twenty-two years:

Smallpox in Boston, Massachusetts[1].

	Population, whites and blacks	Attacked by smallpox	Died of smallpox	Had smallpox before	Moved out of town
1721	10,565	5989	844	All the rest less 750	—
1752	15,684	5545	569	5598	1843

These enormous mortalities in Boston were comparable to those of the old plague itself in European cities, not only in falling upon all ages but also in doubling or trebling for a single year at long intervals the annual average of deaths:

	Deaths of whites	Deaths of blacks	Total
1701	146	—	146
*1702	441	—	441
1720	261	68	329
*1721	968	134	1102
1722	240	33	273
*1730	740	160	909
1731	318	90	408
*1752	893	116	1009

* Smallpox years.

[1] The figures for 1721 are cited above (p. 485) from Douglass and others. Those for 1752 are given in the *Gent. Magaz.* 1753, Sept., p. 413, as "collected from the Accounts of the Overseers in the Twelve several Wards," and sent by the Rev. T. Prince.

Just as smallpox in its first great outbursts in the London of the Stuarts, or in its rare outbreaks in the American colonies in the 18th century, fell impartially upon children and adults, so in its last outbursts in the London of Victoria it fell upon persons at all ages. The notable thing is, not that smallpox should have of late been attacking adults, for that it has ever done except in times and places in which there were few or no adults who had not been through the disease in childhood ; but that it should have ceased to so large an extent to attack infants and children. It has ceased to attack infants and children because other infective and non-infective diseases more appropriate to the modern conditions of the population are attacking them instead. These are measles and whooping-cough, scarlatina and diphtheria, infantile diarrhoea, and the more chronic after-effects of these. The annual death-rate from all diseases under the age of five has fluctuated somewhat per million living from 1837 to the present time, but it can hardly be said that it has fallen much or steadily[1].

Keeping still to the epidemic of 1871–72, let us consider whether there was any natural or epidemiological reason for its cutting off a smaller ratio of infants and children in its whole mortality than that of 1837–40 did. There had been a most disastrous epidemic of scarlatina for three years just before, which had caused 21,912 deaths in 1868, 27,641 in 1869, and 32,543 in 1870, a total of 82,096 in three years, about two-thirds of which were under the age of five, or at the age-period which smallpox used to be fatal to almost exclusively and to be the greatest single epidemic scourge of. Even in the two smallpox years themselves the scarlatinal deaths were 18,567 and 11,922, of which the share that fell to children under five was one and a half times the deaths in that age-period from the co-existing smallpox. The three years of excessive scarlatina, before the epidemic of smallpox began, had removed large numbers of the class of infants and children who succumb to any infectious disease ; if we cannot give the whole *rationale* of one infection dispossessing or anticipating another, we can at least understand that the earlier and more dominant infection takes off the likely subjects. What scarlatina did egregiously during the three years just

---

[1] *Supplementary Report of the Registrar-General*, 1883. The mean death rate per 1000 living, for the period 1838–82, has been 71·0 males, and 61·2 females under five years of age; but as late as 1878 the annual average was the mean of the period, namely 71·2 males and 61·1 females.

before the great explosion of smallpox, it had been doing
steadily (along with measles, &c.) throughout a whole generation
since the last great sacrifice of infants and children by smallpox
in 1837–40. But the fact that scarlatina had in great part
dispossessed smallpox among the factors of mortality under the
age of five, did not prevent the latter infection from attacking
those of the higher ages who were susceptible of it and were at
the same time unvexed by any other great epidemic malady
proper to their time of life. If the epidemic of smallpox in
1871–72 had cut off as large a ratio under the age of five years
as its immediate predecessor in 1837–40 did, its whole mortality
would have been about 70,000 more than it actually was. But
in no state of the population or of the public health can we
suppose that three years of excessive mortality of children by
one kind of contagion would be followed immediately by two
years of equally special mortality at the same ages by contagion
of another kind. It is not only epidemiological science that
tells us this, but also common sense—*est modus in rebus.*

The saving of life by checking the prevalence of smallpox
was a favourite rhetorical topic in the 18th century. Voltaire,
La Condamine, Bernoulli, Watson, Haygarth and others, were
fond of estimating how many thousands of lives might be saved
in a year if inoculation were thoroughly carried out. Dr
Lettsom, Sir Thomas Bernard and Mr James Neild, who were
interested in prison reforms and in whatever else would reduce
the prevalence of typhus, reckoned the possible saving of life
under that head as almost equal to the possible saving from
smallpox[1]. For typhus there was no artificial means of
restraint; it had to decline before natural causes, if it declined
at all,—which, indeed, it has done. But no one at that time
thought of keeping down smallpox except by the inoculation of
itself or of cowpox. The economists and statisticians treated
each of these artifices in its turn as a factor having a certain

---

[1] Lettsom (*Gent. Magaz.* 1804, Aug. p. 701), in a preface to Neild's papers on
the state of the prisons, estimated that 40,000 lives might be saved every year in
England by preventing infectious fevers, "for in this metropolis my respectable friend
Thomas Bernard, Esq., whose caution and accuracy no person will doubt, calculates
the number of victims at 3000 each year [doubtless from the London Bills of
Mortality]....If to this pleasing view we add the preservation of 48,000 victims to the
smallpox, which may now be preferred by the cowpox, we have in our power to
possess the sublime contemplation of forming a saving fund of human life of nearly
88,000 persons annually in this empire, by the exercise of reason, philanthropy and
judicious policy."

absolute value, which they might use like the *a* and *b* of a problem in algebra. This they did, of course, in deference to medical authority. What Bernoulli had worked out for the old inoculation, Duvillard did for the new, in his "Tables showing the Influence of Smallpox on the Mortality of each period of Life, and the Influence that such a preservative as Vaccine may have on the Population and on Longevity[1]." Malthus fell into the conventional way of thinking when he assumed that smallpox alone among the epidemic checks of population was to be controlled artificially; but he introduced an important new consideration. "For my own part," he wrote in 1803, "I feel not the slightest doubt, that if the introduction of the cowpox should extirpate the smallpox, and yet the number of marriages continue the same, we shall find a very perceptible difference in the increased mortality of some other diseases[2]."

Five years after this was written, there came, in 1808, the disastrous epidemic of measles, which in Glasgow killed more infants in a few months than smallpox had ever done at its worst in the same city. In the winter of 1811–12 there was another severe epidemic of measles in Glasgow; and in 1813, Dr Watt, a leading physician of the place, and a man now famous in all countries for his vast labours as a bibliographer, gave to the world his statistical proof, from the Glasgow burial registers, of that law of substitution which Malthus had found necessary in his deduced principles.

"The first thing," said Watt, "that strikes the mind in surveying the preceding Table (1783–1812), is the vast diminution in the proportion of deaths by the smallpox, a reduction from 19·55 to 3·90. But the increase in the subsequent column [measles] is still more remarkable, an increase from 0·95 to 10·76. In the smallpox we have the deaths reduced to nearly a fifth of what they were twenty-five years ago [in ratio of the deaths from all causes]; in the same period the deaths by measles have increased more than eleven times. This is a fact so striking that I am astonished it has not attracted the notice of older practitioners, who have had it in their power to compare the mortality by measles in former periods with what all of them must have experienced during the last five years[3]."

The high ratio of measles and the low ratio of smallpox did not remain as Watt's researches left them. When Cowan resumed the tabulation of figures from 1835 to 1839 he found the ratios of those two infantile infections almost equal, and the

---

[1] Duvillard, *Tableaux etc.* Paris, 1806.
[2] *Essay on the Principle of Population.* Bk. IV. chap. 5.
[3] Robert Watt, M.D. *Treatise on Chincough, with Inquiry into the Relative Mortality of the Diseases of Children in Glasgow.* Glasgow, 1813.

two together contributing to the whole mortality of Glasgow only a little more than half their joint share in the end of the 18th century. The substitution which Watt saw during a few years was only the most dramatic part of a general movement forwards of measles among the causes of infantile mortality. He supposed, as everyone did at that time, that smallpox was forcibly repressed, and that another infectious disease had seized the opportunity to become exuberant. The most relevant thing in the whole situation was urged by those who thought, with Jenner, that the doctrine of substitution had an " evil tendency " as detracting from the absolute value of the inoculation principle. In order to discredit Dr Watt altogether, they pointed out that his ratios of smallpox and measles took no account of the diminished death-rate of Glasgow by all diseases in the earlier years of the 19th century.

Great changes were proceeding in the old city, the Glasgow of ' Rob Roy.' The population which was reckoned at 45,889 in the year 1785, had increased to 66,578 in the year 1791, and thereafter, at a slower rate, to 83,769 in 1801 and to 100,749 in 1811. The first great increase after the American War meant overcrowding; but in a short time new suburbs spread over such an extent that, in the year 1798, more than half the burials were in the graveyards attached to chapels-of-ease and meeting-houses outside the original parishes. The modern expansion of Glasgow, like that of London and of all other large cities, has been an increase of area still more than an increase of numbers. The public health improved steadily, at all events until 1817, the improvement being shown first in the increasing number of infants that survived their second year. That rise in the probability of life corresponded to the substitution of measles for smallpox, and in part depended upon the ascendancy of the milder infection. Still more remarkable was the rise of scarlatina, which Dr Watt did not live to see; so little was made of it at the date of his writing that he found " scarlatina, typhus, &c., all comprehended under the same head." The seeds of measles and scarlatina had long existed beside the seeds of smallpox, but the ascendancy of each of the two former had to wait events. Said Banquo to the witches who hailed Macbeth as king and himself as the sire of later kings :

> " If you can look into the seeds of time,
> And say which grain will grow, and which will not—"

The succession of reigning infections is the same problem. All we can say is that each new predominant type is somehow suited to the changed conditions. In the long period covered by this history we have seen much coming and going among the epidemic infections, in some cases a dramatic and abrupt entrance or exit, in other cases a gradual and unperceived substitution. Some of the greatest of those changes have fallen within the two hundred years since Sydenham kept notes of the prevalent epidemics of London. We are that posterity, or a generation of it, which he expected would have its own proper experiences of epidemics and at the same time would know all that had passed meanwhile—"posteris quibus integrum epidemicorum curriculum venientibus annis sibi invicem succedentium intueri dabitur."

CHAPTER V.

MEASLES.

IN the earliest English writings on medicine, measles is the inseparable companion of smallpox; so closely are they joined in pathology and treatment that even the statements as to the pustules and scars of the eruption are in some compends made to apply to both without distinction. This singular conjunction of two diseases came originally from the Arabian teaching, which was everywhere authoritative in the medieval period, and especially authoritative in all that related to smallpox. In the Latin compends based upon Avicenna or other Arabic writers, the two names were *variolae* and *morbilli*, the former being as it were the *morbus* proper and the latter its diminutive. It can hardly be doubted that we owe the English name of measles as the equivalent of *morbilli* to John of Gaddesden. Originally the English word meant the leprous, first in the Latin form *miselli* and *misellae* (diminutive of *miser*), as in the histories of Matthew Paris, and later in the Norman-French form of *mesles*, as in the Acts of Parliament of Edward I. and in the 'Vision of Piers the Ploughman.' In the 15th century the leper-houses in the suburbs of London were called the "lazarcotes" or "meselcotes."

Gaddesden, by some unaccountable stretch of similarity, coupled the sores or tubercular nodules on the legs of "pauperes vel consumptivi," who were called "*anglicé* mesles," with the spotted rash of the Arabian "morbilli"; and it was doubtless this haphazard bracketting of two unlike diseases that led in course of time to the name of mesles being disjoined from its original sense of the leprous and restricted to the second member of Gaddesden's strangely assorted couple. In the time of Henry VIII. smallpox and mezils are familiarly named together just as *variolae et morbilli* are an inseparable pair in the treatises of the Arabistic writers. A still more singular usurpation by " mezils " or " maysilles " or " measles " is met with in the Elizabethan period. In the vocabulary of Levins, a schoolmaster who was also a medical graduate of Oxford, the word *variolae* is rendered by " ye maysilles," while *morbilli* is omitted altogether among the Latin names and smallpox among the English ; and in the English translation of Latin aphorisms appended to one of the works of William Clowes, surgeon to St Bartholomew's Hospital, *variolae* is in like manner translated " measles " on every occasion. In the English dictionary by Baret, belonging to the same period, measles is defined as " a disease with many reddish spottes or speckles in the face and bodie, much like freckles in colour "—which seems to exclude the possibility of a pustular disease having been part of the Elizabethan notion of measles.

Notwithstanding this singular usage of the vocabularies and dictionaries, the name of smallpox occurs by itself in letters or other memorials of the Elizabethan period, having been doubtless correctly applied to the true pustular *variola*. In the short essay on smallpox by Kellwaye, appended to his book on the plague (1593), measles and smallpox are distinguished on the whole clearly, according to the definitions of Fracastori or other foreign writers of the 16th century. The association between measles and smallpox that survived longest was a peculiar and somewhat uncommon one ; certain cases of smallpox, in which the pustules were wholly or partially represented by, or changed into, broad spots level with the skin, red or livid in colour, and in which haemorrhages occurred from the nose, lungs, bowels or kidneys, that is to say, cases of haemorrhagic smallpox, were apt to be called, from the time of James I. until as late as the case of Queen Mary in 1694, by the name of " smallpox and measles mingled."

From the date of the annual bills of mortality by the Parish Clerks of London, the year 1629, it is improbable that there was any real confusion between smallpox and measles ; there was certainly some ambiguity in the entry of measles long after, but that later confusion, especially in the second half of the 18th century, was with scarlatina[1]. The entry of measles is in

[1] John Graunt, *Natural and Political Observations upon the Bills of Mortality*, London, 1662, says : " The original entries in the Hall books were as exact in the

the bills from the first, apart from that of "flox and small-pox:"

Year	Measles deaths	Smallpox deaths	Year	Measles deaths	Smallpox deaths
1629	42	72	1650	33	184
1630	2	40	1651	33	525
1631	3	58	1652	62	1279
1632	80	531	1653	8	139
1633	21	72	1654	52	832
1634	33	1354	1655	11	1294
1635	27	293	1656	153	823
1636	12	127	1657	15	835
1647	5	139	1658	80	409
1648	92	401	1659	6	1523
1649	3	1190	1660	74	354

In the great epidemic of smallpox in 1628, the year before the bills begin, Thomas Alured wrote to Sir John Coke that his house in London had been visited "once with the measles and twice with the smallpox, though I thank God we are now free; and I know not how many households have run the same hazard[1]." In the year 1656, which has the highest total in the above table, two cases of measles are mentioned in a letter of 31st May: "Young Sir Charles Sedley is at this time very sick of a feaver and the meazells, of which Sir William dyed"— Charles Sedley being then in his seventeenth year[2]. An instance parallel to that of 1628, of measles and smallpox co-existing in the same household, occurred in the royal palace at Whitehall in December, 1660. The princess of Orange, sister of the king, died of smallpox on the 23rd; on that day, or a day or two before, her sister the princess Henrietta, who had come from France on a visit with the queen-mother, Henrietta Maria, removed from Whitehall to St James's, "for fear of infection." After a few days she embarked on board the 'London' at Portsmouth to return to France, but the ship had to come to anchor again owing to the princess being attacked with "the measles." Her illness, which delayed the sailing of the vessel until the 24th of January, 1661, is uniformly spoken of as the measles in the various letters which make mention of

very first year [he probably means 1629, which is the first year of his own extracts from them, but the classification of deaths began in 1604] as to all particulars, as now; and the specifying of casualties and diseases was probably more." The searchers, he explains, were in many cases able to report the opinions of the physicians, receiving the same from the friends of the deceased; while for certain causes of death, among which he includes smallpox, "their own senses are sufficient."

[1] *Cal. Coke MSS.* (Hist. MSS. Commis.) I. 21 June, 1628.
[2] Sutherland Letters, in *Rep. Hist. MSS. Com.* v. 152.

it[1]. In that year, and in several of the next ten years, the measles deaths in London reached a considerable total:

Year	Measles deaths		Year	Measles deaths
1661	188		1666	3
1662	20		1667	83
1663	42		1668	200
1664	311		1669	15
1665	7		1670	295

The epidemic of 1670 is the subject of a description by Sydenham, the diagnostic points of which were doubtless those current at the time.

Sydenham's description of Measles in London, 1670 and 1674.

Sydenham's account of the epidemic of 1670 is full enough to leave no doubt that it was measles of the ordinary kind; the details, indeed, are as minute for all essential points as they would be in a modern text-book[2]:

Measles, he says, is a disease mainly of young children (*infantes*), and is apt to run through all that are under one roof. It begins with a rigor, followed by heats and chills during the first day. On the second day there is fever, with intense malaise, thirst, loss of appetite, white tongue (not actually dry), slight cough, heaviness of the head and eyes, and constant drowsiness. In most cases a humour distils from the nose and eyes, the effusion or suffusion of tears being the most certain sign of sickening for measles, more certain indeed than the exanthem. The child sneezes as if it had taken cold, the eyelids swell, there may be vomiting, more usually there are loose green stools (especially during dentition), and there is excessive fretfulness. On the fourth or fifth day small red maculae, like fleabites, begin to appear on the forehead and the rest of the face, which coalesce, as they continue to come out in increasing numbers, so as to form racemose clusters. These maculae will be found by the touch to be slightly elevated, although they seem level to the eye. On the trunk and limbs, to which they gradually extend, they are not elevated. About the sixth day the maculae begin to roughen and scale, from the face downwards, and by the eighth day are scarcely discernible anywhere. On the ninth day the whole body is as if dusted with bran. The common people say that the spots had "turned inwards," by which they mean that, if it had been smallpox, they would have remained out longer, and have proceeded to suppuration or maturation. The rash having thus "gone in," there is an access of fever, attended with laboured breathing and cough, the latter being so incessant as to keep the children from sleep day or night. If they had been treated by the heating regimen, they are apt to have the chest troubles

[1] *Cal. State Papers, Domestic. Charles II.* s. d. It appears from the *Pyretologia* by Drage, of Hitchin (1665), that the natural history of measles must have been familiar, for he mentions that its incubation period was from fourteen to fifteen days: p. 20.
[2] *Obs. Med.* 3rd ed. (1675), Bk. IV. chap. 5.

pass into peripneumonia, by which complication measles becomes more destructive than smallpox itself, although there is no danger in it if it be rightly treated. When peripneumonia threatens, the patient should be bled, even if it be a tender infant. Diarrhoea, which sometimes continues for weeks after an attack of measles, may be cut short by blood-letting, and so also may whooping-cough.

This epidemic, says Sydenham, began in January, and was almost ended in July, which agrees exactly with the rise and decline of measles deaths in the weekly bills of the Parish Clerks.

His account of the epidemic of 1674 is still more important to be set beside the figures in the bills ; for the type, according to Sydenham, was anomalous, and the total of deaths entered by the Parish Clerks (795) is exceptionally large. Like the epidemic four years before, it began in January, came to a height about the vernal equinox, and was nearly over at the summer solstice[1].

Weekly Deaths in London in the first six months of 1674.
(*Epidemic of Measles.*)

1674

Week ending	Fever	Smallpox	Griping in the guts	Measles	Convulsions	Teeth	Consumption	All causes
Jan. 6	35	13	35	0	37	15	78	332
13	35	19	32	1	32	22	65	369
20	37	12	29	0	39	18	65	327
27	34	15	38	0	38	17	68	354
Feb. 3	32	23	39	7	45	26	75	418
10	47	18	35	4	48	35	86	430
17	55	21	46	15	70	38	98	537
24	62	17	45	28	54	44	97	510
March 3	58	31	28	59	48	49	87	547
10	55	22	31	87	85	58	122	688
17	63	15	46	95	79	57	113	695
24	59	23	44	65	57	39	96	568
31	51	19	49	60	77	51	105	622
April 7	44	13	40	43	65	48	118	547
14	53	20	32	31	60	50	98	535
21	40	17	43	38	55	42	106	517
28	50	17	44	53	67	34	87	520
May 5	51	31	28	30	56	24	75	452
12	38	26	47	30	54	37	79	479
19	50	35	33	26	47	28	82	461
26	67	27	33	13	45	28	63	415
June 2	48	24	28	14	41	26	77	365
9	35	26	38	15	48	27	66	369
16	64	34	38	19	38	22	70	419
23	34	33	34	9	52	15	71	368
30	37	39	30	9	30	21	59	343

[1] Sydenham, *Obs. Med.* 1675, v. 3. "Morbilli anni 1674." It entered almost every household, as on the last occasion, attacking infants more especially. It had

It will be seen that the highest weekly mortality from measles is only 95, in the week ending 17th May. But in that week the deaths from all causes reached the enormous total of 695, which was nearly three hundred above the weekly average of the time. This appears to have been the epidemic of measles which Morton declares to have destroyed three hundred in a week, a mode of reckoning which would claim for measles, directly or indirectly, the excess of mortality from all causes during the height of the epidemic[1].

These high weekly mortalities in February, March, April and May are remarkable for the season of the year. Usually when the weekly figures reach six or seven hundred, it is in a hot autumn, and the cause is infantile diarrhoea, represented in the bills by the excessive number of deaths from "griping in the guts" and "convulsions;" more rarely, and then only for three or four weeks, correspondingly high figures are reached in a season of influenza. But in this case the epidemic measles is the only relevant thing. The measles deaths by themselves do by no means account for the enormous weekly totals; but two of the three columns of figures which help them, and indeed keep pace with the rise of the measles deaths, namely, "convulsions" and "teeth," are infantile deaths obviously related to the prevailing epidemic; while the third column, "consumption," which contributes most of all, did not in the London

some points of difference from the measles of 1670. The rash was less uniformly on the fourth day, now sooner, now later; it would come on the arms or trunk before the face; nor was it followed by the branny powdering which was as obvious in the measles of 1670 as it was usual to see it after scarlatina. Along with these anomalies of the rash, the consecutive fever and peripneumonia were also more severe, and a more frequent cause of death. But in the principal characters of measles the disease of 1674 was the same as that of 1670, and called for no fresh description. Among Sydenham's patients were the children of the Countess of Salisbury, who all took measles in turn, and all passed through the attack and its sequelae without danger, under a particular regimen which is detailed. It is of great interest to see how this season of anomalous measles looks in the weekly bills, as in the above table.

[1] Richard Morton, M.D. *Pyretologia.* 2 vols. Lond. 1692–94, I. 427. He places it in the year 1672 and in the six months of autumn and winter; and in another place (II. 71), where he cites clinical cases, he again gives the year 1672 as that in which measles "epidemice Londini publice grassabantur." He compares the epidemic to a *pestis mitior*, and says that the disease had never been epidemic again to the date of his writing (1692–94). It is tolerably clear that, in writing twenty years after, he had forgotten the year and even the season—not the only error in dates in his work. Sydenham's account of the great measles epidemic of spring and summer, 1674, was published the year after, and is exactly borne out by the weekly bills of mortality. Morton's obvious mistake of the date is the subject of a refutation four pages long by Thomas Dickson, M.D., F.R.S., physician to the London Hospital, in *Med. Obs. and Inquiries*, IV. (1771), p. 266.

bills mean pulmonary consumption exclusively, but also the wasting or marasmus which followed or attended acute fevers in general, and was specially apt to follow or attend measles[1].

Sydenham gives no indication that the spring of 1674 was unusually productive of pneumonia or pleurisy among adults; the winter, he says, was unusually warm, the weather in spring turning colder. But, as to the measles, he does say that the epidemic was anomalous or irregular; while both he and Morton refer the fatalities more especially to the sequelae of measles,—to the "suffocation" of infants and children by the bronchitis or peripneumonia, or to "angina," as Morton says, meaning perhaps the same as in Scotland was understood by "closing" in infants. Measles itself was a milder disease than smallpox, according to the experience of all times; and yet, by its sequelae (bronchitis, capillary bronchitis and pneumonia, including what Morton calls "angina," and excluding, for the present, whooping-cough), it raised the weekly mortalities of February, March, April and May, 1674, to far above the average. Sydenham said, with reference to the much milder epidemic of 1670, that these after-effects of measles "destroyed more than even smallpox itself" (*quae [peripneumonia] plures jugulat quam aut variolae ipsae*). We shall not correctly understand the part played by measles among the infective maladies of children unless we keep that grand character of it in mind—that its effects upon the mortality of infancy and childhood are only in part expressed by the deaths actually appearing under its name.

The London bills for 1674 afford us the opportunity of testing Sydenham's paradox that measles, by its after-effects, destroyed more than smallpox itself. The epidemic of measles was nearly over in June; and immediately thereafter an epidemic of smallpox began (not of course from zero but from the usual level of the disease), which reached a maximum of 122

[1] Fothergill (*Gentleman's Magazine*, Dec. 1751) says, in a criticism of the Bills of Mortality: "If the body is emaciated, which may happen even from an acute fever, 'tis enough for them to place it to the article of consumption." And of course they would do so the more readily if the acute fever, say measles, were past, and its sequelae had been the cause of death. Referring to Kidderminster in 1756, Johnstone says: "Measles at this time went through our town and neighbourhood: vast numbers of children died tabid." It is to be remarked that the fever column is augmented but little during the measles of 1674, a fact which shows that the inflammatory causes of death, such as capillary bronchitis and pneumonia (specially recorded by Sydenham for this epidemic), were more apt to be entered under "consumption" than under "fevers."

deaths in the week ending 20th October. The second half of the year was thus marked by a sharp outburst of smallpox, as the first half was marked by a sharp outburst of measles; and those two diseases were the only epidemic maladies that gave character to the respective seasons, each being in its proper season, according to Sydenham—measles in the spring, smallpox in the autumn. Although the measles deaths were only 795 for the whole year, the smallpox deaths being 2507, yet the former epidemic was attended by so great an excess of deaths under various other heads that the half of the year in which it fell was far more unhealthy than the succeeding half in which the smallpox mainly fell, the weekly average of the first six months having been 468 deaths, and of the second six months 349 deaths. The following table shows the weekly mortalities for the second half of the year; it will be observed that no column of figures keeps pace with the rise of the smallpox deaths, as three columns had kept pace with the rise of the measles deaths in the first six months of the year.

Weekly Deaths in London in the last six months of 1674.
(Epidemic of Smallpox.)

1674

Week ending		Fever	Smallpox	Griping in the guts	Measles	Convulsions	Teeth	Consumption	All causes
July	7	31	44	35	9	44	24	69	351
	14	38	55	34	5	37	17	54	353
	21	40	71	47	6	42	25	56	395
	28	43	71	37	3	49	18	48	367
Aug.	4	38	68	39	6	31	23	47	347
	11	33	66	48	–	18	8	45	324
	18	49	86	41	1	26	20	48	374
	25	35	85	23	3	32	10	46	328
Sept.	1	60	96	41	–	32	18	57	414
	8	32	99	48	3	22	16	32	374
	15	28	102	38	2	30	19	55	362
	22	27	72	32	3	29	11	57	327
	29	39	81	34	2	41	9	53	358
Oct.	6	37	98	29	–	34	10	63	391
	13	36	75	25	–	35	17	49	311
	20	42	122	35	1	34	10	68	402
	27	24	75	36	–	38	15	45	294
Nov.	3	34	83	21	–	30	11	41	322
	10	30	81	15	–	31	12	49	321
	17	31	70	16	–	24	10	58	304
	24	35	70	28	–	38	14	57	344
Dec.	1	33	85	29	–	32	14	68	378
	8	33	66	28	–	36	11	53	327
	15	29	61	26	–	39	16	49	339
	22	34	68	21	–	32	11	52	335
	29	41	41	19	–	33	7	74	337

The total of deaths by smallpox for the year, 2507 was the highest since the bills began, and remained the highest until 1681. It is open to us to suppose that it would not have been so high but for the epidemic of measles preceding. The measles not only made the first half of the year far more deadly than the second, within which most of the smallpox fell, but its effects may have aided the high mortality of smallpox itself, according to the experience of later times that infants and young children recovering from measles in a greatly weakened condition fell an easier prey to smallpox coming after[1].

Morton passes from the fatal epidemic of 1674 (or, as he says, 1672), with the remark that the malady had not been epidemic again in London from that time until the date of his writing, 1692–94, a period of nearly twenty years; and that is on the whole borne out by the London bills and by Syden-ham's records so far as they extend. From 1687 to 1700, inclusive, the London bills grouped the measles deaths along with the deaths from smallpox, under the heading, "Flox, Smallpox and Measles"; in 1701 the total of measles, 4 deaths, is given as a separate item in the same bracket with smallpox; and in 1702 the heading of "Measles," is restored to the place in the alphabetical list which it had held, except for that un-accountable break, from the beginning of the published bills in 1629. The following are the annual totals from and including the great epidemic of 1674:

Year	Death from measles		Year	Death from measles
1674	795		1681	121
1675	1		1682	50
1676	83		1683	39
1677	87		1684	6
1678	93		1685	197
1679	117		1686	25
1680	49			

Thus for a good many years after the general prevalence of measles in 1674 the deaths from it in London averaged only about one and a half in the week, while in no year until 1705–6 is there an epidemic comparable to that of 1674. It is clear that the severe epidemics of measles came at first at very long intervals, and that the years between had a very moderate mortality from that disease.

[1] See Watson's account of smallpox following measles at the Foundling Hospital, *supra,* p. 550.

Measles in the 18th century.

There is hardly a reference to be found to measles in medical or other writings until the annual accounts of the public health at Ripon, York, Plymouth, etc. in the third decade of the 18th century. The annual deaths from it in London, according to the bills, were as follows, from 1701, when the disease was restored to its separate place in the classification:

Year	Measles deaths	Year	Measles deaths	Year	Measles deaths
1701	4	1715	30	1728	82
1702	27	1716	270	1729	41
1703	51	1717	35	1730	311
1704	12	1718	492	1731	102
1705	319	1719	243	1732	30
1706	361	1720	213	1733	605
1707	37	1721	238	1734	20
1708	126	1722	114	1735	10
1709	89	1723	231	1736	169
1710	181	1724	118	1737	127
1711	97	1725	70	1738	216
1712	77	1726	256	1739	326
1713	61	1727	72	1740	46
1714	139				

The high mortalities of 1705 and 1706 belonged to one continuous epidemic from October, 1705, to April, 1706 (Sir David Hamilton says that smallpox was common in London in July, 1705, but the deaths in the bills are not excessive). The epidemic followed a great prevalence of the autumnal diarrhoea of infants, so that it is probable the high mortality was due as much to a greater fatality of cases from the antecedent weakening, as to an unusual number of cases[1]. The following were the weekly deaths in a population about one-sixth that of London now:

1705—1706

Week ending	Measles deaths	Week ending	Measles deaths
Oct. 16	9	Jan. 15	28
23	9	22	20
30	12	29	18
Nov. 6	10	Feb. 5	27
13	30	12	11
20	34	19	26
27	29	26	28
Dec. 4	37	Mar. 5	10
11	46	12	10
18	44	19	9
25	22	26	13
Jan. 1	35	Apr. 2	9
8	33	9	9

[1] It may have been this high mortality that Dover had in mind when he wrote, in

The unusually large mortalities from measles in 1718–19 and in 1733 were again associated with a "constitution" otherwise sickly. The epidemic in the latter year, from the middle of March to the end of July, which had a maximum of 47 deaths in each of the two middle weeks of May, followed close upon a severe influenza. Like the epidemic of 1674, it was attended by a high mortality from other causes, especially "convulsions" and "consumption"; and, as the bills had now begun to give the ages at death, it is no longer doubtful, or merely conjectural, that the great excess of deaths under these and other heads was really among infants, or that a rise in "consumption" at that time of the year meant an increase in the wasting diseases of infancy. This was a period when any epidemic malady among London children was sure to go hard with many of them, the period, namely, when spirit drinking, besides ruining the health of the parents, rendered them, in the opinion of the College of Physicians, "too often the cause of weak, feeble and distémpered children[1]."

The intervals between epidemics of measles in London having been so considerable as the table shows, it is not surprising to find but casual mention of the disease in the chronicles of Wintringham, Hillary, and Huxham for England, of Rogers, O'Connell and Rutty for Ireland, and of the Edinburgh annalists. Wintringham, of York, whose annals extend from 1715 to 1730, records an epidemic of measles in 1721, which began in April and lasted all the summer, being for the most part of a bad type, attended with continual cough and inflammation of the lungs. Hillary, of Ripon, enters measles in 1726, "very common but mild," autumn and winter being the season of it. Wintringham briefly mentions the same epidemic. Huxham of Plymouth has an entry of measles in the first year of his annals, 1727, in the month of July, followed by whooping-cough in December. Wintringham again enters measles at York in 1730 in the company of smallpox. In the annual accounts of the disease at Edinburgh, for a series of years beginning with 1731, measles is first mentioned in 1735[2]. The epidemic

1733: "I do not remember I ever heard of anyone's dying of this disease [measles] till about twenty-five years since; but of late, by the help of Gascoin's powder and bezoartic bolusses, together with blisters and a hot regimen, the blood is so highly inflamed and the fever encreased to that degree that it is become equally mortal with the smallpox." *Physician's Legacy*, 1733, p. 116.

[1] Memorial to the House of Commons, *supra*, p. 84.

[2] *Edin. Med. Essays and Obs.* v. 26.

began in June and became universal in December: "The progress of these measles along the west road of England towards Edinburgh was very remarkable, for they could be traced from village to village; and it was singular that the first person in Edinburgh who was seized with them was a lady in childbed, who saw nobody but her nurse and a friend who lived in the house with her"—an argument, apparently, for the doctrine of an epidemic "morbillous" constitution of the air. Five years after, we obtain the mortality statistics of Edinburgh, in the two great years of scarcity, typhus fever and sicknesses of all kinds, the years 1740 and 1741: in those two years measles must have been as general as smallpox if it were half as mortal, for the deaths set down to it in each year are 110 and 112, as compared with 274 and 206 from the more usual infantile infection. In like manner the second year of the disastrous epidemic of typhus in 1741–42, had the highest total of measles deaths in London until the great epidemic of 1808. While the high mortality of that year was due to special causes, it is at the same time clear from the following table that measles had not yet become a steady or perennial cause of death to the infancy of the capital:

Year	Measles deaths	Year	Measles deaths	Year	Measles deaths
1741	42	1761	394	1781	201
1742	981	1762	122	1782	170
1743	17	1763	610	1783	185
1744	5	1764	65	1784	29
1745	14	1765	54	1785	20
1746	250	1766	482	1786	793*
1747	81	1767	80	1787	84
1748	10	1768	409	1788	55
1749	106	1769	90	1789	534
1750	321	1770	325	1790	119
1751	21	1771	115	1791	156
1752	111	1772	211	1792	450
1753	253	1773	199	1793	248
1754	12	1774	121	1794	172
1755	423	1775	283	1795	328
1756	156	1776	153	1796	307
1757	24	1777	145	1797	222
1758	696	1778	388	1798	196
1759	316	1779	99	1799	223
1760	175	1780	272	1800	395

* Pronounced by Sims to have been wholly scarlatina, and by Willan to have been in part that disease.

The considerable epidemic of 1755 is thus referred to by Fothergill in his monthly notes:

41—2

May: the measles more common than for some years, adults, who had not before had it, rarely escaping. *June:* measles common, smallpox rare. *September and October:* no epidemic disease but measles; few perished in proportion to all who took it[1]. The epidemic of 1758 was more fatal, but Fothergill's notes are not continued to that year. The elder Heberden says that measles was remarkably epidemical (in London) in 1753, which year has only 253 deaths in the bills, whereas the year 1755 has 423 deaths and the year 1758 has 696; but, as he implies that the type was mild, there would have been a multitude of cases to produce that number of deaths. It was a peculiarity of that epidemic, he says, that the cough preceded the outbreak of measles by seven or eight days, whereas it was usually but two or three days in advance of the eruption[2].

At that period there would have been an epidemic of measles in London every other year, or once in three years, with a fatality from the direct effects seldom more than a sixth part that of an epidemic of smallpox. A London writer some twenty years after said that few escaped measles in infancy or childhood, while the deaths put down to it were only a tenth part of those due to smallpox on an average of years[3]. The proportion of measles deaths to smallpox deaths was nearly the same in Manchester for twenty years from 1754 to 1774, according to Percival's table of the burials in the register of the Collegiate Church where most of the poorer class were buried[4]:

Annual averages of Burials from Measles etc. at the Collegiate Church, Manchester.

Period	Measles	Smallpox	All deaths under two	Deaths at all ages	Baptisms
1754–58	21	64	209	651	678
1759–63*	10·6	95	213	639	731
1764–69	9·6	98	229	659	827
1770–74	21·6	102	242	651	1062

* Omitting the year 1760.

The ages of those who died of measles "in six years from 1768 to 1774," to the number of 91, were as follows:

Total	3 mo.	-6 mo.	-12 mo.	-2 years	-3	-4	-5	-10	-20	-30
91	2	3	10	31	25	7	9	2	1	1

Fifty were males, forty-one females—a preponderance of males which is according to rule. Of the whole ninety-one, no fewer than fifty-one died in June of the several years.

[1] Monthly reports in the *Gentleman's Magazine*, under the dates.
[2] Heberden's paper on measles in *Trans. Col. Phys.* III. (1785), pp. 389, 395.
[3] W. Black, M.D., *Obs. Med. and Political on the Smallpox, &c.* London, 1781, p. 207: "Few escape measles in infancy or childhood, and as we find one-tenth fewer to die of measles than of smallpox, etc.... In their future consequences, measles, especially in cities, are not without hazard, and are not unfrequently followed by hecticks."
[4] Percival, in *Med. Obs. and Inquiries*, v. (1776), p. 282.

In the smaller and more healthy towns, such as Northampton, the epidemics of measles came at long intervals and caused but few deaths :

Infantile Causes of Death, All Saints, Northampton[1].

Year	Measles	Whooping-cough	Convulsions	Teething
1742	3	1	10	8
1743	–	–	21	2
1744	–	3	14	4
1745	–	–	22	7
1746	–	3	19	3
1747	7	–	29	–
1748	–	–	24	4
1749	–	6	15	4
1750	1	–	17	1
1751	–	–	14	6
1752	–	1	13	6
1753} 1754}	not published			
1755	–	1	8	1
1756	–	2	10	2
1757	1	1	28	4

In the parish of Holy Cross, a suburb of Shrewsbury, there were 4 deaths from measles in the ten years 1750-60, and 15 in the ten years 1760-70, the smallpox deaths having been respectively 33 and 46. Ackworth, in Yorkshire, may represent the country parishes. It had no deaths from measles from 1747 to 1757, two deaths from 1757 to 1767. At Kilmarnock during thirty-six years from 1728 to 1764, there were 93 deaths from measles, 52 of them in the period 1747-52, and only 11 in the next twelve years. Sims, of Tyrone, having described an epidemic of smallpox which desolated the close of 1766 and spring of 1767 with unheard of havoc (it had been out of the country for some years), mentions farther that an epidemic of measles followed immediately : " Before the close of the summer solstice the measles sprang up with a most luxuriant growth," and was followed in harvest by whooping-cough.

Wherever we have the means of comparison by figures, it appears that measles caused by its direct fatality not more than a sixth part of the deaths by smallpox in Britain generally. But in the colonies, where an epidemic of smallpox was a rare event of the great seaports, and as much an affair of adults as of children, measles seems to have been more fatal, dividing with diphtheria or scarlatina the great bulk of the infectious mortality of childhood. Thus Webster enters under 1772: " In this year the measles appeared in all parts of America with unusual mortality. In Charleston died 800 or 900 children"; and under 1773: " In America the measles finished its course and was followed by disorders in the throat"—especially in 1775[2]. It is

[1] Compiled from the tables in the *Gentleman's Magazine*, 1742–57. All Saints parish contained more than half the population.
[2] Pearce, writing from St Croix, West Indies, 12 Oct. 1782, to Lettsom (*Memoirs*, III. 429), says the measles had been " very rife and fatal" there.

only among the children of public institutions in England that we find in the corresponding period a similar predominance of measles and scarlatina over smallpox. In the Infirmary Books of the Foundling Hospital the more general outbreaks of small-pox cease after 1765, while epidemics of measles, extending to perhaps a third or more of the inmates, as well as great epidemics of scarlatina, begin after that date to be common[1].

In the Infirmary Book from which the following extracts are taken, the number of deaths is not stated. The number of children in the Hospital was 312 in 1763, 368 in 1766 and 438 in 1768.

1763. Before the date of the Infirmary Book, Watson records an epidemic of putrid measles from 21 April to 9 June, 1763, which attacked 180 and caused 19 immediate deaths.

Nov. 19. Nine in the infirmary with "morbillous fever"; many cases of "fever" until the 17th December.

1766. May to July. Many entries in the book; Watson says: "Seventy-four had benign measles, and all recovered."

1768. Great epidemic, May to July; one hundred and twelve in the infirmary with measles on June 4th; Watson gives the total cases at 139, of which 6 were fatal.

1773. Nov. and Dec. Great epidemic: maximum of 130 cases of measles in the infirmary on 27th November. Next week there were 40 with measles, and 90 convalescing therefrom.

1774. May. A slight outbreak (8 cases at one time).

(Records from 1776–1782 not seen.)

1783. March and April. Great epidemic: maximum number of cases in the infirmary with measles 94, on March 22nd.

1784. June. Eleven cases of measles at once.

1786. March and April. Maximum on April 5th—measles 47, recovering from measles 19.

The records from 1789 to 1805 have not been seen, but Willan gives the following dates and numbers, on the information of Dr Stanger, physician to the charity[2].

1794. 28 had measles, all recovered.
1798. 69 had measles, 6 girls died.
1800. 66 had measles, 4 boys died.
1802. 8 had measles, one died.

The general testimony in the last quarter of the 18th century is that measles, if a common affection, was not usually a severe one. Heysham, of Carlisle, says that measles came thither in 1786 from the south-west of Northumberland, "where, I am informed, they proved very fatal"; the epidemic began at Carlisle in August, and continued very general until January, 1787, but extremely mild and favourable, only 28 having died (26 under five years, 2 from five to ten), out of "some six or seven hundred, I suppose." The previous epidemic of measles

---

[1] MS. Apothecary's Books at the Foundling Hospital.
[2] R. Willan, M.D., *On Cutaneous Diseases.* Vol. I. 1808, p. 244.

at Carlisle in 1780 (mortality not stated), had followed a most fatal epidemic of smallpox in 1779; and although the epidemic of mild measles in 1786 did not follow a great epidemic of smallpox, it followed a high and steady annual average of deaths of infants and young children from that cause year after year[1]. In both years of the measles at Carlisle, there were no deaths from smallpox. In like manner at Leeds, in 1790, measles followed smallpox, and was extremely mild; Lucas wrote of it, "I have not seen one instance of a fatal termination[2]." This was the time (1785) when Heberden said of the disease in London, just as Willis, Harris and others had said of it and of smallpox together a century before: "The measles being usually attended with very little danger, it is not often that a physician is employed in this distemper."

Increasing mortality from Measles at the end of the 18th century.

There were epidemics of measles with high mortality in the 17th and 18th centuries, occurring in special circumstances of time and place, of which instances have been given. But in general the position of measles was not then so high among the causes of death in infancy and childhood as it afterwards became. It is not easy to demonstrate the exact proportions by figures, even for London; the bills of the Parish Clerks are less trustworthy for measles than for smallpox, for the reason that deaths from scarlatina were probably included among the former (see under Scarlatina). For example, the ratio of 1·10 per cent. measles deaths for the ten years 1781–90 in the following table should be only 0·70 if the 793 deaths in 1786, supposed scarlatinal, be left out. But, taking the bills as they stand, they show an increasing ratio of measles (as well as of whooping-cough) among the deaths from all causes towards the end of the 18th century.

Percentage of Measles and Whooping-cough in all London deaths, 1731–1830.

Ten-year periods	Share of measles	Share of whooping-cough	Ten-year periods	Share of measles	Share of whooping-cough
1731–40	0·70	0·41	1781–90	1·10	1·32
1741–50	0·68	0·40	1791–1800	1·34	1·97
1751–60	1·15	1·03	1801–10	3·11	3·14
1761–70	1·11	1·12	1811–20	3·52	3·49
1771–80	0·93	1·66	1821–30	3·17	3·13

[1] Heysham, u. s., p. 538.
[2] James Lucas, "On Measles." *Lond. Med. Journ.* XI. 325, dated 22 Aug. 1790.

During the same period, the ratio of deaths from all causes under two years of age had decreased, while the ratio of deaths from two to five, and at all ages above five, had increased as in the following table, also compiled from the London bills beginning with the year 1728 when the ages at death were first published.

Ratios of Deaths from all causes under two years, from two to five, and above five, London, 1728–1830.

Period	Total deaths	Ratio under Two years	Ratio from Two to Five	Ratio of all ages above Five
1728–30 (3 yrs.)	84,293	36·7	8·7	54·6
1731–40	246,925	38·6	8·9	52·5
1741–50	254,717	33·6	7·9	58·5
1751–60	204,617	30·9	9·3	59·8
1761–70	234,412	34·1	9·1	56·8
1771–80	214,605	34·4	9·6	56·0
1781–90	192,690	32·5	9·5	58·0
1791–1800	196,801	31·8	10·9	57·3
1801–10	185,823	29·3	11·5	59·2
1811–20	190,768	27·7	9·8	62·5
1821–30	209,094	28·0	9·7	62·3

Thus, while measles (with whooping-cough) was usurping, so to speak, a larger share of all the deaths, the two first years of life were claiming a smaller share of the deaths from all causes as the probability of life was improving. The saving of infant life was due to various things, but especially due to the decline of smallpox, as described in another chapter. We may now turn to consider, by a less abstract method, the increase of measles mortality from the last years of the 18th century.

In Willan's periodical reports of the prevailing diseases of London[1], scarlatina declined in 1795 and became sporadic, after having been extremely fatal for a long period, while measles and smallpox began to extend about the end of that year, the former being for the most part mild in its symptoms and favourable in its termination, the latter often confluent, and fatal to children. The report for March and April, 1796, is that measles had become more severe, and had been followed by obstinate coughs; for May, that "smallpox and measles have prevailed more during this spring than has been known for many years past." However, it was smallpox that occasioned the larger share of the deaths among infants and children. The

---

[1] *Reports on the Diseases of London*, 1796–1800. Lond. 1801, pp. 2, 13, 18, 32, 229.

next general view that Willan gives us of the relative importance of measles among the infectious diseases is under Oct.–Nov. 1799 : " The measles, though extensively diffused, have continued mild and moderate. The scarlet fever has increased, since the last report, both in extent and in the violence of its symptoms; but the contagious malignant fever [typhus] has been the most frequent, as well as the most fatal, of all acute diseases." There is little sign of fatal measles in the London bills during the years of distress, 1799–1801 ; but we hear of it in Scotland and Ireland, where there was probably less scarlatina. An Edinburgh observer of the prevailing diseases says that " several hundreds" died of measles there in the winter of 1799[1]. In the Irish emigration to America, which took one of its periodic starts owing to the repressive measures following the rebellion of 1798 and the union with England, measles appears to have been the fatal form of infection among the children on board ship. A medical letter from Philadelphia, 10 December, 1801, says that measles had been imported to Newcastle and Wilmington in the summer of 1801 by some vessels from Ireland, on board which a great many children died during the voyage ; the epidemic at length reached Philadelphia and had become general throughout the city[2]. At Whitehaven large numbers of infants were attended in measles from the Dispensary in 1796 and 1799, but the deaths (2 in 202 cases, and 2 in 266 cases) are probably only a few that came to the knowledge of the visiting physician. An epidemic at Uxbridge, Middlesex, in the winter of 1801–2 was certainly malignant or fatal more than ordinary, whatever its anomalous type may have meant.

The epidemic began in September, and was at first of so mild a type as to need no medical assistance. Towards November the cases increased in number and severity, but still, says the narrator, " I believe every case terminated favourably, not in my practice only, but in that of other gentlemen also." Towards the middle of November, the attacks were more sudden and more violent while they lasted, and were soon over either in death or recovery. In some the eyes became all at once as red as blood, the pulse full, quick and hard, the cough incessant, with a rattling noise in the throat and quick laboured breathing, the skin hot and parched.

---

[1] John Roberton, in *Med. and Phys. Journ.* XIX. 185. Measles seems to have been more usual than scarlatina in Scotland as well as in Ireland. In the accounts of the several parishes written for the *Statistical Account*, about 1791–99, measles is often mentioned (and would appear at that time to have been more usual in country districts than smallpox), while hardly anything is said of scarlatina under that name, and not much of sore-throat.

[2] *Med. and Phys. Journ.* VII. (1802), p. 316.

" Another peculiarity in this epidemic was that the cuticle in many children did not separate after the disappearance of the eruption, and in several others that I particularly noticed, it came off in large flakes instead of branny scales; and the appearance of the rash in others assumed so striking a resemblance to the scarlet fever that, had it not been for the violent cough and other measly symptoms, many such cases occurring singly might, upon a superficial view, have been considered and treated as that disorder." The various forms occurred in the same family; thus, of four children, one had typical measles, ending in a branny scurf, two others had the sneezing and the watery inflamed eyes, but the eruption in the form of an universal red fiery rash, after which the skin peeled in large flakes, while the fourth had the disease of a low typhoid type and recovered with difficulty. The epidemic "continued its destructive career" through December and January, after which the type became as mild as it had been at first. If the author had not discussed the diagnosis as between measles and scarlatina, deciding in favour of the former, one might have suspected that there were cases of both. But even the sphacelation that followed the application of blisters, the pemphigus-like eruption turning gangrenous, and the petechiae, were signs of malignancy in more than one of the exanthematous fevers. The sequelae of this epidemic of measles were as anomalous as the symptoms themselves; instead of the inflamed eyes, and the distressing cough (some-times ending in consumption) there were aphthous fever and dysenteric purging[1].

The deaths in the London bills for the first twelve years of the century will be found in the table on p. 655. We find the measles deaths for the first time equalling the smallpox deaths in 1804, and in 1808 surpassing them, and we may take it that the deaths so entered were almost wholly of measles proper. The epidemic of measles in 1807–8 was, in fact, a great and clearly defined event in British epidemiology, the first of a series of epidemics in which that disease established not only its equality with smallpox as a cause of infantile deaths but even its supremacy over the latter. It would appear, also, to have been more malignant than the scarlatina that coexisted with it. Thus, Bateman, of London, at the outset of the great measles epidemic of 1807–8, says: " The most prominent acute disorders have been eruptive fevers and particularly the measles, which during October and November have been very prevalent, and, when occurring in young children, have proved very fatal by terminating in violent inflammation of the organs of respira-tion...The scarlatina was generally mild, presenting the eruption with a slight sore-throat[2]."

---

[1] "Observations on Measles." By Mr Edlin, surgeon, Uxbridge. *Med. and Phys. Journ.* VIII. (July–Dec. 1802), p. 28. An earlier epidemic of anomalous eruptive fever ("dark coloured eruption of the neck and breast which spread at length over the whole body") was described for Uxbridge and its vicinity in the summer and autumn of 1799, in an essay reviewed in *British Critic,* XV. 435.
[2] T. Bateman, M.D., *Report on the Diseases of London,* 1804–16. Lond. 1819, p. 90-91.

Other accounts of the epidemic in London show it to have been of the type which Sydenham, in 1674, called anomalous or malignant.

The epidemic began in October–November, 1807, and was remarked as unusually fatal[1].

Several children in the same family had fallen victims to it. Some cases were fatal in a few days, either from the intensity of the fever or from pneumonic complication. "But when these symptoms have been less violent, and the patient has passed without much alarm through the different stages of the disorder, and even after all apprehension of danger in the mind of parents or friends has been dismissed, a continuance or recurrence of pneumonic symptoms has laid a foundation for phthisis pulmonalis." In some cases attended from the Westminster Dispensary, death followed from effusion into the chest or from membranous inflammation of the trachea. Numbers who recovered from the measles were afterwards affected with debility, cough, emaciation and oedematous swellings of the face and extremities which proved very difficult to remove. These particulars are given mostly for the end of 1807, but it is under the year 1808 that the great rise in the measles deaths appears in the London bills of mortality.

Besides these accounts for London, we have some details of the same epidemic at Edinburgh and Aberdeen and exact figures for Glasgow. It began at Edinburgh in the winter of 1807, and at Aberdeen (as at Glasgow) in the spring of 1808. At both places it was remarked as unusually fatal, chiefly from a complication of bowel complaint in children and from pulmonary affections in adults.

The Aberdeen observer says that in town (the disease being milder in the country) there were troublesome symptoms in almost every case—a violent pain in the belly, frequently accompanied with diarrhoea (and even with vomiting), and with the dysenteric symptoms of tenesmus and mucus in the stools. This bowel complaint usually lasted three or four days, and wasted the patients remarkably. There was also the usual catarrh with violent tickling cough, and, after the acute attack, a tendency to sudden dyspnoea and "fatal coughs." In some the convalescence was lingering and very distressing to the patient: "it consists in a slow kind of fever, with evening exacerbations[2]."

The observers at Edinburgh and Aberdeen agree that the epidemic was the worst that had been seen for many years. Says the former[3]: "I believe that the present epidemic has been more general in this place and its vicinity than ever happened within the remembrance of any medical man at present living,

---

[1] Samuel Fothergill, M.D., and others, in *Med. and Phys. Journ.* XVIII. (Dec. 1807), pp. 569, 572 ; XIX. 91, 185.
[2] "The Epidemic Measles of 1808." By Dr Ferguson. *Med. and Phys. Journ.* XXI. 359.
[3] John Roberton, *Med. and Phys. Journ.* XIX. 182, 272, 278, 471.

and I am sorry to say it has been very fatal." The Aberdeen chronicler says the mortality was "greater than we have witnessed for a long period," and that the epidemic was general throughout the whole of England and Scotland. But, besides this direct testimony, there is a not less indirectly significant fact of the epidemic. It affected many adults—"persons of all ages, who had never had them," says the Aberdeen writer: few persons escaped, says the Edinburgh observer, "who had been previously unaffected by this disease." The deaths from pulmonic complaints did not often happen among children, but among people somewhat advanced in life. Significant also was the outbreak in the Invernessshire Militia, which marched into Edinburgh in March while the epidemic was raging. Fifty men, all young recruits newly joined, were attacked in the course of a few days, the others escaping the disease though equally ·exposed to it; in some of those who died in the regiment there were found, on opening the thorax, fibrinous pleurisy and pericarditis, with effusion of fluid, as well as evidences of bronchial catarrh[1]. The Aberdeen writer says: "I always observed that in full-grown persons the eruptions were more numerous, quicker in appearing, and longer in going off than in young subjects.... Many full-grown persons were very ill, yet the measles were more fatal to the young." The implication of so many adults in the severe epidemic of 1808 would of itself show that measles had not been for some time before a steady and universal affection of infancy and childhood[2].

Measles in Glasgow in 1808 and 1811–12: Researches of Watt.

The measles epidemic of 1808, which appears to have been somewhat general in England and Scotland, made an extraordinary impression in Glasgow. That disease had never before been nearly so mortal there, nor had any infection since the time of the plague, not even smallpox itself, engrossed the burial registers so much as measles did in the months of May and

---

[1] Roberton, *loc. cit.* XIX. 471.
[2] In the earlier period, according to Grainger, Lind and others, numerous cases of measles sometimes occurred on board ships of war.

June, 1808. Glasgow had been the worst city in the kingdom for smallpox; by a somewhat sudden transition the infancy of the city died for a few months in larger numbers by the new disease than by the old. The highest monthly mortalities from smallpox had been 114 in October and 113 in November, 1791, the population being 66,578; but in 1808, the population having increased to 100,749 by the census of 1811, measles carried off 259 children in May and 260 in June, and in the months before and after as follows:

Measles in Glasgow, 1808.

Month	Deaths	Month	Deaths	Month	Deaths
Jan.	2	May	259	Sept.	22
Feb.	2	June	260	Oct.	10
March	5	July	118	Nov.	4
April	71	Aug.	32	Dec.	2

The figures were not known at the time; but every doctor in Glasgow, as well as the whole populace, knew that measles was cutting off the infants, while smallpox had fallen to insignificance. So dramatic was this turn in the public health that the common people set it down to the new practice of inoculating children with cowpox : ready to believe anything of vaccination, they concluded that, if it kept off smallpox, it brought on measles. Dr Robert Watt took the trouble to refute this singular notion; he found in his own practice that three children in one family, and in another two, had died of measles who had neither been vaccinated nor had smallpox before. Another great epidemic of measles arose in Glasgow three years after, in the winter of 1811–12:

1811	Measles deaths		1812	Measles deaths
October	12		January	130
November	76		February	61
December	161		March	30
			April	19
			May	15
			June	18

Those two great epidemics of measles in Glasgow, in 1808 and 1811–12, were the occasion of one of the earliest and most memorable inquiries in vital statistics in this country, the research by Dr Robert Watt on "the Relative Mortality of the Principal Diseases of Children, and the numbers who have died

under ten years of age in Glasgow during the last thirty years[1]."
Having begun with a search of the principal Glasgow burial-
registers for deaths by whooping-cough, he extended it to sixteen
folio volumes of the registers of all the burial-grounds, old and
new, and included the mortalities from all causes with the ages
at death, and from fevers and the principal diseases of infancy
and childhood. The increase of population from 1783, when his
figures begin, to 1812, the date of his writing, was known to
him; but as the numbers living at the respective periods of life
were not known, he was obliged to state the change in the
mortalities at the various ages, and from the various diseases, in
ratios of the annual deaths from all causes,—a perfectly scientific
comparison so long as the nature of the ratios compared was
clearly stated. It would have been more satisfactory, of course,
if the comparison could have been made in terms of the annual
death-rate, which was much lower (for reasons already explained), in the second half of his period than in the first; but,
in the circumstances, that was impracticable, and Watt did the
next best thing. The following is the principal part of his table
of ratios in five successive periods of six years each:

Vital Statistics of Glasgow in sexennial periods, 1783–1812. (*Watt.*)

Period	Sum of all deaths	Per cent. under Two	Per cent. from Two to Five	Per cent. from Five to Ten	Per cent. of Smallpox	Per cent. of Measles	Per cent. of Whooping-cough	Per cent. of "Bowel-hive"
1783–88	9994	39·40	10·66	3·42	19·55	0·93	4·51	6·72
1789–94	11103	42·38	11·90	3·79	18·22	1·17	5·13	6·43
1795–1800	9991	38·82	12·21	3·45	18·70	2·10	5·36	6·47
1801–06	10304	33·50	13·43	5·10	8·90	3·92	6·12	7·27
1807–12	13354	35·89	14·22	5·58	3·90	10·76	5·57	9·26

The actual deaths from smallpox, measles and whooping-
cough are shown in the next table, which includes for comparison the corresponding figures from the London bills of
mortality:

---

[1] Published as an Appendix to his *Treatise on the History, Nature and Treatment
of Chincough.* Glasgow, 1813. Reprinted by John Thomson, Glasgow, 1888.
Dr Watt is best known by his *Bibliotheca Britannica* (Edinburgh, 1819. 4 vols.
4to.), a wonderfully complete bibliography under the dual arrangement of subjects
and authors, which is still indispensable for research in every branch of knowledge.
Perhaps the many who use it are not all aware that it was the labour of a physician
in Glasgow (originally a surgeon at Paisley), who died (in 1819) at the age of forty-
five, having reached such professional distinction in his own city as to be elected
President of the Faculty of Physicians and Surgeons.

Smallpox, Measles and Whooping-cough in London and Glasgow,
1783–1812.

	London			Glasgow		
Year	Smallpox	Measles	Whooping-cough	Smallpox	Measles	Whooping-cough
1783	1550	185	268	155	66	153
1784	1759	29	457	425	1	41
1785	1999	20	194	218	0	34
1786	1210	793	200	348	2	173
1787	2418	84	228	410	23	57
1788	1101	55	298	399	1	17
1789	2077	534	374	366	23	45
1790	1617	119	391	336	33	177
1791	1747	156	279	607	4	117
1792	1568	450	311	202	58	68
1793	2382	248	352	389	5	112
1794	1913	172	469	235	7	51
1795	1040	328	311	402	46	180
1796	3548	307	536	177	92	60
1797	522	222	567	354	5	76
1798	2237	196	418	309	3	98
1799	1111	223	451	370	43	95
1800	2409	395	380	257	21	27
1801	1461	136	428	245	8	125
1802	1579	559	1004	156	168	90
1803	1202	438	586	194	45	60
1804	622	619	697	213	27	52
1805	1685	523	703	56	90	129
1806	1158	530	623	28	56	162
1807	1297	452	439	97	16	85
1808	1169	1386	326	51	787	92
1809	1163	106	591	159	44	259
1810	1198	1031	449	28	19	147
1811	751	235	486	109	267	62
1812	1287	427	508	78	304	103

The ratio of deaths under the age of two had decreased greatly in Glasgow, while the ratios from two to five and from five to ten had increased. At the same time smallpox had almost ceased (but only temporarily, as it appeared) to be the great infectious scourge of infancy, while measles had come in its place. "Now that the smallpox are in great measure expelled," (Watt believed that cowpox inoculation had done this), "the measles are gradually coming to occupy the same ground which they formerly occupied. I am sorry to make this statement, but the facts, at least with regard to Glasgow, are too strong to admit of doubt."

In order to explain the enormous increase of deaths by measles, he had recourse to the following argument. Formerly nearly all children, say nine-tenths, had both smallpox and measles, the attack of smallpox in most cases coming first. Children who had survived smallpox were fortified by that ordeal, not merely as selected lives, but positively fortified, so that measles, when it assailed them in due time afterwards, was taken mildly or was "modified," not one in a hundred cases proving fatal. But now (1813), when so few children have been through the smallpox, measles has become ten times more fatal to them, although it could hardly be more common than it used to be. Having found it necessary to assume that children in former times took smallpox before they took measles, nine-tenths of them taking both, he qualifies this in another passage : "Still, however, as the measles came round now and then, as a very general epidemic, they must occasionally have had the precedence, and it was perhaps chiefly among such patients that the disease proved fatal."

The measles which came round now and then as a general epidemic was nearly the whole of it ; even in London there were intervals of several years with only a few annual deaths, and in smaller towns or country districts the clear intervals were longer. The prevalence of measles on the great scale being more casual than that of smallpox, it is likely that most children had taken smallpox before they incurred measles. But it is clear from such instances as the London epidemic of 1674, and the epidemic in the Foundling Hospital in 1763, that measles might attack children just before smallpox, and by its weakening effects, increase the number of victims of the latter. As to the fatality of measles itself in the 17th and 18th centuries, the statement of Watt that it did not amount to one death in a hundred attacks, while it can neither be proved nor disproved by an array of figures, can be shown to be inconsistent with the language of annalists. The epidemics of measles varied in severity then as afterwards : that of 1670 in London was regular and mild, that of 1674 in the very same months of the year was anomalous and fatal ; Huxham characterizes the measles at Plymouth in the winter of 1749-50 as "maximé epidemici, imo et saepe pestiferi"; at Kidderminster, in 1756, after fevers had been very fatal to adults, the measles went through the town so that an immense number of children "died tabid"; in the West of England about 1760 a disease called measles made "a melancholy carnage amongst children."

While Watt's theory of the working of this principle of substitution is open to criticism on some points of detail, the law itself, as enunciated by him, remains to the present time one of the soundest and most instructive generalities in epidemiology. He based it upon a laborious search of the burial registers, such as no one before him in this country had undertaken. Next he saw correctly that a great rise in the deaths of infants by such a disease as measles could only be accounted for by a great increase in the rate of fatality. Thirdly, he connected the loss from measles with the saving from smallpox. Adopting an old opinion, which may be discovered in Willis[1], he argued that smallpox, when taken first, served to fortify children so that they passed easily through the measles afterwards; but in the following passage he indicated a better reason why the absence of smallpox gave measles the chance of proving more fatal : " In this point of view we are not to consider the smallpox as so peculiarly

[1] *De Febribus*, 1659. Cap. xv.

fatal in their nature. They perhaps prove so fatal merely by having the start of other diseases. The measles, the chincough, the croup, the scarlet fever, and perhaps many others, would have proved equally fatal had they occurred first." The principle is true to this extent, that a certain proportion of weakly infants, or children of poor stamina, will succumb to almost any disease —if not to smallpox, then to measles, and if not to measles directly, then to the sequelae of measles. This was perceived in the form of a necessary truth by Haygarth in 1793: "A considerable number of those who now die of the smallpox would die in childhood of other diseases if this distemper were exterminated[1]." It was commonly believed that smallpox had at length found its real artificial check, not in the inoculation of itself, but in the inoculation of cowpox. At all events it had declined greatly in Glasgow. During the three years before the measles epidemic of 1808, there could hardly have been more than a thousand children attacked by smallpox, or not one in ten of all the children born. During several years the infancy of the city had been spared any great ordeal of infectious disease; the first epidemic that came along happened to be measles, so that it fell to that infection to take off the weaklings. In the economy of nature it is impossible to rear all the young of a species, nor would it be good for the species if it were possible. It is among the birds that the principle of population, or of the survival of the fittest, is seen working in the most admirable way : the annual migration of many species to breed in a remote country brings with it an ordeal for the birds of the year in finding their way to the winter feeding-grounds—an ordeal which only the strongest come through. For some unexplained reason, the young of the human species are peculiarly tried by infectious diseases, which multitudes pass through safely, while many of poor stamina or of ill tending are cut off.

Dr Watt's teaching as to the displacement of one infectious cause of death by another was resisted at the time as being of "evil tendency" for the pretensions of vaccination, although Watt believed as firmly in the virtues of cowpox as Jenner himself did. Writing to James Moore on 6 Dec. 1813, Jenner says of Watt's essay (Baron, II. 392): "There is nothing in its title that developes its purport or *evil tendency....* Is not this very shocking? Here is a new and unexpected twig shot forth for the sinking anti-vaccinist to cling to." Sir Gilbert Blane, who was then president of the Medical and Chirurgical Society, having a natural fondness for ideas of all kinds expressed in a paper to that society rather more approval of Watt's

[1] *Sketch of a Plan to exterminate the Casual Smallpox, &c.* London, 1793, p. 152.

view than was thought prudent : " An ingenious friend of mine has remarked
to me in conversation that some light is thrown on this subject by considering
that whichever of the epidemic maladies attack children first, it will be the
most fatal, inasmuch as all feeble constitutions will fall in its way while the
stronger will be left to encounter the attacks of the others ; and that the
smallpox, owing probably to the greater abundance and rankness of their
effluvia, are generally caught in a casual way before measles, hooping cough
and scarlet fever, and are therefore reckoned more fatal than any of these.
But, a new field of research being opened," etc.   Efforts were made to correct
the effect of this, by showing that measles in some parts of the country had
not been more fatal than usual.   Holland, of Knutsford, attributed the
fatality of the epidemic in 1808 to a change of the wind to the east.   Writers
in the *Edinburgh Med. and Surg. Journal*, pointed out that Watt had
compared the absolute deaths by smallpox at one time and by measles at
another without taking account of the increase of population, and the rates
of mortality from each disease.   The best criticism of Watt was by Roberton
in his *Mortality of Children*, 1827, p. 49.   He offers the following considerations, without seeming to know that they were really to be found in
Watt's own essay : Smallpox used to be caught first ; it swept off the feeble
and sickly, leaving the strong and vigorous *only* to encounter the attacks of
other diseases.   "That infectious febrile disease to which in early infancy
there is the strongest predisposition will of course in general make the first
attack and prove the most fatal of any."   There were reasons why measles
used to have comparatively few victims, "and why, when they now prevail
epidemically, they, as was the case with smallpox, are caught at an earlier
age than other diseases in general and prove so very fatal : which happens
not more from their priority in attack than from being in their nature what
they were ever considered—a severe and dangerous disease.   We are to
recollect, however, that measles do not in general attack at so early an age
as smallpox ; nor ever, like the latter, destroy eight or nine-tenths of all the
children that die in the place where they happen to prevail, as was the case
in the variolous epidemics of Chester and Warrington [this is an error, *vide
supra*, p. 554] ; consequently we have reason to hope that neither measles
nor any other infantile disease will, as Dr Watt imagined, 'come to occupy
the place which smallpox once occupied,'" (p. 58).   A feeble echo of
Roberton's criticism, with all its scientific candour left out and its points
against Watt emphasized in a spirit of paltry cavilling, was heard next year
in the Goulstonian Lectures of Bisset Hawkins on *Elements of Medical
Statistics*, 1829.

Many years after, when the enormous increase of deaths by scarlatina
was illustrating the doctrine of displacement in a new way, Dr Farr gave a
full analysis of Watt's essay in his annual Letter to the Registrar-General
for the year 1867, and endorsed the Glasgow teaching of 1813 with more
heartiness than it had hitherto received.   Although Farr did not take the
Malthusian view that the loss of weakly children by one means or another
was inevitable, yet he could not help seeing, in his work upon the registration
returns from 1837 onwards, that one infection had been taking what
another spared.   He recurred to Watt's doctrine time after time in his
annual reports, and in that of 1872 (p. 224), expressed his belief thus plainly :
" The zymotic diseases replace each other ; and when one is rooted out, it is
apt to be replaced by others which ravage the human race indifferently
whenever the conditions of healthy life are wanting.   They have this
property in common with weeds and other forms of life : as one species
recedes, another advances."

Two remarks remain to be made under the doctrine of
displacement.   The first is that the substitution of measles for

smallpox was one of a series of such changes in the public health of Britain. The great infective scourge of medieval and early modern periods had been plague, which destroyed at times immense numbers of the valuable or mature lives. Its successor was typhus fever, which also cut off the parents more than the children, but did not retard population as the plague had done. The saving of life by the extinction of plague was in great part balanced by the loss from smallpox, which fell, however, more and more upon the earliest years of life until at length it was almost confined to them. The first great decline of smallpox itself corresponded to a great decline of typhus fever during the second half of the French war; but while there was no great infectious disease in those years to thin the ranks of the adults, measles took the place of the more loathsome smallpox in cutting off a certain number of young lives. While the older types of infection have disappeared, the incidence has shifted from mature lives to children, so much so that at the present time enteric fever, and occasional choleras and influenzas, are almost the only infections that correspond to the old plague and to typhus fever in their age-incidence.

The other remark is that the greater prevalence or fatality of measles, as if in lieu of smallpox, meant a good deal more for the bills of mortality than actually appeared under the name of measles. Smallpox was not an infection that did much consti-tutional damage to those that came through it, although it sometimes destroyed the vision and spoiled the beauty of the face. On the contrary, it was held by many that the general health was better after an attack of smallpox than before; and, if personal experience can justify an opinion, that ought to be my own view of the matter[1]. But measles is an infection peculiarly apt to leave mischief behind. The bronchial catarrh, which is an integral part of the malady, and is often the cause of death in the second stage of the attack, may so affect weakly children that the respiratory organs are permanently damaged. Tuberculosis of the lungs is apt to follow measles. Some children, again, fall into mesenteric disease after measles, and die

---

[1] It was believed that smallpox left ill effects in some constitutions. William III. is said to have had the dregs of smallpox in his lungs. Roberton (u. s.) cites Saunders as teaching that smallpox caused scrofula, and he is himself doubtful whether an attack of it ever improved the constitution. Dr Moses Younghusband, of New Lebanon Springs, *Med. Phys. Journ.* XI. (1804), 317, wrote: "I see no more of the glandular suppurations formerly so frequent and unavoidable" after smallpox.

tabid, the intestinal catarrh being as dangerous in one way as the bronchial is in another. Another large proportion of the subjects of measles take whooping-cough[1]. While smallpox did its work summarily, the full effects of measles were longer in being realized. This may in part explain the fact brought out by Watt, that while fewer children died under two years of age, measles being the dominant epidemic disease, there was an increase in the ratio of deaths from all causes between the years of two and five and from five to ten.

Measles in the Period of Statistics.

The history of measles for nearly a generation after the great epidemics of 1808 and 1811–12 is little known. No one in Glasgow continued Watt's laborious tabulation of the causes of deaths in the numerous burial registers[2]; nor was any regular account kept elsewhere except by the Parish Clerks of London. The following deaths by measles in their bills from 1813 to 1837, when the modern registration began, were probably no more than from a third to a half of the deaths in all London :

Year	Measles deaths	Year	Measles deaths	Year	Measles deaths
1813	550	1822	712	1830	479
1814	817	1823	573	1831	750
1815	711	1824	966	1832	675
1816	1106	1825	743	1833	524
1817	725	1826	774	1834	528
1818	728	1827	525	1835	734
1819	695	1828	736	1836	404
1820	720	1829	578	1837	577
1821	547				

The inadequacy of these figures to the whole of London will appear from the fact that the registration returns under the new Act gave for the last six months of 1837 the measles deaths at 1354, while the bills of the Parish Clerks gave them at 577 for the whole year. But the old bills enable us to compare the deaths from different diseases within the same area and under

[1] Johnstone, *Malignant Epidemic Fever of* 1756, London, 1757, says of Kidderminster during a season of high mortality from fever and other diseases: "The measles at this time went through our town and neighbourhood. The children commonly got over the usual course of this distemper; but vast numbers died tabid of its consequences. The chincough succeeded the measles."

[2] The *Edin. Med. and Surg. Journ.* XXVI. 177, cites from Cleland, with a reference which I have not succeeded in verifying, the following Glasgow figures for the period 1813–19: all deaths 22,060, smallpox 236 (1·07 per cent.), measles 614 (3·69 per cent.). But see Cowan, *Glas. Med. Journ.* v. 358, *supra*, p. 597.

the same system of collection, and to compare the deaths " within the bills " in a series of years since the last of the new parishes were taken in about the middle of the 18th century. Using the bills so far legitimately, we find that measles at length came to be of equal importance with smallpox itself as a cause of death in childhood, and that it had become a larger and steadier total from year to year.

So far as concerns Glasgow, the high mortality from 1807 to 1812, making 10·76 on an annual average of the deaths from all causes, was not maintained. When the tabulation of the causes of death was resumed from 1835, the annual average of measles for the five years ending 1839 was found to be only 6 per cent. of the deaths from all causes, the average of smallpox having come back to 5·3 per cent. During that unwholesome period, in which there was much distress among the working class and a great epidemic of typhus, measles and smallpox were dividing the infectious mortality of childhood somewhat equally, the age-incidence of measles being only a little lower than that of smallpox :

Ages of the Fatal Cases of Measles in Glasgow, 1835–39[1].

	Under one	1–2	2–5	5–10	10–20	20–30	30–40	40–50	Total
1835	116	141	121	34	10	4	–	–	426
1836	86	209	183	38	1	1	–	–	518
1837	77	133	122	16	2	1			350
1838	76	124	161	39	3	1	1		405
1839	165	259	275	73	7	2		1	783
	520	866	863	200	23	9	1	1	2482

In Limerick, which may stand for a typically unhealthy Irish city in the worst period of over-population, there were many more deaths from smallpox among children than from measles, the age-incidence being nearly the same, according to the following dispensary statistics for a number of years before 1840[2] :

Limerick Dispensary Deaths.

	Age 0–5	5–10	10–15	15–20	Total
Smallpox	333	55	5	0	393
Measles	187	32	6	1	226
Scarlatina	8	2			10

Although it is impossible to prove it, yet the indications all point to measles having kept for a whole generation after 1808 the leading place among infantile causes of death which it then

[1] Cowan, *Journ. Statist. Soc.* III.
[2] Griffin, *ibid.* III.

for the first time definitely took[1]. Almost the only direct
references to the subject were made by way of controverting the
doctrine of Watt; but these are too meagre, or too general in
their terms, to be of any use[2]. The epidemics of measles seem
to have travelled then, as they do now, from county to county in
successive years. Thus in 1818, while most parts of England
were or had recently been suffering from smallpox, the Eastern
counties were suffering from measles "very frequent and fatal."
Smallpox at length reached Norwich in 1819, and became the
reigning epidemic in the place of measles, which was "hardly
met with" so long as the enormous mortality of the other
disease proceeded[3]. At Exeter in the spring of 1824 measles
became epidemic after a long interval; many susceptible children
had accumulated, and of these few escaped. The mortality was
very great, and was caused by severe pulmonary inflammation,
the catarrhal symptoms being mild. In one day seventeen
children were buried in one of the five parish churchyards of the
city; but that high mortality, according to the parochial
surgeon, did not on an average stand for more than four deaths
in one hundred cases[4].

When the curtain rises, in the summer of 1837, upon the
prevalence and distribution of diseases in England, as ascertained
by the new system of registration of the causes of death, measles
is found in the first place among the infectious maladies of
childhood, thereafter yielding its place to smallpox for a year
or more, and taking the lead again until it was passed by
scarlatina.

Deaths by Measles and Smallpox in London, 1837–39.

	1837		1838			1839	
	3rd Qr.	4th Qr.	1st Qr.	2nd Qr.	3rd Qr.	4th Qr.	(four quarters)
Measles	822	532	173	96	94	225	2036
Smallpox	257	506	753	1145	1061	858	634

The epidemic of smallpox hardly touched the Eastern counties
until 1839; so that while the home counties in that year had

[1] Macmichael, in an essay on scarlatina and other contagions, 1822, says:
"Parents considering the measles as a disease almost inevitable have wisely chosen to
expose their children to the contagion at such auspicious times [summer season]; so
that the disorder may be once well over, and all further anxiety at an end." p. 30.

[2] P. Macgregor, *Med. Chir. Trans.* v. 436, obtained from Henry, of Manchester,
the burials from measles at the Collegiate Church and St John's Church for two years,
1812–13, which when compared with those abstracted by Percival from the former
register for twenty years, 1754–74, showed a higher ratio of measles to the burials
from all causes.

[3] Cross, u. s.   [4] Delagarde, *Med. Chir. Trans.* XIII. 163.

far more deaths by measles than by smallpox, Norfolk had only
72 deaths by the former against 820 deaths by the latter. In
the same year measles took the lead in four out of six great
English towns, scarlatina being the· dominant infection in one
(Sheffield), and smallpox in one (Bradford):

Deaths in 1839 *by the three chief infections of Childhood.*

	Liverpool	Manchester	Leeds	Birmingham	Sheffield	Bradford
Measles	401	773	383	170	33	70
Scarlatina	374	264	35	133	419	7
Smallpox	259	237	171	56	16	208

In all England and Wales during fully half-a-century of
registration, measles has fluctuated somewhat from year to year
but has not experienced a notable decline among the causes of
infantile mortality (see the table at p. 614). In the decennial
period 1871–80, its annual average death-rate was 377 per
million living; in the next decennium it rose to 441, the previously
high rates of scarlatina having fallen greatly. Among the
highest rates for the ten years 1871–80, were those of Plymouth,
1·13 per 1000, East Stonehouse 1·79, and Devonport 1·19
(owing to a great epidemic in 1879–80), Exeter, 0·82, Liverpool
·91, Bedwelty (Tredegar and Aberystruth collieries) 0·88, Wigan
0·74, Whitehaven 0·71, Alverstoke 0·81. In the most recent
period there have been some very high death-rates ; thus at
Jarrow the annual rate, which was only ·27 per 1000 from 1871
to 1880, rose in the nine years 1881 to 1889 to an annual
average of ·94, having been made up almost wholly by great
epidemics every other year—in 1883 (2·9), 1885 (2·4), 1887 (1·4),
and 1889 (·9)[1]. In the year 1888, an epidemic at Stoke-on-
Trent, Hanley, &c. with 342 deaths, made a rate of 2·8 for the
year ; in Wolstanton, Burslem, &c., 221 deaths were equivalent
to a rate of 2·6.

The latest reports of the Registrar-General have traced a
progression of the epidemic of measles from county to county or
from district to district in successive years, such as was
remarked, both for smallpox and measles, by some of the 18th
century epidemiologists in England, Scotland and Ireland.

Thus in 1890, measles was epidemic in Cheshire, South Lancashire and
North Staffordshire ; in 1891 it ceased in these, but became epidemic in
North Lancashire, South Staffordshire and the West Riding ; in 1892 it

---

[1] A. Campbell Monro, M.D., "Measles: an Epidemiological Study." Chiefly
from the Jarrow statistics. *Trans. Epid. Soc.* N. S. X. (1890–91), p. 94. The author
connects the recent increase with the greater concourse of children to infant and
elementary schools under the Education Act.

ceased in its last-mentioned area, and became epidemic in Warwickshire, Leicestershire, Derbyshire, the East and North Ridings, Westmoreland and Durham. During the same three years a similar progression or cycle was observable (on looking over the tables) in the South-west of England. The epidemic year of measles in Devonshire was 1889. It ceased there, and became epidemic in 1890 in Cornwall on the one side and in Somerset on the other, sparing Dorset. In 1891 it ceased to be epidemic in those parts of Cornwall and Somerset which it occupied in 1890, and became prevalent in the extreme west of Cornwall, in parts of Somerset, in Wiltshire and in Gloucestershire. In 1892 it ceased in all the last-mentioned excepting Gloucestershire, and became epidemic in Dorset, where there had been no severe prevalence of measles since 1888[1].

Measles has no such decided preference for a season of the year as scarlatina and enteric fever have for autumn or infantile diarrhoea has for summer. But it often happens that most deaths are recorded from May to July, owing, doubtless, to the greater number of attacks in summer and not to any excessive fatality of that season. In London and the great industrial towns the deaths are spread somewhat uniformly over the year; or, in the language of statisticians, the maxima do not rise far above the mean of the year. In a tabulation of the weekly deaths in London from 1845 to 1874[2], it appears that they touch a higher point in mid-winter (Nov.–Jan.) than in summer, a fact which may be readily accounted for by the injurious effects of the London air in winter upon a disease which is largely a trouble of the respiratory organs. In the great industrial populations of Lancashire, which resemble London in their high death-rate from measles, the rise of the deaths in mid-winter is almost the same as the summer increase[3].

Most of the deaths from measles fall at present upon the ages from six months to three years, just as they did when the deaths were comparatively few, as at Manchester from 1768 to 1774. Deaths of adults, which were not altogether rare in the first great epidemic of modern times in 1808, are seldom heard of at present, for the same reason that adult deaths used to be uncommon in smallpox, namely, that the disease is passed by almost everyone in infancy or childhood. Although the deaths from measles sometimes reach large totals—in London during

---

[1] *Rep. Reg.-Genl.* LIV. p. xviii, and LV. p. xi. The explanation given is as follows: " When a county or other area has been visited by a severe epidemic [of measles] there is for several succeeding years scarcely sufficient material, in the shape of unprotected children, for another considerable outbreak, unless it be in very populous areas such as London or Liverpool; and in such places the disease is endemic."

[2] Buchan and Mitchell, *Journ. Scot. Meteor. Soc.* July, 1874, p. 194.

[3] Ogle, in the 47th Report of the Registrar-General (for 1884), p. xv.

the spring of 1894 they were in some weeks as high as one hundred and fifty—yet it is the common experience of practitioners that a strong or healthy child rarely dies of measles, that the fatalities occur among the infants of weakly constitution, and especially in the numerous families of the working class in the most populous centres of mining, manufactures and shipping.

To bring these various characteristics of measles together in a concrete instance, I shall give briefly the facts of a recent epidemic in a town in Scotland of some twelve thousand inhabitants. There had been only five deaths from measles for two years. There had not been a case of smallpox for at least ten years. The measles epidemic, when its triennial opportunity came, reached a height in July, on a certain day of which month there were seven or eight burials from measles or its direct sequelae. Nearly all the children in the place who had not been through the measles in the corresponding epidemics of 1889 or 1887 suffered from it on this occasion, excepting the class of very young infants. The deaths in the whole epidemic numbered about fifty, which would not all be registered, however, as from measles. Yet this high mortality was not due to any unusual malignancy of the disease, but to the feeble stamina of a certain number of infants, or to the indifferent housing and tending of the poorer class. One did not hear of a death in the well-to-do families (probably there was none), although they had their full share of attacks. The frequency of the burials for a short time, and the effects of the epidemic on the mortality from first to last, must have been very nearly the same as in an epidemic of smallpox a century before, when the population was only a third or fourth part as large. But in the period when smallpox was in the ascendant, having few rivals among the infective causes of death in childhood, the general conditions of health in this town were altogether different. One or two specimens of the thatched huts of the poorer class had been left standing into the era of photography, so that we could compare past with present, in externals at least ; also, of the houses of the richer class some still remained, perhaps turned into tenement-houses, with small windows, low doorways, and crow steps on their gables ; and it was on record by the parish minister at the end of the 18th century, that within the memory of that generation there had been peat stacks and dunghills before the doors on the High Street of the burgh.

CHAPTER VI.

WHOOPING-COUGH.

IT is singular that a malady so distinctively marked as whooping-cough is should figure so little in the records of disease from former times. Astruc could find no traces of it in the medical writings of antiquity or of the Arabian period. In modern times the first known account of an epidemic of it is under the year 1578, when Baillou of Paris included a prevalent convulsive cough as part of the epidemic constitution of that year, remarking in the same context that he knew of no author who had hitherto written of the malady[1]. Yet, if whooping-cough had been as common in former times as it has been in quite recent times, it deserved a high place among the causes of infantile mortality. Doubtless it occurred in former times in the same circumstances in which it occurs now. Baillou in 1578 speaks of it as a familiar. thing; and it can be shown from an English prescription-book of the medieval period that remedies were in request for a malady called " the kink," a name which survives in Scotland (like other obsolete English words of the 15th century) in the form of " kink host[2]."

In Phaer's *Booke of Children* (1553) chincough is not named. It is perhaps more singular that the disease should be omitted from the list in Sir Thomas Elyot's *Castel of Health* (1541), of maladies proper to three periods of childhood; for that list has every appearance of being an exhaustive enumeration[3]. Still, it would be erroneous to suppose that the convulsive cough of

---

[1] Cited by Hirsch, *Geogr. and Histor. Pathology.* Eng. transl. III. 28.

[2] *Harl. MSS.* No. 2378. Moulton's *This is the Myrour or Glasse of Health*, circa 1540, is in the main a printed reproduction of this manuscript prescription-book. The same receipt which is "for ye kink" in the one, is "for the chyncough" in the other (formula LXXIX.).

[3] "Sycknesses happenynge to children :—When they be new borne, there do happen to them sores of the mouth called aphte, vometyng, coughes, watchinge, fearefulness, inflamations of the nauelle, moysture of the eares. When they brede

children which is so common an epidemic incident in our time, and in some impressionable subjects is the almost necessary sequel of a coryza or catarrh, did not then occur in the same circumstances as now. When Willis, in his *Pharmaceutice Rationalis* of 1674, remarks that pertussis was left to the management of old women and empirics, he suggests the real reason why so little is said of it in the medical compends. Sydenham mentions it twice, and on both occasions in a significant context. Under the name of pertussis, "quem nostrates vocant *Hooping Cough*," he brings it in at the end of his account of the measles epidemic of 1670, without actually saying that it was a sequel of the measles. His other reference to it, under the name of the convulsive cough of children, comes in his account of the influenza of 1679. In both contexts it is adduced as an instance of a malady much more amenable to bloodletting than to pectoral remedies, the depletion being a sure means of cutting short an attack that was else very apt to be protracted, if not altogether uncontrollable[1]. One glimpse of it we get among the children of a squire's family in Rutlandshire in the summer of 1661. On the 26th of May the mother of the children writes to her husband then on a visit to London[2]:

"I am in a sad condition for my pore children, who are all so trobled with the chincofe that I am afraid it will kill them. There is many dy out in this town, and many abroad that we heare of. I am fane to have a candell stand by me to goo in too them when the fitt comes." On 2 June, the children are still "all sadly trobeled with the chincofe. Moll is much the worst. They have such fits that it stopes theare wind, and puts me to such frits and feares that I am not myselfe." In a third letter, the children "are getting over the chincofe. I desire a paper of lozenges for them"; and on 30 June, the children are better, but the smallpox is still in the village. It was probably from the latter disease that many were dying.

In Dr Walter Harris's *Acute Diseases of Infants*[3], the convulsive or suffocative coughs are mentioned in one place without being identified as chincough, while in two or three other places the malady is briefly referred to under its name. Thus, "corpulent and fat infants troubled with defluxions, and having an

tethe, ytchinge of the gummes, fevers, crampes and laskes. When they waxe elder, than be they greved with kernelles, opennesse of the mould of the head, shortnesse of wynde, the stone of the bladder, wormes of the bealy, waters, swellynges under the chynne, and in Englande commonly purpyles, measels and small pockes."

[1] *Obs. Med.* 3rd ed. Bk. IV. chap. v. § 8; *Epist. Respons.* I. § 42.

[2] Mary Barker at Hambleton, to Abel Barker at the Dog and Ball in Fleet Street. *Hist. MSS. Commis.* v. 398.

[3] *Tractatus de morbis acutis infantum.* Lond. 1689. Englished by W. Cockburn, M.D. London, 1693, pp. 38, 78, 87.

open mould, are most subject to the rickets, chincough, king's evil, and almost incurable thrushes." Again, chincough of infants is one of the inflammatory diseases that are "not altogether free from contagion"; and again: "Albeit that any notable translation of the subject matter of the fever into the lungs, and chincoughs, do advise bloodletting for the youngest infants, yet it is most evident that it is not a remedy naturally convenient for them....And therefore its help is not to be invoked for all the diseases of infants except in the chincough or any other coughs that do attend and are concomitants of fevers that do suddenly begin"—showing his deference to Sydenham, his master.

Probably the "any other coughs" are those that he thus describes in another place (p. 26):

> "Moreover he is often troubled with a slight, dry cough, though sometimes it is strangling and suffocative : with a dry cough because of the sharpness and acrimony of the humours that continually prickle the most sensible branches of the windpipe ; but the choaking doth proceed from the abundance of serous and watry humours that so fill up and burden the small vesicles of the lungs that it cannot be cast off and discharged. But also they being endued with a great debility and weakness of nerves, and a superlative softness and delicacy of constitution, they are not able to subsist with that violent trouble of coughing, but do succumb under that unnatural and excessive motion of their breast, and their face is blackish as that of strangled people."

These were cases of whooping-cough, although they are not so called. Among his eleven cases, Harris gives two in infants of the Marquis of Worcester; one had been "very often troubled with an acute fever," and was found to be much weakened by a chincough when the physician was called to him; the other, an infant of eleven months, had at the same time an acute fever "and a cough almost convulsive."

This inclusion, under the generic name of cough, of cases that had all the signs of whooping-cough, namely, the paroxysmal seizures, choking fits, and blackness of the face, is found also in the London bills of mortality. Although "coughs" are entered as the cause of a not very large number of deaths in the earlier annual bills, with an occasional special mention of whooping-cough among them, it is not until 1701 that "hooping cough and chincough" becomes a separate item, with six deaths in the year; next year the entry is "hooping cough" alone, with a single death, and so on for a number of years in which the deaths are counted by units; in 1716 they rise to eleven, and continue to be counted by tens until 1730, when 152 deaths are set down to "cough, chincough, and whooping-cough." It would be a mistake to suppose that these figures during the first thirty years of the 18th century are anything like a correct measure of the number of infants in London who suffered from whooping-cough, or are at all near the number who might have reasonably been returned as dying from it. It was in that generation that the entries of the Parish Clerks became most indefinite as to the causes of death in infants, five-sixths of the enormous total of deaths under two years being entered under the generic head of "convulsions" and "teeth," while the item "chrysoms" received the deaths under one month old.

The increase of whooping-cough in the following table, from units to tens, from tens to hundreds, and thereafter to a somewhat steady total of hundreds year after year, can hardly be explained except on the hypothesis of more exact classification of infantile deaths, corresponding to the actual decline of the article "convulsions" in the second half of the century.

Years	Whooping-cough	Years	Whooping-cough	Years	Whooping-cough
1701	6	1731	33	1761	197
1702	1	1732	65	1762	300
1703	5	1733	97	1763	291
1704	0	1734	139	1764	251
1705	0	1735	81	1765	225
1706	2	1736	130	1766	213
1707	3	1737	160	1767	364
1708	3	1738	69	1768	262
1709	1	1739	72	1769	318
1710	5	1740	280	1770	218
1711	7	1741	109	1771	249
1712	3	1742	122	1772	385
1713	6	1743	92	1773	235
1714	6	1744	46	1774	554
1715	7	1745	135	1775	206
1716	11	1746	95	1776	181
1717	15	1747	151	1777	529
1718	24	1748	150	1778	379
1719	17	1749	82	1779	268
1720	33	1750	55	1780	573
1721	20	1751	275	1781	165
1722	21	1752	188	1782	78
1723	38	1753	65		
1724	25	1754	336	(Continued in the table	
1725	53	1755	93	of measles deaths, p.	
1726	37	1756	199	655)	
1727	67	1757	239		
1728	21	1758	84		
1729	35	1759	227		
1730	152	1760	414		

(Continued in the table of measles deaths, p. 655)

It is not without significance that the vital statistics of Sweden were the first to give whooping-cough something like its rightful place among infantile causes of death : from 1749 to 1764 the deaths set down to that cause were 42,393, or an annual average of 2600, the epidemic year 1755 having 5832. In this we should find merely the influence of systematic nomenclature. Nosology, or the scientific classification of diseases, may be said to have begun under Linnaeus, who was for many years professor of medicine at Upsala before he became professor of botany, and was teaching a somewhat rudimentary nosology to the Swedish students of medicine before the great work of his friend and correspondent Sauvages made classifications general.

Concerning the year 1751, which has 275 deaths from whooping-cough in the London bills, Fothergill writes in May : "Great numbers of children had the hooping cough, both in London and several adjacent villages, in a violent degree. Strong, sanguine, healthy children seemed to suffer most by it ; and to some of them it proved fatal where it was neglected or improperly managed"—the deaths having become more numerous towards the end of the year[1]. At Edinburgh, during the second year of high mortalities in the famine-period 1740–41, whooping-cough has 101 deaths to 112 from measles, having had only a fourth part as many the year before (see p. 523). In the Kilmarnock register from 1728 to 1763, "kinkhost" is credited with a total of 116 deaths, about 3 on an annual average, measles having a total of 93 during the same thirty-six years. In Holy Cross parish, a suburb of Shrewsbury, chincough has 9 deaths in the ten years 1750–60, and 6 in the next ten years, measles having 4 and 15 in the respective periods, and convulsions 9 and 31. In Ackworth parish, chincough has no deaths in the ten years 1747–57, and 2 in the next ten years, "infancy" having 13 in each decade, "convulsions" and measles none in the first, 6 and 2 respectively in the second. Warrington, in the disastrous smallpox year, 1773, had 16 deaths from chincough and 34 from convulsions. In the two years 1772 and 1773, Chester had 33 and 10 deaths from chincough, 70 and 69 from convulsions, 17 and 13 from "weakness of infancy."

Watt's researches in the registers of all the Glasgow burial-grounds brought out the fact that whooping-cough during a

---

[1] *Gent. Magaz.* 1751, pp. 195, 578.

period of thirty years, 1783 to 1812, had been a common and somewhat steady cause of death among infants, having made 4·51 per cent. of the annual total of deaths at all ages in the first six years of the period, and 5·57 per cent. in the last six years[1]. This was a higher annual average ratio than in the London bills for the same period (see the tables at p. 647 and p. 655), and was probably the maximum in Britain, inasmuch as the Glasgow death-rate of infants was the worst from all causes.

Whooping-Cough in Modern Times.

When the causes of death began to be registered, in July, 1837, whooping-cough was found to have the following relative place among the principal maladies of children during the latter six months of the year in London and in all England and Wales.

Mortality by diseases oj Children, last six months of 1837.

	London	England and Wales
Convulsions	1717	10729
Measles	1354	4732
Whooping-Cough	1066	3044
Smallpox	763	5811
Scarlatina	418	2550

Throughout the whole registration period, whooping-cough has kept its place steadily among the chief causes of infant mortality, neither decreasing nor increasing notably in the successive periods from 1837 to the present time. Its mortality has varied a good deal from year to year, owing to occasional great epidemic years such as 1866 and 1878; but on the mean annual average of decennial periods, it has varied little :

Annual Deaths by Whooping-cough per million living at all ages.

	Males	Females	Both sexes
1851–60	460	545	503
1861–70	487	566	527
1871–80	474	547	512
1881–90	—	—	451

No other epidemic malady has shown the same excess of female deaths in proportion to the numbers of the sex living, diphtheria being the only other that shows an excess at all

[1] *Treatise on Chincough.* Glasgow, 1813.

The excess of deaths by whooping-cough among female infants was roughly shown by Watt in 1813, viz. 975 females to 842 males in the registers of the Glasgow High Church, College Church and the North-Western Cemetery, the relative numbers of the sexes living at the respective ages being then unknown. In all Scotland in 1889 the ratio was 1043 male deaths to 1225 female. The singular difference between the sexes in this respect is almost certainly related to the corresponding differences in the formation and development of the larynx, the organ which gives character, at least, to the convulsive cough of children. The expansion of the larynx in boys, which becomes so obvious at puberty and remains so distinctive of the male sex, is one of those secondary sexual characters which begin to differentiate quite early in life, and are probably congenital to some extent. It is not known whether female children are more often attacked than males; but it is probable that they are predisposed both to acquire coughs of the convulsive suffocative kind and to have their lives shattered by the attack—for the same anatomical and physiological reasons, namely, the imperfect development of the posterior space of the glottis with the spasmodic closure by reflex action[1]. The deaths have been nearly all under the age of five.

Deaths by Whooping-cough per million living at the respective age-periods.

	0—5	5—10
1851–60	3624	174
1861–70	3766	152
1871–80	3652	135

These proportions are almost the same as those given by Watt in 1813 from three of the Glasgow registers.

Period	Deaths by whooping-cough	Under five	Five to ten	Above ten
1783–1812	1817	1713	98	3

[1] Vierordt, *Physiologie des Kindesalters*, Tübingen, 1877, p. 82, without adducing evidence that the larynx is congenitally different in the two sexes (a matter of very nice measurements which even Beneke does not appear to have attempted), says that the development of the posterior glottidean space has advanced before puberty much more in boys than in girls. Stark, a former Superintendent of Statistics for Scotland (*Rep. Reg. Gen. Scot. for* 1856, p. xxxviii), has raised the question thus : "The causes of this greater liability of the female sex to death while suffering from whooping-cough are worthy of being investigated. So far as one's own limited experience goes, it would appear to be produced by the greater tendency which the female sex exhibits to have fits or convulsions when attacked by a paroxysm or fit of coughing in that disease."

Most of the deaths are in the first year, and in a rapidly declining ratio until the fifth, according to the following rates per million of male children living at each age-period (these figures are for a single year, 1882):

Under one	One to two	Two to three	Three to four	Four to five
3039	2115	826	433	248

The mortality from whooping-cough falls very unequally on town and country. Thus, in Scotland in 1889, it caused 2268 deaths, being 3·13 per cent. of the deaths from all causes, and equivalent to a rate of ·58 per 1000 living. The death-rate varied as follows: ·91 in the eight principal towns, ·46 in the group of large towns, ·45 in the group of small towns, ·25 in the mainland rural districts, and ·08 in the insular rural districts. In England, the capital has more than its share of deaths from whooping-cough, Lancashire coming next, while the death-rates of Monmouthshire, Cornwall and Warwickshire are also a good deal above the mean of the whole country. The lowest death-rates are found in the purely agricultural counties.

During the last half-century there has been a decline in the death-rate from all causes, including the infectious diseases as a group; but it can hardly be said that whooping cough has had a due share in this decline. Notably in Ireland, where the decline of infectious disease has been most marked, it has been, as it were, pushed to the front of its class by the shrinkage of the other items. In Scotland it is now decidedly at the head of the list, and in England it has shared the first place with measles since the great diminution of scarlatina deaths.

Annual average Death-rates per 100,000 living.

		Whooping-cough	Measles	Scarlatina
England	1871–80	51·2	37·7	71·6
	1881–90	45·1	44·1	33·8
Scotland	1871–80	63·1	37·0	79·5
	1881–90	60·7	38·3	28·8
Ireland	1871–80	34·8	21·0	43·5
	1881–90	28·5	19·2	20·8

There is a small decrease in the death-rate of whooping-cough within the last decennial period, whereas in that of measles there is a slight increase (except in Ireland). The comparative steadiness of whooping-cough among the causes of death is doubtless owing to the fact that the bulk of its fatalities

C. II. 43

are among infants, and that there appears to be an irreducible minimum of the deaths from all causes at that age-period.

Whooping-Cough as a Sequel of other Maladies.

Although it is convenient to group whooping-cough among the infectious diseases, and although it is a clear case of a malady that comes in epidemics, yet its pathology is peculiar. It seems to be more a sequel of other diseases than an independent or primary affection. The whoop of the breath, from which it is named, is really proper to any convulsive cough of some infants or children. Adults, having undergone the change in the form and relative size of the larynx at puberty, have the convulsive cough usually without the whoop if they have it at all. After the successive influenzas of recent years (1889–92), many adults suffered from convulsive paroxysmal cough which was whooping-cough in all respects but the whoop, the choking fits, the blackness of the face, and the vomiting being, of course, all kept in subjection by the greater control of adults over their reflex actions.

It has been often remarked that the ordinary whooping-cough of children has followed epidemics of influenza, or widely prevalent catarrhs. Thus, Hillary records in July, 1753, an epidemic of whooping-cough, or "the fertussis," all over the island of Barbados following the epidemic catarrh which was at a height in January of the same year. Whooping-cough had not been known in the island for many years past, "neither could I find by the strictest inquiry that I could make that any child or elder person did bring it hither[1]." Willan, in his corresponding records of the succession of diseases at the Carey Street Dispensary, London, from 1796 to 1800, has the following :

"There was also among infants and children during the month of January [1796], an epidemic catarrh attended with a watery discharge from the eyes and nostrils, a frequent though slight cough, a shortness of breath, or rather panting, a flushing of the cheeks, great languor with disposition to sleep, and a quick small irregular pulse.... It was succeeded in February by the hooping cough."

Measles, which is usually a catarrhal malady, has undoubtedly been followed by whooping-cough in many individual cases and in epidemics as a whole ; and it may be that there is a closer association of whooping-cough with measles than with any other

---

[1] *Changes in the Air, &c....in Barbadoes.* Lond. 1760.

infectious disease. In the table on p. 647, the deaths by whooping cough in London from 1731 to 1830 have been reduced to ratios per cent. of the deaths from all causes, in a parallel column with the ratios of measles; it will be seen that the increase of both is equally remarkable towards the end of the table. But the Glasgow ratios abstracted by Watt show no such decided increase of whooping-cough from 1783 to 1812, side by side with the astonishing increase of measles; while his annual bills for the same period show that there were many deaths from whooping-cough in Glasgow for years before measles began to replace smallpox or to divide the mortality with it. The first high monthly mortalities from whooping-cough in Watt's bills were from November, 1785, to the end of 1786; but there had been so little measles for twenty-four months before that epidemic began, that only one death from it is recorded all the time. Again, the great measles epidemic of 1808 in Glasgow was indeed followed by many deaths from whooping-cough in 1809; but, while the height of the measles epidemic was in May and June, 1808, it was not until April, 1809, that whooping-cough began to cause many deaths.

Glasgow: Deaths by measles and whooping-cough.

	Whooping-cough	Measles		Whooping cough	Measles
1807			**1809**		
Nov.	18	2	Jan.	7	4
Dec.	18	1	Feb.	6	4
			March	7	2
1808			April	16	1
Jan.	10	2	May	22	4
Feb.	20	2	June	25	4
March	12	5	July	22	6
April	18	71	Aug.	15	2
May	9	259	Sept.	35	4
June	9	260	Oct.	23	1
July	2	118	Nov.	36	2
Aug.	2	32	Dec.	45	10
Sept.	2	22	**1810**		
Oct.	2	10	Jan.	33	4
Nov.	4	4	Feb.	32	4
Dec.	2	2	March	19	3

Whatever correspondence or relation there may be between measles and whooping-cough, (and it has been remarked by many in the ordinary way of experience), it eludes the method

of statistics[1].   As for the catarrhs of infants and children other
than those which are part of the actual attack of measles or
influenza, they are so common from year to year, and even
from month to month, (perhaps coincident with teething, or
with chicken-pox or other slight febrile disturbance), that a
statistical study of whooping-cough in relation to them could
lead only to an empirical, and possibly bewildering, result.   It
may be more useful to consider the antecedent probability of
some such relationship, arising out of the pathology of the
convulsive cough.

Whooping-cough is not only a paroxysmal cough coming on
in convulsive fits at intervals, but the paroxysms, as they recur
for many weeks, or, as they say in Japan, "for a hundred days,"
have none of the obvious occasions of coughing, such as catarrh
of the mucous membrane, congestion of the lungs from hot or
close air, irritation of the bronchial tubes from dusty particles or
vapours, or the presence of tubercles in the substance of the
lungs.   Such irritants can, indeed, produce whooping-cough, as
in the following instance of "artificial chincough" related by
Watt:

> Two children having quarrelled in their play, one of them thrust a handful
> of sawdust into the mouth of the other.   Some of the sawdust passed
> into the windpipe.   After a short time the child began to have violent
> convulsive fits of coughing, in which the whoop was very distinctly formed.
> Expectoration in the course of a few hours removed all the irritation, and the
> coughing thereupon ceased.

But in natural or ordinary whooping-cough there is no
mechanical irritation, there is nothing to cough up, the reflex
action, violent and paroxysmal though it be, has apparently no
motive.   I have, in another work, offered an original explanation
of the paroxysmal cough of children as being the deferred
reaction, the postponed liability, the stored-up memory, of some
past catarrhal or otherwise irritated state of the respiratory
organs, to which I refer without attempting to summarize it
here[2].

[1] In the Irish Decennial Summary for 1871–80 (*Suppl. to 17th Report of Reg.-Gen. Ireland*, 1884) it is said : " A general relation has been noticed by many observers between the prevalence of whooping-cough and measles, and there is no doubt that in many localities an epidemic of measles is frequently accompanied by or followed by a prevalence of whooping-cough.   A comparison of the figures in Table XV. does not point to any very close relationship.   Whooping-cough was a much more fatal disease than measles, but it is more than probable that measles was equally prevalent."
[2] *Illustrations of Unconscious Memory in Disease.*   London, 1886 [1885]. Chapter VI. pp. 64–83.

The epidemicity of whooping-cough presents no more difficulty if the malady be viewed as the sequel or dregs of something else than if it be taken for an independent primary affection. The many infants and children that suffer from it together may have equally been suffering together from one or other of the various things of which it is assumed to be the sequel—influenza, measles, sore-throat, the bronchitis of rickets, simple bronchial catarrh of the winter, simple coryza. Again, it may be a secondary or residual affection with many, but a communicable disease to others. Much of the whooping-cough of an epidemic is believed by good authorities, such as Bouchut and Struges[1], to be simply mimetic, or a habit of coughing acquired by hearing other children coughing in a particular way, just as chorea is sometimes acquired in schools or hospital-wards through the mere spectacle of it. But it may be doubted whether much of the whooping-cough which swells the bills of mortality is acquired in that way. The children that die of it are probably most of them such as had only escaped dying of the measles or other infective disease, or of the non-specific catarrh, which had preceded the whooping-cough.

[1] *Med. Times and Gaz.* 1885, II. p. 6.

CHAPTER VII.

SCARLATINA AND DIPHTHERIA.

SCARLATINA and diphtheria have to be taken together in a historical work for the reason that certain important epidemics of the 18th century, both in Britain and in the American colonies, which were indeed the first of the kind in modern English experience, cannot now be placed definitely under the one head or the other, nor divided between the two. It may be that this ambiguity lies actually in the complex or undifferentiated nature of the throat-distemper at that time, or that it arises out of the contemporary manner of making and recording observations upon the prevalent maladies of seasons. The older or Hippocratic method was not unlike the mason's rule of lead, said to have been in use in the island of Lesbos for measuring uneven stones; it took account of gradations, modifications, affinities, being careless of symmetry, of definitions or clean-cut nosological ideas, or the dividing lines of a classification. Sydenham was the great English exponent of this method; but, in one of his more discursive passages, he sketched out another method of describing diseases as if they were species or natural kinds[1]. He did no more than indicate this analogy, at the same time declining to put it in practice; so that Sauvages correctly described his great Nosology of 1763 as being constructed "juxta Sydenhami mentem et Botanicorum ordinem." The identification of scarlatina in its modern sense, including scarlatina simplex and scarlatina anginosa, falls really in the time of the nosologies in the generation following the work of Sauvages, although both the name and definition in the modern

---

[1] Preface to 3rd ed. of *Obs. Med.*, Greenhill's ed. p. 16.

sense were used in England as early as 1749. On the other hand, the name and definition of diphtheria were little known until about the years 1856–59, when the form of throat-distemper which is now quite definitely joined to that name became suddenly common, having been almost unheard of for at least two generations before. The only English writer who has attempted to unravel the accounts of the 18th century epidemics of throat-disease was Dr Willan in his unfinished work on Cutaneous Diseases, 1808; he swept the whole of those epidemic types into the species of scarlatina, to which also he reduced the great Spanish epidemics of "garrotillo" in the 16th and 17th centuries. Whether he would have used so summary a method if he had seen the sudden return of diphtheria in 1856, may well be doubted; at all events the German writers who brought their erudition to bear upon the question of identity some thirty years ago have discovered true diphtheria among the 18th century throat-distempers, although no two of them agree as to which of these should be called diphtheria and which scarlatina anginosa. It is one advantage of a historical method that the complexities of things may be stated just as they are, with due criticism, naturally, of the matters of fact and of the relative credit of observers. The result is more an impression than a logical conclusion,—an impression which will take a colour from the pre-existing views or theoretical preferences of individual readers on such points as fixity of type or the incompetence of the earlier observers. An author who has puzzled over these difficulties in detail can hardly help having a tolerably definite impression of the real state of the case; and I do not seek to conceal mine, namely, that scarlatina anginosa and diphtheria were not in nature so sharply differentiated in the 18th century as they have been since 1856.

The significant name of *pestis gutturuosa* or plague of the throat is given by the St Albans chronicler to the great pestilence, or some part of it, in 1315–16, during one of the worst periods of famine and murrain in the whole English history. But those two words being all that we have to base upon, there is no use speculating whether the disease was scarlatina anginosa, or diphtheria, or something different from either. This is perhaps the only reference to an epidemic throat-distemper in England for several centuries in which bubo-plague was the grand infection. In the popular medical handbooks of the Tudor period one naturally looks for scarlatina among the diseases of children.   In Elyot's *Castel of Health* (1541), "the purpyles" is mentioned among children's maladies in company with smallpox and measles, and the same name is in the London bills of mortality from their beginning in 1629, although it does not appear whether the deaths assigned to it were of children or adults.   Perhaps the most common use of purples in the 17th and 18th centuries was for a form of childbed fever often attended with discoloured miliary vesicles.   In Scotland, according to Sibbald (1684), "the fevers called purple" were any fevers, even measles or smallpox, in which livid or dark spots occurred as an occasional thing.   Unless a few scarlatinal deaths are included under "purples" in the London bills (they could not have been many in any case), there is no other evidence of their existence until 1703, when the entry of scarlet fever appears for the first time, with seven deaths to it in the year.   The heading remains in the bills until 1730 (the deaths never more than one figure), after which it is merged with fevers in general.   The same indications of the insignificance of scarlatina among the causes of death in the 17th century may be got from the medical writers in London.

Sydenham introduced into the third edition (1675) of his *Observationes Medicae* a short chapter entitled "Febris Scarlatina[1]."   It was a disease that might occur at any time of the year, but occurred mostly in the end of summer, sometimes infesting whole families, the children more than the elders.   It began with a rigor, as other fevers did, the malaise being but slight.   Then the whole skin became interspersed with small red spots, more numerous, broader, redder and less uniform than in measles; they persisted for two or three days and then vanished, and, as the cuticle returned to its natural state, there were successive desquamations of fine branny scales, which he compares elsewhere to those following the measles of 1670. Sydenham took it to be a moderate effervescence of the blood from the heat of the summer just over, or from some such excitement.   It was a mild affair, not calling for blood-letting nor cardiac remedies, and requiring no other regimen than abstinence from flesh and spirituous liquors, and that the patient should keep in doors, but not all day in bed.   The disease, he says, amounted to hardly more than a name (*hoc morbi nomen,*

[1] *Sydenhami Opera*, ed. Greenhill, 1844, p. 243.

vix enim altius assurgit); but it appears that it was sometimes fatal; and in those cases Sydenham was inclined, after his wont, to blame the fussiness of the medical attendant (*nimia medici diligentia*). If convulsions or coma preceded the eruption, a large epispastic should be applied to the back of the neck and paregoric administered. Whether Sydenham was describing true scarlatina simplex, or a "scarlatiniform variety of contagious roseola," it is from him that we derive the name of scarlatina by continuous usage to the present time[1].

A few years after Sydenham had thus described scarlatina, Sir Robert Sibbald, physician and naturalist of Edinburgh, professed to have discovered the same as a new species of disease. "Just as the luxury of men," he says, "increases every day, so there grow up new diseases, if not unknown to former generations, yet untreated of by them. Nor is this surprising, since new depravations of the humours arise from unwonted diets and from various mixtures of the same. Among the many diseases which owe their origin to this age, there has been most recently (*nuperrime*) observed a fever which is called *Scarlatina*, from the carmine colour (named by our people in the vernacular *scarlet*) with which almost the whole skin is tinged. Of this disease the observations are not so many that an accurate theory can be delivered or a method of cure constructed." He proceeds to append one case—a child of eight, daughter of one of the senators of the College of Justice, who fell ill with redness of the face (thought at first to indicate smallpox coming on), became delirious and restless, then had the redness all over, which disappeared and left the child well about the fifth day. He had heard from some of his colleagues that the scarlet rash was sometimes interspersed with vesicles—perhaps the *miliaria* so much in evidence a generation or two later. In adults, Sibbald had seen the cuticle fall from nearly the whole body. But extremely few (*paucissimi*) had died of this fever. Like Sydenham, he omits to mention sore-throat and dropsy[2].

[1] Maton, *Med. Trans. Col. Phys.* v., having seen an extensive epidemic attended by a red rash in one of the great public schools, was disposed to erect it into a new type of roseola, owing to its mildness, while he admitted that it was the same as Sydenham's scarlatina simplex. Macmichael (*New View of the Infection of Scarlet Fever*, 1822, p. 78) thought that this was "rather a proof of extreme refinement," and that there was no need to give it a new designation. Gee, *Brit. Med. Journ.*, 1883, II. 236, cites this "refinement" of Maton's as one of the noteworthy things in the history of the diseases of children in this country.

[2] Sir Robert Sibbald, M.D., *Scotia Illustrata, sive Prodromus Historiae Naturalis.* Edin. 1684. Lib. II. cap. 5, p. 55.

Another 17th century reference is by Morton, who practised in London, in Newgate Street, from about 1667 to the end of the century, and was frequently called to consult with apothecaries or other physicians in cases of sickness in middle-class families.   In the second volume of his *Pyretologia*, published in 1694, he has a chapter " De Morbillis et Febre Scarlatina," and a separate chapter "De Febre Scarlatina."   His position towards scarlet fever is peculiar.   He uses the name, he says, in deference to the common consent of physicians, but, for his own part, he thinks scarlatina different from measles only in the form of the rash, so-called scarlatina being confluent measles just as there is a confluent smallpox.   Except in that sense he sees no reason for retaining scarlatina in the catalogue of diseases.   Both arise from the same cause, both have hacking cough, heaviness of the brain, sneezing, diarrhoea; the single difference is that in scarlatina the rash is continuous.   He gives eleven cases, most of which are clearly enough cases of measles; but the fourth case, that of his own daughter, Marcia, aged seven, in 1689, " in quo febris dicta Scarlatina, tempore praesertim aestivo, quadantenus publice grassabatur," had no cough, nor redness of the eyes, nor diarrhoea, nor any other catarrhal symptoms (such as her sister had in 1685), but on the fourth day a continuous scarlet rash over the whole skin, which ended, not in a desquamation of fine branny scales, but in parchment-like peeling. The eleventh instance is complex enough to show that Morton had some reason, at that early stage in the history of scarlatina, for hesitating to make the disease a distinct type under a name of its own.

About midsummer, 1689, he was called to the house of his friend Mr Hook, merchant, of Pye Alley, Fenchurch Street, and found the whole household, three young girls, one little boy, and their aunt Mrs Barnardiston, a matron aged seventy, all suffering from the effects of some infection of as deleterious a kind as synochus, the symptoms being hacking cough, coma, delirium, and other signs of malignity.   But on the 4th, 5th, or 6th day, each had a scarlatinal rash all over the skin, which lasted until the 7th, 8th or 10th day.   Two of the girls, and the boy, had " on the 4th or 5th day of the efflorescence" extensive parotid swellings, difficulty of swallowing, vibrating arteries, and other urgent symptoms, for which they were blooded. The parotid abscesses burst, and discharged a copious acrid, corrosive pus by the nostrils, ears and throat, for the space of thirty days, during which the patients gradually got well.   The third girl had, on the 3rd or 4th day of the rash, a painful swelling in the left armpit, not unlike a bubo ; she also was blooded, and recovered completely, the swelling having broken and discharged pus for many days.   The case of the aunt, aged seventy, was somewhat different ; she neglected her medicines, acquired a " carcinoma" or slough over the pubes, which became gangrenous, recovered with difficulty, and lived three years longer.

Morton calls these cases a veritable *pestis* or plague; and he goes on in the same context to say: "what swellings have I seen of the uvula, fauces, nares, and how protracted! At other times, what turgid lips, covered with sordid crusts and ulcerated!"—instancing the child of Mr Blaney, who had these symptoms long after the efflorescence, together with fever and coma[1]. These cases, all given under the eleventh history illustrating the chapter on Scarlatina, are perhaps not different from those which Huxham, next in order, described in 1735, but not under the same name. It would appear from a reference in Hamilton's essay on Miliary Fever, published in 1710, that scarlet fever continued to be seen in London: "If, in a scarlet fever, miliary pustules should arise, dying away with a red colour, they promise safety[2]."

Several of the annalists of epidemic constitutions agree as to fatal anginas in the year 1727, with an exanthem of the miliary kind. Wintringham, of York, mentions the two things apart—in one place a putrid fever with cutaneous eruptions of a fuscous colour, sometimes dry, sometimes filled with a clear serum; in another place, "about this time many anginas were prevalent, attended with extreme suffocation, which proved fatal unless they were speedily relieved." He mentions the same putrid fever in the summer of 1728, and again anginae. Hillary, who was then at Ripon, gives the same fever in 1727 (or perhaps in 1726) with miliary eruption, and chronicles "a fatal suffocative quinsey" in the winter of 1727–28, of which many died, especially those that had been reduced by the fever. Huxham's account of an epidemic malady of the throat and neck at Plymouth in January and February, 1728, might relate to mumps (which Hillary and an Edinburgh observer describe clearly enough under 1731); and under October, 1728, he describes an erysipelatous and petechial fever, often relieved by an eruption of red miliary vesicles accompanied by sweats, the same miliary fever being again common in the autumn of 1729. This association

---

[1] Richard Morton, M.D. *Pyretologia.* 2 vols. London, 1692–94, II. 69.

[2] Engl. transl. 1737, p. 80. The reference by Dover (*Ancient Physician's Legacy,* 1732, p. 117), is almost in the words of Sydenham, his master: "This is a fever of a milder kind than the measles [of which latter he did not remember anyone's dying till about twenty-five years since], and does not want the assistance of a doctor. The skin seems to be universally inflamed, but the inflammation goes off in forty-eight hours."

of "putrid" fever with sore-throat became still more notable in the period 1750–60.

These anginas of 1727–28 are unimportant compared with the outbreak a few years later. We hear first from Edinburgh in June, 1733, of scarlet fever and sore throats frequent in several parts of the country near the city, and continuing all through the summer into the winter and spring of 1734[1]. Then in April, 1734, begins a series of important notes by Huxham at Plymouth[2]. In that month, he says, there began a certain anginose fever ("for so I shall call it"), raging more and more every day. It mostly affected children and young people. Among other symptoms were vomiting and diarrhœa, pain and swelling of the fauces, languor, anxiety, delirium or stupor, a favourable issue being attended with sweats and red pustules. In May it was raging worse, with more severe angina and most troublesome "aphthae." In June it was now miliary-pustular, and not seldom erysipelatous, while the throat was "less oppressed." On the 6th or 7th day the cuticle looked rough and broken as if thickly sprinkled with bran; at length the whole desquamated—sometimes the entire skin of the sole of the foot coming off. The more copious the rash, the better the chance for life. It was contagious, affecting several in the same house. In July it cut off several within six days of the onset. Huxham's references to this putrid miliary fever in Devon and Cornwall go on for some time, without farther mention of the throat complication. In April, 1735, "raro nunc adest strangulans faucium dolor, paucaeque nunc erumpunt pustulae." But, in September, 1736, he enters again, "febres miliares, scarlatinae, pustulosae," often attended with swelling of the parotid glands and of the fauces, and with profuse sweats.

The most important scene of fatal angina with rash in the same period (1734–35) was the North American colonies. Before coming to that remarkable outburst, I shall mention one curious coincident outbreak in the island of Barbados. Dr Warren, who occupies his pen chiefly with yellow fever, says[3]: "In this space of time [1734 to 1738], there arose here a few other diseases, that were really epidemical and of the contagious kind too, few escaping them in families where they had once got

---

[1] *Edin. Med. Essays and Obs.* III. 26.
[2] *Obs. de aere et morb. epid.*
[3] H. Warren, M.D., *On the Malignant Fever in Barbados.* London, 1740, p. 73.

a footing. The first was an obstinate and ill-favour'd erysipe-latous quinsey. The second a very anomalous scarlet fever, in which almost all the skin, even of the hands and feet, peeled off,"—just as Huxham described for Devonshire.

It is beyond our purpose to include the evidence from foreign countries; but it may be noted in this context that Le Cat, in tracing the antecedents of the great Rouen fever in his paper of 1754, refers to many fatal anginas in that city about twenty years before[1]. Thus we find about the year 1735 evidence of the beginning of a remarkable "constitution" of throat-disease both in the old world and in the new. But the facts in America stand out with peculiar prominence, and shall be given on the threshold of the subject as fully as possible.

The Throat-distemper of New England, 1735–36.

The accounts of the great wave of "throat-distemper" that spread over the towns and villages of New England in 1735 are singularly clear and even numerically precise. The arrival of this sickness is one of the most definite incidents in the whole history of epidemics; it was hardly possible for the common belief, whether popular or professional, to have been mistaken about it. Just a hundred years had passed since the first settlement of the Puritans on Massachusetts Bay and along the Connecticut river; Boston had grown to a town of some 12,000 inhabitants, and many small towns and townships had sprung up along the coast and in the interior. The population was still sparse, although it was growing rapidly from within; it is difficult to believe that even the largest towns could then have deserved the strictures which Noah Webster passed upon them two generations later[2].

In the mother country at that time, smallpox was the great infectious malady of infancy and childhood. It was not unknown in the colonies, Boston having had epidemics in 1721,

---

[1] Le Cat, in *Phil. Trans.* XLIX. 49: In 1736 and 1737, a prevalence of gangrenous sore-throats which chiefly attacked children. They reappeared in 1748 in young persons of the first distinction, not only at Rouen, but also at St Cyr, near Versailles, and at Paris.

[2] Webster, *Brief History of Epidemick and Pestilential Diseases.* Hartford, 1799, II. 253: "Away, then, with crowded cities—the thirty feet lots and alleys, the artificial reservoirs of filth, the hot-beds of atmospheric poison! Such are our cities—they are great prisons, built with immense labour to breed infection and hurrying mankind prematurely to the grave."

1730 and 1752, and Charleston an epidemic in 1738 after an almost free interval of thirty years. Even in the chief cities of the colonies such epidemics were only occasional, affecting adults and adolescents perhaps more than infants and as much as children; while in such a town as Hampton, for which the register was well kept from 1735, it is known that there were no smallpox deaths in the twenty years following, or until the period 1755–63, when four died of the disease, and that only one death from it occurred in the next recorded period of ten years, 1767 to 1776. It was in these circumstances of a growing population, almost untouched, at least in the inland towns, by the great infantile infectious malady of the old country, that the throat-distemper broke out and raged in the manner now to be described.

The disease "did emerge," as Douglass says, on the 20th of May, 1735, at Kingston township, some fifty miles to the east of Boston[1]. The first child seized died in three days; in about a week after three children in a family some four miles distant were successively seized, and all died on the third day; it continued to spread through the township, and Douglass was informed that of the first forty cases none recovered. It was vulgarly called the "throat illness" or "plague in the throat." Some died quickly as if from prostration, but most had "a symptomatic affection of the fauces or neck: that is, a sphacelation or corrosive ulceration in the fauces, or an infiltration and tumefaction in the chops and forepart of the neck, so turgid as to bring all upon a level between the chin and sternum, occasioning a strangulation of the patient in a very short time." In August it was at Exeter, a town six miles distant, but it did not appear at Chester, six miles to the westward, until October. After the first fatal outburst in Kingston township it became somewhat milder; but in the country districts of New Hampshire it was fatal to 1 in 3, or 1 in 4 of the sick, and in scarce any place to less than 1 in 6. This average was made up by its excessive fatality in some families; Boynton of Newbury Falls lost his eight children; at Hampton Falls twenty-seven died in five families. The following table, compiled by Fitch, minister of Portsmouth, shows the deaths from it in various

---

[1] W. Douglass, M.D., *The Practical History of a New Epidemical Eruptive Miliary Fever, with an Angina Ulcusculosa, which prevailed in New England in the years* 1735 *and* 1736. Boston, N.E. 1736. This rare essay was reprinted in the *New England Journ. of Med. and Surg.* XIV. 1 (Jan. 1825).

towns and townships of New Hampshire during fourteen months from May, 1735, to 26 July, 1736, with the ages[1]:

Deaths from the throat-distemper in 14 months, 1735–36 (Fitch).

	Under ten years	Ten to twenty	Twenty to thirty	Thirty to forty	Above forty	Total
Portsmouth	81	15	1	—	2	99
Dover	77	8	3	—	—	88
Hampton	37	8	8	1	1	55
Hampton Falls	160	40	9	1	—	220
Exeter	105	18	4	—	—	127
Newcastle	11	—	—	—	—	11
Gosport	34	2	—	—	1	37
Rye	34	10	—	—	—	44
Greenland	13	2	3	—	—	18
Newington	16	5	—	—	—	21
Newmarket	20	1	—	1	—	22
Stretham	18	—	—	—	—	18
Kingston	96	15	1	1	—	113
Durham	79	15	6	—	—	100
Chester	21	—	—	—	—	21
	802	139	35	4	4	984

The meaning of these figures in the townships of New Hampshire will appear from the case of Hampton. In the year 1736 its burials from all causes were 69, and its baptisms 50; while the throat-distemper alone, during fourteen months of that and the previous year, cut off 55. As we have seen, Hampton had no smallpox to ravage its children; but the throat-disease of 1735–36 had almost the same effect as the occasional disastrous epidemics of smallpox had upon English towns of a corresponding population or annual average of births.

This plague in the throat attacked the children of the most sequestered houses, especially those situated near rivers or lakes. It was least fatal to those who lived well, both Douglass and Colden assigning the salt diet, and other things likely to produce *psora*, as the reason of its greater severity. In the country districts or townships, in which the fatalities were most numerous, it would appear that an eruption, scarlet or other, was not only not the rule but even something of a rarity. Douglass, who was familiar with the exanthem in the Boston cases, assigns its absence in the country to a mistaken evacuant treatment, by which "the laudable and salutary cuticular eruption has been so perverted as to be noticeable only in a few, and in these it was called a scarlet fever."

[1] In Belknap's *History of New Hampshire.* Boston, 1791.

When the disease broke out in due course at Boston it proved much less malignant than in the country. The first case, on the 20th August, had white specks in the throat and an efflorescence of the skin. A few more soon followed in the same locality, of which none were fatal; they had soreness in the throat, the tonsils swelled and speckt, the uvula relaxed, a slight fever, a flush in the face and an erysipelas-like efflorescence on the neck and extremities. The first death was not until October, the disease becoming more frequent and more fatal in November, and reaching its worst in the second week of March, when the burials from all causes rose to 24, the average per week in an ordinary season being 10. The fatalities in Boston were so few for the enormous number of cases that many could scarce be persuaded that it was the same disease as in the Townships. In the corresponding weeks (1 Oct. to 11 May) of eight ordinary years preceding, the average deaths were 268, whites and slaves; during this sickness they were 382, or an excess of 114, which were probably all due to the throat-distemper, as many as 76 fatal cases having come to the knowledge of Douglass himself. He estimates the whole number of attacks at 4000, giving a ratio of one death in thirty-five cases; but it is clear that very slight cases of sore-throat were counted in.

The fatal cases in Boston seem to have shown a great range of malignant symptoms : "We have anatomically inspected persons who died of it with so intense a foetor from the violence of the disease that some practitioners could not continue in the room." Among the bad symptoms were the coming and going of the miliary eruption, dark livid colour of the same, the vesicles large, distinct and pale, like crystalline smallpox; an ichorous discharge from the nose; many mucous linings expectorated, resembling the cuticle raised by blisters; pus brought up where no sloughs could be seen in the fauces; extension to the bronchi, with symptoms of a New England quinsey (? croup); in some children, spreading ulcers behind the ears; the tongue throwing off a complete slough with marks of the papillae. Among the after-effects in severe cases were anasarca or dropsy of the skin, haemorrhages, urtications, serpiginous eruptions chiefly in the face, purulent pustules, boils, or imposthumations in the groins, armpits and other parts of the body, indurations of the front of the neck (the same by which many in the country were suffocated, and a few in Boston), hysteric symptoms in women, and epileptic fits.

Douglass gives special attention to the eruption, which he calls miliary in his title-page. Some had a sore-throat without any eruption, and a very few had an eruption with no affection of the throat beyond the tonsils and uvula swollen. In some the eruption preceded the soreness of the throat, in some the two came together, but in the general case the eruption was a little later than the affection in the throat. The ordinary course was a chill and shivering, spasmodic wandering pains, vomiting or at least nausea, pain, swelling and redness of the tonsils and uvula, with some white specks : then followed a flush in the face, with some miliary eruptions, attended by a benign mild fever; soon after, the miliary efflorescence appears on the neck, chest and extremities; on the third or fourth day the rash is at its height and well defined, with fair intervals; the flushing goes off gradually with a general itching, and in a day or two more the cuticle scales or peels off, especially in the extremities. At the same time the cream-coloured sloughs or specks on the fauces become loose and are cast off, and the swelling goes down. Where the miliary eruptions were considerable, the extremities peeled in scraps or strips like *exuviae*; in one or two, the nails of the fingers and toes were shed. Some who had little or no obvious eruption underwent a scaling or peeling of the cuticle.

The epidemic having spent its force upon the New England towns from the autumn of 1735 until the summer of 1736, gradually travelled westward, and was two years in reaching the Hudson River, distant only two hundred miles in a straight line from Kingston, where it first appeared in May, 1735. It continued its progress, with some interruptions, until it spread over the colonies from Pemaquid in 44° N. latitude to Carolina; and as Douglass, writing in 1736, had heard that "it is in our West India Islands," it was probably the same disease that Warren recorded for Barbados in the same years under the names of "an obstinate and ill-favour'd erysipelatous quinsey," and "a very anomalous scarlet fever"; and the same as the epidemic "sore-throats" that another records for the Virgin Islands in 1737[1].

Although it usually attacked several children in the same house, it did not seem to be communicable, like smallpox, from person to person or by the medium of infected clothes. The Boston physicians held a consultation on the point, and published their opinion that it proceeded entirely from "some occult quality of the air."

This was the first appearance of sore-throat with efflorescence of the skin among the English colonists of North America. For at least two generations after, the disease remained in the country, breaking out unaccountably from time to time at one place or another and often cutting off many children, but never so malignantly as at first[2]. Colden, writing from near New York in 1753, says:[3]

[1] *Gent. Magaz.* Feb. 1752, p. 73.
[2] The account by Kearsley, of Philadelphia, written about 1769 (*Gent. Magaz.* XXXIX. 251), refers to a great epidemic of throat-disease in New England in the spring, summer and autumn of 1746; but the date is almost certainly a mistake for 1736, as no such epidemic is known on contemporary authority.
[3] Cadwallader Colden, M.D. "Letter to Dr Fothergill on the Throat Distemper," dated New York, 1 Oct. 1753, in *Med. Obs. and Inquiries*, I. 211.

"Ever since I came into this part of the country where I live (now about fourteen years), it frequently breaks out in different families and places, without any previous observable cause, but does not spread as it did at first. Sometimes a few only have it in a considerable neighbourhood. It seems as if some seeds or leaven or secret cause remains wherever it goes; for I hear of the like observations in other parts of the country. Several have been observed to have it more than once... In different years and different persons the symptoms are various. In some seasons it has been accompanied with miliary eruptions all over the skin; and at such times the symptoms about the throat have been mild and the disease generally without danger if not ill treated. Some have had sores, like those on the tonsils, with a corrosive humour behind their ears, on the private and other parts of the body, sometimes without any ulceration in the throat" (case given of a child of ten with sores on the pudenda).

It was in 1754, the very next year after Colden wrote as above, that the second great epidemic of throat-distemper arose in New Hampshire and the neighbouring parts of Massachusetts. The figures of its mortality which have been preserved for the town of Hampton, New Hampshire, may serve as a sample of its prevalence subsequent to the original explosion of 1735–36. In the first epidemic, 1735–36, there died at Hampton of the throat-distemper, 55 persons, mostly children. In the second, from January 1754 to July 1755, there died of it 51 persons. The deaths from all causes in those two years were 85, and the births 70.

The following table shows the proportion of deaths from throat-distemper to the deaths from all causes in Hampton from 1735 to 1791[1].

Period	Deaths from throat-distemper	Deaths from all causes
1735–44	91	216
1745–54	60	221
1755–63	30	187
1764–66	—	—
1767–76	3	115
1777–86	7	99
1787–91	0	46

It was once more described, for New York city, by Dr Samuel Bard in 1771[2]. He identifies it with the disease described by Douglass in 1735, and gives an account of it on the whole like Colden's.

[1] Belknap, III. 421.

[2] Samuel Bard, M.D. "An Inquiry into the Nature, Cause and Cure of the Angina Suffocativa, or Sore throat Distemper, as it is commonly called by the inhabitants of this city and colony." *Trans. Amer. Philos. Soc.* I. (1769–1771). Philad. 1771, p. 322. What purports to be a translation of this, is given in Reutte's *Recueil d'Obs. sur le Croup* (Paris, 1810), the name of "croup" being introduced into the title, and some strange liberties taken with the text.

It was "uncommon and very dangerous," mostly a malady of children under ten. They drooped for several days, had a watery eye, then a bloated livid countenance, and a few red eruptions here and there on the face. This went on for three or four days, the throat meanwhile showing white specks on the tonsils. Sudden and great prostration ensued, with a peculiar hollow cough and tone of voice, or loss of voice, constant fever, especially nocturnal, and a degree of drowsiness. In fatal cases there was great restlessness and tossing of the limbs towards the end. In one family all the seven children took it one after another; three died out of the four elder; the three younger recovered, having had ulceration behind the ears, which continued for several weeks and rendered an acrid, corrosive ichor. Many other children had these ulcerations behind the ears, sometimes with swelling of the parotid and sublingual glands. The same ulcerations might occur also "in different parts of the body." Sloughs of the fauces and epiglottis extended as a membranous exudation into the trachea. Two cases occurred in women, one of them having assisted to lay out two children dead of the distemper.

The last time of its general spreading (within the period covered by Belknap's *History of New Hampshire,* 1791) was in 1784–85–86 and –87. It was first seen at Sandford in the county of York, and thence diffused itself very slowly through most of the towns of New England; but its virulence and the mortality which it caused were comparatively small[1].

Angina maligna in England from 1739.

Although there had been an extensive prevalence of angina with miliary or scarlet or erysipelatous rash in Devon and Cornwall in 1734 and following years, a slight amount of sore-throat with scarlet fever in and near Edinburgh in 1733, a great prevalence of throat-distemper with scarlet or miliary rash in the North American colonies in 1735–37, and an ill-favoured erysipelatous quinsy as well as an anomalous scarlet fever in Barbados, St Christopher, &c., during the same period, yet it

---

[1] The impression made upon modern historians by these American accounts of the throat-distemper has not always been the same. Hecker finds in the malady described by Douglass the form of *Frieselbräune*, or miliary diphtheria, a somewhat rare and sporadic malady; in the account by Bard, he finds *häutige Brandbräune*, or membranous angina maligna; while he finds in an account by Chalmers for Charleston, S. Carolina, in 1770, a third variety, *Friesel-Scharlachbräune*, or miliary scarlet angina. Again, Jaffe finds in the account by Bard "many analogies with the diphtheria of our own day." Hirsch identifies the throat-distemper of Douglass and Colden as "exquisite scarlet fever" and the disease described by Bard as diphtheria. Häser identifies the epidemic described by Douglass as diphtheria. Bard himself did not doubt that the disease which he saw in New York previous to 1771 was the same that Douglass saw at Boston in 1735–36. Hecker, *Geschichte der neueren Heilkunde.* Bk. I. chap. 8. Max Jaffe, "Die Diphtherie in epidemiol. u. nosol. Beziehung, &c." Original paper in *Schmidt's Jahrbücher,* CXIII. (1862), p. 97. Hirsch, 1st ed. of *Handb. der histor. geogr. Pathol.* I. 237, note 6; II. 125, note 4; and 2nd ed. III. 80. Eng. transl. Häser, *Geschichte, &c.* III. 471.

was not until the end of the year 1739 that cases more or less similar occurred in London. The incident that first drew attention to the throat-distemper in the capital was the death of the two sons of Henry Pelham, the colleague of his relative the Duke of Newcastle in the premiership[1]. Horace Walpole, writing twenty years after concerning similar calamities in the family of the Earl of Bessborough, says that not only Mr Pelham's two sons, but also two daughters and a daughter of the Duke of Rutland all died together. Chandler, writing in 1761, says that he well remembered the disease at the end of 1739. Early in 1740 he had in his own practice as an apothecary two cases of children sick in one family; the first died, and as he was at a loss to account for the death, there being "something in the whole of the case quite new and unknown to me," he called in Dr Letherland to see the other, who declared that the child would die also, as it did. Letherland then spoke to Chandler of the death of the two Pelhams shortly before, "of the alarm it caused all over this great city, both from its novelty and fatality," and of his own care and pains in turning over ancient and modern writers to see if he could trace any footsteps of this remarkable and terrible disease: at last, after long search, he had been so happy as to discover the identical disease circumstantially described in the Spanish writers[2].

The identification of the English throat-distemper of the 18th century with the *garrotillo* of Spain in the 16th and 17th centuries was thus undoubtedly due to Letherland, so far as English learning was concerned, and he received due credit for it in the Harveian Oration at the College of Physicians on the first occasion after his death[3].

Chandler thus described the state of the disease at its first breaking out in 1739:

"The first and common appearances are feverishness, sickness, vomiting or purging; the proper and diagnostic signs which follow are an ulcerous slough in some part of the fauces, discharging a fœtid matter....The nostrils are glandered....From the absorption of the fœtid pus, the blood is contami-

[1] *Gent. Magaz.* IX. Nov. 1739, p. 606:—Died, "Nov. 27, the eldest and youngest son of Henry Pelham, Esq. of sore throats."

[2] John Chandler, F.R.S., *A Treatise of the Disease called a Cold. Also a Short Description of the Genuine nature and seat of the Putrid Sore-Throat.* London, 1761, p. 55.

[3] Munk, *Roll of the College of Physicians.* Fothergill cites Spanish and other foreign writers on *garrotillo* in the historical introduction to his essay on the Sore-Throat (1748), without mentioning the fact that Letherland had been before him in that field.

nated; crimson efflorescences and small putrid pustules break out on the skin of the neck and breast, a quick depressed pulse, with a tendency rather to stupor than violent perturbations accompanying all, and, if not relieved, terminate in delirium, languor, clammy sweats and death."

Fothergill, whose name is so closely associated with the outbreak of gangrenous sore-throat a few years after, makes little of the earlier epidemic in London; besides the cases in the Pelham family and some others in the same part of the town, there were, he says, very few observed, so that "the disease and the remembrance of it"—including Letherland's priority— "seemed to vanish altogether." The winter of 1739–40, in which these cases had occurred, was one of intense frost and the beginning of a two years' sickly period in which typhus in Britain, dysentery and typhus in Ireland, reached a height unprecedented in the 18th century.

An epidemic of Throat-disease in Ireland, 1743.

In Ireland the dysenteries, typhus and relapsing fevers, attendant on and following the famine, were hardly over when the plague of the throat began among the children. It was seen first in the summer of 1743 (an influenza having preceded in May and June), it raged through the autumn and winter, and was not extinct for many years after. There were but few instances of it in Dublin, but it was prevalent in the adjoining counties, and exceedingly so in Wicklow, Carlow, Queen's County, Kilkenny, Cavan, Roscommon, Leitrim, Sligo "and perhaps many others, carrying off incredible numbers, and sweeping away the children of whole villages in a few days." The country doctors, who knew most of it, were not apt to record their experiences; so that the following account, which Rutty extracted from Dr Molloy, is all the record that remains of an epidemic concerning which one would wish to have known more[1]:

"It is peculiar to children, and those chiefly of from a month to three, four, five, six, eight or nine years old. They commonly for a day or two, or more, had a little hoarseness, sometimes a little cough; then in an instant they were seized with a great suffocation lasting a minute or two, and their face became livid; they have frequent returns of these fits of suffocation like asthmatic persons. The said suffocation is ever followed by one symptom which continues till they die, viz. a prodigious rattling in the upper part of

[1] John Rutty, M.D., *Chronological History of the Weather and Seasons, and prevailing Diseases in Dublin, during forty years.* London, 1770, p. 108.

the aspera arteria [windpipe] resembling that sound which attends colds when there is phlegm that cannot be got up. It is scarce sensible when they are awake but very great when they are asleep."

While there is little in this account to suggest the malignant sore-throat, and no mention of a miliary or scarlet rash, yet Rutty made no doubt that it was the malignant angina, comparing it rather to that described by Starr for Cornwall in 1748 than to that of Fothergill's description. He adds, from some other source of information, that children had generally clammy sweats upon them, with foetor of the breath. Many died in twenty-four hours; none lived above five days. Some had tumours behind the ears, which mortified. Many had a prodigious weeping behind the ears, which was very corrosive. A case is given of a child recovering after a profuse sweat, which suggested diaphoretic treatment by warm baths and sack-whey. Swellings of the tonsils and uvula were not observed.

It will be convenient to give here what remains to be said of the 18th century history of sore-throat in Ireland. In 1744 Rutty enters "mortal anginas" in Dublin. In March, 1751, tumours of the face, jaws, and throat, following an epidemic among horses in December, 1750. In the spring of 1752 "the pestilential angina" made great havoc among children. In the spring of 1755, "the gangrenous sore-throat" (same as in 1743) was fatal to some children. In the winter of 1759—60 he records "scarlet fever," and a singular form of the same in May, 1762, noticed under Influenza (p. 356). This must serve for the Irish experiences, although it is far from satisfactory. But it should be added that Dr James Sims, of Tyrone, who came to London afterwards and there wrote on the Scarlatina Anginosa (1786), says in an account of his Irish practice : "During all my practice here I have not seen one instance of the malignant ulcerous sore-throat as described by authors" (*op. cit.* 1773, p. 86).

Malignant Sore-throat in Cornwall, 1748.

Dr Starr, of Liskeard, calls the Cornish throat-disease the Morbus Strangulatorius. Writing in January, 1750, he said it had raged in several parts of Cornwall "within a few years," with great severity[1]: "Many parishes have felt its cruelty, and whole families of children been swept off: few, very few, have escaped." Cases given by himself belong to the year 1748; and Huxham, who did not meet with it at Plymouth until 1750–51, says that it had been raging with great fatality for a year or two before in and about Lostwithiel, St Austel, Fowey and Liskeard. In the account of the Cornish epidemic the emphasis falls upon

[1] John Starr, M.D., "Account of the Morbus Strangulatorius." *Phil. Trans.* XLVI. 435, dated Liskeard, Jan. 10, 17⁴⁸⁄₄₉.

the affection of the larynx and trachea; while there are so many other symptoms enumerated, including eruptions and brawny swelling of the neck, that it is clearly impossible to distinguish between exanthematous fever with sore-throat and laryngeal diphtheria pure and simple. Starr says: "Dr Fothergill's sore-throat with ulcers and Dr Cotton's St Albans scarlet fever are, in my opinion, but its shadows."

The symptoms generally pointed to the glottis.

Agonized breathing for a time was followed by the spitting up of jelly-like, glairy and somewhat transparent matter, mixed with white opaque thready matter, which might resemble more or less a rotten body or slough. The paroxysm returned, and the patient either died suddenly or sank away gradually, and died worn out, with or without convulsions. A plate is given of a whitish membrane loosened from the velum by means of hydrochloric acid on a silver probe ; it was not a slough, but a strong tenacious membrane which would bear handling and stretching without breaking. In the same case, the child's father afterwards pulled from the mouth a complete cast of the trachea including the bifurcation of the bronchi, of which a figure is given : "what sweated from it was as sticking as bird-lime"; he lived twenty-one hours after this second cast was drawn from him and died somewhat suddenly in his perfect senses. Such formations Starr clearly believed to be the essence of the disease ; but he gives many variations of it. The train of symptoms was not the same in every subject : "Some, I am informed, have had corrosive pustules in the groin and about the anus, eating quick and deep, and threatening a mortification even in the beginning [as Colden described for the sore-throat in New York State]. Others after a few days' illness have had numbers of the worst and deepest petechiae break out in various parts of their body : such I have not seen." But he gives cases of his own at Liskeard in 1748: "A child here and there had red pustules which broke out in the nape of the neck and threw off a surprising quantity of thin transparent ichor"; these pustules sloughed when poulticed; in another case sloughs followed where blisters had been applied to the neck and arm. Many had swelling of the tonsils, parotids, submaxillary and sublingual glands. A few had oedema from the chin to the thyroid, and up the side of the face. In one case, a tumour of the fauces broke and yielded some ounces of coffee-coloured foetid matter, to the patient's relief and ultimate recovery. Not a few had gangrenous sloughs in the mouth, which formed quickly. Some had foetor of the breath as an early symptom, but others had it not. Some were merely feverish and hoarse.

When Huxham came to describe the disease at Plymouth a year or two later, he laid the emphasis on other symptoms than those mostly dwelt upon by Starr, describing really a sloughing sore-throat with rash. But he has this also : "The windpipe itself was sometimes much corroded by it, and pieces of its internal membrane were spit up, with much blood and corruption ; and the patients lingered on for a considerable time, and at length died tabid."

Fothergill's Sore-throat with Ulcers, 1746–48.

Meanwhile we have to overtake Fothergill's history of the ulcerous sore-throat in or near London[1]. It broke out at Bromley, near Bow, Middlesex, in the winter of 1746 (Short says that it was in Sheffield in 1745). So many children died suddenly, some losing all and others the greater part of their families, that people were reminded of the plague.

It began with a chill and rigor, followed by heat. The throat became sore, and there were nausea, vomiting and purging. The face turned red and swollen, the eyes were inflamed and watery, the patient was restless, anxious and prostrated. The seizure was often in the forenoon, and in all cases the symptoms became much worse towards night, to be relieved by a sweat in the morning, as in an intermittent fever. The uvula, tonsils, velum, inside of the cheeks, and the pharynx, were florid red, with a broad spot or patch, irregular in figure, of pale white colour like the blanched appearance of the gums when they have been pressed by the finger. Usually on the second day of the disease, the face, neck, breast and hands to the tips of the fingers became of a deep erysipelatous colour with perceptible swelling, the fingers in particular being often of so characteristic a tint as at once to suggest an examination of the throat. A great number of small pimples, of a deeper red than the skin around them, appear on the arms and other parts ; they are larger and more prominent in those subjects, and in those parts of the same subject, where the redness is least intense, which is generally on the arms, the breast, and lower extremities. With the coming out of this rash, the sickness, vomiting and purging cease. The white spot or spots on the throat are now seen to be sloughs ; they come first usually in the angles above the tonsils. They are not formed of any foreign matter covering the parts but are real mortifications of substance leaving an ulcer with corrosive discharge behind. The nocturnal exacerbation now takes the form of delirium and incoherent talking. The parotids are commonly swelled and painful ; and if the disease be violent, the neck and throat are surrounded with a large oedematous tumour threatening suffocation. The pulse is 120, perhaps hard and small. The urine is at first crude and pale like whey ; afterwards it is more yellow, as if from bile ; and towards recovery it is turbid and deposits a "farinaceous" sediment. The initial purging having ceased, the bowels become irregular. The disease had no crisis, but in general, if the patient were to recover, the amendment began on the third, fourth or fifth day, when the redness disappeared and the sloughs in the throat were cast off.

Such is the main outline ; the following symptoms have less general value.

At the outset, the patient complained of a putrid smell in the throat and nostrils, which caused nausea. The nostrils were often inflamed, yielding a sanies, and the inside of the lips covered with vesicles filled with an excoriating ichor. Some had the parts about the anus excoriated. Fothergill was inclined to think that either the excoriations or the ichor from them extended down the whole intestinal tract, and accounted for the purging,

[1] John Fothergill, M.D., *An Account of the Sore Throat attended with Ulcers ; a Disease which hath of late years appeared in this City and the parts adjacent.* London, 1748.

with other bowel symptoms, which sometimes remained for weeks after the primary disease and caused death by emaciation[1]. In some there was bleeding at the nose, or mouth, which might be fatal ; in one case there was a like accident from the ear. Several cases are given in which there were no sloughs of the throat, but a dry glossy redness or lividity ; in these cases, there was a general brawny swelling of the neck, a coldness of the hands and feet, involuntary evacuations, a glassy eye and certain death. Three of Fothergill's five briefly reported cases are of that variety. In one of them, a boy of 14 years, he says there was "deep redness of the face, hands and arms, with a plentiful eruption of small pimples, which induced those about him to apprehend it was a scarlet fever."

That is the only reference to a possible diagnosis of scarlet fever in the whole essay. In the New England throat-distemper of 1735, "scarlet fever" was in like manner the name given by the laity, and disapproved by the profession. Fothergill, adopting the erudition of Letherland, identified the ulcerous or gangrenous sore-throat of London in 1746–48 with the *garrotillo* of Spain in the 16th and 17th centuries, the famous throat-plague of Naples and other places in Italy and Sicily from 1618 onwards, and the "plague in the throat" mentioned by a traveller, Tournefort, in 1701 as occurring among children in the island of Milo, (Douglass having already identified the Levantine plague in the throat with the throat-distemper of New England in 1735.)

After the outbreak at Bromley and Bow in the winter of 1746, the ulcerous, or putrid or gangrenous angina continued in London and the villages near until the date of Fothergill's writing (1748). By credible accounts, he says, it was also "in several other parts of this nation." Short, of Rotherham, a professed epidemiologist, says that the malignant angina "never left Sheffield entirely since the year 1745[2]." Fothergill himself, in his monthly accounts of the weather and diseases of London from 1751 to 1755, refers to the sore-throat once or twice ; thus, in October, 1751 : "epidemic sore-throat, in both children and adults"; and again, in July, 1755 : "The ulcerated sore-throat likewise appears in many families, with the greatest part of its usual symptoms, but gives way without much difficulty, if no improper evacuations have been made, to the method heretofore recommended (XXI. 497)[3]."

---

[1] Sir Thomas Watson (*Lectures*, II. 817), who mentions excoriations of the anus, carried Fothergill's idea of an absorption of the acrid matter to an extreme length in explaining the irritation of the alimentary canal in scarlet fever.
[2] Letter to Rutty, *Chronol. Hist.* 1770, p. 117.
[3] *Gent. Magaz.* Oct. 1751, and July, 1755, p. 343.

"Scarlet Fever" at St Albans, 1748.

The same disease that Fothergill described for London and villages near was seen at St Albans in the autumn of 1748, and described as "a particular kind of scarlet fever," by Dr Nathaniel Cotton, who kept a madhouse there. Among his friends were the poet Cowper (at one time his patient), and Young, of the 'Night Thoughts.' Cotton himself had the same melancholy cast of mind, and found the same solace in making verses, which have probably served more to keep his memory green than his essay in medicine[1]. He professes to describe " a particular kind of scarlet fever" in his title-page ; and in the text he has this remark: " From this diversity of symptoms, I have found some practitioners inclined to think that this disease could not with propriety be called a scarlet fever. But I imagine that such disputes are about words only." It is, indeed, difficult to find any real difference between his particular kind of scarlet fever and the "sore-throat with ulcers" which Fothergill wrote upon a few months before, or, again, between his scarlet fever and that of Withering thirty years after.

The sickness began about the end of September, 1748, in St Albans and some towns adjacent. At first it attacked children only, afterwards also adults. The symptoms given are just those detailed by Fothergill, as well as by Douglass for New England :

Sickness with purging at the outset, rapid swelling of the tonsils and (or) the parotids and maxillary glands, whitish sloughs on the tonsils, small ulcers up and down the fauces, the eyelids puffed as in measles, swelling of the neck, arms and hands in many, in some swelling of the body also, intense red efflorescence, coming on either suddenly or tardily, with thick spots as if dipped in blood. On the face, neck and breast, the rash was even with the surface, elsewhere it was miliary or shagreen. Some were restless or anxious, and delirious, others so drowsy that when awakened to receive a draught or the like, they relapsed at once into stupor. The attack, if not violent, ended on the fourth or fifth day ; there were few in whom the fever did not return on one, two or more evenings thereafter, so going off gradually. In one or two, the parotids swelled after the fever was gone, continuing hard

---

[1] Nathaniel Cotton, M.D. *Observations on a particular kind of Scarlet Fever that lately prevailed in and about St Albans.* In a Letter to Dr Mead. London, 1749 (12th February). The copy in the British Museum library has a written note signed R. W. (Robert Willan, M.D.): "The only just and correct account ; but was not noticed during the author's lifetime, and it has since been consigned to oblivion." In his work *On Cutaneous Diseases* (1808), Willan sarcastically contrasts the means by which Fothergill gained fame while Cotton escaped notice ; of the latter he says: " But, as he gave an old appellation to a disease certainly not new, his work attracted little attention, and procured him no emolument."

for a fortnight and then suppurating.   In nearly all, the cuticle peeled off "as in other scarlet fevers."   In some the nervous system was much shaken; in particular they dreaded the approach of evening with an unusual kind of horror, and started at the shadows of the candles on the wall.   In convalescence some complained of universal soreness.   The spots where blisters had been applied continued to discharge in some cases eight or ten days or more.

Besides the reference to swelling of the neck, arms or body among the early symptoms, there is no reference to oedema, while the pallid dropsy of convalescence, which Withering described in 1779, is not mentioned.   It is noteworthy that Cotton, who lays the emphasis on the scarlatina, and not on the throat-disease, was of opinion that the copiousness of the eruption was not a measure of the security of the patient, although that was clearly the opinion of Huxham and others, who laid the emphasis on the sore-throat.

Epidemics of Sore-throat with Scarlet rash in the period between Fothergill and Withering.

The years 1751–52, and indeed the whole of that decade, saw a good deal of the same diseases, after which little is heard of them until 1778.   Huxham's accounts for Plymouth, which are of the first importance, begin with 1751[1].   They are of importance because his memory went back to the anginose fever of 1734, in which the miliary eruptions, with sweats, were critical or relieving to the throat, and because he could not clearly distinguish between them and the sore-throats of 1751–52, although he follows Fothergill in identifying the latter with the Spanish *garrotillo*.   The throat affection began in the end of 1751, and became most severe in October, November and December, 1752, in Plymouth and at the Dock and all around, carrying off a great many adults as well as children.   It ceased in May, 1753.   He describes the sloughing patches in the throat, the excoriated nostrils with acrid dripping discharge, the swelling of the parotids and sometimes of the whole neck, just as other writers had done; and gives the account of laryngeal or tracheal membranes already cited (p. 695).   It is perhaps more important to dwell upon his account of the rash.   Most commonly the angina came on before the efflorescence, but in many instances the cuticular eruption appeared before the sore-throat.

[1] John Huxham, M.D., *A Dissertation on the Malignant Ulcerous Sore-Throat.* London, 1757.

" A very severe angina seized some patients that had no manner of eruption, and yet even in these a very great itching and desquamation of the skin sometimes ensued; but this was chiefly in grown persons, very rarely in children." Commonly there was a rash, general or partial, on the second, third or fourth day.

" Sometimes it was of an erysipelatous kind, sometimes more pustular ; the pustules were frequently very eminent, and of a deep fiery-red colour, particularly in the breast and arms, but oftentimes they were very small and might be better felt than seen, and gave a very odd kind of roughness to the skin. The colour of the efflorescence was commonly of a crimson hue, or as if the skin had been smeared over with the juice of raspberries, and this even to the fingers' ends ; and the skin appeared inflamed and swollen, as it were; the arms, hands and fingers were often evidently so, and very stiff and some- what painful. This crimson colour of the skin seemed indeed peculiar to this disease." The eruption seldom failed to give relief ; but there were also cases of an universal fiery exanthem which proved fatal. An early and kindly eruption, when succeeded by a very copious desquamation of the cuticle, was one of the most favourable symptoms.

Comparing it with the *febris anginosa* which he had entered in his annals under the year 1734, at a time when the ulcerous or malignant sore-throat was still unheard of, he says that the earlier type differed from the later in being more inflammatory, and less putrid ; the sore-throat of 1751–52 might seem to be a disease *sui generis*, but it differed from the anginose fever of 1734 only in the above respect : " In a word, the high inflamma- tory smallpox differs as much, or more, from the low malignant kind, as the *febris anginosa* from the pestilential ulcerous sore- throat." In the latter he found the remarkable evidences of putridity already cited in connexion with putrid fevers[1]. He gives the case of a boy of twelve whose tongue, fauces and tonsils were as black as ink; he swallowed with difficulty, and continually spat off immense quantities of a black, sanious and very foetid matter for at least eight or ten days; about the seventh day, his fever being abated, he fell into a bloody dysentery, but recovered eventually. In a few the face before death became bloated, sallow, shining and as if greasy, and the whole neck swollen. Even the whole body might be oedematous in some degree, retaining the impression of the finger.

Perhaps it may be said that Huxham had really to do with two diseases; and he does in one place say: " The anginose fever still continued, and we had several of the malignant sore-

---

[1] *Supra*, p. 125.

throats in September, many more in October, &c."—as if the two were not the same. But he generalized the "epidemic constitution" of 1751–52, in another way: "In all sorts of fevers there was a surprising disposition to eruptions of some kind or other, to sweats, soreness of the throat and aphthae. The smallpox were more fatal in August, and sometimes attended with a very dangerous ulceration in the throat and difficulty of swallowing. Indeed the malignant ulcerous sore-throat was now also frequent, probably sometimes complicated with the smallpox." Even pleuritic and peripneumonic disorders were attended during this constitution with a sore-throat, aphthae, and some kind of cuticular eruption.

Some facts about the throat-disease at Kidderminster and other places in Worcestershire will complete this part of the somewhat perplexing history. Dr Wall says it appeared about the beginning of 1748 chiefly in low situations[1]: "It then went generally under the name of scarlet fever, the complaint in the throat not being much attended to, or at least looked upon only as an accidental symptom." His first cases were at Stratford-on-Avon— a young lady who recovered with difficulty, and then two sisters who died, all three having been treated by blood-letting and the cooling regimen. By these cases Wall was convinced that the disease was more putrid than inflammatory, that it was infectious, that the antiphlogistic treatment was a mistake, that bark was the grand remedy, that the throat was the principal seat, and that the scarlet efflorescence was rather an accidental symptom than essential to the disease, some having petechiae and purple spots. He adopts Mead's name of *angina gangraenosa*. The malady had been rife in the city of Worcester, and most of all at Kidderminster, where it was in a manner epidemical. He was told that nine or ten poor persons had died of it there one after another. Having been called to the child of a respectable tradesman, he treated the case with bark and the cordial regimen. He persuaded the Kidderminster surgeons and apothecaries to adopt the same method, which they did with such success that, as he found afterwards in the books of one of them, there were only 7 deaths in 242 cases of the disease, while Dr Cameron did not fail once, and Wall himself had fifty recoveries and only two deaths. It is said, however, on the authority of the parish

---

[1] John Wall, M.D. "Bark in the Ulcerated Sore Throat." *Gent. Magaz.* 1751, Nov. p. 497. Dated Worcester, 15 Oct. 1751.

register, that a hundred persons died at Kidderminster of the malignant sore-throat in 1750, "in the months of October and November only[1]." Dr Wall goes on to say that the "Kidderminster sore-throat" had a vast variety of symptoms, the only certain ones being aphthous ulcers and sloughs on the tonsils and parts about the pharynx. "Very few here [which may mean Worcester] have had the scarlet efflorescence on the skin." Dr Johnstone, senior, confirms this in a measure for Kidderminster[2]: "The anginous fever was not always, though often, attended with cutaneous eruptions; and these, for the most part red, were sometimes also of the christalline miliary kind." And in writing again in 1779, when Withering's scarlet fever was dominant in place of Fothergill's sore-throat, Dr Johnstone said: "A scarlet eruption was a much more frequent symptom of this disease than it used to be when I first became acquainted with it nearly thirty years ago." But, as it is known that the rash of true scarlet fever is far less constant in adults than in children, and as many of the attacks referred to by Wall and Johnstone were in adults, the so-called Kidderminster sore-throat may have been a fairly uniform scarlatina. Still, it is clear that all the leading writers, excepting Cotton, of St Albans, distinguished between sore-throat (gangrenous, malignant, or ulcerous) and scarlatina, identifying the former with the old *garrotillo* of Spain and Italy[3]. The distinction may have been really between scarlatina simplex and scarlatina anginosa, as Willan believed; but, whether the disease were malignant scarlatina, or diphtheria, or a mixture of the two (as in Cornwall), or an undifferentiated type with the characters of both, it was certainly new as a whole to British experience in that generation, and, if we except the reference by Morton to certain cases which may have been sporadic, it was a disease hitherto unheard of in England since systematic medical writings began. We may realize the impression which it made, both in the American colonies and in England in the middle third of the 18th century, by recalling the sudden appearance of diphtheria some thirty-five years ago;

[1] Nash, *History of Worcestershire*, II. 39.
[2] James Johnstone, M.D., *Malignant Epidemic Fever of* 1756. London, 1758.
[3] To those who explicitly distinguished the sore-throat or angina maligna from scarlatina may be added Dr Richard Russell: "In hoc quidem morbi statu mitissimo, si ad quartum vel quintum usque diem eruptiones in cute superstites sint, paulatim recedant, et desquamationes furfuraceae, perinde ut in febre scarlatina, post se reliquant, ibi crisis integra et perfectissima est." *Œconomia Naturæ in Morbis Acutis et Chronicis Glandularum.* Lond. 1755, p. 105 seq.

but, whereas the diphtheria of 1856–58 came upon a generation of practitioners who had seen much of the very worst kinds of scarlatina for twenty years or more, the contemporaries of Huxham, Letherland, Fothergill, Johnstone and Wall in England, or of Douglass, Colden and Bard in America, knew no scarlet fever but scarlatina simplex. The outbreaks of the 18th century throat-distemper in certain families were of the same tragic kind as diphtherial outbreaks in our own time. Instances of whole families swept away have been cited from the New Hampshire epidemic of 1735. Horace Walpole gives the following instance of a noble family in London :

> "There is a horrid scene of distress in the family of Cavendish; the Duke's sister, Lady Bessborough, died this morning of the same fever and sore throat of which she lost four children four years ago. It looks as if it was a plague fixed in the walls of their house ; it broke out again among their servants, and carried off two a year and a half after the children. About ten days ago Lord Bessborough was seized with it and escaped with difficulty ; then the eldest daughter had it, though slightly : my lady attending them is dead of it in three days. It is the same sore throat which carried off Mr Pelham's two only sons....The physicians, I think, don't know what to make of it [1]."

The medical accounts of the sore-throat of those years are none the easier to interpret in a modern sense owing to the frequent use of the term "miliary" to describe the rash. Douglass had used this term in the title of his Boston essay in 1736. Bisset applies it to a Yorkshire epidemic some twenty years after[2]. The disease began among adults at Whitby in September and October, 1759, and spread over the country between the coast and Guisborough in the spring of 1760, as well as in some places to the westward of the latter ; afterwards it became epidemic in all the western parts of Cleveland in August and September of 1760, the summer months having been almost a clear interval. It was remarkable, he says, that some persons in the eastern parts of Cleveland who had escaped it when it was epidemical in the spring, were attacked by it in the autumn after it "had got a good way to the westward of them." This epidemic progression is spoken of as of a single but composite disease,—"the epidemic throat-distemper and miliary fever that appeared in the Duchy of Cleveland in 1760." In adults it was mostly an affection of the throat, few having the miliary eruption, and only one adult

[1] *Letters of Horace Walpole,* ed. Cunningham, III. 280, letter to Mann, 20 Jan. 1760.
[2] Charles Bisset, *Essay on the Medical Constitution of Great Britain, with obs. on the weather and diseases in* 1758–60. London, 1762.

dying "within the circle of my observations." But in children the fever with miliary rash was predominant, and of it the fatality is put at one death in every thirty cases. There is no discussion as between the names of scarlet fever and miliary fever; but the following on the peeling of the skin is significant: "From the ninth to the thirteenth day the scarf-skin begins to peel off in cases that were attended by a copious rash; and that of the hands and feet sometimes came off almost entire." Soreness of throat often happened in this fever of children; and, to repeat, the sore-throat of adults and the miliary fever of children are described as parts of one and the same epidemic[1]. An account which probably relates to the same disease comes from Rotherham or Sheffield in a letter by Dr Short, the epidemiologist, to Rutty, of Dublin. It was very violent, he says, in July, 1759, and cut off whole families of children. The attack was attended with diarrhoea, swelled tonsils, oedema of the face, an eruption like measles all over the body, and a discharge of sanious humour from the nostrils. "In some there was an efflorescence on the skin like the scarlet fever, and these recovered[2]."

Another complication arises owing to the prevalence, in the same period, of putrid or miliary fevers, which had sometimes an anginous or "throaty" character. This source of perplexity extends from near the beginning to near the end of the 18th century, but it is greatest in the middle period, when the "constitution" was most decidedly "putrid[3]." The relationship was most definitely expressed by Johnstone, of Kidderminster: "This malignant fever (*vide supra*, p. 123) was very often, though not constantly, complicated with, and in general had great analogy with the malignant sore-throat which at this time prevailed in many parts of England." An Oxford practitioner, in 1766, actually wrote a dissertation to distinguish the "putrid sore-throat" which attended the "putrid" continued fever of the

---

[1] Hecker (u. s.) identified Bisset's epidemic disease in Cleveland with Douglass's in New England. Merely because they used the term "miliary," he erects their epidemics into an imaginary class of *angina miliaris* which was not scarlatina.

[2] Short to Rutty, Rotherham, 26 March, 1760, in Rutty's *Chronol. Hist. of Weather, &c. and Diseases in Dublin.* London, 1770, p. 117.

[3] Sir David Hamilton, *Tractatus Duplex, &c.* London, 1710 (Engl. transl. 1737, p. 84), says that, in 1704, several in the "miliary fever" had "a pain in the jaws resembling that of the squinsy," which killed many suddenly. At the other end of the century, Willan (*Cutaneous Diseases*, 1808, p. 333) said of fever in 1786: "The title 'angina maligna' would have applied with equal, if not with more propriety, to the sore-throat connected with a different species of contagion, namely, that of the typhus or malignant fever originating in the habitations of the poor where no attention is paid to cleanliness or ventilation."

time, from the "gangrenous sore-throat" of Fothergill, Huxham and others: in the former, the aphthae and sloughs of the tonsils and uvula, as well as of the mouth, were only symptomatic of the putrid fever, and late in showing themselves; in the latter, the throat affection was the primary and dominant one, present from the beginning of the illness[1].

The last complication of the highly complex circumstances in which scarlatina first became a great disease in England is with "putrid" or malignant measles. In the same years as the epidemic described above for Yorkshire, namely, 1759 and 1760, there occurred an "anomalous malignant measles," which for some months had made a melancholy carnage amongst children in the west of England. The symptoms were difficult breathing, an amazingly rapid pulse, white or brown tongue, and "some red eruptions which run in irregular groups and splatches on the surface of the skin." The attack was apt to be attended by colliquative diarrhoea. A fatal issue was indicated by a sunken and very quick pulse, the abatement of the dyspnoea, and the eruption coming and going. Some rapid cases in infants ended in convulsions on the third day. Children from one to six years were attacked most[2]. Perhaps the only reason for not including this among epidemics of measles is the author's remark: "I look upon the poison of the disease to be a good deal akin to that of the ulcerated sore-throat so very rife and fatal some years since," although he does not allege throat-complications in the malady which he describes.

Three years later, in 1763, there was an epidemic at the Foundling Hospital, London, which Watson, the physician to the charity, described in a special essay as one of "putrid measles." Willan, writing in 1808, challenged the diagnosis on the ground both of the symptoms as given by Watson, and of the names given to the malady in the Infirmary Book at the time. The first entry in the apothecary's book is on 23 April, 1763, a case of "fever with a rash," the next on 30 April, a case of "scarlet fever," then on 7 May, ten cases of "eruptive fever," and, for the rest of May and all June, very long lists of "eruptive fever," the name of measles not occurring at all in that outbreak,

---

[1] Francis Penrose, *A Dissertation on the Inflammatory, Gangrenous and Putrid Sore-Throat. Also on the Putrid Fever.* Oxford, 1766.
[2] *Some Thoughts on the Anomalous Malignant Measles lately peculiarly prevalent in the Western Parts of England.* London, 1760. And to be sold at Bath and Exeter.

while the names of " morbillous fever" and " fever" are given to
a smaller but still considerable outbreak in November of the
same year.　Among the symptoms, Watson mentions that the
fauces were of a deep red colour, that the rash came out on the
second day, and that there was no cough.　The most remarkable
character of the epidemic as a whole was a tendency to sloughing
in various parts:

> " Of those who died some sank under laborious respiration : more from
> dysenteric purging, the disease having attacked the bowels; and of these
> one died of mortification in the rectum.　Besides this, six others died
> sphacelated in some one or more parts of the body.　The girls who died
> most usually became mortified in the pudendum.　Two had ulcers in their
> mouth and cheek, which last was so covered by them that the cheek, from the
> ulcers within, sphacelated externally before they died.　Of these one had the
> gums and jawbone corroded to so great a degree that most of the teeth on
> one side came out before she died.　The lips and mouth of many who
> recovered were ulcerated, and continued so for a long time."　The anatomical
> examination of those who died showed the bronchitic affection, in one case
> pleurisy, and in some a gangrenous condition of the lungs.　One died of
> emaciation six weeks after the attack.　Eleven others succumbed shortly
> after to smallpox, out of eighteen who caught the latter during recovery from
> the preceding epidemic disease[1].

Long after, in 1808, when the diagnosis between measles and
scarlatina was fixed, Dr James Clarke saw at Nottingham in
several cases of measles "a great tendency to gangrene," the
sites of blisters having mortified in two (as in scarlet fever) and
two having gangrene of the cheek and mortification of the upper
jaw[2].　Huxham, he says, saw such cases, Willan never; and
that was one of the reasons why Willan claimed the Foundling
cases as scarlatina.　The diagnosis is important; for, in the
same year, 1763, the bills of mortality record 610 deaths from
measles in London, and Watson expressly includes the 19
deaths in the Foundling Hospital (in 180 attacks) as part of
the general epidemic in London.

The confusion between measles and scarlatina is farther
shown by the entries in the Infirmary Book of the Foundling
Hospital from the beginning to the end of an extensive epidemic
in 1770: On 31 March, 23 children are in the infirmary with
"measles," and on 7 April, 37 children still with "measles"; on
12 May the long list is headed "measles and ulcerated sore-

---

[1] William Watson, M.D.　"An Account of the Putrid Measles as they were
observed at London in the years 1763 and 1768."　*Med. Obs. and Inquiries*, IV.
(1771), p. 132.
[2] James Clarke, M.D.　"Medical Report for Nottingham from March, 1807, to
March, 1808."　*Edin. Med. Surg. Journ.* IV. 425.

throat," on 19 May, "putrid fever," and on 26 May, "fever and ulcerated sore-throat[1]."

Whether or not we agree with Willan in taking the Foundling epidemic of 1763 (and perhaps with it the general epidemic in London) for one of scarlatina, it can hardly be doubted that the Foundling epidemic of 1770 was the latter disease, the names of "measles with ulcerated sore-throat," "putrid fever," and "fever and ulcerated sore-throat" clearly indicating scarlatina anginosa. Grant also records the prevalence of epidemic sore-throat in London in 1770[2], and Dr William Fordyce, writing in 1773, dealt with the "ulcerated and malignant sore-throat" as a question of the day[3].

It was not until forty years ago, he says, that they had become acquainted in England with ulcerated and malignant sore-throat, while "both kinds" are now very common. His aim is to separate the ulcerated from the malignant, and he instances an outbreak in a gentleman's house at Islington, where the worst symptoms of the malignant occurred in the children, while only the ulcerous prevailed among the servant maids. In 1769 it was reported to be seldom fatal in London and Westminster, and in the villages around; but within these last twelve months (1773) it had appeared of a bad type in high situations such as Harrow, in the months of June and July. In a later note, he adds that "it still continues to make a havock so considerable as to keep up the alarm about it both in the metropolis and all over England," his own last experience of it having been two fatal cases in a noble family a few miles to the west of London. Fordyce identified this disease with Fothergill's sore-throat, and described the eruption as "the general erysipelatous colour that comes about the second day on the face, neck, breast and hands to the finger ends, which last are tinged in so remarkable a manner that the seeing of them only is sufficiently pathognomonic of the malady [this is a repetition of Huxham and Fothergill]; and finally a great number of small pimples, of a colour more intense than that which surrounds them, appearing in the arms and other parts of the body." He gives the following as a case of the malignant sore-throat in a young gentleman five or six years

[1] These changes of the name from week to week represent probably the independent judgment of the apothecary more than the modified opinions of Watson the physician. The views which the latter expressed in his paper of 1771, are clearly reechoed in the following anonymous paragraph in the *Gent. Magaz.* XLII. (1772), Nov. p. 541: "The measles have lately been very rife and fatal in this metropolis. They are of a very different kind from those described by the great Doctor Sydenham, being of a malignant putrid nature, such as visited London in 1763 and 1768, where bleeding seemed of so little service, but small does of emetic tartar, cordial medicines and blisters, were very efficacious. The above disorder was epidemic at Plymouth and parts adjacent in the years 1745 and 1750, and so long since as the year 1762 [1672] was described by Dr Morton, who says it raged so severely during the autumn of that year that it appeared like a gentle kind of plague, sparing neither sex nor age, and that 300 died weekly of it."
[2] W. Grant, M.D., *Account of a Fever and Sore Throat in London, September,* 1776. London, 1777.
[3] W. Fordyce, M.D., *A new Inquiry into the Causes, Symptoms and Cure of Putrid and Inflammatory Fevers; with an Appendix on the Hectic Fever, and on the Ulcerated and Malignant Sore Throat.* London, 1773. The appendix on Sore-throat is pp. 209–222.

old: "Every part of the body that bore its own weight was gangrened, as well as the orifices where he had been blooded twice before I saw him (which was three days after the seizure); the parotid glands were very much swelled, the whole body was more or less oedematous, and the skin throughout of an erysipelatous purple; he died the third day after I saw him."

Although Fordyce, and probably most others, still adhered to Fothergill's view of the sore-throat with ulcers as a disease apart, yet there appear to have been at this date some who followed the line taken with regard to it by Dr Cotton in 1749. Sometime about the end of 1771 or beginning of 1772, a physician at Ipswich sent to a London physician, who sent it to the *Gentleman's Magazine*, an account of a " Successful Method of treating the Ulcerated Sore Throat and Scarlet Fever," by tartar emetic, calomel &c.[1] He begins: " The ulcerated sore-throat and scarlet fever has been very rife in this place and the neighbourhood for some months past, and has been in a considerable number of instances fatal. It has in every respect answered the description given of it by Dr Fothergill "— so much so that he does not give the symptoms, but only the treatment, which, in his own hands, had been singularly successful: " I have had considerably more than one hundred patients, and have not buried one," his cases, between the writing and printing of the paper (3 June) having " increased to near three hundred with the same success." This must have been an interval of mild scarlatina, during which the prevalence of the malady, however extensive, had attracted little notice. The outburst in 1777–78, from which the diagnosis and naming of scarlatina anginosa properly date, was obviously an interruption of a quiet time of the disease.

Scarlatina anginosa in its modern form, 1777–78.

Dr Levison[2], who was physician to a London charity called the General Medical Asylum located at No. 4, Tottenham Court-road (afterwards in Welbeck Street), observed the outbreak, on 15 July, 1777, of a malignant sore-throat, "nearly such as described by Dr Fothergill and Dr Huxham (only without the efflorescence and attended with costiveness)," among children from three to seven years, by which many were cut off in the space of six to eight days, some by suffocation and others by

---

[1] *Gent. Magaz.* XLII. (1772), June, p. 258.
[2] G. Levison, M.D., *An Account of the Epidemical Sore-Throat.* 2nd ed. corrected. London, 1778 (1st ed. 1778).

vomiting of blood.   It became more general in August, and in
some was very malignant, being joined with an erysipelatous
inflammation and a diarrhoea.   It raged with great fury in
Kentish Town, and at Enfield Chase it swept away many in
twenty-four hours.   But on the high ground about London, as at
Hampstead and Highgate, it was of a benign type.   It was worse
in the villages round than in the capital itself.

In the milder form, there was only a superficial whiteness of the uvula,
tonsils and velum ; in the more severe, the same parts were beset with thick
ulcerations, running very deep in the fauces.   Both in the milder and in the
more severe cases the neck became swollen on the second or third day.
The commencement was usually with shivering and nausea, followed by
heat, and an efflorescence over the breast, the limbs, and often the whole
body, of a crimson red.   "Some were spread over with a kind of little
millets, similar to that in the miliary fevers, and which scaled off the skin
the sixth or seventh day ; in which cases the ulcerations were very slight, as
also all other symptoms of malignancy."   The mouth was apt to be full of
sloughs, the teeth covered with black crusts.   The urine was scanty, high-
coloured, with a thin suspended cloud.   Some bled from the nose.   The
nostrils were apt to be stuffed with greenish sanies, which dropped out
continually.   The efflorescence and sore-throat were often met with separately.   Most had cough throughout, great dejection of spirits, and oppressed
breathing.   The disease had no regular progress and no crisis ; the whole of
the symptoms would often cease suddenly about the eighth or ninth day.
In one case there was recovery after three weeks' illness.   Several cases had
suppuration of the glands of the neck.   In one fatal case, a tumour behind
the right tonsil was found to contain three ounces of foetid pus.

Oedema was frequent after recovery—the lips, nose and face
bloated, sallow, shining and greasy ; the belly also might be
swollen.   This, says Levison, was a peculiar kind of dropsy ;
and as he adds that it had not been remarked by Huxham he
intends to distinguish it from the bloated greasy appearance
which Huxham did remark.   Some died of it a month after the
fever ; many recovered from it by the aid of calomel, rhubarb
and diuretics—the treatment for the scarlatinal dropsy—and
full doses of bark.   In the acute disease blisters were sometimes
tried, in compliance with custom ; but they did no good, and
occasioned a great discharge of thick matter.   Bleeding and
antiphlogistics were seldom called for.   This outbreak, which
began in July 1777, abated in November.   Next year it came
back about the middle of March, but in a benign form, and
unattended with either the efflorescence or the diarrhoea, and so
continued until the date of writing, the 11th May, 1778.   Levison
distinguishes two or three types—a malignant sore-throat at the
outset early in summer, 1777, to which in autumn two other
epidemics were joined, namely, on the one hand, scarlet fever

(or miliary fever), and on the other hand, a purging like autumnal dysentery.

The second season of the epidemic in London[1], the spring and summer of 1778, saw the outbreak of malignant sore-throat, with rash, in the Midlands. It appeared in Birmingham about the middle of May, and in June it was frequent in many of the towns and villages in the neighbourhood. It continued to the end of October, and revived a little during mild weather after the middle of November. It seems to have reached Worcester-shire in the autumn, cases having been seen first at Stourbridge and afterwards at Kidderminster and Cleobury. According to Johnstone, the younger, it broke out first in schools, and spread very rapidly among children, attacking adults sometimes. The summer of 1778 was remarkable for heat, which is described as West Indian in its intensity.

The account of this epidemic which has attracted most attention (and deservedly) is that of Withering, of Birmingham, who had written his thesis at Edinburgh twelve years before (1766) on *angina gangraenosa*. He calls it definitely by the name of "scarlet fever and sore-throat, or *scarlatina anginosa*," explaining that it was "preceded by some cases of the true ulcerated sore-throat," by which he meant the disease described by Fothergill in 1748. The elder Johnstone, then of Worcester, who had described the Kidderminster sore-throat of 1750--51, declared that the scarlet eruption was a more common symptom of this 1778 disease than it used to be when he first became acquainted with it near thirty years before; and dealing with the same epidemic as Withering, he makes out three varie-ties:—namely, first the scarlatina simplex of Sydenham, with no sore-throat, second, the scarlatina anginosa, and third, the ulcerated sore-throat[2]. His son, who also wrote upon the epidemic of 1778 as he saw it at Worcester, having written his Edinburgh thesis upon malignant sore-throat several years before, says: "The disease which now prevails is the ulcerous malignant sore-throat, combined with the scarlet fever of Sydenham[3]." Saunders, a retired East Indian surgeon,

---

[1] It might have been the third, as Grant (u.s.) says there was fever with sore-throat in London in September, 1776.

[2] "Angina and Scarlet Fever of 1778." *Mem. Med. Soc.* III. 355.

[3] James Johnstone, junr. M.D., *A Treatise on the Malignant Angina or Putrid and Ulcerous Sore-Throat, &c.* Worcester, 1779.

described the corresponding epidemic in the north of Scotland as one of sore-throat and fever[1].

Withering's account of the symptoms differs little from that given by Levison the year before, and is chiefly noteworthy for confirming that writer as to the occurrence of scanty urine and oedema[2]:

> The rash came out on the third day, continued scarlet, the colour of a boiled lobster, for two or three days, then turned to brown colour, and desquamated in small branny scales.   He had been told of three instances in which the desquamation was so complete that even the nails separated from the fingers.   In the colder weather of October the scarlet colour was less frequent and less permanent.   Many had no appearance of it at all ; while others, especially adults, had on tender parts of the skin a very few minute red pimples crowned with white pellucid heads.   The worst cases fell into delirium at the outset, had the scarlet rash on the first or second day, and might die as early as the second day ; if they survived, the rash turned to brown, and they would lie prostrate for several days, nothing seeming to afford them any relief.   " At length a clear amber-coloured matter discharges in great quantities from the nostrils, or the ears, or both, and continues so to discharge for many days.   Sometimes this discharge has more the appearance of pus mixed with mucus.   Under these circumstances, when the patients do recover, it is very slowly ; but they generally linger for a month or six weeks from the first attack, and die at length of extreme debility."   These discharges, compared by a writer a generation before to glandered secretions, are not to be confused, says Withering, with the matter from abscesses on both sides of the neck, under the ears, which " heal in a few days without much trouble."   The submaxillary glands were generally enlarged.   Adults usually had a ferretty look of the eyes, and sometimes small circular livid spots about the breast, knees and elbows.   Some had a succession of boils.   One man had " lock-jaw."   Most patients had the fauces, particularly the tonsils, covered with sloughs, which separated and left the parts raw, as if divested of their outer membrane.   The most troublesome symptom was exulcerations at the sides and towards the root of the tongue ; these were painful and made it impossible to swallow solid food. Some threw out several white ash-coloured sloughs, though no such sloughs were visible upon inspecting the throat.

With reference to the diagnosis between scarlatina anginosa and angina gangraenosa (of Fothergill) Withering says: " They are both epidemic, they are both contagious ; the mode of seizure, the first appearances in the throat, are nearly the same in both; a red efflorescence upon the skin, a great tendency to delirium and a· frequent small unsteady pulse are likewise common to both.   With features so strikingly alike, and these, too, of the most obvious kind, is it to be wondered that many practitioners considered them the same disease ? "   And again : " But perhaps

[1] Robert Saunders, *Observations on the Sore-Throat and Fever in the North of Scotland in* 1777.   London, 1778.   ·
[2] William Withering, M.D., *Account of the Scarlet Fever and Sore-Throat, particularly as it appeared at Birmingham in* 1778.   London, 1779; preface dated 1st January.

he will never be able precisely to draw the line where the light begins and where the penumbra ends[1]."

The extent of the epidemic of scarlatinal sore-throat, of which we have particulars from Middlesex, Warwickshire and Worcestershire in 1778, cannot be ascertained. It is heard of, as we saw, in the north of Scotland in 1777. According to Barker, of Coleshill, the scarlet fever which "in a manner raged in the neighbouring town of Birmingham," occurred in only a few cases in his own parish, and these mild[2]. It appears to have been in Carlisle the year after, 1779, under which date Heysham says that "two epidemics swept off a great number of children— smallpox and a species of scarlet fever[3]." Nothing more is heard of it in Carlisle for the next eight years, during which Heysham kept an account of the diseases. The epidemic of 1778–9 fell also upon Newcastle:

---

[1] Withering was perhaps too desirous to be thought the first in England to have described scarlatina anginosa. "The scarlet fever in its simple state," he says, "is not a very uncommon disease in England, but its combination with a sore-throat, as described above, the violence of its attack, and the train of fatal symptoms that follow, are circumstances hitherto unnoticed by English writers." It is probable from this that he had not seen Levison's essay, with preface dated 11 May, 1778, his own being dated 1 January, 1779; but Cotton's essay of 1749 actually bore the name of scarlet fever on its title-page, and described the throat-affection, glandular swellings, and the like quite correctly.

The name of the elder Heberden is frequently brought into the history of the identification of scarlatina, with a reference to his *Commentaries on Diseases,* which were not published until 1802, some time after his death at a very advanced age. The following are among his remarks: "In the fever which has just been described there is always some degree of redness in the skin, and the throat is not without an uneasy sensation. Where it happens that the throat is full of little ulcers attended with considerable pain, there the disease, though the skin be ever so red, is not denominated from the colour, but from the soreness of the throat, and obtains the name of *malignant sore-throat*; and many suppose that the two disorders differ in nature as well as in name," p. 23. "The enfeebled and disordered state of all the functions of the body evidently points out such a malignity of the fever as cannot be owing to the affection of the uvula or tonsils, which in other distempers we often see ulcerated and eaten away, without any danger of the patient's life. These sores, therefore, like pestilential buboes, point out the nature of the disorder; but the danger arises, not from them, but from the fever," p. 25.

In 1790 an elaborate attempt was made by William Lee Perkins, M.D. (dating from Hampton Court, 1 March) to distinguish between cynanche maligna and scarlatina anginosa, in *An Essay for a Nosological and Comparative View of the Cynanche Maligna or Putrid Sore-Throat, and the Scarlatina Anginosa.* London, 1790. He proceeds by the nosological method of Sauvages and Cullen, erecting genera, species and varieties. The result is not clear after all; for on p. 43 (note) we read that *scarlatina* is frequently accompanied with inflammatory and ulcerous appearances in the fauces or throat, and that *angina maligna* or ulcerated sore-throat is often attended with red efflorescence on the skin; this had led to their being regarded as one and the same, and treated by the same method of cure.

[2] J. Barker, *A Treatise on the Putrid Constitution of 1777 and the preceding years, and the Pestilential one of 1778.* London, 1779 (of inferior value beside Withering's).

[3] Heysham, in Hutchinson's *Hist. of Cumberland,* u. s.

From the month of June, 1778, until the 1st September, 1779, there were treated 146 cases of "ulcerated sore-throat," of which 18 were fatal. The epidemic was at its height in September and October. The ages were: under ten years, 98, ten to twenty, 25, twenty to thirty, 18, above thirty, 5. Dropsy followed in 23; 75 were mild scarlatina and sore-throat, 33 were angina maligna. During the ten years following, until 1789, only 57 more cases were treated from the Newcastle Dispensary, of which 8 were fatal[1].

History of Scarlatina after the Epidemic of 1778.

In London, according to Dr James Sims, scarlatina with sore-throat occasioned a great mortality in the latter half of 1786. The bills of mortality assign only 19 deaths to sore-throat, while they give 793 for the year to measles. But Sims says that "measles were not present in London during the whole year; at least I saw none, and I saw about two thousand cases in private and at the General Dispensary."

The deaths from scarlet fever, he thinks, had been given under measles and also under "fevers," which were a large total for the year. The epidemic was very virulent, going through families; many lost two children, some a larger number; many adults fell victims to it who were supposed to die of common fever.

Sims' first case was of a youth at Camberwell, in March, with scarlet rash and sloughs of the throat. He saw no more cases for several weeks, and then, on 1 May, he was called to a case of sore-throat in a school at Hampstead; the illness was slight, and there was no efflorescence; but in June there occurred in the same school an explosion of scarlatina, twenty of the girls being seized within a short time. It was in other suburban villages in the summer, but did not enter London until August, after which Sims saw three hundred cases of it; of some two hundred treated by him in a certain way, only two died. The symptoms of the epidemic were the usual ones of scarlet fever with ulcerated or sloughing throat. In November and December, swelling attacked the face and extremities, which were painful but not oedematous. The parotids were swollen. Several had the angina without the rash; others the rash without the angina[2].

The same epidemic in London was one of the early medical experiences of Dr Robert Willan, who gave some account of it in the volume 'On Cutaneous Diseases' which he published in

---

[1] John Clark, M.D., *Obs. on Fevers, and on the Scarlet Fever with Ulcerated Sore-Throat at Newcastle in* 1778. Lond. 1780; *Account of the Newcastle Dispensary from its commencement in* 1777 *to Michaelmas*, 1789. Newcastle, 1789 (also by Clark).

[2] James Sims, M.D. "Scarlatina Anginosa as it appeared in London in 1786." *Mem. Med. Soc. Lond.* I. 388. Willan, however, says that measles was the epidemic in the winter and spring of 1785–86; while the epidemic at the Foundling Hospital was "measles" in March and April, 1786, "fever" in June and July, and "scarlet fever" in 1787.

1808, shortly before his death[1]. It began in the autumn of 1785, was superseded by measles for a time, and revived again in 1786, to last into 1787. It was most malignant in the narrow courts, alleys and close crowded streets of London, but existed also in the villages near. While admitting the existence of measles in the winter of 1785–86, he confirms Sims in saying that it was not measles (as in the Bills) but scarlatina that caused the high mortality in 1786: "The cases of scarlatina during the year 1786 exceeded in number the sum of all other febrile diseases within the same period." The deaths were mostly between the seventh and eighteenth day of the fever. The following is his classification of over two hundred cases seen by himself:

1786

	Scarlatina simplex	Scarlatina anginosa	Scarlatina maligna	Sore-throat without eruption
April	—	3	—	—
May	6	10	2	—
June	4	12	1	4
July	2	11	1	3
August	1	17	4	4
Sept.	2	29	9	12
Oct.	3	24	5	7
Nov.	0	38	12	10
Dec.	0	8	5	2
	18	152	39	42

The infirmary book of the Foundling Hospital has long lists of patients sick of "scarlet fever with sore-throat" in August and September, 1787, as many as 76 being under treatment in one week, the next week 39 sick of scarlet fever, besides 45 recovering from it. This is the first unambiguous entry of an epidemic of scarlet fever in the Foundling Hospital records[2]. Under the same year, 1787, Barker, of Coleshill, records "scarlet fever, smallpox, and chincough" in a neighbouring city, as well as pestilential sore-throats "epidemical everywhere in the terrible foul weather of winter." His next entry of "scarlet fever and sore-throat" is under the year 1791[3].

An account by Dr Denman, of London, dated 28 November, 1790, of "a disease lately observed in infants," but otherwise unnamed, appears to relate to diphtheria. Eight cases in young infants were seen, one per month from April to October, of which six proved fatal. The signs were "thrush in the nose," fulness of the throat and neck, the tonsils red, swelled, and covered by ash-coloured sloughs or extensive ulcerations. The skin sloughed at places where blisters were applied. Nothing is said of a scarlet rash[4].

[1] *On Cutaneous Diseases.* Vol. I. London, 1808, pp. 262, 277, 345.
[2] I have not succeeded in finding the apothecary's book for the years 1776–82, within which the great London epidemic of 1777–78 fell; but Willan, who may have had the complete set of books before him, says (*op. cit.* 1808, p. 245) "the denomination 'scarlet fever and sore-throat' first occurs in the weekly report, 1st September, 1787." I am indebted to the courtesy of Mr Swift, M.R.C.S. for a sight of the books.
[3] J. Barker, *Epidemicks, or General Observations on the Air and Diseases from the year 1740 to 1777 inclusive, and particular ones from that time to the beginning of 1795.* Birmingham (no date).
[4] *Lond. Med. Journ.* XI. 374.

Scarlatina (1788) and Diphtheria (1793–94) described by the same observer.

One good observer at the end of the 18th century, Rumsey, a surgeon at Chesham, in Bucks, has left full accounts of two epidemics in his district, one in 1788, which he calls "epidemic sore-throat[1]" and the other in 1793–94, which he calls "the croup[2]." The one corresponds to scarlet fever, the other to diphtheria. The author does not think it necessary to enlarge on the distinction between the "epidemic sore-throat" and "the croup" as it was so obvious; yet the former was "Fothergill's sore-throat," which some English writers of the present time assume to have been diphtheria; while the disease which Rumsey calls "the croup" corresponds with laryngeal and tracheal diphtheria, not unmixed with diphtheritis of the tonsils, uvula and velum. There is hardly anything in the history of scarlatina and diphtheria more instructive than the juxtaposition of those two excellent descriptions by Rumsey, who grudged the name of scarlatina to the former epidemic because the rash was not invariable, and called the latter by the name of croup although it was not confined to the larynx and trachea, and was epidemic in the summer months.

The epidemic of "sore-throat" in 1788 began in April and lasted until November, attacking those of every age except the very old, but especially children, and mostly women among adults.

The throat was slightly sore for twelve or twenty-four hours; it then became fiery red, the uvula and tonsils being much swelled. About the second or third day there were whitish or yellowish sloughs on the tonsils and uvula, which in many cases left deep, ragged ulcers. It was many days before the sloughs were all exfoliated. Some spat up an astonishing quantity of mucus; in young children there was apt to be a discharge of mucus from the nostrils, and in a few cases from the eyes. The parotid and submaxillary glands were often enlarged, sometimes suppurating or sloughing. A white crust separated from the tongue on the third or fourth day, leaving it raw and red. In some cases there was sickness with vomiting, in some diarrhoea. In many cases there was a scarlet eruption over the whole body, usually on the second or third day. The fatal cases had all a very red eruption, and the skin burning to the touch. In some the eruption was so rough as to be

[1] H. Rumsey, "Epidemic Sore-Throat at Chesham in 1788." *Lond. Med. Journal*, x. 7, dated 14 Dec. 1788.
[2] H. Rumsey, "An Account of the Croup as it appeared in the Town and Neighbourhood of Chesham, in Buckinghamshire, in the years 1793 and 1794." *Trans. of a Soc. for Improving Med. and Chirurg. Knowledge*, II. (1800), 25. Read 1 July, 1794.

plainly felt. In a few cases, after the efflorescence broke out, a number of little pustules made their appearance about the breast, arms, &c., of about the size of millet seeds, which died away in twenty-four or thirty-six hours. This was not common; but in one family the mother and three of the four ailing children had pustules. One young man had large white vesicles on the sixth day; another young man, in November, had vesicles on the arms, thighs and legs as large as a half-crown piece, filled with yellow serous fluid, or gelatinous substance, with a good deal of erysipelas round them. The red efflorescence was always followed by peeling. Many had the throat-disease without rash, but none had the efflorescence without the sore-throat.

Rumsey decides against two distinct types of disease; it was the same contagion acting on different constitutions; yet he could not help thinking that scarlatina anginosa was an improper term for it, inasmuch as the rash was not constant. It was a less putrid disease than that described by Fordyce in 1773 (*supra*, p. 707), and carried off but few considering the great numbers who were affected by it. Two of the fatalities in children were from the anasarca of the whole body, with scanty urine, which came on a week or two after. He bled only once, applied leeches to the temples in several, and saw many recoveries with no treatment but topical applications.

The epidemic five or six years after in the same town in a valley of Buckinghamshire and on the hills for some six miles round was something unusual. Rumsey had about forty cases of " the croup" from March, 1793, until January, 1794; whereas his father, who had practised there above forty years, could not recall more than eight or ten cases of " croup" in all his experience. The cases were all in children from one to fourteen years; there were sometimes three attacked in one family; most of the fatal cases occurred in summer; the epidemic was distributed impartially in the valley where Chesham stands and upon the hills enclosing it. Rumsey gives full details of seventeen cases, eight that died and nine that recovered, with post-mortem notes for some.

His first case was in March, 1793; then came a succession of cases about June and July, of which four that proved fatal were in children just recovered from measles. All those earlier cases had the disease coming on insidiously, then the peculiar cough and tone of voice, if any voice remained, paroxysms of choking, expectoration of shreds of membrane, giving relief to the distress, and the trachea found after death lined with a coagulated matter[1]. Among

---

[1] " Several children brought up portions of a film, or membrane of a whitish colour, resembling the coagulated matter which was found in the trachea of those children whose bodies were opened. This was thrown off by violent coughing or retching; and the efforts made to dislodge it were often so distressing that the child appeared almost in a state of strangulation."

these summer cases were three children in one family, of whom two died, both being just out of the measles. The later series of cases in the winter of 1793–94 were less often fatal; the epidemic constitution, he says, became less severe towards the end; he also used mercurials freely on the later cases; but it is farther noteworthy that "most of the cases which occurred in November and afterwards, were attended with inflammation and swelling of the tonsils, uvula and velum pendulum palati, and frequently large films of a whitish substance were found on the tonsils"—so that the disease was in its extension more than cynanche trachealis, or croup, even if it had not been also an epidemic infection.

In only one case, the eighth recorded, does he seem to have hesitated between "the croup" and sore-throat: "ulcerated sore-throats being at this time [6 Sept. 1793] somewhat prevalent, induced me to inspect the fauces, and I observed a swelling and no inconsiderable ulcer on the left tonsil." It was in the autumn and winter that these throat complications of "the croup" mostly appeared; and it was because he found "so much disease about the tonsils" in the tracheal and laryngeal cases that he forebore to bleed, and used mercurials. Also in the same season when "the croup" was joined to disease of the tonsils, uvula and velum, there was a certain epidemic constitution prevalent: "In the autumn, likewise, and winter, many children suffered by erysipelatous inflammation behind the ears, in the groins, on the labia of girls, or wherever the skin folded, attended with a very acrid discharge"—precisely the complication of the "throat-distemper" of America described by Douglass and Colden as well as by Bard, also of the Irish throat-epidemic in 1743 mentioned by Rutty, of the morbus strangulatorius in Cornwall described by Starr, and of the sore-throat described by Fothergill. In systematic nosology, do the corrosive pustules behind the ears, in the groins, labia, &c., belong to scarlatina or to diphtheria?

It is perhaps the same juxtaposition, or intermixture of scarlatina anginosa and diphtheria, that we find in the north of Scotland about the same time of the 18th century. Various parish ministers who contributed to the first edition of the *Statistical Account* make mention of "the putrid sore-throat" about 1790 and 1791, without any reference to fever or scarlet rash. The following relates to three localities in Aberdeenshire:

New Deer: "In the autumn of 1791, a putrid kind of sore-throat, which first made its appearance about the coast side, found its way into this parish. Since that, it has continued to rage in different places with great virulence and little intermission, and is peculiarly fatal to the young and people of a full constitution[1]." Crimond, a coast parish: "The putrid sore-throat raged with great violence two or three years ago [1790 or 1791] in most parishes in the neighbourhood, and carried off great numbers : but though a few were seized with it in Crimond, none died of that disorder[2]." Fyvie, an upland parish :—"There has been no prevalent distemper for some time except the putrid sore-throat, which raged about two years ago [probably 1791] and proved fatal to several people. It has appeared this winter, but is not so violent as formerly[3]."

From Aberdeen the epidemic is reported in a letter by one of the physicians, in May, 1790, in such terms as not to imply that it was scarlatina: "The malignant sore-throat has been most prevalent and very fatal, no period of life being exempted." In children from six months to three years there was observed a livid appearance behind the ears which, in seven or eight cases, spread over the external ear, causing the latter on one or both sides to drop off by sloughing before death[4].

The scarlet fever, with sore-throat, which reappeared in London about 1786–87 (and at Chesham in 1788) is said to have been somewhat steady until 1794. Willan, who began his exact records in 1796, says retrospectively that the scarlet fever with an ulcerated sore-throat had been prevalent every autumn from the year 1785 to 1794, "and proved extremely fatal[5]." Lettsom gave a particular account of it in the spring of 1793[6]; it was seen first in the higher villages about London, gradually descended into lower situations, and visited the metropolis pretty generally about the end of February. "It has been remarked for many years that this disease appears in the vicinity of London before it visits the metropolis," beginning often among the numerous boarding-schools in the suburbs, to be carried thence by the dispersion of pupils to their homes. In some villages private families suffered greatly ; in a few Lettsom heard of half the children dying, as well as of deaths among the domestics and other adults. The same epidemic of 1793 also called forth one of the numerous essays of Dr Rowley, who had written on the "malignant ulcerated sore-throat" in 1788[7].

---

[1] Sinclair's *Statist. Account of Scotland*, IX. 190.
[2] *Ibid.* II. 412.　　　　　[3] *Ibid.* IX. 461.
[4] Livingston to Lettsom, Aberdeen, 13 May, 1790, in *Memoirs of Dr Lettsom*, III.
[5] R. Willan, M.D., *Reports on the Diseases in London*, 1796–1800. Lond. 1801, p. 2.
[6] "Cursory Remarks on the Appearance of the Angina Scarlatina in the Spring of 1793." *Mem. Med. Soc. Lond.* IV. (1795), p. 280.
[7] W. Rowley, M.D., *An Essay on the Malignant ulcerated Sore-Throat, containing reflections on its causes and fatal effects in 1787, etc.*, London, 1788; *The Causes of the Great Numbers of Deaths...in Putrid Scarlet Fevers and Ulcerated Sore-Throats explained,etc.*, London, 1793. Based on the practice of the St Marylebone Infirmary.

Scarlatinal Epidemics, 1796–1805.

The history of scarlatina in London, as of most epidemic maladies, is enriched for a few years by Willan's monthly or quarterly accounts of the cases treated at the Carey Street Dispensary. From the beginning of 1796 to the end of 1800, scarlet fever is hardly ever wanting, and is occasionally the principal epidemic. It is only now and then, however, that a death from it appears in the Parish Clerks' bills of mortality. Willan remarks that they gave only one death from that cause between the 8th and 29th November, 1796, "a period during which there occurred many fatal cases of that disease." The bills have only three deaths from it in the quarter 27 Sept.–27 Dec. 1796. The Parish Clerks did not adopt scarlet fever fully into their classification until 1830; long after it had become an important factor in the mortality, they placed the deaths from it under "fevers" or under "measles." According to Willan's experience, it must have been as common as measles from 1796 to 1801. It was, he says, always most virulent and dangerous in the month of October and November, but generally ceased on the first appearance of frost. He records a spring epidemic as an exceptional thing in 1797 : "Since the beginning of May, the scarlatina anginosa has become more frequent than any other contagious disease, both in town and in many parts of the country ; the disease has generally occurred in its malignant and fatal form, which, at this season of the year, is very unusual." The bills give only one death from 18th April to 18th May. Willan says that it was rife again in the autumn of 1797 and of 1798. Dr James Sims, who had described the scarlatina of London in 1786, found the epidemic in the end of 1798 so different from the former, and attended with so great fatality, that he made it the subject of a second paper[1]. It was preceded in the winter and spring of 1797–98 by a remarkable epidemic among the cats of London (an angina, with sanious discharge from the nostrils and running at the eyes), which killed "myriads" of them[2]. In Sept.–Oct. 1798, he heard that a scarlet fever

---

[1] James Sims, M.D. "Sketch of a Description of a Species of Scarlatina Anginosa which occurred in the Autumn of 1798." *Mem. Med. Soc. Lond.* v. (1799), p. 415.

[2] This is the source of Noah Webster's information for London ; he adds that the "cat distemper" appeared in Philadelphia in June, and was very fatal in New York and over the Northern States.

had been fatal to some adults about South Lambeth, and afterwards to several children there, five dying in one family and three in another. The swellings on each side under the jaw were so great as to force the chin up into the horizontal; there was much acrid foetid discharge from the nostrils, the pulse sank about the seventh day, and the scarlet eruption remained out until near death, which took place usually about the ninth or tenth day. Along with this malignant type, a mild or simple scarlatina was also prevalent. Sims wrote when the epidemic seemed to be "in its infancy," and so it proved; for Willan describes it as prevailing to the end of 1798 and rising still higher in the first months of 1799, his report for February and March being: "Scarlatina anginosa in its malignant form has been very prevalent, and has proved in many instances fatal; and in those who recovered, it produced after the cessation of the fever, anasarca, swelling of the abdomen, swelling of the lips and parotid glands, strumous ophthalmia, with an eruption of the favus, and hectical symptoms of long duration. The disease spread from London to the adjacent villages, and was almost universal in Somers Town during the month of February." It continued throughout the year, and into 1800, being second in importance among the epidemic maladies only to typhus, which, in that time of distress, was the grand trouble of the poorer classes in London. Willan's reports cease with the year 1800; but it appears from other sources that a very malignant scarlet fever and sore-throat prevailed in London in the summers and autumns of 1801 and 1802, becoming milder in 1803[1], and in various parts of England during the same three years. The provincial accounts for those years give the impression that this was the first general outbreak for some time, perhaps since the one described by Withering and others in 1778; and that is also suggested by the statistics of the Newcastle Dispensary: in the two first years of its practice, from 1 October, 1777, it treated 146 cases, with 18 deaths; in the next ten years 1779–1789, it treated only 57 cases, with 8 deaths; and from 1790 to 1802, it treated 152 cases, with 7 deaths[2]. Accounts of very general

---

[1] E. Peart, M.D., *Practical Information on the Malignant Scarlet Fever and Sore-Throat.* London, 1802. See also *Med. and Phys. Journ.* IX. 16, report for Dec. 1802: "so very general that few of those who have continued in the same house have entirely escaped it"; and the reports, *ibid.* X. 76, 276.

[2] Clark, u.s. Monteith, *Report of the Newcastle Dispensary from its Foundation,* 1878.

scarlatina come from various parts of England. In the summer and autumn of 1801 it ran through many parishes of Cornwall, sparing others. In the parish of Manaccan, twelve out of the twenty-five burials in the year 1801 were from scarlatina—the malignant or putrid form, which was often fatal before the third day. In many other cases, the first untoward symptom was the dropsical swelling which came on as the fever went off. Three years after, in 1804, there was much scarlatina in and around Falmouth[1]. In 1805 it caused 12 in a total of 20 deaths in Revelstoke parish, South Devon.

In Northamptonshire in 1801 it was observed "in a form similar to the epidemic described by Dr Withering[2]." At Cheltenham in 1802 it was also compared to the epidemic described by Withering: "in consequence of the number of persons who have gone through the disease, it has for this month past (20th December) been gradually on the decline[3]." At Derby, in 1802, it had been the prevailing complaint in the last eight months of the year[4]. In the district of Framlingham, Suffolk, in 1802–3, it had proved very malignant and fatal in many families[5]. It is heard of also from Lancaster[6], and from various other parts of England, being casually mentioned in reports on the influenza of 1803.

To this period also belong several incidents of a kind that had attended scarlatina from its first appearance, namely, school epidemics of it. One of these was an outbreak in the Quaker boarding-school for boys and girls at Ackworth, in Yorkshire, in 1803. Although many of the children dispersed, yet no fewer than 171, in a total of 298 on the roll, were attacked with scarlatina in the course of four months, of whom seven died[7]. In the same year Dr Blackburne published a treatise on the preventive aspect of the disease, with directions for checking the spread of it "in schools and families[8]." It broke out in 1804 among the boys in Heriot's Hospital, Edinburgh, and in the city generally in 1805[9]. Ferrier makes mention of a "destruc-

---

[1] Polwhele's *Cornwall.* Part VII. *Diseases*, p. 59.

[2] F. Skirmshire, *Med. Phys. Journ.* VI. 424.

[3] R. Freeman, *ibid.* IX. 157. [4] H. Gilbert, *ibid.* IX. 249.

[5] Goodwin, *ibid.* IX. 509. [6] Braithwaite, *ibid.* XI.

[7] Willan, *Cutan. Dis.* 1808, p. 379, particulars from Dr Binns, with full discussion of the methods of treatment. Willan was told by Dr Stanger that there were 71 cases in the Foundling Hospital from June to October, 1804, with 4 deaths.

[8] W. Blackburne, M.D., *Facts and Observations concerning the Prevention and Cure of Scarlet Fever, &c.* London, 1803.

[9] James Hamilton, M.D., *Obs. on the Utility, &c. of Purgative Medicines.*

tive epidemic of scarlet fever" in Manchester in 1805, which he supposed to have been introduced from Liverpool[1].

The general prevalence of malignant scarlet fever in the first years of the 19th century is farther shown by the accounts from Ireland, which were recalled by Graves in a clinical lecture of the session 1834–35, during the prevalence of a scarlet fever as malignant as that of thirty years before[2].

"In the year 1801," he says, "in the months of September, October, November and December, scarlet fever committed great ravages in Dublin, and continued its destructive progress during the spring of 1802. It ceased in summer, but returned at intervals during the years 1803–4, when the disease changed its character ; and although scarlatina epidemics recurred very frequently during the next twenty-seven years, yet it was always in the simple or mild form, so that I have known an instance where not a single death occurred among eighty boys attacked in a public institution. The epidemic of 1801-2-3-4, on the contrary, was extremely fatal, sometimes terminating in death (as appears by the notes of Dr Percival kindly communicated to me) so early as the second day. It thinned many families in the middle and upper classes of society, and even left not a few parents childless. Its characters seem to have answered to the definition of the scarlatina maligna of authors."

The long immunity from malignant scarlatina which Graves asserts for Ireland after 1804, is made probable also for England and Scotland after 1805, by the fewness of the references to it in medical writings. Bateman in 1804 resumed the regular reports on the prevalent diseases of London, which Willan had left off at the end of 1800, and continued them until 1816[3]; but he makes very few references to scarlatina compared with his predecessor. The two occasions when it is said to have been somewhat common were in 1807–8, during the severe epidemic of measles (and then it was "generally mild, presenting the eruption with a slight sore-throat"), and in 1814 when it was "very prevalent" along with measles. In Scotland during the same epidemic of malignant measles, in 1808, scarlatina was only occasional, and mild. It is heard of in its old malignant form from two localities of England, during the time of distress and typhus fever in 1810–11. At Nottingham it was "very prevalent, passing through whole families," in September, 1810, and in October became more violent and often fatal[4]. In the

4th ed. Edin. 1811. App. III. p. 66 (three boys in Heriot's Hospital died of dropsy). Autenrieth, *Account of the State of Medicine in Great Britain.* Extracts translated by Graves, u. i.

[1] Ferriar, *Med. Hist. and Reflect.* III. 128.
[2] R. J. Graves, M.D., *A System of Clinical Medicine.* Dublin, 1843, p. 493.
[3] T. Bateman, M.D., *Reports on the Diseases of London, and the State of the Weather, from 1804 to 1816.* London, 1819.
[4] Clarke, *Ed. Med. and Surg. Journ.* XXX.

district around Debenham, in Suffolk, where it was last reported by the same observer in 1803, it made its appearance in February, 1810, in its very worst forms, causing deaths of children and adults in many houses, and destroying some children within forty-eight hours from the first attack. "All the surgeons for ten miles round have had to attend to scarlatina maligna in a variety of cases in all ages, from infants to fifty and sixty years." It was still raging in October, 1810, and was breaking out "in different spots around this country, that appear to have had no communication with the afflicted[1]."

It is not until 1831 that we begin to hear much of malignant scarlatina again. But it is clear that scarlet fever was common enough all through that interval, probably in its milder form. It was now the usual epidemic trouble of schools. In September and October, 1814, there were fifty-five cases, mostly mild, in children and two in adults in the Asylum for Female Orphans at Westminster[2]. In 1812 it was among the cadets in the Royal Military College at Marlow, having been followed by anasarca in only one instance[3]. Heysham, whose exact records of epidemics at Carlisle were made twenty or thirty years earlier, mentions casually in 1814 that scarlet fever had been "more frequent of late," but that it did not spread as formerly[4]. Other references to it in this interval are to show how seldom fatal it was under the cold water treatment or the lowering regimen[5]. At the Newcastle Dispensary fully twice as many cases of scarlatina were attended in the twenty-five years 1803–27 (795 cases) as in the twenty-five years 1777–1802 (355 cases); but in the larger total, which an increasing population might account for, there were actually fewer fatalities (30) than in the smaller (33); the highest number in any one year was 71 in 1824, of which every one is entered as having recovered. This is the impression derived from various sources—that the scarlatina from about 1803 until about 1830 may have been frequent, but that it was mild, or easily treated, or not often fatal. Mac-michael, writing in 1822, not only testified that the "scarlatina

---

[1] Goodwin, of Earlsoham, *Med. and Phys. Journ.* XXIV. 465.
[2] Samuel Fothergill, M.D. *Med. and Phys. Journ.* XXXII. 481.
[3] N. Bruce, *Med. Chir. Trans.* IX. 273.
[4] Heysham to Joshua Milne, in the latter's *Treatise on the Valuation of Annuities.* Lond. 1815. App. p. 755.
[5] Currie, *Med. Reports*, 1805, II. 458 ; Armstrong, *Pract. Illustr. of the Scarlet Fever, Measles, &c.* Lond. 1818 ; Lodge, of Preston, in *Med. and Phys. Journ.* XXXIII. (1815), p. 358.

of last summer was very mild," but argued that the malady in general was taken by many in those years in so mild a form that it was not recognized as scarlatina, "a name that sounds so fearfully in the ears of mothers," and a rare disease in families compared w th measles or even with smallpox. His point is that scarlet ever was in fact as nearly universal as measles, but that, as it v as often extremely slight, it passed for rose rash or the like; at the same time he identified these slighter forms with true scarlatina by simply pointing to the oedema which might follow them[1].

The testimony of Graves, of Dublin, who occupies many pages of his 'Clinical Medicine' with the disastrous scarlatina in various parts of Ireland about 1834, is conclusive that the severe type was new in the experience of that generation :

> "I have already mentioned that the disease called scarlet fever assumed a very benign type in Dublin soon after the year 1804, and continued to be seldom attended with danger until the year 1831, when we began to perceive a notable alteration in its character, and remarked that the usual undisguised and inflammatory nature of the attack was replaced by a concealed and insidious form of fever, attended with great debility. We now began occasionally to hear of cases which proved unexpectedly fatal, and of families in which several children were carried off; still, it was not until the year 1834 that the disease spread far and wide, assuming the form of a destructive epidemic[2]....Many parents lost three of their children, some four, and in one instance which came to my knowledge, five very fine children were carried off." The severe cases were mixed with others of scarlatina simplex. The violence of the attack lay in the throat-affection, the congestion of the brain, or the irritability of the stomach and bowels, nausea, vomiting and diarrhoea being early symptoms, as in the malignant sore-throat with rash a century before.

Graves proceeds, with much candour, to show how mistaken had been the reasons assigned equally for the mild type of scarlatina between 1804 and 1831 and for the severe type of it previous to 1804 :

---

[1] W. Macmichael, M.D., *A New View of the Infection of Scarlet Fever, &c.* London, 1822, pp. 30, 59, 78, 81–2. The title of another essay appears to reflect the same ideas, *Caution to the Public, or hints upon the nature of Scarlet Fever, designed to show that this disease arises from a peculiar and absolute virus, and is specifically infectious in its mildest as well as in its most malignant form.* By William Cooke, London, 1831.

[2] Kreysig, "Ueber das Scharlachfieber," *Hecker's Annalen,* IV. 273, 401, 1826, says that scarlatina had been "not only almost uninterrupted in all Europe since twenty-six or twenty-seven years [1799 or 1800], but also frightfully fatal." The period in which this was written appears to have been one of fatal scarlatina in some parts of Germany; so also the years 1817–19, and the years 1799–1805 (as in Great Britain and Ireland). But the sweeping assertion as to frightful scarlatina mortality in all Europe without interruption since 1799 is clearly a flight of rhetoric, and is as nearly as possible the reverse of the truth so far as concerns Britain and Ireland.

" The long continuance of the period during which the character of scarlet fever was either so mild as to require little care, or so purely inflammatory as to yield readily to the judicious employment of antiphlogistic treatment, led many to believe that the fatality of the former epidemic was chiefly, if not altogether, owing to the erroneous method of cure then resorted to by the physicians of Dublin, who counted among their numbers not a few disciples of the Brunonian school ; indeed, this opinion was so prevalent, that all those whose medical education commenced at a much later period, were taught to believe that the diminished mortality of scarlet fever was entirely attributable to the cooling regimen and to the timely use of the lancet and aperients, remedies interdicted by our predecessors.   This was taught in the schools, and scarlet fever was every day quoted as exhibiting one of the most triumphant examples of the efficacy of the new doctrines.   This I myself learned—this I taught : how erroneously will appear from the sequel.   It was argued, that had the cases which proved fatal in 1801–2 been treated by copious depletion in their very commencement, the fatal debility would never have set in, for we all regarded this debility as a mere consequence of previous excessive reaction.   The experience derived from the present [1834–35] epidemic has completely refuted this reasoning, and has proved that, in spite of our boasted improvements, we have not been more successful in 1834–5 than were our predecessors in 1801–2."

From 1829 to 1833 there are numerous references to the scarlatina maligna in England and Scotland : at Plymouth[1] in 1829, Bridlington[2] in 1831, Baddeley Green, Brown Edge, and other places in Staffordshire[3] in the summer of 1831, Beaconsfield, Bucks[4], in 1832, Edinburgh[5] in 1832–1833. It is in 1830 that scarlet fever begins to have a line to itself in the old and inadequate bills of the Parish Clerks of London, the deaths that year being 94 ; in the next seven years they are 143, 388, 481, 523, 445, 261 and 189. In 1835 we begin to have statistics of the deaths from it in Glasgow[6] for five years, during which they fell much below the deaths from either measles or smallpox.

Deaths from Scarlatina in Glasgow.

	Under one	1–2	2–5	5–10	10–20	20–30	30–40	40 and up.	Total
1835	27	50	89	73	23	7	2	2	273
1836	34	57	136	86	25	9	5	3	355
1837	4	9	34	22	5	3	1	1	79
1838	3	15	42	17	7	1	1	1	87
1839	29	45	104	74	10	—	—	—	262

The two first years of this period, which had the most scarlatina deaths, correspond to the years of the Dublin

[1] Blackmore, *Lond. Med. Gaz.* VI. 114.
[2] Sandwith, *Edin. Med. and Surg. Journ.* XI. 249.
[3] Aulsebrook, *Lancet*, 12 Nov. 1831, p. 217 : cases of very malignant suddenly fatal scarlatina in infants and young persons up to the age of twenty-two. In the house of a canal boatman a son and two daughters, from 21 to 13 years, died in the course of two days after a very sudden and brief illness.
[4] Rumsey, *Trans. Prov. Med. Assoc.* III. 194.
[5] Hamilton, *Edin. Med. Surg. Journ.* XXXIX. 140.
[6] Cowan, *Journ. Statist. Soc.* III.

epidemic, and were also the years when it was common in Edinburgh[1]. Probably the smaller mortality of Glasgow in 1837 and 1838 was general; for, when registration of the causes of death began in England and Wales in the latter half of 1837, it found the scarlatina mortality at a much lower figure than it reached in 1839 and continued to keep thereafter.

Scarlatina since the beginning of Registration, 1837.

The first returns of the causes of death under the new Registration Act happened to correspond with a great epidemic of typhus fever, and with an equally great epidemic of smallpox which took its victims in largest part among infants and young children. The deaths from scarlatina were also considerable during those two years and a half; but in 1840 scarlatina nearly doubled its mortality, and continued year after year for a whole generation to be the leading cause of death among the infectious maladies of childhood. The figures for England and Wales are given in a table at p. 614, in comparison with the annual deaths by smallpox, measles, and diphtheria. The enormous number of deaths from scarlatina during some thirty or forty years in the middle of the 19th century will appear in the history as one of the most remarkable things in our epidemiology. There can be no reasonable doubt that this scarlatinal period was preceded by a whole generation with moderate or small mortality from that disease, just as it is now being followed by annual death-rates which are less than a half, perhaps not more than a third, of the average during forty years before 1880.

The first great epidemic all over England was in 1840 (it had reached a maximum in London the year before), another came in 1844, a third in 1848 (in which the London death-rate was 2·12 per thousand living). In the next decennial period, 1851–60, the worst years for scarlatina were 1858–59, which were also the years of the return of diphtheria; in the period 1861–70, the great scarlatinal years were 1863–64 and 1868–70; in the period 1871–80, the year 1874 was the epidemic year. The annual average death-rates per million inhabitants in all England and Wales were as follows in four decennial periods:

---

[1] Sidey, Stark and others in *Edin. Med. and Surg. Journ.* 1835–36. H. Kennedy, M.D., *Account of the Epidemic of Scarlatina in Dublin from 1834 to 1842.* Dublin, 1843.

| 1851–60 | 832 | | 1871–80 | 716 |
| 1861–70 | 972 | | 1881–90 | 338 |

In the greatest epidemic years since 1863 the death-rates per million for the whole country have been:

1863	1498		1869	1275
1864	1443		1870	1461
1868	1020		1874	1062

In those years scarlatina made from four to six and a half per cent. of the deaths from all causes.

While no county of England has been free from this infection, the bulk of the deaths have fallen upon the capital, the great Lancashire and West Riding towns, the Black Country of Staffordshire with Warwickshire, the mining districts of Durham and South Wales, and, in the earlier part of the period, upon the south-western counties.

Highest Mortalities by Scarlatina in three Epidemics.

	1863	1864	1868	1869	1870	1874
England and Wales	30475	29700	21912	27641	32543	24922
London	4955	3244	2916	5841	6040	2648
Lancashire	4580	4854	4445	4890	3702	6404
West Riding	2218	3135	1676	2870	3718	3779
Durham	1216	403	2678	1512	983	1941
South Wales	501	1990	285	804	1370	1388
Staffordshire	1147	1134	943	1198	1064	1270
Devonshire	778	1054	60	155	646	72
Cornwall	995	572	254	161	587	50
Somerset	773	1013	55	154	584	173

In Lancashire and South Staffordshire there has been less fluctuation of the mortality from year to year than elsewhere. The stress of an epidemic has not fallen equally on all the principal centres in the same year or years: thus Durham has had the epidemic in advance of other centres, while South Wales has had it in arrear. The decline of the south-western counties from their leading position in 1863–64 has been remarkable. Plymouth, Devonport and Stonehouse, which had contributed most to the high scarlatinal death-rate of Devonshire in 1863–64, were found on the average of the next decennial period to have low rates from scarlatina, but death-rates from measles which were unapproached in any other region of England. In the following table four Devonshire towns are

compared with certain Staffordshire registration districts in
which the scarlatinal death-rate has remained high.

Annual average Death-rates per 1000 *living*, 1871–80.

	All causes	Scarlatina	Measles
Plymouth	22·63	·25	1·13
E. Stonehouse	28·23	·33	1·79
Stoke Damerel	20·42	·37	1·19
Exeter	24·99	·50	·82
Stoke-on-Trent	25·80	1·22	·49
Wolverhampton	22·78	1·05	·35
Walsall	22·82	1·21	·30
Dudley	24·24	1·18	·59

This looks like a correlation between measles and scarlatina.
The excessive death-rate from measles in Plymouth, Stonehouse
and Devonport was due to a disastrous epidemic in the last two
years of the decennium, 1879 and 1880 (338 deaths at Plymouth,
121 at Stonehouse, and 235 at Devonport). Measles remained
high in Plymouth all through the next decennium, scarlatina
still continuing low until the very end of it, when in 1889 there
was a mortality of 270, equal to a death-rate of 3·39 per 1000
living. In like manner Stoke-on-Trent had its great epidemic
of measles in 1888, causing 342 deaths, or a rate of 2·8. The
high Plymouth death-rate, after nearly twenty years with
extremely little scarlet fever, was surpassed in 1882 by an
epidemic of 346 deaths in the colliery townships of Aberystruth
and Tredegar, Monmouthshire, equal to a death-rate of 6·1 per
1000. Other high death-rates for single years were at Wakefield
and Swansea in 1889 and at Neath in 1890. The highest
death-rates from scarlatina on an average of ten years, 1871–80,
were at Durham 1·70, Todmorden 1·64, Auckland 1·63, Gateshead 1·60, Sheffield 1·49, Leigh 1·41, Wigan 1·30, Newcastle
1·28. The purely agricultural counties have the lowest death-
rates[1].

[1] The principal epidemics of scarlatina which have been inquired into by
inspectors of the medical department since 1870 have been the following:
In 1870, Camborne, Wing.
    1873, Fleetwood-on-Wyre.
    1874, Hetton (Durham).
    1877, Massingham, Portsmouth.
    1879, Pontypool, Easington (Durham), Fallowfield (near Manchester), Yeadon.
    1880, Bedlington (near Morpeth), Stourbridge, Swindon, Castleford, Llanelly,
      Huntingdon, Barkingside (Orphans' Home near Romford).
    1881, Durham, Halifax, Thame.
    1882, Bedwelty (Tredegar and Aberystruth), Potton.
    1883, Sutton in Ashfield, Thorne, Donington and Moulton (Spalding).
    1885, Sandal (near Wakefield).
    1886, Atherton, Hayfield, Hindley, Wombwell.
    1889, Spennymoor (Durham), Macclesfield, Faringdon, Brixham.

As to age-incidence, the proportion of deaths under five has been almost exactly two-thirds steadily for the last four decennial periods (supra p. 625). The following table by Dr Ogle, the Superintendent of Statistics, shows both age and sex of the scarlatina mortality[1]:

Mean annual Mortality from Scarlet Fever per million living at successive age-periods 1859–85. England and Wales.

Age	Males	Females
0—1	1664	1384
1—2	4170	3874
2—3	4676	4491
3—4	4484	4332
4—5	3642	3556
0— 5	3681	3482
5—10	1667	1613
10—15	346	381
15—20	111	113
20—25	59	77
25—35	36	58
35 and upwards	13	15
All ages	778	717

From certain hospital statistics on a large scale, and some figures of cases and deaths at Christiania, it was also found that the attacks of scarlatina were much more fatal in the first years of life, the fatality decreasing rapidly after five. This was only to be expected. But it was somewhat surprising to find that more girls were attacked than boys, while the fatalities among boys were more than among an equal number of girls at all ages until womanhood, when the few females attacked by scarlatina had more fatalities among them than the somewhat fewer males of the same ages. A slight excess of fatality in the female sex over the male between the ages of ten and twenty years, is shown also for smallpox by the table at p. 618. Recent notifications of infectious diseases to medical officers of health have enabled a comparison to be made between the number of cases of scarlatina notified, with age and sex, and the number of deaths certified in the corresponding time and place to the Registrar-General ; from which the above generalities as to the proportions of fatal cases in the several age-periods of either sex have been confirmed[2].

---

[1] William Ogle, M.D., in the 49*th* *Report of the Registrar-General* (*for* 1886), p. xiv.
[2] See a paper, with Tables, on "Age, Sex and Season in relation to Scarlet Fever," by Arthur Whitelegge, M.D. in *Trans. Epidemid. Soc.* N.S. VII. p. 153, for Nottingham and some other towns. A paper by Dr Ballard, "On the Prevalence

The enormous mortalities of some years may be taken to have depended in part upon an increased prevalence of the disease, but still more upon an increased fatality among the subjects of it. Since the establishment of the Metropolitan Fever Hospitals in 1870 the percentage of deaths to cases has ranged from 15·3 in 1879 to 6·6 in 1873 and 6·7 in 1891. Among the smaller totals of the London Fever Hospital the percentage of deaths has ranged even more widely from year to year[1]. What is thus statistically proved is also a matter of common experience; there have been whole epidemics, extending perhaps over two or three years, marked by high malignancy, and epidemics just as uniformly marked by mildness of type. The severe type has usually been made by the sloughing in the neck or throat; but there has also been a class of cases tending to a fatal issue early in the attack by a sunken pulse and with few external manifestations. The cause of these variations in the severity of scarlatina is the old problem of epidemic constitutions: sometimes the constitution is "putrid" or "pestilential" or malignant, sometimes it is mild or benign.

Graves, in the passage above cited, has sufficiently exposed the fallacy of attributing changes of type to modes of treatment. On the other hand there is reason to think that the percentage of deaths (by which the "type" is usually judged) is higher in children carried off to hospitals than in those treated at home. As the same fact has been uniformly observed in epidemics of Asiatic cholera, when the ambulances have been almost as busy as those of the Metropolitan Asylums Board during an ordinary autumnal rise of scarlatina, it is probable that the reasons which used to be given in the former case hold good also in the latter.

Scarlet Fever in London, 1890 *and* 1891.

Year	All Cases Notified	Treated at Home	Treated in Hospital	Fatalities at Home	Fatalities in Hospital
1890	15330	8793	6537	348 or 3·95%	510 or 7·8%
1891	11398	6136	5267	232 or 3·8%	357 or 6·8%

and Fatality of Scarlatina as influenced by Sex, Age and Season," which was written twenty years before but left unpublished, follows Whitelegge's in the *Trans. Epidem. Soc.* N.S. VII. (1887–8).

[1] A table of figures showing this will be found in Dr B. A. Whitelegge's second lecture on "Changes of Type in Epidemic Diseases." *Brit. Med. Journ.* 4 March, 1893.

This is a comparison of two parts of the same epidemic, which had a very moderate fatality in any case. The real problem of malignity or severity of type arises over such epidemics as those of 1840, 1848, 1858–59, 1868–70 and 1874, in which the doubling of the deaths, for one year, or for two or even three consecutive years, had depended less upon an increased number of seizures than upon a higher ratio of fatalities. An explanation for each occasion will have to be sought either in the condition of the patients, or in the inherent properties or external favouring circumstances of the virus. As to the former, the most fatal epidemic years of scarlet fever have not been marked in any such uniform way as the great seasons of typhus or relapsing fever; nor is scarlatina an infection that keeps mainly within the poorer classes. Among factors of the external kind, a rainfall below the average has been thought a relevant thing: thus in the three years 1862–64, the annual average rainfall at Greenwich was only 20·6 inches, the scarlatina death-rate in London for the same years reaching the high figure of 1·33 per 1000 inhabitants; in the next three years, 1865–67, the death-rate fell to ·56 (it would have fallen in any case), while the rainfall reached the very high average of 29 inches; in the three years following, 1868–70, the death-rate reached the excessive annual average of 1·5 per 1000 in London, the rainfall of the same period averaging only 22·3 inches. Thereafter for a number of years the rainfall was moderate and the scarlatina death-rate low; but in the years 1883–87, they were both low together, the scarlatina death-rate of ·26 being lower than it had ever been since registration began[1].

Although an empirical correspondence between the great scarlatina periods and a series of dry years has not been made out without important exceptions, hitherto unexplained, yet there is a very obvious correspondence between the great rise of scarlatina deaths in London every year and the season of late autumn, which is the season when the ground-water touches its lowest level or begins to rise therefrom to the high water-mark of spring. Of all the curves of seasonal rise and fall constructed by Buchan and Mitchell from the weekly bills of mortality in London from 1845 to 1874, that of scarlatina is the most

---

[1] Longstaff, *Trans. Epid. Soc.* N.S. IV. (1880), 421, and *Studies in Statistics.* London, 1891, p. 310. D. A. Gresswell, *Contribution to the Natural History of Scarlatina.* Oxford, 1890, p. 193.

decided next to that of infantile diarrhoea, the deaths rising in October and November far above the mean line of the year, and falling farthest below the mean in spring and early summer[1]. This was an old observation—by Sydenham for the scarlatina simplex of that age, by Willan in the end of the 18th century (one or two spring epidemics being remarked upon as exceptional). It is a very curious fact, and one that is as certain (for London at least) as it is curious. Sydenham explained it by the doctrine of his time, that the favouring things were in the human body, namely, some susceptibility of the humours owing to the heat of the preceding summer; but, according to modern views, it should bring scarlatina into the same class with the soil-poisons of enteric fever, yellow fever and cholera, which are believed to become more rife owing to the greater activity of their respective miasmatic viruses when the pores of the ground are occupied to the greatest depth with air in place of water.

It would be singular indeed if, after all, we should have to include scarlatina among the miasmatic diseases; for it is an exquisite instance of an infection which is passed from person to person, or by the agency of volatile contagion, or by fomites in clothes, bed-linen, house-furnishings and the like. The controversy which has raged so keenly in the past between contagionists and non-contagionists over the instances of plague, yellow fever and Asiatic cholera, would become still more keen over scarlatina—and be still more confused if it were not stated in more correct terms at the outset. What we all find so hard to learn is, that the one way of infection does not exclude the other. Plague was for the most part a miasmatic infection in the air of a plague-stricken town; but it could be conveyed in clothes or bales, while it was prudent to remain not too long in the company of a plague-patient. In like manner contagion from the person was, as Rush said and Blane confirmed, a "contingency" in yellow fever; and there are some authentic cases of Asiatic cholera which cannot well be explained except on the hypothesis of contact with the persons of those sick or dead of the disease. Scarlatina is more contagious than any of these, because it shows so much on the surface of the body and scatters its infective matter into the atmosphere of a room with the fine scales or dust of desquamation. Still, there are conditions for the contagiousness of scarlatina, just as there are for the rarer event of

[1] *Journ. Scot. Meteorol. Soc.* July, 1874, p. 195.

contagion from the persons of the sick in the plague, yellow fever and cholera. It is a remarkable fact that scarlet fever should ever be sporadic, or that a single case should appear in the midst of a crowded population (as I have seen in a coast town filled with strangers during the herring fishery to the extent of one-half more than its usual numbers), and no other cases follow for months after, although there had been not the smallest attempt at isolation. Every medical practitioner knows, if some laymen and legislators do not, that scarlatina is sometimes highly contagious, and sometimes hardly contagious at all; and who can say whether the mechanical routine of "stamping out" contagion, which certain persons pursue with more zeal than knowledge, may not be the means of turning a mere potency into an actuality? The tact of individuals rather than the grinding machinery of an Act of Parliament is needed in dealing with vagaries such as Willan thus describes:

"I have seen in numerous families one child have scarlatina without communicating it to any of the rest; yet, perhaps, in the succeeding autumn, several of them were infected by only passing near a patient recovering from the disease, or by touching those who had a little time before visited some persons affected with it[1]."

There are two special forms of epidemic scarlatina which may prove to be finger-post instances for the general pathology. It happens from time to time in the surgical wards of hospitals for children, where many cases of suppurating diseases (especially of the bones or joints) are aggregated and kept together perhaps for months, that groups of the patients acquire a scarlet rash, or an erysipelatous rash, or a hybrid form of rash, along with the constitutional symptoms of scarlatina. Whether it be from the suppuration, or from the blood of operations, this disease must be reckoned a product of so-called "hospitalism." It is not without significance that there may be an element of erysipelas in such cases. They are probably cases of "blood poisoning," in a double meaning of the term—poisoning of the living blood by dead blood or by pus which is closely allied to blood[2].

---

[1] *Cutaneous Diseases.* Vol. I. 1808, p. 254.

[2] An unfortunate event that came under the writer's notice some years ago may be illustrative of this. Two women with cancer of the breast were operated on, the one after the other, in the same operating theatre. Their beds were in the same hospital ward, but separated by the whole length of the ward. A few days after the operations, one of the women developed erysipelas, which was most extensive on the back; very soon after the other woman got the disease in a precisely similar way; they both died of it. As it seemed improbable that No. 1 had been infected in the ward, or that No. 2 had been infected from No. 1, (some dozen surgical cases

The other special kind of epidemic scarlatina is that which has broken out among the inmates of houses supplied with milk from a common source.   There have been many such outbreaks, including one most remarkable instance in which a large number of guests at an evening party, who had partaken of cream with strawberries, were shortly thereafter attacked by scarlet fever at their widely scattered homes.   There can be no question that milk, or cream, has been the vehicle of scarlatinal infection. The first hypothesis tried was that of scarlatina on the dairy-man's premises; the effluvia of a scarlatinal patient might have become mixed with the milk.   In some instances, it was actually shown that there had been a case or cases of scarlet fever among the dairyman's children; but there were other instances in which that could not be shown, and it was, of course, possible to refer the cases, where they did occur, to a common cause in the milk used at the dairy and in the milk distributed from it.   As more and more outbreaks of the kind came to be investigated, it was indeed made probable that the infection had got into the milk from the cow[1].   Someone threw out the suggestion that the cow suffered from scarlet fever, the sign of it being soreness of the paps.   Without taking seriously so random a hypothesis as that, we find much agreement as to the fact that the cows, to which the contaminated milk has been traced, were affected, one or more of them, with sore paps.   In some cases the disease of the teats had been admitted to be the same as cowpox; in other cases that has been denied; in a third variety, a cow has had cowpox on one teat and something else on another.   It matters little what name be given to the affection of the cow's paps. All soreness of the skin of the teats has the same effect so far as concerns the purity of the milk.   Unless the milk be drawn off by a catheter (according to a German practice), the paps are necessarily made to bleed by being "stripped"; it has been

between them escaping,) the suggestion arises of a common source of both infections in the operating theatre.   The operating table was covered by a woollen cloth, of red colour so as not to show blood stains; it must have contained a good deal of putrid invisible blood from former operations.

[1] The first instance showing this came from a dairy at Hendon.   See James Cameron, M.D. *Trans. Epid. Soc.* v. (1885–6), p. 104; and *ibid.* VIII. 40.   One of the latest and most fully investigated came from a dairy near Glasgow, J. B. Russell, M.D., LL.D., and A. K. Chalmers, M.D. *Glas. Med. Journ.* Jan. 1893, p. 1.   An outbreak at Wimbledon and Merton is described, *Rep. Med. Off. Loc. Gov. Bd.* for 1886, p. 327.   See also *ibid.* for 1882, p. 63.   The scarlatina caused by cream (with strawberries) is traced, *ibid.* for 1875, p. 72.   A very clear case of scarlatinal epidemic due to contaminated milk occurred at Blackheath, both among children and adults, in April, 1894.

admitted by milkers that the blood, pus, and scabs are apt to become mixed with the milk; and the discharges from the sore paps have actually been seen, by a scientific witness, to trickle over the fingers of the milkers into the milk-pail[1]. The contamination of the milk which produces scarlatina in those who use it is neither more nor less specific than that. The disease is blood poisoning in the double sense of the term— poisoning of the living blood by dead blood. Blood is a peculiar fluid, and so is milk. When the two come together the result is peculiar. Both are animal fluids that curdle by some peculiar ferment-change in their constituents. Again, milk is peculiar in its property of taking up organic effluvia; thus the milk standing in shallow vessels has been known to acquire the taste and odour of tar from a tarpaulin in the adjoining farm-yard. With such properties of the milk, a small quantity of blood or pus in it will go a long way.

The one thing that connects the scarlatina of surgical wards in children's hospitals and the scarlatina of the milk-pail is putrefying blood or pus: the disease is a septic effect of blood, just as a scarlet rash is known to be a toxic effect of very various drugs in peculiarly susceptible subjects. The obviously septic varieties of scarlatina make but an insignificant part of the whole; but they may be finger-post instances. Thus, if we assume that the infection may be miasmatic from the ground as well as contagious from the person, there are certain facts, or suspicions, that will fit the hypothesis of putrefying blood. A theory of scarlatina was put forward in 1871, on the basis of observations near Croydon, that its virus came from the blood and offal of slaughter-houses collected at particular spots to be used as manure[2]. The first death in a recent small epidemic within the writer's knowledge was of a school-girl who lived just across the road from a slaughter-house. The septic hypothesis of scarlatina might be made to include other corrupting animal matters. Some practitioners have a suspicion that scarlet fever is bred in the atmosphere of a horse-mews. On the greater scale, others have traced a connexion between the more signal outbreaks of angina maligna and preceding murrains

[1] E. M. Crookshank, *Path. Trans.* XXXIX. 382, in an extensive prevalence of cowpox on a dairy farm near Cricklade. No scarlatina could be traced in the neighbourhood.
[2] Alfred Carpenter, M.D. *Lancet*, 28 Jan. and 4 Feb. 1871.

of cattle[1]. The animal matters which may become toxic to man, in miasmatic or other form, are indeed many. If scarlatinal drug-eruptions are any clue to the mystery of scarlet fever, we need not be surprised to find a somewhat uniform disease-effect produced by a variety of septic agents[2]. But, in that hypothesis, the refuse of the shambles will merit most attention. This was thought the one great nuisance of London in the sanitary ordinances of Edward III., Richard II. and Henry VII.; it was then considered a danger to health in the measure of its offensiveness to sight and smell, but there may still be dangers from it which are subtle and unperceived.

Reappearance of Diphtheria in 1856–59.

The memorable outburst of epidemic throat-disease in Britain about the years 1858–59 was part of a sudden uprising of the malady all over the globe—in Europe, America, North Africa, India, China, and the Pacific[3]. It was only in some parts of France, and of Norway and Denmark, that "diphtheria" had been epidemic in the generation before. Of its novelty to nearly the whole British profession in 1858, familiar as they were with the angina of scarlet fever, there can be no question. Its appearance among diseases coincided with the publication of Darwin's hypothesis of the origin of species by natural selection ; and it was in the terms of that hypothesis that Farr, of the Registration Department, spoke of the phenomenon of diphtheria. New diseases, he said, "are only recognized as distinct species when they have existed for some time. Diphtheria is an example. It obtains a distinct line in the Tables of this year [1859] for the first time"—with a total of 9587 deaths. For four years before that, it had been in a " provisional table " under the names of " diphtheria " and " cynanche maligna " ; but in the general table, the deaths under these names had been merged with the scarlatinal deaths. This inclusion for a time of diphtheria under scarlatina could not have been because practitioners had any difficulty in diagnosing the one from the other,

---

[1] Wall, *Gent. Magaz.* 1751, p. 71, 501. He quotes Severinus to the effect that the great epidemic of *garrotillo* in the province of Naples in 1618 was preceded by a murrain.

[2] Prince A. Morrow, " Drug Eruptions," edited for the New Sydenham Society by T. Colcott Fox, in *Selected Monographs on Dermatology*. London, 1893.

[3] Hirsch, III. 87.

but probably because scarlatina anginosa seemed the nearest affinity in the nosological system. Diphtheria in 1858 had no scarlet rash, and yet it was supposed to be the same disease that had made so much commotion in England about the middle of the 18th century: "In Fothergill's account," says Farr, "the symptoms are confused by the introduction of the eruption of scarlatina into his description"—as if his description had been a patchwork of his fancy, with some characters taken from "diphtheria" and some from scarlet fever. The greatest of our nosologists, Cullen, had long before that separated "cynanche maligna" from "scarlatina anginosa," but the separation was not made on the ground of absent or present rash. Both had the rash, the cynanche having, besides a general exanthem, very distinctively the peculiar scarlet redness, with swelling and stiffness, of the fingers which Fothergill described, while the scarlatina rash was "commonly more considerable and universal." Both also might have a discharge from the nose; but when the coryza did occur in scarlatina, "it is less acrid, and has not the foetid smell which it has in the other disease." It was really on the ground of malignancy or fatality that Cullen separated them. In forty years he had seen scarlatina anginosa six or seven times prevailing as an epidemic in Scotland, and he had seen two or three epidemics of cynanche maligna. He had seen mild cases in the latter, as well as in the former; but whereas there would be only one or two malignant cases in a hundred of scarlatina anginosa, the malignant or putrid cases in an epidemic of cynanche were four-fifths of the whole[1]. On the other hand Willan, writing just fifty years before the modern diphtheria made its appearance, maintained that "no British author has yet described any epidemical and contagious sore-throat except that which attends the scarlet fever," not even Starr, whose "morbus strangulatorius" he held to be "the most virulent form of scarlatina[2]."

[1] Cullen, *First Lines of the Practice of Physic*, Part I., Book II. chap. 5, § 2, and Book III. chap. 4.

[2] *On Cutaneous Diseases*, vol. I., London, 1808, pp. 319, 326, 333. He included also the *garrotillo* of Spain and the throat-plague of Naples (1618) among the "varieties of scarlatina," inasmuch as they had not unfrequently a rash which was of the erysipelatous kind. Hirsch (u. s.) and Max Jaffe ("Die Diphtherie in epidemiologischer und nosologischer Beziehung vornehmlich nach Französischen und Englischen Autoren zusammengestellt," Originalabhandlung in *Schmidt's Jahrbücher*, CXIII., 1862, pp. 97–120) do not seem to doubt the diphtheritic nature of the *garrotillos* of Spain and Italy in the 16th and 17th centuries, but they agree with Willan in classing most of the 18th century throat-distempers of English and American writers as scarlatinal,

The name diphtheria, which appeared for the first time among the classified causes of death in England in the report for the year 1855 (published two years after), had been given originally in 1826, with the termination *itis* according to the then Broussaisian fashion, by Bretonneau in his account of epidemics at Tours in 1818–21 and at La Ferrière in 1824–25[1]. It was in January, 1855, or just before the disease became general in Europe, that he changed the termination to *diphtherie*[2]. This name was taken from διφθέρα, a prepared skin or hide, suggesting in strict correctness, a certain toughness and texture which were actually found in only a small proportion of all the diphtheritic deposits or exudations or sloughing infiltrations in the first great epidemic and subsequently.

The interval between 1793–94, the date of Rumsey's diphtheria or "croup" at Chesham, and the outbreak of diphtheria in England in 1856–59, affords several instances of the disease, some of which were contemporaneous with Bretonneau's in France, but were still called "croup" in this country. These I shall merely enumerate in a note, passing at once to the beginnings of the great outbreak[3].

The first public notice of the reappearance of a fatal throat epidemic in England appears to have been in the Registrar-

reserving as diphtheritic, or as more nearly allied to diphtheria, Starr's "morbus strangulatorius" of Cornwall, some cases of infants recorded by Denman (*supra*, p. 714), Rumsey's cases of "croup" (*supra*, p. 716), and the epidemic described by Bard, of New York (*supra*, p. 690). These matters of identification appear to be like matters of taste, for which the best rule is *non disputandum*. I have already pointed out that Bard himself did not hesitate to identify the epidemic throat-disease of his time with that which Douglass had described in New England thirty years before.

[1] P. Bretonneau, *Des inflammations spéciales du tissu muqueux et en particulier de la Diphthérite*, Paris, 1826, with supplement in 1827.

[2] Id. *Arch. gén. de méd.*, Jan., 1855.

[3] Mackenzie, *Ed. Med. and Surg. Journ.*, April, 1825, p. 294, and *Med. Chir. Rev.*, 1827, p. 289, for Glasgow in 1819. The disease which Mackenzie called croup, was generally known in Glasgow at that time as "croupy sore throat." It was very fatal, attacking several children in the same family, was reckoned contagious, was not a modification of scarlatina, was very different from idiopathic croup as it began on the tonsils and descended to the larynx and trachea, and, lastly, was sometimes marked by gangrenous foetor.

Robertson, *Edin. Med. and Surg. Journ.* (1826) XXV. 279, for Kelso in 1825.

Bewley, *Dub. Journ. of Med. Sci.* VIII. 401, for Dublin in 1835–36. An outbreak observed by Brown, at Haverfordwest, in 1849–50, involving some 200 cases and 40 deaths, was identified in 1858 with diphtheria (*Med. Times and Gaz.*, May, 1858, p. 566, see also *Med. Chir. Trans.* XL. 49). Outbreaks more vaguely recalled in 1858 as diphtheria occurred at Ashford in 1817, and at Leatherhead (30 deaths in the workhouse) at an uncertain date (*2nd Rep.* (1859) *Med. Offices Privy Council*, pp. 244, 320). F. Ryland, *Diseases and Injuries of the Larynx and Trachea*, London, 1837, pp. 161–175, described a similar disease as a complication of measles at Birmingham in 1835.

General's third quarterly report of the year 1857, when attention was drawn to the remarks by various local registrars (Thame, Billericay, Maldon, Liskeard, Truro and Chesterfield) as to fatalities from "inflammation of the throat," "putrid sore throat," "malignant sore throat," "disease in the throat," and "throat-fever." About this time it was also called the "Boulogne sore throat." There had been an epidemic at Launceston from 30 September, 1855, which had come to a height in August, 1856; several deaths had occurred near Spalding, in Lincolnshire, in July, 1856, and the disease had been seen at Ash, in Kent, in November, 1856. When the registered causes of death during the year 1855 were classified (in 1857), "diphtheria" was credited with 186 deaths, in the Supplementary Table then first introduced, "cynanche maligna" having 199 deaths. The following shows the progress of the epidemic during the four first years, and the mode of entry:

Year	Cynanche maligna	Diphtheria	Scarlatina (inclusive of columns 1 and 2 in the general table)
1855	199	186	17,314
1856	374	229	14,160
1857	1273	310	14,229
1858	1770	4836	30,317

In 1857 and 1858 the deaths from croup were above the average, and probably included some of the new disease.

Accounts of the epidemic began to come into the medical journals[1] from various localities in the course of 1858,—from Lincolnshire, Essex, Kent, Sussex, etc. A systematic inquiry, conducted by Greenhow and Sanderson for the Medical Department, under the direction of Simon, gave an exact picture of the several degrees of throat-distemper that constituted the epidemic in the year 1858, in certain of the more severely visited centres of Lincolnshire, South Staffordshire, Cornwall, Kent, and other counties[2]. The numerous cases of throat disease occurred often in the midst of scarlatina, but sometimes also where there was no scarlatina. One of the worst centres was in

---

[1] *Med. Times and Gazette, Lancet, British Med. Journal, &c.* for 1858 and 1859. See references in Hirsch, III. 89.
[2] *Second Report* (for 1859) *by the Medical Officer of the Privy Council*, London, 1860, p. 161 *seq.* Dr Greenhow published an essay on Diphtheria in 1860. Lectures important for the nosological definition were published by Sir William Jenner in 1861 (reprinted in 1893). Other essays called forth by the epidemic were by W. F. Wade (1858), Ernest Hart (1859), Edward Copeman (Norwich, 1859). Christison, J. W. Begbie and others wrote upon it in Scotland.

and around Spalding, a market town situated in a flat grazing
country within the fen district of Lincolnshire. A thousand
cases were counted in and near Spalding, many of them mild, a
small ratio of them gangrenous and mortal; one practitioner
had 200 cases with 5 deaths, another 200 cases with 2 deaths,
another 160 cases with 17 deaths (of 65 tabulated with 9 deaths,
which occurred in 35 houses, the first four all died from gangrene
in June, 1858). The doctor at Pinchbeck, in the same district,
had some 500 cases of which 300 occurred in the space of about
six weeks; most of the 19 deaths in his extensive series happened
in the first cases (this was observed also in the New Hampshire
epidemic of 1735). At Launceston, in Cornwall, there were
about a thousand cases known, the height of the epidemic
having been in the summer and autumn of 1856; among 126
taken as they came in 98 families, 18 died. The mildest and
the most severe cases were equally parts of the epidemic constitution, and occurred side by side in the same households; many
of them were quinsies, ulcerated sore-throats, or the like, others
were gangrenous. In this great variety, only a part could be
reckoned "true diphtheria." From the first, the remarkable
sequel of paralysis, not only of deglutition but of the motor
powers generally, was remarked here and there. Sometimes an
eruption of the skin was seen, but desquamation did not occur[1].
Albumen in the urine was somewhat constant. It is noteworthy,
the more so that the coincidence was not remarked at the time,
that the true diphtheritic pellicle,—tough, leathery, elastic,—was
found most distinctively, if not exclusively, where it was found
in 1748, namely in Cornwall[2].

Although the epidemic was not confined to low and damp
situations, yet there was no mistaking the severity of it in
Lincolnshire; and although it fell upon both clean and filthy
houses, yet it is probable that the cases with most pronounced

[1] Mr Jones, of Fletching, Sussex, wrote that scores of cases (probably at least 50
or 60) have had more or less eruption. In one case it was general and bright...It was
like scarlatina...but the whole surface was covered with minute miliary vesicles of
clear fluid, 'one mass of small vesications.' There was a great deal of itching and no
subsequent dropsy. In other cases the eruption was partial. *Rep. Med. Off. Privy
Council*, II. (1859), p. 284.

[2] Starr's description for 1748 is referred to *supra*, p. 695. Sanderson, *Report*, u. s.
p. 263, says of the disease in 1858: "At Launceston the diphtheritic pellicle was
tough, leathery, and highly elastic; and on the mucous surface of the fauces and
pharynx it attained so great thickness (from one-tenth to one-eighth of an inch) that it
was compared by several practitioners to the coriaceous lichens which grow on rotten
bark. In the other districts this was never observed."

gangrene or foetor happened amidst the most unwholesome surroundings. The disease was very general in England in 1858. When the deaths from it in 1859 (9587) were tabulated for the first time according to counties, it was found that they came from every part of England and Wales. The highest death-rate was in Lincolnshire, 1·2 per 1000 on the annual average of 1859 and 1860 (995 deaths in the two years). Sussex, Kent, Essex and Norfolk had also high death-rates, the agricultural counties in general having somewhat more than their usual share of an infective mortality as compared with the industrial centres. But it would be erroneous to suppose that diphtheria was at all specially a country disease. The mining districts of Staffordshire, Durham and South Wales had considerable mortalities, and so had Lancashire and the West Riding. But the North Riding and East Riding had their full share or even more than their share; whereas, if it had been scarlatina or enteric fever, they would have been far behind the great industrial division of Yorkshire in ratio of their populations. In the more recent prevalence of diphtheria the country districts have lost their preeminence, according to the following table of death-rates per million living in registration districts classified roughly as sparse, dense and medium[1]:

Diphtheria Death-rates per million, according to density of population.

Period	Dense	Medium	Sparse
1855–60	123	182	248
1861–70	163	164	223
1871–80	114	125	132

In Scotland, also, the incidence was the same: e.g. in 1862, of 997 deaths, 360 were in the towns, 617 in the mainland rural and 20 in the insular districts[2].

The law of incidence of diphtheria upon town and country respectively has become a good deal confused by the extraordinary severity with which diphtheria has fallen in the last two or three years upon most parts of London and upon the

---

[1] G. B. Longstaff, M.D., "The Geographical Distribution of Diphtheria in England and Wales," in *Supplement to the 17th Annual Report of Loc. Gov. Board*, 1887–8, p. 135. See also Downes, *Trans. Epid. Soc.* N. S. VII. 193. Farr, *Rep. Reg. Genl.* for 1874, p. 219, gave the following illustration: "It is remarkable that of diphtheria, out of the same number born, more die in the healthy districts of England than in Liverpool; the proportions are 1029 in the healthy districts and 442 in Liverpool of 100,000 born. The deaths from scarlet fever are 2140 in the healthy districts to 3830 in Liverpool."

[2] *8th Detailed Report of the Reg. Gen. Scot.*, p. xxxix.

adjoining municipal boroughs of Croydon and West Ham. The following table compares the annual death-rates per million in all England and Wales and in London from the year of the first recognition of diphtheria to the present time.

Death-rates from Diphtheria per million, in all England and in London.

Year	England	London	Year	England	London
1855	20	—	1875	142	167
1856	32	—	1876	129	109
1857	82	—	1877	111	88
1858	339	—	1878	140	155
1859	517	284	1879	120	155
1860	261	174	1880	109	144
1861	225	239	1881	121	171
1862	241	288	1882	151	220
1863	315	275	1883	158	241
1864	261	207	1884	185	236
1865	126	144	1885	163	221
1866	140	152	1886	147	205
1867	120	145	1887	157	226
1868	137	155	1888	168	305
1869	47	107	1889	185	371
1870	120	104	1890	179	330
1871	111	105	1891	173	340
1872	93	80	1892	222	460
1873	108	95	1893	302	740
1874	150	122			

The deaths in London in 1893 were 3196, having been 1962 the year before, but never more than half the latter total in any year previous to 1888. Besides Croydon and West Ham, Cardiff is the great town which has come nearest the London rate, having had 0·68 deaths from diphtheria per 1000 living in 1892, while Swansea had only 0·05, Wolverhampton (including Bilston and Willenhall) only 0·06, Huddersfield 0·03 and Blackburn 0·02. In London the very high death-rate of 1893 was distributed not unequally over all the divisions, the highest mortality corresponding to the highest fecundity.

Diphtheria in London in 1893.

District	Death-rate from all causes	Birth-rate	Diphtheria death-rate
Eastern	25·1	37·3	1·00
Central	26·6	29·0	0·82
Southern	19·9	31·7	0·73
Northern	20·0	29·3	0·73
Western	18·7	26·4	0·52

Diphtheria shows no such decided preference for the late autumnal or early winter season as scarlatina, but the winter is on the whole its most fatal season, according to the following annual averages of the quarters of the year for twenty years from 1870 to 1889 (total of 67,676 deaths in England and Wales).

Annual average of Diphtheria deaths in the quarters of the year.

1st qr.	2nd qr.	3rd qr.	4th qr.
903	713	730	1025

According to some recent returns under the Notification Act, which are of doubtful value owing to the laxity of diagnosis (greater perhaps in throat-disorders than in any other class of diseases), the second and third quarters of the year have also the lowest mortality in proportion to the number of attacks[1]. As to the ages at which diphtheria proves fatal, they are somewhat similar to those of fatal scarlatina, but slightly higher all over ; thus, while two-thirds of the deaths from scarlatina are of infants and children under five years, only one-half of the deaths from diphtheria are under that age. In the first epidemic period, 1855–61, Farr reckoned that 1553 adults had died of diphtheria above the age of twenty-five, while the deaths under that age had been 28,216. In its age-incidence diphtheria is very different from croup, which attacks chiefly children of one, two, and three years of age, the boys dying in greater numbers than the girls[2]. But in all comparisons between diphtheria and croup, as regards sex and age, it should be kept in mind that many cases of angina of the throat, which end in death by extension to the larynx and trachea, are registered as croup, even in epidemics. Diphtheria is the only epidemic disease besides whooping-cough which is more fatal to female children than to males in proportion to the numbers of each sex living. The following annual average death-rates per million for the period 1855–80 show the higher death-rates of females at certain age periods[3]:

	All ages	0–	1–	2–	3–	4–	5–	10–	15–20
Males	157	490	724	617	667	589	325	107	50
Females	168	377	673	668	746	694	413	159	57

It is not until the third year that female children begin to die of diphtheria in excess of males; which means that the

---

[1] R. T. Thorne, M.B., *Diphtheria: its Natural History and Prevention.* Milroy Lectures for 1891. London, 1891.
[2] Farr, *Rep. Reg.-Genl.* XXIV. (1861), p. 217.
[3] Longstaff, u. s.

usually greater risk to male infants holds good also in this disease for the two first years, while some difference between the sexes becomes thereafter so marked as to turn the balance of fatality to the side of the females. Something of the same kind happens in whooping-cough; and it is probable that in both maladies the cause lies in the earlier acquisition by the male of secondary sexual characters in the throat and larynx, as suggested in the chapter on whooping-cough.

Conditions Favouring Diphtheria.

The circumstances of the great and sudden explosion of diphtheria in 1858 and 1859 are as likely as any to throw light on the causes or determining conditions of the disease. Those two years were remarkable for the Thames running so low in summer as to give out a stench, which was thought to forebode much fever[1]. The expected epidemic of fever did not come; on the contrary the fever deaths in London were much lower than usual in 1858 and 1859, and, to judge from the few admissions of each kind to the London Fever Hospital, enteric fever declined as well as typhus[2]. It was diphtheria that came. The lowness of the rivers was due to a succession of years with rainfall below the average:

Low rainfall			High rainfall		
1855	21·1	inches	1865	29·0	inches
1856	22·2	,,	1866	30·7	,,
1857	21·4	,,	1867	28·4	,,
1858	17·8	,,	1868	25·2	,,
1859	25·9	,,	1869	24·0	,,
Average	21·7	,,	Average	27·4	,,

The low state of the rivers was an index of a low level of the ground-water. If diphtheria is to be included among the infections that have the habitat of their virus in the soil, it will probably be found to be affected by irregularities in the movements of the subsoil water. A series of observations have been made which seem to favour that hypothesis.

At Maidstone in each of the three years 1885, 1886 and 1887, the ground-water rose with the greatest regularity and steadiness to its highest point

---

[1] G. Budd, M.D., "Obs. on Typhoid or Intestinal Fever." *Brit. Med Journ.*, 9 Nov. 1861, p. 485.

[2] *Supra*, pp. 210, 213.

towards the end of the first quarter of the year, and fell with equal steadiness to its lowest point in the autumn. During two of the years there was little diphtheria, and in one of them none. But, in the next two years, 1888 and 1889, "the levels of the ground-water oscillated to and fro with unwonted frequence," having several maxima in 1888, and a somewhat uniform high level all through 1889; and during those two years there was a severe outbreak of diphtheria, as well as an excessive number of deaths registered as "croup[1]."

The relationship with the ground-water, if any, will probably be found to be more than ordinarily complex; but some connexion is indicated by the remarkable selection of the Fen country of Lincolnshire in 1858. Among the 18th century observations, it was remarked in New England in 1735—36 that the throat distemper was worst near lakes or rivers, as at Newbury Falls, Hampton Falls, and the like. The ill-reputed "Kidderminster sore throat," was associated with the low situation of weavers' houses in the valley of the Stour, subject to inundations. Practitioners in many parts of England and Scotland have suspected an association with water, even if it were only a mill dam, in the more recent prevalence of diphtheria[2].

Diphtheria has affinities in its pathological nature with enteric fever on the one hand and with scarlatina on the other. The process in the throat and pharynx is comparable to the typhoid process in the ileum, which is often a truly diphtheritic process in the second half of the fever[3]. The affinities to scarlatina are shown best of all in the real ambiguity of diagnosis in some whole epidemics of the 18th century, if not also in the great epidemics of *garrotillo* in the 16th and 17th centuries. Another singular affinity both to scarlatina and to enteric fever lies in the fact that diphtheria, as well as each of these, has been distributed in milk from some particular dairy, and that contamination of the milk by the products of disease upon the cows' teats has been found to be the relevant thing both for the scarlatina and the diphtheria[4]. Again, whatever suspicion pertains to slaughter-houses or animal offal for the production of a scarlatinal miasm, pertains to them also for the diphtherial. With such more or less real affinities in the pathology and etiology, it may be made a question whether the recent increase of the death-rate by diphtheria in London and some other places has depended, as if in the way of correlation, upon the decrease in the

---

[1] Matthew A. Adams, cited by Thorne, u. s. with diagram.
[2] M. W. Taylor, M.D., "Diphtheria in connection with Damp and Mould Fungi." *Trans. Epic. Soc.* N. S. VI. (1886–7), p. 104. Thorne, u. s. gives instances in which diphtheria seemed to choose out wet and impervious soils.
[3] L. Traube, *Gesammelte Beiträge, &c.*, Berlin, 1871, II. 11.
[4] Thorne, u. s. has collected and analysed very fully the instances of diphtherial epidemics traced to cows' milk. It is commonly assumed that the epidemics are either wholly diphtherial or wholly scarlatinal, but not a mixture of the two diseases.

death-rates of scarlatina and of enteric fever[1]. Diphtheria is
perhaps the most obscure and complex of all the infective
diseases in its causes and favouring conditions.   A certain
explanation may seem to suit one outbreak and be wholly
irrelevant for another.   More particularly there have been
innumerable cases for which insanitary surroundings cannot be
alleged in any ordinary meaning of the term.

[1] W. N. Thursfield, *Lancet*, 3 Aug. 1878, p. 180, has contended for some such
correlation between diphtheria and enteric fever in their respective preferences, at that
time, for rural and urban districts.

CHAPTER VIII.

INFANTILE DIARRHOEA, CHOLERA NOSTRAS, AND DYSENTERY.

INFANTILE diarrhoea and the cholera nostras of adults are closely allied in symptoms and pathology, but they are so unlike in their fatality that they are best considered apart. Dysentery is sufficiently distinguished from choleraic disorders even in nosological respects; and except in Ireland, where its history (already given) has been somewhat special, it might have been made the subject of a separate chapter in British epidemiology. But, for the same reason as in the case of influenzas and epidemic agues and of scarlatina and diphtheria, it is necessary in a historical review to include infantile diarrhoea, cholera nostras of adults, and dysentery in one chapter, the reason being, that they are not clearly separated in the earlier records. So little are they separated in the London bills of mortality that the younger Heberden, in his fragment upon 'The Increase and Decrease of Diseases[1],' has understood the name of "griping in the guts," under which enormous totals of deaths are entered in the bills for many years of the earlier period, to mean dysentery alone: having assigned that meaning to the name, and having observed, as everyone must, the very palpable fact that "griping in the guts" steadily declined in the bills from the end of the 17th century until it had almost disappeared from them in his own time, he has elaborately proved from the figures that dysentery was at one time among the most important causes of death in London, that it declined in the most regular way, and at length became all but extinct. This illustration of the increase or decrease of diseases has seemed so apt, the statistical demonstration so complete, that it has become a favourite example of those broad contrasts between

---

[1] William Heberden, M.D. junior. *Observations on the Increase and Decrease of Diseases, particularly the Plague.* Lond. 1801.

the public health of past and present times which are not less pleasing in rhetoric than they are on the whole true in fact[1]. But it happens that the particular instance is wholly fallacious and erroneous. It was not dysentery that the article "griping in the guts" meant for the most part, it was infantile diarrhoea; which has not only not ceased in our own time, but is commonly believed to be distinctively a product of the industrial town life of the present age. I shall show that it was one of the most important causes of London mortality from the Restoration onwards, and that although it is still one of the great causes of death in infants, yet that it had weekly mortalities in some of the hot summers of former times which were far higher in ratio of the numbers living than the diarrhoeal death-rates of our own time. So far as concerns dysentery itself, it is indeed now rare in England and Scotland, and not common in Ireland; but the real history of its decrease has been altogether different, both in the period of it and in the extent of it, from what Heberden supposed. There are two reasons for the fallacy and error of that writer: the first, that he overlooked the question of age-incidence in "griping in the guts"; the second, that he failed to observe that enormous annual totals of deaths under that head had been gradually transferred in the bills of the Parish Clerks to the head of "convulsions," until there were only a few of the old name left[2].

Summer Diarrhoea of Infants in London, 17th century.

In the period of twenty-five years which Sydenham's epidemic constitutions cover (1661–1686), the first distinctively choleraic season was the late summer and autumn of 1669. It was the first of a series of such seasons, in one or more of which there occurred dysentery, cholera morbus and bilious colic. In the context of the bilious colic of the years 1670–72, Sydenham

---

[1] Among the numerous medical writers who have used it are Macmichael, Watson and Chevers. Among historians Lecky (I. 573) has thought it worthy of mention among the progressive improvements of the 18th century.

[2] Heberden (l. c. p. 42) accounted for the enormous increase of the article "convulsions" in the Bills by the inclusion under that term of most of the deaths originally entered under "chrisomes and infants," which were infants under one month. But the latter had been mostly transferred at an early period while convulsions was still a small total; and even at the worst period of the public health in London, about 1730–40, they would not have accounted for a sixth part of the deaths under convulsions. The probability of the deaths from "griping in the guts" having been transferred to "convulsions" was pointed out in a review of Heberden's essay in the *British Critic* on its appearance, without reasons given such as I adduce in the sequel.

remarks that this was a disease which attacked chiefly the young of a hot and bilious temperament, and was most rife in the summer season[1]. It is in connexion with the smallpox of 1667–69 that he speaks of diarrhoea in infants; in that malady, he says, diarrhoea is as natural to infants as salivation to adults, and he blames the imprudent efforts of nurses to check the diarrhoea for the deaths of "many thousands of infants[2]." This is perhaps all that can be found in Sydenham to show that infants did in fact suffer from diarrhoea, and that it was fatal to them in large numbers. Equally indirect is the testimony of Willis. Speaking of convulsions, he says they occur at two special periods of life,—within one month of birth (the "fits of the mother" of 18th century writers), and during teething; and with reference to the cause he says: "As often as the cause of the convulsive distemper seems to be in the viscera, either worms or sharp humours, stirring up to torments of the belly, are understood to be at fault[3]." It may be thought singular that Sydenham and Willis should not have enlarged upon the infantile age at which the summer diarrhoea of London mostly proved fatal, or that Sydenham should not have elucidated by some comment the enormous weekly totals of deaths by "griping in the guts" in the Parish Clerks' bills during many of the summers and autumns that came within the period of his epidemic constitutions.

It should be kept in mind, however, that it was from the populous liberties and outparishes occupied by the working class,—from Cripplegate, Shoreditch, Spitalfields, Whitechapel, St Olave's, Southwark, Newington and Lambeth,—that the largest totals in the bills came. Sydenham in Pall Mall, Willis in St Martin's Lane, and Morton in Newgate Street, were not likely to see much of the maladies of the poorest class, least of all the infantile part of these; and the fact that their illustrative cases of choleraic disease are mostly of adults should not mean that the age of infancy did not then furnish most of the deaths, as it certainly did in later times.

Whatever may have been the reason of their saying so little of infantile diarrhoea, its great frequency or fatality in London in the end of the 17th century rests upon the explicit testimony of Doctor Walter Harris, in his book on the Acute Diseases of

---

[1] *Observ. Med.* IV. cap. 7, § 2.   [2] *Ibid.* III. cap. 2, § 54.
[3] *Pathol. Cerebri.* Pordage's Transl. p. 25.

Infants, written in 1689[1]: "From the middle of July to the middle of September these epidemic gripes of infants are so common (being the annual heat of the season doth entirely exhaust their strength) that more infants, affected with these, do die in one month than in other three that are gentle." It was probably this remarkable fatality of the summer diarrhoea of infants that led Sydenham to say that the cholera morbus of August differed *toto caelo* from the disease with the same symptoms at any other time of the year[2].

The summer of 1669 was excessively hot; it was a season of enormous mortality from fevers in Holland, of a type very difficult to understand, and in New England it was remarkable for fluxes, agues and other fevers. In that summer, as well as in the following, Sydenham lays stress upon the amount of choleraic and dysenteric sickness, without saying that it was specially fatal to children. The following Tables, compiled from the weekly bills of the Parish Clerks for each of the two summers, show the enormous rise of the total deaths in August and September, "griping in the guts" accounting for almost the whole of the increase.

Weekly Mortalities supposed of Infantile Diarrhoea in London.

Summer and Autumn of 1669				Summer and Autumn of 1670			
Week ending	Convulsions	Griping in the guts	All causes	Week ending	Convulsions	Griping in the guts	All causes
June 29	30	42	283	July 5	37	41	318
July 6	49	74	365	12	40	51	320
13	48	105	391	19	43	76	351
20	53	119	389	26	40	77	372
27	36	122	368	Aug. 2	49	113	470
Aug. 3	28	96	340	9	38	160	485
10	22	129	437	16	44	189	555
17	43	173	510	23	47	222	629
24	31	182	482	30	42	250	629
31	42	269	665	Sept. 6	31	253	617
Sept. 7	45	318	707	13	24	239	586
14	34	277	619	20	38	225	575
21	33	231	524	27	27	150	474
28	29	232	570	Oct. 4	16	130	401
Oct. 5	38	185	553	11	13	104	376
12	30	172	518	18	17	78	325
19	25	156	473	25	15	75	336
26	16	146	421	Nov. 1	19	46	283
Nov. 2	14	89	372				

[1] Walter Harris, M.D., *Tractatus de Morbis Acutis Infantum.* Lond. 1689. Engl. Transl. by Cockburn, 1693, p. 39.

[2] *Obs. Med.* IV. cap. 2, § 7 : "haud aliter ac si in aëre peculiaris mensis hujus [Augusti] lateat reconditum ac peculiare quiddam, quod specificam hujus modi alterationem, soli huic morbo adaptatam, vel cruori vel ventriculi fermento valeat imprimere."

These are the characteristic London bills of a hot autumn ; they recur sometimes two or three years in succession, and on an average perhaps once or twice in a decennium. Any year with an unusually high total of deaths from all causes is almost certain to show a large part of its excess of deaths in the weekly bills of summer and autumn. The proof that these enormous weekly totals under the head of "griping in the guts" were infantile deaths lies in the fact that they were gradually transferred to "convulsions," as will appear in the tables of future autumnal epidemics showing the transference half made and wholly made. The transference to "convulsions" was almost complete before the year 1728, when the ages at deaths from all causes were first published in the weekly bills. After that year it is obvious that any excessive mortality of the six or eight hot weeks of late summer or autumn corresponds to a great increase of the deaths under two years, which is also the increase of deaths from convulsions. But those were the "convulsions" of a particular season, occupying exactly the place which "griping in the guts" held in the weekly bills of certain years in the earlier period. As most of the deaths from infantile diarrhoea are really from convulsions, it is easy to see that high weekly totals of deaths under that generic name must have been from infantile diarrhoea—when they began to rise in August far above the ordinary level of convulsions to fall to the level again in October. It is by precisely the same reading between the lines that we discover, under the head of "diarrhoea and dysentery" in the modern registration returns, that there is hardly any fatal dysentery, not much fatal diarrhoea of adults, but an enormous fatality from the diarrhoea of infants, especially in summer.

The sickness of the latter half of 1669, and of the years following to 1672, which we know from Sydenham and Morton to have been choleraic and dysenteric, was not special to London. The following abstracts of the burial registers of country parishes,

Deaths in Country Parishes of England.

Years	Registers examined	With excess of burials over baptisms	Baptisms in these	Burials in these
1669	118	33	685	878
1670	119	53	781	1403
1671	121	36	668	1051
1672	121	28	555	741
1673	124	16	365	487

by Short, show an excessive mortality in those years, which would have been in part caused by bowel complaints, as in the general " choleric lasks" of the 16th century.

In the summers of 1671 and 1672 the article of "griping in the guts" continues high in the London bills. It rises again decidedly in the summer of 1675, reaching a maximum of 129 deaths in the week ending 24 August, the deaths from all causes being 460. In the summer of 1676 it almost equals the high mortality of 1669 and 1670, reaching a maximum of 238 deaths in the week ending 22 August, the deaths from all causes being 607. In 1678 and 1679 there were epidemic agues, complicated with choleraic flux and gripes, which undoubtedly affected many adults[1]. The deaths from "griping in the guts" continue high in the summers of 1680 and 1681. But by that time the article "convulsions" had steadily increased in the bills; and in the next great season of bowel complaint, the excessively hot and dry summer of 1684, the high mortality of the season is divided more equally between "griping in the guts" and "convulsions," a sufficient indication of the age-incidence of the former:

London Weekly Mortalities.

1684

Week ending	Griping in the guts	Convulsions	All deaths
July 1	56	98	454
8	71	92	404
15	65	79	364
22	74	89	420
29	116	84	503
Aug. 5	154	180	720
12	—	—	—
19	186	100	609
26	—	—	—
Sept. 2	171	95	585
9	144	82	564
16	103	58	471
23	91	59	464

The summers and autumns of 1688 and 1689 were again characteristic seasons of infantile diarrhoea. The deaths rose in August and September almost as in 1669 and 1670; but now the article of convulsions has actually more of the mortality of the season assigned to it than the original article of "griping in the guts."

[1] See the reference to Simpson's essay, *supra*, p. 333.

London Weekly Mortalities.

	Summer and Autumn of 1688				Summer and Autumn of 1689		
Week ending	Convulsions	Griping in the guts	All causes	Week ending	Convulsions	Griping in the guts	All causes
July 10	84	28	353	July 16	108	60	486
17	94	35	388	23	109	65	463
24	90	80	491	30	121	69	504
31	108	86	510	Aug. 6	147	102	576
Aug. 7	122	119	557	13	121	130	631
14	141	136	630	20	140	150	662
21	130	113	518	27	150	190	726
28	120	90	483	Sept. 3	150	170	733
Sept. 4	109	98	532	10	108	156	693
11	112	119	547	17	110	117	630
18	90	102	474	24	95	90	558
25	102	76	476	Oct. 1	104	89	540
Oct. 2	71	65	380	9	76	78	486
9	67	43	362				

The following table from the annual bills will serve to show the summers most fatal to infants in London, and at the same time the gradual usurpation of the place of "griping in the guts" by "convulsions."

Annual deaths from Infantile Diarrhoea, etc., in London.

	Griping in the guts	Convulsions		Griping in the guts	Convulsions
1667	2108	1210	1694	1443	5024
1668	2415	1417	1695	1115	4496
1669	4385	1730	1696	1187	4480
1670	3690	1695	1697	1136	4944
1671	2537	1650	1698	1165	4480
1672	2645	1965	1699	1225	4513
1673	2624	1761	1700	1004	4631
1674	1777	2256	1701	1136	5532
1675	3231	1961	1702	1189	5639
1676	2083	2363	1703	985	5493
1677	2602	2357	1704	1134	5987
1678	3150	2525	1705	1021	6248
1679	2996	2837	1706	948	5961
1680	3271	3055	1707	883	5948
1681	2827	3270	1708	768	5902
1682	2631	3404	1709	812	5892
1683	2438	3235	1710	707	6046
1684	2981	3772	1711	614	5516
1685	2203	3420	1712	575	6156
1686	2605	3731	1713	581	5779
1687	2542	3967	1714	670	7161
1688	2393	4438	1715	589	6818
1689	2804	4452	1716	709	7114
1690	2269	3830	1717	653	7147
1691	2511	4132	1718	801	8055
1692	1756	3942	1719	826	7690
1693	1871	4218	1720	731	6787

Summer Diarrhoea of Infants, 18th century.

The first series of unhealthy summers in the 18th century is from 1717 to 1729 (the summer of 1715 having had also high "convulsions"). In the week ending 17th September, 1717, the article of "convulsions" rises to 187, while that of griping in the guts is only 13, the deaths from all causes being 522. For the next two years, the highest mortalities of the autumn were these:

London Weekly Mortalities.

Week ending	Griping in the guts	Convulsions	All deaths	Births
1718				
Aug. 12	34	226	653	355
19	23	239	645	383
26	25	256	693	347
Sept. 2	28	265	668	350
9	27	245	725	388
16	26	221	653	336
23	27	213	639	367
30	24	182	632	361
1719				
Aug. 11	32	215	688	354
18	29	243	670	342
25	28	245	755	371
Sept. 1	27	233	726	362
8	17	229	735	393
15	22	218	728	379
22	14	202	663	360
29	17	161	639	372

If these two tables be compared with the tables already given for the summers and autumns of 1669 and 1670, it will be found that the figures under "griping in the guts" and under "convulsions" have exactly changed places, the hundreds of the former in 1669–70 becoming tens in 1718–19, and the tens of the latter in 1669–70 becoming hundreds in 1718–19.

In those two years the article of fever was very high, contributing largely to the weekly totals of deaths from all causes, especially in the summer and autumn. In 1720 "fever" and "convulsions" again reached a maximum in September, the deaths from all causes in the week ending 20th September being 592. The winter of 1721 (February) is the first of a series when the weekly deaths of the cold season reach the enormous height of the most unwholesome summers, the causes being "fever," "aged," "consumption," "dropsy," and the like, with a due proportion of infantile deaths. The fatal winters following are 1723 (January), 1726 (Jan.—March), 1728 (Feb.—March, the end of a great epidemic of fever), 1729 (Nov.—Dec., still fever), 1732—33 (Dec.—Feb.) and 1738 (November). This was the great period of spirit-drinking, crime, and general demoralization in London. In the week ending 30th Jan. 1733, the deaths from "dropsy" were 64: it was in the midst of an influenza.

The next characteristic weekly bills of autumn are found in the year 1723, when the following enormous mortalities occurred in three successive weeks:

1723

Week ending	Griping in the guts	Convulsions	All deaths	Births
Sept. 3	23	308	761	396
10	32	251	705	339
17	33	262	768	390

Then comes a succession of four summers and autumns, 1726–29, in which the weekly mortalities are of the same kind— high totals from all causes and high "convulsions," while "fevers" are high in several seasons of the period, perhaps from influenzas. Strother, writing in the summer of 1728, says there was much diarrhoea in London "last autumn [1727] and this summer," the effects of which upon the bills of mortality are nowhere visible except under the enormous weekly totals of "convulsions."

I shall take one more example of a season fatal to infants, the autumn of 1734, by which time we find recorded the ages at death:

London Weekly Mortalities, with the numbers under five years.

1734

Week ending	Convulsions	All deaths under two	All deaths from two to five	Total of deaths at all ages
Aug. 13	218	240	71	558
20	217	284	76	547
27	240	297	80	573
Sept. 3	260	331	59	638
10	226	283	61	593
17	209	253	43	528
24	169	225	46	515
Oct. 1	158	224	59	510
8	190	236	61	558
15	136	172	42	464

In those nine mortal weeks of 1734, it will be seen that the deaths under two years were about 45 per cent. of the deaths at all ages; they were at the same time considerably more than half the recorded births. That was the characteristic mortality of an unhealthy summer and autumn. It was chiefly caused by the same cholera infantum or summer diarrhoea which raises the weekly bills of London in our own time, and the occasions of it recurred in a series of hot summers, or at intervals, just as they do now. I shall not seek to illustrate this point for the rest of the 18th century, and down to the beginning of registration in

1837. The history of infantile diarrhoea is a continuous and uniform one, with indications of greatest severity in the first half of the 18th century. Sir William Fordyce, whose general theme is what he calls the hectic fever of children (rickets), thus reveals some reasons why that should have been the worst period of infantile diarrhoea[1]:

"I speak within the bounds of truth when, judging from the Bills of Mortality and the numbers in such circumstances who have been brought to my door since the year 1750, I assert that there must be very near 20,000 children in London, and Westminster and the suburbs (if this be questioned, examine the public charity schools and workhouses, the purlieus of St Giles's and Drury Lane, and satisfy yourselves) ill at this moment of the hectic fever, attended with tun-bellies, swelled wrists and ancles, or crooked limbs, owing to the impure air which they breathe, the improper food on which they live, or the improper manner in which their fond parents or nurses rear them up: for they live in hotbed chambers or nurseries, they are fed even on meat before they have got their teeth, and, what is if possible still worse, on biscuits not fermented, or buttered rolls, or tough muffins floated in oiled butter, or calves-feet jellies, or strong broths yet more calculated to load all their powers of digestion ; or are totally neglected."

Mistaken regimen among the more comfortable, total neglect among the lowest class—these general causes of infantile mortality reached their highest point in London under George I. and George II., at the time of the disastrous mania for spirit-drinking. But the broken constitutions of the parents were probably a more telling thing for the poor stamina of the children than close nurseries, injudicious food or even total neglect[2].

While the article "Convulsions" in the London bills gradually swallowed up nearly all the deaths of infants under two years, and so far extinguished the article "griping in the guts" that the latter in the year 1739 had fallen to the merely nominal figure of 280 deaths in the year, yet it should be borne in mind that there must have been in the same period an excessive mortality from convulsions not specially related to cholera infantum. For example, the kind of convulsions in new-born infants which nurses called the "nine-day fits," produced the following mortalities in the Lying-in Hospital of Dublin : Of 17,650 infants born alive in the hospital from 8 Dec. 1757 to 31 Dec. 1782, there died 2944 within a fortnight of birth, or 17 per cent. The disease of perhaps nineteen in twenty was "general convulsions, or what our nurses have been long in the habit of calling the nine-day fits[3]." Corresponding deaths in London would have been included under "chrisoms and infants" in the earlier period ; but as that article gradually ceased, they were naturally transferred to the article "convulsions."

[1] W. Fordyce, M.D. *A new inquiry into the Causes, Symptoms and Cure of Putrid and Inflammatory Fevers: with an Appendix on the Hectic Fever and on the Ulcerated and Malignant Sore Throat.* London, 1773, p. 207.
[2] See the Representation of the College of Physicians on Drink in 1726, cited at p. 84.
[3] Joseph Clarke, M.D. "Nine-day Fits in the Lying-in Hospital of Dublin." *Trans. Royal Irish Academy* (in *Med. Facts and Obs.* III. 1792).

The sacrifice of infants' lives in London by the diarrhoea of summer having been so enormous as the preceding tables show, the question arises whether the same disease was a chief factor in the mortality of provincial cities and towns. There is little positive evidence for, and there is a good deal of probability against, its having been so important anywhere as in London. In the second quarter of the 18th century, when London had 700,000 inhabitants, the larger provincial towns such as Edinburgh, Glasgow, Manchester, Newcastle had not more than 30,000 to 40,000. A Liverpool writer in 1784, by which time the population had grown much, does indeed say that young children in large towns during the hot summer months are apt to be fretful and peevish, and that they should have a change to the air of the country[1]. But it is inconceivable that Manchester, with such vital statistics as are shown at p. 644 could have had the same death-rates from convulsions in general or from the summer-diarrhoea kind of them in particular, that London then had. Still it had at least a local predisposition, then as now, to epidemic diarrhoea. Thus Ferriar, having described certain flagrant nuisances in the town, goes on to say that the burning summer of 1794 was followed by wet warm weather, that a bilious colic raged among all ranks of the people, and that thereafter "the usual epidemic fever" became very prevalent among the poor[2].

The bills of mortality for occasional years at Chester, Warrington, Northampton, Carlisle and Edinburgh, which have been cited before in various contexts, throw hardly any light upon this question of infantile diarrhoea. The records of the Newcastle dispensary in the end of the 18th century do show a good many cases of diarrhoea to have been attended, with a proportion of fatalities which suggests that some, at least, were in infants. Newcastle, as will appear in the sequel, was certainly much subject to dysentery and the diarrhoea of adults in the 18th century, and was as likely a place as any in England for cholera infantum. In the records of two towns of Scotland it seems probable that a good deal of infantile diarrhoea had been entered in the burial registers under the name of "bowel-hive."

---

[1] Moss, u. s. He makes out that the infants of the poorer class were much neglected by their drunken parents.
[2] John Ferriar, M.D., *Medical Histories and Reflections.* 2 vols. Lond. 1810. II. 213 seq. "On the Prevention of Fevers in Great Towns."

At Kilmarnock, from 1728 to 1764, and at Glasgow from 1783 to 1800, the principal causes of death in infancy had the following annual average ratios per cent. of the deaths from all causes :

	Kilmarnock 1728–64		Glasgow 1783–1800	
Smallpox	16	per cent.	18·8	per cent.
Bowel-hive	7·0	„	6·5	„
Chincough	3·0	„	5·0	„
Closing	2·8	„	2·7	„
Measles	2·4	„	1·3	„
Teething	1·4	„	3·5	„

The article " bowel-hive " has a somewhat higher ratio of the deaths from all causes at Kilmarnock, with about 4000 population, than at Glasgow with some 80,000, and was probably a very comprehensive term[1].

So far as concerns systematic medical description, an article by Dr Benjamin Rush, of Philadelphia, written in 1773, is the first expressly on the theme of cholera infantum or the summer diarrhoea of children ; but, as Hirsch correctly remarks, the popular names of the disease then current in American towns, such as "disease of the season," " summer complaint," or " April-and-May disease " (Southern States), indicate that it was well known before the profession began to write upon it[2]. So far as concerns London, I am disposed to infer that it was more common, relatively to the population, in the end of the 17th century and throughout the 18th than in our own time. I shall come back to that after giving the modern statistics of the malady for the capital and other English towns.

Modern Statistics of Infantile Diarrhoea.

The first six months of registration of the causes of death in England and Wales, July—December, 1837, brought to light the following highest mortalities from diarrhoea, which are mostly in manufacturing towns, and especially in those of Lancashire and Yorkshire :

[1] Watt, u. s., says that "bowel-hive" at Glasgow included, along with teething, "a promiscuous mass which may be considered nearly in the same light as the great number of deaths in the London bills of mortality ranked under the terms convulsions, gripes of the guts, &c.... If the patient dies in a state of convulsions, this, we are told, is owing to the hives having gone in about the heart, or their having seized the bowels."

[2] Hirsch, *Geographical and Historical Pathology*, Engl. Transl. III. 376.

1837

Deaths by Diarrhoea	3rd qr.	4th qr.	Deaths by Diarrhoea	3rd qr.	4th qr.
Manchester	164	47	Wolverhampton	37	32
Salford	26	15	Bolton	40	27
Chorlton	63	14	Newcastle	35	25
Liverpool	142	49	Sheffield	30	23
West Derby	53	15	Stockport	28	23
Leeds	52	37	Preston	21	20
Nottingham	43	4	Wakefield	22	10
(besides dysentery	25	2)	Cockermouth	12	14
Dudley	45	52			

The returns were incomplete at first; and, for London, the figures of only three parishes are given:

	3rd qr.	4th qr.
Shoreditch	73	15
Greenwich	43	19
Kensington	35	13

Apart from the imperfect machinery of registration in the first years, the figures of mortality by infantile diarrhoea are incorrect owing to many such deaths having been certified as from "convulsions," according to the old tradition of the Parish Clerks' bills. Doubtless this goes on still to a considerable extent; but it will appear from the following comparative table for London that it masked the real amount of infantile diarrhoea to a much greater extent at the beginning of registration than afterwards.

London Mortalities from the beginning of Registration.

Years	Diarrhoea	Dysentery	Cholera	Gastritis and Enteritis	Convulsions
1838	393	105	15	881	3419
1839	376	79	36	843	2961
1840	452	70	60	977	2983
1841	465	78	28	957	2778
1842	704	151	118	996	2773
1843	834	271	85	874	2701
1844	705	125	65	818	2736
1845	841	99	43	707	2395
1846	2152	156	228	648	2086
1847	1976	—	—	—	2258

There is a progressive decline under "convulsions" and a progressive increase under diarrhoea. The year 1846 was undoubtedly marked by an unusual amount of choleraic disease; but the high level of the diarrhoeal deaths was maintained from that year, so that it is probable that some radical change had been made in the mode of entry. The nearly equal proportion of deaths from diarrhoea and from convulsions in London has continued since that time to the present, the former falling mostly in the third quarter of the year, the latter not unequally on all the quarters.

In all England and Wales during the first five and a half years of registration the deaths from diarrhoea were few compared with the numbers relative to population in later periods:

England and Wales

Years	1837 (6 mo.)	1838	1839	1840	1841	1842
Deaths from Diarrhoea	2755	2482	2562	3469	3240	5241

There is a break in the annual tabulations of the returns for four years from 1843 to 1846; when they are resumed in 1847, the diarrhoeal death-rate per million living is found to have apparently risen to an enormous height, at which it remained somewhat steady for a whole generation.

Annual average Mortalities per million living from Diarrhoea (and Dysentery).

England and Wales		London	
1838–42	254	1838–40	274
1847–50	900	1841–50	782
1851–60	918	1851–60	1030
1861–70	968	1861–70	1040
1871–80	917	1871–80	949
1881–90	662	1881–90	749

From year to year the mortality has fluctuated enormously, as in the following list, the rise or fall depending for the most part on the kind of summer: e.g. that of 1893 was hot, and had an excessive mortality from infantile diarrhoea.

1866	18266	1876	22417	1886	24748
1867	20813	1877	15282	1887	20242
1868	30929	1878	25103	1888	12839
1869	20775	1879	11463	1889	18434
1870	26126	1880	30185	1890	17429
1871	24937	1881	14536	1891	13962
1872	23034	1882	17185	1892	15336
1873	22514	1883	15983	1893	28755
1874	21888	1884	26412		
1875	24729	1885	13398		

These large annual totals stand almost wholly for deaths of infants, according to the following table of rates per million living at the respective ages:

Mortality from Diarrhoeal diseases per million living at the age-periods.

	All ages	0—5	5—10
1851–60	1080	5263	229
1861–70	1076	5985	160
1871–80	935	5728	69

Three-fourths of the deaths are of infants in their first year. The middle period of life is comparatively free from this cause of death, but at fifty-five the ratio begins to rise again, and at seventy-five and upwards is almost as high, among the comparatively small number living in extreme age, as it was in infancy. Male infants die of it in excess of females, according to a very general rule of sex mortality. It is also according to rule that the ratio of female deaths approximates to that of males in middle life and old age.

The deaths from infantile diarrhoea fall in great excess upon the towns, and most of all upon the manufacturing towns and certain seaports. London, which almost certainly had a great pre-eminence in the 18th century in the matter of infantile deaths by summer diarrhoea, has lost it to a number of provincial towns, of which the following is a list in the order of the percentage ratios of their diarrhoeal death-rate per 1000 living under five years to their death-rates from all causes under five years (Decennial Period, 1871–80):

Percentages of Diarrhoeal death-rate in the death-rates from all causes under five years.

Yarmouth	19·4	Wigan	12·7
Leicester	19·2	Hartlepool	12·5
Preston	16	Nottingham	12·4
Worcester	16	Sheffield	12
Sculcoates	16	Hunslet	12
Hull	14	Bolton	11·6
Northampton	15	Holbeck	11·6
Coventry	15	Stoke-on-Trent	11·3
Goole	14	Stockport	11·2
Leeds	13·7	Liverpool	11
Birmingham	13·5	Blackburn	10
Manchester	13	London, St Giles's	10
Salford	13	London, Whitechapel	9·6
Norwich	13		

The reasons for placing the towns in the above order will be found in the Table that follows, the significance of which will be pointed out after some other matters have been disposed of. Meanwhile it may be said that all these have diarrhoeal death-rates under five years greatly in excess of all England and of all London.

Table of English Towns with highest death-rates from Infantile Diarrhoea.

	Death-rate from all causes under five per 1000 living at the age-period	Death-rate from diarrhoea under five per 1000 living at the age-period	Deaths of infants under one to 1000 births	Birth-rate per 1000	Death-rate per 1000
Liverpool	119·29	14·13	217	35·08	33·57
Manchester					
(1871–73 incl. Prestwick)	103·82	18·84	207	38·97	31·46
Manchester (1874–80)	103·52	11·23	190	40·78	32·16
Preston	97·85	15·61	212	37·86	28·05
Salford	95·96	12·44	184	42·39	27·65
London, Whitechapel	95·83	9·24	181	36·42	33·03
Holbeck	94·00	10·93	196	42·63	26·64
London, St Giles's	92·69	9·42	176	34·05	23·42
Leicester	92·52	17·81	214	41·44	24·46
Sheffield	91·22	10·96	183	42·50	27·41
Blackburn	90·33	9·02	191	39·30	25·29
Hunslet	88·35	10·75	192	44·52	25·49
Leeds	87·47	12·02	188	39·33	26·04
Wigan	87·28	11·13	172	45·70	25·77
Stoke-on-Trent	86·76	9·91	189	43·29	25·80
Birmingham	86·10	11·78	179	39·89	25·82
Stockport	80·33	9·05	182	35·79	24·73
Nottingham	79·30	9·86	184	32·58	22·55
Bolton	78·54	9·13	167	39·20	24·34
Yarmouth	75·37	14·38	199	32·45	22·94
Hartlepool	75·26	9·43	166	43·36	22·49
{Hull	77·89	11·02	178	37·88	24·52
{Sculcoates	71·53	11·64	170	39·46	21·66
Norwich	72·29	9·78	188	32·86	23·32
Northampton	71·41	10·85	173	37·48	22·65
Worcester	68·24	11·10	176	32·00	22·13
Coventry	68·09	10·06	164	35·17	21·59
Goole	64·58	9·20	166	36·47	21·39

The deaths by infantile diarrhoea have a seasonal rise more marked than that of any other malady. In the curves formed by Buchan and Mitchell of the rise and fall of the deaths by various diseases in London throughout the year, that of diarrhoea was the sharpest, rising to a high peak in the third quarter of the year (July—Sept.). "Speaking generally," says Dr Ogle, "it appears from the returns of mortality in London that the diarrhoeal mortality becomes high when the mean weekly temperature rises to about 63° F.[1]" The season is practically the same

---

[1] Supplement to the 45th Annual Report of the Registrar-General. London, 1885, p. xiii. Ballard, following the method of Pfeiffer (1871) for Asiatic cholera, has shown that the correspondence is closest with the temperature of the ground four feet deep.

throughout the British Isles. But in warmer countries, such as the more southern of the United States of America, infantile diarrhoea is "the April and May disease." It is not the fatalities only, but the cases as a whole, that fall decidedly upon the third quarter of the year[1].

Causes of the high death-rates from Infantile Diarrhoea.

Sydenham said that the diarrhoea or bilious colic of London in the month of August differed *toto coelo* from that of other seasons of the year; and Harris, writing in the year of Sydenham's death (1689), said that more infants, affected with the epidemic gripes, died in one month of the hot season, from mid-July to mid-September, than in other three that are gentle. If this were taken to mean that the infantile mortality from all causes was trebled by the prevalence of diarrhoea during the eight warmest weeks of the year, it would be nearly borne out by the weekly bills of mortality, according to the examples given of them from the more fatal years. So far from the deaths of infants in London by summer diarrhoea having increased in the present century, they would appear to have diminished greatly. The two worst weeks of an unhealthy summer or autumn raised the London deaths in former times relatively as much as the whole diarrhoeal season would do now. If this great change for the better be admitted as correct, it may throw some light upon the causes of excessive infantile diarrhoeal mortality in London in former times, and in some other English towns at the present time.

The London populace in the 17th and 18th centuries were not only the single great urban community in the kingdom, but they were far more "urban" than now, in Milton's sense of being

> "long in populous city pent,
> Where houses thick and sewers annoy the air."

The houses stood closer together, many of them back to back in courts and alleys. The streets were narrower. The inhabited area had few or no open spaces besides the bed of the Thames. Not only the City and Liberties, but also the out-parishes were

---

[1] Ballard, *Report to the Local Government Board upon the Causation of Summer Diarrhoea,* 1889, p. 32.

compact, as if within a ring fence, joining on to the open country abruptly, and not as now in straggling suburbs. It was hardly possible to take children out for an airing, except in the west end. When Lettsom about 1770 applied the fresh-air treatment to convalescent cases of typhus, he had to send the patients to loiter on the bridges spanning the Thames. As Cobbett said, London was a "great wen," in the correct sense of a shut sac which grew by distension. The soil was full of organic impurities, including the decompositions of many generations of the dead. A hot summer in former times raised effluvia from the ground such as the modern residents have no experience of. The life indoors was equally adverse to infants. Fustiness was favoured by the window-tax; a tenement-house was apt to be pervaded by the excremental effluvia from the "vault" at the bottom of the stair. The worst time of all in London was the great drunken period from about 1720 onwards. Doubtless drink was then used, as it is sometimes now, to drug the fretful infants into torpor; but it told also upon them indirectly, inasmuch as dissolute parents would have bred children with *mala stamina vitae*[1]. In all these respects there has been so great an improvement in London that, although its population now exceeds four millions, its death-rate from infantile diarrhoea, a distinctively urban disease, exceeds only by a little the mean of all England and Wales.

While the mortality from infantile diarrhoea in London has undoubtedly decreased since the 17th and 18th centuries per head of the population, it is equally certain that there has been within the present century a great relative increase of the deaths from that cause in the country generally. The reason is that there has been an enormous increase of population and that the increase has been almost wholly urban. The rise of new manufacturing towns, with the great extension of the borders of old towns, as in Lancashire and Yorkshire, has inevitably brought to the front this distinctive fatality of town-bred infants. If the additional millions had been dispersed in village communities over the face of the country, as in Bengal, the mere density of population per square mile would have had its effect on the

[1] Willis mentions an instance (*Pathol. Cerebri*, Pordage's transl. p. 25) which can hardly mean anything but congenital feebleness as a cause of infantile convulsions. A neighbour of his (in St Martin's Lane) had lost all his children by convulsions within the space of three months. Another child was born, and Willis was sent for to advise what regimen should be followed so as to save it from the same fate.

public health, but not the same effect. There are now two or three provincial cities comparable in size to 18th century London, and there are some twenty more large enough to be in the same group. In most of these the mortality from infantile diarrhoea has held its ground, for all the improvements in sanitation and in well-being whereby the death-rate from all causes has been considerably reduced. It is mainly owing to that disease, and to whooping-cough, that the death-rate in the first year of life, although it has ranged widely from year to year, has fallen but little in the successive decennial periods. The bad eminence of some towns in the list already given is probably due to a composition of causes, among which the situation, soil, depth of ground-water, and the like, would count. It is remarkable, however, that there are only a few of them, such as Liverpool and Hull, that have been the chosen seats of great epidemics of Asiatic cholera. On the other hand, Leicester and Birmingham never had an epidemic of that disease, while Preston and the cotton-weaving towns of Lancashire generally have had but slight outbreaks of it. Again, the deaths from diarrhoea have been more purely infantile in the group of towns which have had little or no Asiatic cholera[1].

That which distinguishes the Lancashire and West Riding towns with highest proportions of diarrhoeal death-rates in their infantile death-rates generally, as well as such towns as Leicester, Worcester, Northampton, Coventry and Norwich, Birmingham, Nottingham and Stoke-on-Trent, is the extensive employment of women in factory work and other labour of the factory kind. The Census returns do not adequately show this for married women, who may be returned simply as of the married rank whether they be wage-earners or not; but it is well known that the female labour of industrial towns is to a large extent the labour of child-bearing women. Among the towns that stand highest for infantile diarrhoea, Preston, in the Census of 1881, had 32 per cent. of its adult female population occupied in the cotton mills; Leicester had 20 per cent. of all its women occupied in

---

[1] This is clearly seen in comparing ages at death in Liverpool, and in Preston or Salford. Again in the ten years 1871–80, there were 4530 deaths from diarrhoea in the group of shipping towns, Yarmouth, Hull (with Sculcoates), Goole and Hartlepool, of which 70 per cent. were under one year, 19 per cent. from one to five, and 11 per cent. above five, chiefly in old age. In the group of Leicester, Worcester, Northampton and Coventry in the same period, there were 5001 deaths, of which 74 per cent. were under one year, 17 per cent. from one to five, and 9 per cent. above five, chiefly in old age.

various industries, of which the chief are the hosiery and boot-making ; Northampton only 13 per cent., all at boot-making ; Worcester, a percentage, unknown for the city, occupied mostly at glove-making ; Norwich about 10 per cent. of its women returned as employed at boot-making, silk manufacture, and various smaller industries.

One obvious result of married women engaging in factory labour, or piece labour of the same kind at home, is that they do not suckle their infants ; and it has long been known that infants brought up with milk from a feeding-bottle are much more liable to diarrhoea than infants brought up at the breast. But the feeding-bottle is now too universal an appurtenance of infancy among all classes and in all places to be a sufficient explanation without something else, although there is no doubt that feeding-bottles which are not kept very carefully clean are a real danger in the particular way. Again, young children above the age for suckling or feeding by the bottle are attacked by summer diarrhoea in about the same proportions (e.g. at Leicester) as infants under one year, although they do not contribute an equal quota to the death-roll.

In the discussions upon this question it has been commonly assumed that the fault lies with the mother after the birth of her child, and all the remedial measures, such as crèches for the infants of workwomen, have that assumption underlying them[1]. I believe that this is a very inadequate account of the cause of this great modern evil, and that the remedies proposed are mere palliatives which are destined to fail. The importance of the matter may justify me for once in making an excursus into physiology and pathology.

The problem of infantile diarrhoea is in great part the same as the problem of rickets. The peculiar summer disease of town-bred infants is especially apt to assail the rickety: probably a very large number of the

---

[1] Ballard, *Report, &c.* u. s. says that "occupation of females from home," which had been often assigned by medical officers of health and others as a fruitful cause of infantile fatal diarrhoea, "resolves itself mainly into the question of maternal neglect, with the substitution more or less of artificial feeding for feeding at the breast." Tatham, *Brit. Med. Journ.* 1892, II. 277, is of opinion that the rate of infant mortality was considerably increased by the practice, which obtained in most manufacturing towns, of allowing women to return to work within a week or ten days after their confinement, so that the duties of the mother were necessarily delegated. The paper by Dr G. Reid, *ibid.* p. 275, which called forth that and similar opinions as to the kind of maternal neglect that favoured the mortality by infantile diarrhoea, bore the title, "Legal restraint upon the employment of women in factories before and after childbirth"; but the emphasis falls almost wholly upon restraint of the mother's industrial occupation after the child is born.

infants under one who are cut off by it would have become obviously rickety if they had lived a few months longer. But even if there were not this well-known correspondence between the subjects of infantile diarrhoea and of rickets, we should find analogies in the pathology of each. Rickets is an exquisitely congenital disease, or a disease acquired by the child in the womb from the kind of intra-uterine nutrition that it receives. In recent times it has been usual to restrict the term congenital in rickets to the very few cases that have rickets developed at birth. This is a typical instance of the peculiar narrowness of view in modern pathology. All rickets is congenital, although it is rare to find the symptoms made manifest until the infant is nearly a year old. Cullen's reasoning on this point a century ago has never been answered nor superseded. The theories of that day to explain rickets by injudicious feeding or regimen after birth seemed to him beside the mark: "Upon the whole I am of opinion that hired nurses seldom occasion this disease unless when a predisposition to it has proceeded from the parents....I am very much persuaded that the circumstances in the rearing of children have less effect in producing rickets than has been imagined....I doubt if any of the former [dietetic errors and the like] would produce it where there was no predisposition in the child's original constitution....So far as I can refer the disease of the children to the state of the parents, it has appeared to me most commonly to arise from some weakness, and pretty frequently from a scrofulous habit, in the mother," (Cullen, *First Lines*, Part III. Bk. II. chapter 4). The chief exponent of the diathetic views on rickets in our time has been Sir William Jenner (*Med. Times and Gaz.*, 1860, I. 466); but I remember at the Pathological Society on 7 Dec., 1880, how unacceptable, or perhaps unintelligible, that part of his exposition was to a younger generation who appeared to have forgotten the meaning of *mala stamina vitae*.

The congenital nature of rickets is not only an empirical fact, based upon experience, but it is a doctrine of rational pathology. The latter aspect of it rests upon the correct physiology of intra-uterine nutrition, for which I refer to my investigations on the structure and function of the placenta (*Journal of Anatomy and Physiology*, July, 1878, and January, 1879). The detailed application of the physiological facts to rickets I have attempted deductively in section 5 of the article "Pathology" in the *Encyclopaedia Britannica*, vol. XVIII., 1884. The building up of the placenta by the mother, and the due performance of function by that great and wonderful extemporised organ, require certain favouring conditions, which have been never unperceived by the common sense of mankind. Those conditions are certainly not to be found in factory labour. A woman who has to be thinking of the time-keeper at the gate and the foreman in the mill, who has ever in her ears the din of belts and wheels and mill-stones, who has dust in her lungs and weariness in her back, can hardly do justice to the child in her womb. The rearing of the child after it is born is of small consequence beside the rearing of it before it is born. The opportunity comes once (heredity apart) of giving it good stamina or bad; and in the circumstances of factory labour the wonder is that breeding women provide so well as they do for their unborn offspring. It is undoubted that they often tax themselves beyond measure to do so, in tacit obedience to the great law of maternity.

While the connexion of rickets in the child with the laborious or anxious preoccupations of the mother during gestation can be followed out in physiological or pathological detail, the connexion with the same of a disposition to summer diarrhoea remains empirical, except in so far as it is a part of the rickety constitution itself. Some congenital weakness, we may suppose, attends the functions of digestion and assimilation, and, under the relaxing influence of continued high temperature, leads to vomiting and purging, to which many infants succumb through the eventual implication of the cerebral functions.

Ballard gives a table to show that of 332 infants (in a total of 340) who died of diarrhoea at Leicester in 1881 and 1882, 141, or 42·5 per cent. were "healthy," and 191, or 57·5 per cent. were "weakly," and other tables to show that "our experience of these Leicester epidemics by no means supports an opinion commonly held that a summer diarrhoeal epidemic makes its first fatal swoop upon the weakliest children[1]." If "weakly" and "healthy" were as determinate as bushels of wheat or barley, there would be some fitness in this resort to numerical precision. But, in the circumstances, common experience will come as near the truth as the statistical method can, and will assign poor stamina to a much larger proportion of the infants that die. The poor stamina may be more a matter of inference than of direct observation. Thus, the last case of a death from infantile summer diarrhoea that came under my notice was in a big-boned and well-grown infant in the country. But it was the twelfth child of an equally large-built country woman, then big with her thirteenth, whose husband, a farm labourer, earned on an average not more than ten shillings a week. The rate of fecundity has, of course, a direct influence upon the stamina of the children. Its bearing upon the death-rate from infantile diarrhoea is shown in one of the columns of the table at p. 762.

Cholera Nostras.

Thus far I have considered diarrhoea as the "disease of the season" for the age of infancy or early childhood; and undoubtedly the large totals of deaths from it in the London bills, whether under the name of "griping in the guts" or afterwards under the generic name of "convulsions" were nearly all infantile deaths, both in earlier and later times. If we had regard only to the statistics of mortality and the effects upon population, we might now pass from the subject of epidemic diarrhoea, having said all that has to be said of it in those respects. But the deaths from epidemic diarrhoea, mostly of the summer and autumn, are far from being a correct measure of its prevalence, whether in our own time or in earlier times. Adults suffered from it in a fair proportion of the numbers living at the higher ages, although few of them died of it, except among the elderly and aged. It is only for modern times that we have any figures of the number of persons attacked at the respective periods of life; and these I shall take first in order, as illustrating the probabilities or generalities that may be collected from earlier writers such as Willis and Sydenham.

[1] L. c. pp. 43–45.

The following Table of the ages attacked at Leicester during a recent series of years shows a smaller proportion of attacks in infancy than some other modern tables do; but it is not misleading for general experience, and it will serve emphatically to correct the illusion that infants, because they contribute the bulk of the deaths, are most obnoxious to the attacks[1]:

44,678 *cases of Summer Diarrhoea at Leicester in seven epidemic seasons*, 1881–87.

Age	Cases	Per cent.
Under one year	2,284	5·2
One year and under five	8,956	20·0
Five years and upwards	33,438	74·8
	44,678	100·0

On the other hand, the fatalities from diarrhoea in all England during the same seven years had the following very different incidence upon the periods of life:

	Under one year	One year and under five	Five years and upwards
1881	9408	2476	2852 = 19·3 per cent.
1882	10680	3555	3050 = 17·6 „
1883	9962	2843	3128 = 19·6 „
1884	17854	4794	3764 = 14·2 „
1885	8821	2023	2524 = 17·9 „
1886	16514	4936	3298 = 13·3 „
1887	14101	2936	3205 = 15·8 „

Annual average per cent. above five   16·8

Thus, while (at Leicester) the attacks above the age of five years were 74·8 per cent. the fatalities above that age (in all England) were only 16·8 per cent. and the greater part of the deaths in that small fraction were of elderly or aged persons. This means that persons attacked by diarrhoea between the ages of five and (say) fifty nearly all recover; on the other hand a large proportion of infants in their first year succumb to the attack, and a considerable proportion of elderly or aged persons succumb to it.

If we were to judge from the direct testimony of Sydenham and Willis, we should say that the cholera nostras of London in the 17th century was chiefly a malady of the higher ages; there is little in their writings to suggest the enormous mortality of infants from that cause, which can be deduced from a close

[1] Ballard, u. s. Table VI.

study of the bills. One reason for this, as already said, was that the ailments of infants and young children in former times came little under the notice of physicians, being left to the "mulierculae" or nurses, and that among the working class, from which most of the deaths in the bills came, there was in those times an almost total lack of the medical experiences now gained through dispensaries, hospitals and other charities or public institutions. With this proviso we may take the accounts of the older writers as giving a correct picture of the epidemic cholera nostras of a hot and close summer or autumn in former times.

The great seasons of choleraic disease in the 16th century were the years 1539–40, (which were remarkable all over Europe for dysentery as well), 1557–58, 1580–82, and probably 1596[1]. The term commonly used in that period was a choleric lask, which meant *profluvium*. In some, if not in all, of those seasons there was unusual heat and drought. It is clear that these were only the years when cholera nostras of the summer season was exceptionally common and severe. According to a medical work of the year 1610, dealing with the indications for the use of tobacco by individuals, including the seasons of the year when it was most admissible, midsummer is characterized in general terms, and perhaps in the stock language of foreign medical treatises, as the season for "continuall and burning fevers, bleareyedness, tertian agues, vomiting of yellow choler, cholericke fluxes of the belly, paines of the eares and ulcerations of the mouth, putrefactions of the lower parts : especially when the summer, besides his heat, is enclined to overmuch moisture, and that no windes blow, and the weather bee darke, foule, close and rainie....So that in this season, and for these remembered griefes, no man, I trust, will grant tobacco to be verie holesome[2]." Consistently with this Sydenham says that, while the cholera morbus of August, 1669, was more general than he had ever known it, yet in every year, at the end of summer and beginning of autumn, there was some of it ; and he compares its regularity to the coming of the swallow in spring or of the cuckoo in early summer. It was marked by enormous vomiting, purging, vehement pain in the bowels, inflation and distension, cardialgia,

[1] See former volume, p. 412.
[2] *The Triall of Tabacco, &c.* by E. G. [Edmund Gardiner], Gent. and Practicioner in Physicke. London, 1610, fol. 11.

thirst, a quick pulse, sometimes small and unequal, heat and anxiety, nausea, sweats, spasms of the arms and legs, faintings, coldness of the extremities, and other symptoms, alarming to the attendants and sometimes causing death within twenty-four hours[1]. Next year, 1670, in the corresponding season, he describes under the name of a bilious colic, a prevalent malady which, he says, should count rather among chronic diseases[2]. It was marked by intolerable pain, the abdomen being now bound as if in a tight bandage, now bored through as if by a gimlet. These pains would remit for a time, and the paroxysm come back, the patient shrinking from the mere idea of it with misery expressed in his face and voice. This was evidently somewhat different from the cholera morbus of the summer of 1669; it was apt to end in inverted peristaltic action, with vomiting of the matters of enemata, or in iliac passion[3]. There was also dysentery in both years, as we shall see.

Morton gives the first choleraic and dysenteric season under the year 1666, and says of its recurrence in the following autumn, that hardly any other disease was to be seen, that the whole town was seized, and that 300, 400 or 500 died of it in a week. This is obviously antedated by two years, just as Morton is two years earlier than Sydenham with the great fatality of measles (1672 instead of 1674). Willis, again, who wrote some twenty years nearer to the events than Morton did, places the great choleraic seasons in 1670 and 1671, instead of 1669 and 1670. Sydenham's dates are undoubtedly correct, both as borne out by the bills of mortality, and as occurring in consecutive order in the annals which he kept for a period of twenty-

---

[1] *Obs. Med.* IV. cap. 2.

[2] *Ibid.* IV. cap. 7.

[3] Dr Andrew Wilson, a pupil of the Edinburgh School in the great period of the first Monro, Whytt and Rutherford, used his Newcastle experiences in 1758 and following years as the basis of two excellent essays, one on Dysentery (1761) and the other upon Autumnal Disorders of the Bowels (1765). In the latter he includes both cholera nostras and bilious colic, (as well as dry colic) as Sydenham had done, and makes the following distinction between the two forms, which "are very nearly allied in their nature":—"The vomiting of bile in the cholera is not so early as it is in the other; neither is it so constant, nor in so large quantities. Though a purging generally attends the bilious colic, yet it does not correspond so regularly as it does in the cholera, in which there generally is a call to stool soon after every paroxysm of vomiting...The bilious colic is not generally so quickly hazardous as the cholera is. The intervals between the sick fits are often longer, and when it is attended with danger, it does not become so suddenly as the cholera does." Bilious colic was not so strictly an autumnal complaint as cholera. It was not so soon relieved by medicines. It resembled cholera in the remarkable character of exciting cramps in other muscles than the abdominal.

Cholera Nostras.

five years. The correctness of his dates apart, Willis may be cited for the symptoms of the London cholera[1].

> The onset was sudden, with vomiting and watery purging, accompanied by prostration : "I knew a great many that, though the day before they were well enough and very hearty, yet within twelve hours were so miserably cast down by the tyranny of this disease that they seemed ready to expire, in that their pulse was weak and slender, a cold sweat came upon them and their breath was short and gasping ; and indeed many of them, that wanted either fit remedies or the help of physicians, died quickly of it. This distemper raged for a whole month, but began to decrease about the middle of October, and before the first of November was almost quite gone." The vomitings and purgings were copious, watery, almost limpid, not bilious. The sickness was peculiar to London or the country within three miles of it. It did not seem to be infectious, but to attack only those predisposed to it ; for it would seize those who kept out of the way of the sick and spare those who attended them. Morton, however, declares that he was infected in two successive seasons, "dum, mense Augusto, sedes dysentericorum minus cauté inspicerem."

These illustrations from the highly choleraic summers of 1669 and 1670 will serve to show the prevalence of cholera nostras among adults in London in former times. Its great seasons were the same as those of cholera infantum, of which numerous instances have been given from the London weekly bills of mortality. The years 1727–29 were specially noted for cholera by the annalists, such as Wintringham, of York. Hillary, of Ripon, having entered in his annals a "cholera morbus" in 1731, adds: "which disease I have observed to appear almost every year towards the latter end of summer[2]." A letter from Darlington, 29 July, 1751, having mentioned the death of the earl of Derby by "the cholera morbus," adds that the disease usually rages at the close of summer and towards the beginning of autumn[3]. Newcastle was much subject to it, as well as to dysentery, Wilson, of that town, devoting an essay to dysentery in 1761 and to cholera in 1765. Lind, who went to Haslar Hospital in the very unwholesome period about 1756–58, found much aguish and choleraic sickness: "Obstinate agues, and what is called the bilious cholic, from being accompanied with vomitings and a purging of supposed bile, but especially the flux, are often at Portsmouth and Gosport in the autumnal season highly epidemical. Since I resided here, I have observed those distempers to rage among the inhabitants, strangers and troops with an uncommon degree of mortality ; while, during

---

[1] *Pharmaceutice rationalis.*
[2] Appendix to *Essay on Smallpox*, 1740.
[3] *Gent. Magaz.*, Sept. 1751, p. 398.

this period of universal distress at land, ten thousand men in the ships at Spithead remained unaffected with them[1]." At Manchester, in the burning summer of 1794, a bilious colic, says Ferriar, "raged among all ranks of people[2]." Clarke, of Nottingham, writing in 1807 of the great prevalence of cholera nostras, calls it "the usual attendant on autumn[3]."

The appearance of Asiatic cholera in England in the end of 1831 gave rise to much controversial writing for a few months, as to whether the epidemic were really the foreign pestilence. Every effort was made by a certain school to find native precedents for a disease equally malignant; which, if they did not prove the point in question, gave more exact particulars of cholera nostras than we might otherwise have received. The only one of these accounts that need concern us here is Thackrah's for Leeds and its vicinity in 1825[4].

The weather had been exceptional. In May, three-eighths more rain fell than usual, the wind being in the east the whole month. June was showery and sultry, the thermometer on the 12th marking 87°. July was sultry, with drought for several weeks to the 3rd of August, when showers fell. There had been a few cases of cholera in May, June and July, but it was not until August that the disease became rife in Leeds and still more in certain villages near it. The symptoms were purging, vomiting, cramps, prostration, coldness of the extremities, shrinking of the features, &c. At Moor Allerton, a parish three or four miles north of Leeds, with a poor scattered population occupied on the farms, there were found in 60 houses, containing 299 persons, no fewer than 114 cases of sickness in July, August and September, 81 of these from cholera, with 3 deaths. Dysentery was common, both as a sequel of the cholera and as a primary malady. At Halton, three or four miles east of Leeds, with a population better off than in the former, there were found in 60 houses, with 298 persons, 74 cases of sickness, of which 63 were choleraic. At Grawthorpe, four miles west of Wakefield, with a weaving population not poor but of filthy habits, there had been for two months before the visit of inspection more sickness than any one remembered. Twenty of all ages had died of the epidemic, there having been 7 corpses in the village on one morning. Of 70 houses inspected, only 7 had been exempt from cholera and dysentery. In one house of 9 persons 7 were ill, 2 with cholera, others with dysentery and typhus. This was one of the most unhealthy villages, supplied with water from ponds only. In Leeds the choleraic epidemic was less than in the adjoining country, and the few deaths that occurred from it were all among the poor and debilitated. The hot summer of 1825 was unusual for the amount of cholera nostras. It prevailed at South Shields that season with unusual severity, the cramps and spasms being peculiarly manifest[5].

---

[1] *Two Papers on Fever and Infection,* 1763, p. 35.
[2] *Med. Hist. and Reflect.* II. 220.
[3] *Ed. Med. Surg. Journ.,* 1807.
[4] Charles Turner Thackrah, *Cholera, its character and treatment, with remarks on the identity of the Indian and English.* Leeds, 1832, p. 24.
[5] W. Horsley, *Med. Phys. Journ.* 24 March, 1832, p. 270.

Dysentery in the 17th and 18th centuries.

The younger Heberden remarks, " There is scarcely any fact to be collected from the bills of mortality more worthy the attention of physicians than the gradual decline of dysentery." I have shown the fallacy of Heberden's proof in the first part of this chapter on Infantile Diarrhoea. It is true that dysentery did decline in London, but not on the evidence adduced by Heberden, nor within the noteworthy limits that he supposed. It was at no time one of the greater causes of death in London, and it had already by the middle of the 18th century reached as low a point as it stood at when Heberden wrote. As it is one of the diseases that have become rare in this country, there is a scientific interest in establishing the fact of its decrease, even although its prevalence had been at no time more than occasional.

Hirsch groups the outbreaks of dysentery as of four degrees of extent: (1) localized in a single town or village, or even a single house, or barrack, or prison, or ship; (2) dispersed over a few neighbouring localities; (3) dispersed over a large tract of country in the same season; (4) simultaneous in many countries, or extending over a great part of the globe, and continuing as a pandemic for several years[1]. The last are the most curious; and of these there are at least two in which Britain had a share, the dysenteries of 1539–40 and of 1780–85. Of the next degree, there have been several in Ireland and Scotland, including those of the great Irish famines of the 18th and 19th centuries, and the " wame-ill" of Scotland in 1439. Of the two minor degrees of extent, there have been, of course, many instances in the towns, counties or provinces of Britain.

A considerable decline of dysentery in London before the end of the 17th century is made probable by various facts that can be gathered from the bills of mortality. When these began to be printed in 1629, dysentery appeared in them under the un-ambiguous name of bloody flux; there were 449 deaths from that cause in 1629, they had decreased to 165 in 1669 (a year re-markable for dysentery and other forms of bowel-complaint), and to 20 in the year 1690, soon after which the article of bloody flux ceased in the bills. But we are not to judge of the amount

---

[1] *Geogr. and Histor. Path.* Engl. transl. III. 315.

of dysentery from the entries under the name of bloody flux alone. In 1650 there began the article of "griping in the guts"; as I have shown, it was mostly infantile diarrhoea of the summer and autumn, but, so long as it lasted, it had probably included some dysentery. Besides the articles of bloody flux and griping in the guts, there was a third article for a time in the bills, namely "surfeit," a term which came at length to mean dysentery[1]. Thus the great plague of 1625 is said to have been preceded by a surfeit in Whitechapel; and it is clear from other uses of that word, for example as applied to slaves shipped on the West Coast of Africa for transport to the West Indies, that it meant dysentery more than any other form of bowel-complaint[2]. Accordingly when we find in the weekly bills of mortality for London that a series of weeks in the dysenteric summer and autumn of 1669 had deaths from "surfeit" to the numbers of 9, 11, 10, 12, 9, 15, &c., we may take it that these were dysenteric rather than choleraic, the more so as the other name "bloody flux" has fewer deaths to it than we might have expected from Sydenham's general language. These various items in the London bills cannot be used for an exact statistical purpose, but only as indications. Perhaps the most trustworthy indication is the total of 449 deaths from bloody flux in the year 1629, being a twentieth part of the mortality from all causes (8771 deaths). That was a prevalence of fatal dysentery in London far in excess of anything that is known in the 18th century, for example in the dysenteric seasons of 1762 and 1781. So long as plague lasted, dysentery seems to have been somewhat common, and probably most so in the plague years; for, besides the surfeit in Whitechapel with which the plague of 1625 is said to have begun, we find many deaths from bloody flux in the year of the Great Plague itself, 1665. As Sydenham and Willis have left good accounts of the London dysentery of 1669–72, it will be convenient to take from these sources our impressions of the disease in the 17th century.

[1] It is probable that the association of surfeit with bowel-complaint in general and at length with dysentery in particular came from the popular belief that these maladies of the autumnal season were due to repletion with fruit. That was the popular belief from an early period, which nearly all the medical writers on autumnal diarrhoea and dysentery took occasion to combat as either inadequate or erroneous.

[2] See Vol. I. of this History, p. 626. The following is in a letter from Charles Bertie to Viscountess Campden, London, 22 Nov. 1681: "I have safely received your choice present of four bottles, three of Plague and the other of Surfeit water, which I shall preserve against the occasion, being confident that better are not made with hands." *Cal. Belvoir MSS.* (Hist. MSS. Com.) II. 60.

Referring to the dysentery of 1669, Sydenham says that there had been comparatively little of it for ten years before, no including, doubtless, the plague-year of 1665, when Sydenham was out of town[1]. Both he and Willis are clear that there was a certain amount of it every year, although it was seldom fatal in ordinary seasons. The ordinary London dysentery, says Willis, though it be horrid or dreadful by reason of its bloody stools, and is most commonly of a long continuance, yet it is not very contagious nor often mortal[2]. Sydenham says that it was fatal more particularly to aged persons, but highly benign in children, who might be subject to it for months *sine quovis incommodo*. However, in certain seasons it became malignant and caused a good many deaths.

It began usually with chills and shiverings, to which succeeded heat of the whole body, and shortly after tormina with dejections; but sometimes the griping and stools were the first symptoms. Always there was intense suffering and "depression of the intestines," with frequent straining at stool. The stools were mucous, not stercoraceous, and with traces of blood. The tongue might be whitish, or dry and black; the strength was prostrated and the spirits faint. After a time the streaks of blood in the motions would be replaced by pure blood, without even mucus, a change which threatened a fatal end. Sometimes the bowel became gangrenous, while aphthae would appear in the mouth and fauces. If the patient were about to recover, the symptoms would gradually be restricted to the rectum, in the form of tenesmus. Willis says that the dysentery of the autumn of 1671 was really a bloody one, and extraordinarily sharp and severe, hurrying many to their graves. At the outset blood was voided plentifully, with griping pains; there might be twenty stools in a day. Some were able to rise after a week; but the malady would go on for several weeks or even months. It was protracted also in fatal cases, the end being marked by watchfulness, roughness of the tongue, thirst and thrush in the mouth. He gives a case of a strong young man who recovered after having had not only terrible bloody stools, but also bloody vomit, which, Willis thought, might have come from ulceration of the stomach. But with good diet and treatment most of those attacked escaped death. Sometimes it became virulent and, as it were, pestilential, destroying many and diffusing its infection very largely by contagion.

It was most common, says Willis, in camps and in prisons, by reason of the stench of the places and the evil diet. From what Sydenham was told by Dr Butler, who accompanied Lord Henry Howard in his embassy to Morocco, the dysentery of North Africa was the same as that which prevailed in London, as an occasional epidemic, in 1669–70.

The dysentery of the siege of Londonderry and of the camp at Dundalk, both in the year 1689, have been described else-

---

[1] *Obs. Med.* IV. cap. 3.
[2] *Pharmaceutice Rationalis*, lib. III. cap. 3.

where. During the same reign, Dr William Cockburn got fame
and wealth by a secret remedy for dysentery, which was tried
first on board the king's ships at Portsmouth[1]. In 1693–99, there
was dysentery in Scotland and in Wales. Of Scotland in 1698,
the climax of the "seven ill years," Fletcher of Saltoun says:
"From unwholesome food diseases are so multiplied among
poor people that, if some course be not taken, this famine may
very probably be followed by a plague[2]." A Welsh practitioner,
who graduated at Dublin in 1697 said, in his thesis, that
dysentery had raged for the space of three years in several
maritime regions of South Wales so severely and had made such
havock that in not a few houses there were hardly one or two
left to bury the dead[3]. Writing before the seven ill years, Sir
Robert Sibbald mentions dysentery as one of the *dira morborum
cohors* that everywhere affected the Scots peasantry in the end
of the 17th century, the causes of which were coarse food and
excesses in spirit-drinking. In the century following we hear of
dysentery in Scotland in particular years, which correspond on
the whole to the unwholesome seasons in England. Thus in
1717, special mention is made of a fatal bloody flux in Lorn,
Argyllshire. In 1731 there were dysenteries in Edinburgh in
autumn, often tedious, rarely mortal. In 1733, during the
harvest months, dysenteries were frequent and mortal in Fife,
especially along the shores of the Firth of Forth. In the
following autumn (1734) many in Edinburgh were seized with a
dysentery, which continued more or less epidemic all the winter:
"It had the ordinary symptoms of slight fever, frequent stools,
for the most part bloody and mucous, violent gripes and an
almost constant tenesmus"—being fatal to some and very tedious
to others[4]. This was a well-marked dysenteric period in
Scotland, but just as much a rare or occasional experience as
the corresponding epidemic a century after in 1827–30. It
appears to have lasted in various parts of Scotland until the end
of 1737. A regimental surgeon, who was stationed at Glasgow
in the end of 1735 and afterwards at Edinburgh, had 190
dysenteric patients (civil and military) from December, 1735, to

---

[1] *Supra*, p. 103.
[2] Andrew Fletcher, *Two Discourses, &c.* No. 2. p. 2, 1698.
[3] John Jones, M.D., *De Morbis Hibernorum specialim vero de Dysenteria Hibernica. Accesserunt nonnulla de Dysenteria Epidemica.* Inaug. Diss. Trin. Col. Dub. Londini, 1698, p. 12.
[4] *Edin. Med. Essays and Obs.* I. (1733) 37, II. 30, IV. V.

February, 1738[1]. The summer and autumn of 1736 appear to have been its more severe seasons; it is heard of at St Andrews and in the country near it, at Kingsbarns and Crail (where "many of the boys" were seized), at Dalkeith, and in Glasgow and the neighbourhood, where one practitioner claims to have treated "some hundreds" with cerate of antimony[2]. In the great period of epidemic fever shortly after, the years 1740 and 1741, flux in the Edinburgh bills of mortality has respectively 3 and 36 deaths, which would probably have meant thirty to fifty times as many cases[3].

The English epidemiographists, Wintringham, Hillary and Huxham, mention dysentery in certain years, which were the seasons of high general mortality. Wintringham's first entry for York is under the year 1717, his second in 1723 (autumnal), a third in 1724 (some fluxus alvi with blood), in 1726 diarrhoeas and dysenteries "called morbus cholera," and the same for two or three weeks of September, 1727. Wintringham was one of the first in England to emphasize the seasonal connexion between dysenteries and agues. There was undoubtedly dysentery among the many forms of sickness in the disastrous years 1727–29. Huxham includes it among the fluxes which were common at Plymouth in 1734–36. A still greater dysenteric period followed the influenza epidemic of 1743, Huxham being again the chief chronicler of it[4].

In the second half of the 18th century, two periods were specially noted for dysentery, the years about 1758–62 and 1780–82. The first of these called forth perhaps the only medical piece written by Dr Mark Akenside, physician to St Thomas's Hospital and author of the 'Pleasures of the Imagination[5],' as well as accounts by Sir G. Baker[6] and Sir W. Watson[7]. All three writers agree that the true epidemic

---

[1] James Stephen, surgeon to Gen. Whetham's regiment, in Pringle's collection of accounts of the "Success of the vitrum Antimonii ceratum." *Ibid.* v. pt. 2, p. 179, 4th ed.

[2] Professor T. Simpson, of St Andrews, Andrew Brown, of Dalkeith, John Paisley and John Gordon, of Glasgow. *Ibid.*

[3] *Gent. Magaz.*, 1741, p. 705.

[4] The "epidemic constitution" of 1743 was so markedly dysenteric after the influenza in the spring that Huxham regarded the dysentery as a sequela of the influenza.

[5] Mark Akenside, M.D., *De Dysenteria Commentarius*, London, 1764.

[6] George Baker, M.D., *De Catarrho et de Dysenteria Londinensi Epidemicis utrisque An.* MDCCLXII. *Libellus*, Lond., 1764.

[7] William Watson, M.D., in *Phil. Trans.* LII. pt. 2 (1762), p. 647.

prevalence occurred in London in the autumn of 1762. It is clear, however, that Akenside had been treating in St Thomas's Hospital since 1759 many cases of true dysentery (which he defines as a bowel complaint with gripes, tenesmus and bloody or mucous evacuations). He had more than one hundred and thirty cases of it described in his ward-books in the five or six years previous to his writing (1764); he had proved the good effects of ipecacuanha on many in 1759; and he had remarked that the autumnal dysenteries of 1760, 1761 and 1762 in each case lasted the whole winter, not abating until the spring. Perhaps this may have been a special experience of the Surrey side of the Thames; for both Watson and Baker are clear that dysentery was something of a novelty to them in the early autumn of 1762. Says the former, writing to Huxham on 9 Dec. 1762: "We have had here this autumn a disease which has not been in my remembrance epidemic at London. Very few of our physicians have seen this disorder as it has appeared of late. You mention it as frequent at Plymouth in the year 1743...." And Baker begins his essay by saying that there became epidemic in London in the end of July, 1762, the disease of dysentery—"morbi genus hac in civitate novum feré, aut nuperis saltem annis inauditum[1]."

The three observers agree that it attacked the poorer classes, children more than adults, convalescents, lying-in women and the like. Akenside says that it was mostly a slow non-febrile disease (in the autumnal outburst of 1762, the subjects of it were more fevered), and that some patients came to him who had been labouring under it for two or three months. His account agrees on the whole with Sydenham's for the years 1669—72: some had vomiting, some had a painless flux following the dysentery, some had dropsy as a sequel. In cases about to end fatally there was a remission of the griping before the end; in some there were aphthae of the mouth, stupor, and somnolence, with cold sweats. Watson saw three children (of four or five years) die from debility a week or more after the gripings and discharges had ceased; they could keep down no food, and were greatly emaciated. In another case, a young child, the motions were pure blood, and death followed on the third day. Baker gives Hewson's notes of the anatomy in a case that was clearly one of follicular dysentery, as well as Charlton Wollaston's account of two other anatomies (mixed catarrhal and follicular), with plates of the dysenteric bowel.

Watson, physician to the Foundling Hospital, says that the dysentery, or dysenteric fever, was very prevalent among the children in 1762, the year of its most general prevalence[2]. It

[1] Pringle also, who was well acquainted with the dysentery of campaigns, speaks of the London epidemic as an exceptional occurrence, and as having caused few deaths.
[2] *Med. Obs. and Inquiries*, IV. (1771), p. 153.

may have been part of that dysenteric "constitution" which caused the following outbreak among the foundlings at the hospital at Westerham, Kent, a branch of the Guilford Street charity: "26 January, 1765. The apothecary visited the children at the hospital at Westerham, January 12th, 1765, and found twenty ill with dysenteries, many of whom had the whooping-cough complicated with it. Two of them are since dead, which, with six that died before he went down, make eight dead of that disease." Two cases of dysentery were in the infirmary of the Foundling Hospital in London on the 2nd of March, 1765[1]. These accounts of dysentery in London in the middle third of the 18th century show it to have been then a very occasional malady and a very small contributor to the bills of mortality.

Next to the capital, the town that seems to have had most dysentery in the 18th century was Newcastle, which had been also the seat of frequent and severe plagues. There was much dysentery in it and in the neighbouring places on Tyneside during the autumns of 1758 and 1759, but the disease was not epidemic in 1762, the season of the malady in London[2]. It was prevalent among the same classes in Newcastle as in London— the poorer households, children, weakly persons. It recurred in the harvest quarter, in fine clear weather, when the days were almost as hot as at midsummer, but the evenings and mornings remarkably cold and the nights frequently foggy. The reason why the lower class of people were most liable to it seemed to be their "negligence in the article of cooling after heats by labour, exercise, &c." But there may have been something also in the soil and situation of Newcastle which made these common risks to be followed by so special an effect.

The Newcastle dysentery of 1758–59, two or three years earlier than the London epidemic, was the occasion of the essay by Dr Andrew Wilson, a work which compares favourably with the writings of the metropolitan physicians. Among the symptoms of true autumnal dysentery he gives the following:

"Constant fever, drought, parchedness of the mouth and throat, dejection of the spirits, prostration of the strength, frequent viscid, acid or bilious vomiting, flatulency in the belly, wringing pain in the lower part of it, and often in the same region of the back; these pains sometimes constant, but always preceding stools; an almost constant pressing to stool, with great pain and irresistible tendency to it at the same time, called a tenesmus; the

[1] MS. Infirmary Book of the Foundling Hospital.
[2] *An Essay on the Autumnal Dysentery.* By a physician (Andrew Wilson, M.D.), Lond., 1761 (Preface dated Newcastle, 25 March, 1760), pp. 1, 23.

stools generally bloody, always slimy, and full of glary stuff, sometimes mixed with a whitish matter of less tenacity, which appears in separate little curdled-like parcels, often with blackish corrupted-like bile ; the stools always odiously fetid ; they are seldom natural without the assistance of purgatives, and then they are often discharged in hard, dry little lumps ; dryness of the skin, except when clammy unbenign sweats are raised by the intenseness of the gripings and tenesmus ; great watchfulness, their sleep, when accidentally they drop into any, being short and broken, with recurring pains which awake them unrefreshed.   These are the principal symptoms which attend a true febrile dysentery.   When such a disease is epidemic there are many slight appearances of it which happily do not extend to all these complaints, and which easily yield to proper applications.

The signs of danger in this disease are the violence with which all the above symptoms appear.   But the signs of immediate danger are, decrease of pain, great sinking of the spirits, lowness of the pulse, beginning coldness of the extremities, parchedness and blackness of the tongue, aphthae ; white scurf or ulceration of the throat and fauces, and constant hiccup.   When there is a cessation of pain, intolerably fetid and involuntary stools, shiverings, with sometimes a sense of coldness in the belly, a slight delirium, and often unaccountable fits of agony, or rather anxiety ; then the case is beyond remedy, and the patient hastens to dissolution.   This stage of the disease is generally attended with a small obscure pulse and cold extremities, but I have seen it in some particular cases otherwise.

...When dysentery is epidemic, it is not uncommon for people who escape the dysentery itself to have their stools altered from their natural colour to sometimes a greenish hue, as if they had eaten much herbs, sometimes of a clay colour, and sometimes quite blackish, as if they had eaten a quantity of blood....In 1759 particularly, it was very common for numbers of people who escaped the dysentery to be troubled with flatulencies, slight gripings and twitchings in the belly, which was generally attended with blackish stools. Stranguaries were likewise pretty frequent, and icteric complaints, or the jaundice.   The stranguary was a very common symptom in many fevers which occurred during the prevalency of the dysentery.   Another complaint which frequently occurred during the last dysenteric season was dry gripes.

The dysentery this last season [1759] differed in many respects from its appearance in the former season.   In the latter season greater numbers had it in that slight degree which was attended with little fever and no danger. In many who were seized with seemingly great violence, it was unexpectedly checked when there appeared all reason to apprehend it would have run to a much greater length.   It was not uncommon to find it complicated with agues, rheumatisms, &c., into the latter of which it frequently degenerated. In the former season the griping pains attending it were confined to the lower belly.   In the latter they were very ordinarily felt also in the back, along, as might be supposed, the windings of the rectum and colon ; yet, after the dysenteric stools were in a great measure gone, and the disease over, these pains often remained, or assumed the appearance of a lumbago or sciatic, with pains striking down the thighs....The more the season advances, and the later in the year it is when persons are seized with this epidemic, the more chronical do the symptoms of it grow."

The last sentence is probably the explanation of Akenside's original point, that dysentery was as much a winter as an autumnal malady, not really abating until the spring.   Wilson himself claims originality in the following point relating to the sluggishness of the bowels in dysentery, his treatment having been largely determined by that view of the pathology:

"During the increase and height of this distemper, it is very improperly called a flux. A proper flux, or diarrhoea, is a constant flow of immoderately liquid but otherwise natural stools, dissolved by too great an irritation upon, or too great a relaxation of, the vessels destined for mollifying the faeces and lubricating the passages by their humours; by which means they are disposed to dismiss a superfluous quantity of them. But in the dysentery the passage of the natural discharges is resisted, and their consistence is often increased to such a degree that, when they are urged along by the assistance of purgatives, they are excluded in unnaturally hard and dry little lumps or balls" (p. 3). The question whether scybala were an essential character of dysentery was often referred to in later writings.

Nothing more is heard of dysentery at Newcastle until the date of the opening of the dispensary there, 1 October, 1777. From that date to 1 September, 1779, when the disease was not epidemic there, 72 cases were treated from the dispensary.

Some importance, as regards priority, attaches to one of Dr Andrew Wilson's observations of the Newcastle dysentery of 1759: "It was not uncommon to find it complicated with agues, rheumatisms, &c., into the latter of which it frequently degenerated." The pains, he says, were not confined to the lower belly, but were felt also in the back; or, after the dysentery was gone, the muscular pains remained as a lumbago or sciatica, striking down the thighs. This curious relationship of dysentery to rheumatism, shadowed forth in the Newcastle essay of 1761 [1760], was formally stated by Akenside in his essay of 1764, being perhaps the best of his various attempted originalities. It was afterwards taken up in Germany by Stoll, Richter, Zimmermann and others in the 18th century, and was illustrated from the Dublin epidemics of the 19th century by O'Brien[1] and Harty[2]. The doctrine of a relationship between dysentery and acute rheumatism has been discovered in the 7th century writer, Alexander of Tralles, but erroneously. The Byzantine writer does indeed introduce into two paragraphs on bowel-complaint the word ῥευματισμός—one of them relating to the alvine profluvium attending fevers or following fevers, the other relating to "dysenteria rheumatica[3]." But it is clear that he is merely ascribing to the diarrhoea in the one case and to the dysentery in the other a rheumy nature, on certain theoretical grounds of humoral pathology; there is no reference to joint pains or muscular pains, or to anything else connoted in the later use of the word rheumatism. The idea is originally an English one, from the middle of the 18th century, and belongs most properly to Akenside, although Wilson, a not less trained and capable observer, had recorded the empirical fact three or four years earlier. Akenside was led to regard dysentery "as a rheumatism of the intestines," and to maintain that "the cause and the *materies* of each disease were similar[4]." Stoll adopted these phrases, adding that dysentery differed from rheumatism of the joints "merely in form and situation." But for a few empirical facts, the relationship would be thought fanciful. These, however, may be finger-post instances, pointing to the true pathology of a somewhat mysterious malady. They are simple enough: e.g. cases of dysentery have "degenerated," as Wilson said, into rheumatism; or cases of acute rheumatism, treated by purging, have

[1] *Trans. K. and Q. Col. Phys.* v. (1828), p. 221.
[2] *Obs. on the History and Treatment of Dysentery and its Combinations, etc.*, 2nd ed., Dublin, 1847.
[3] *Alexandri Tralliani Medici libri duodecim.* Basil, 1556, Lib. VIII. pp. 423, 432.
[4] Akenside, *l. c.* "Ut dysenteriam jam pro rheumatismo intestinorum habeam, et similem utriusque morbi causam et materiem esse contendimus."

developed the gripings, tenesmus and stools of dysentery ; or, in a time of dysentery, cases have occurred in which the symptoms of the latter were joined to those of acute rheumatism, or cases in which the symptoms of the one disease obtained, say for twenty-four hours, to give place to the symptoms of the other. Again there are countries such as Lower Egypt where the frequency of dysentery is not more remarkable than the frequency of rheumatic fever. Harty points out that the rheumatic complications of dysentery seem to have arisen only when the latter malady was improperly treated by opium and astringents ; but, howsoever the signs of affinity were called forth, they may prove to be true indications for the pathology. The circumstances of taking dysentery are those of taking rheumatic fever—exposure to chill after being heated with labour[1]. In rheumatism the effect of the chill falls upon the great groups of voluntary muscles, pain being manifested at the surfaces where the muscular work is applied, namely the joints ; while the redness, heat and swelling are as if restricted to the tissues by which the muscles become effective, namely the tendons, aponeuroses, ligaments and synovial membranes[2]. In dysentery, it may be said, the effect of the chill falls upon the great involuntary muscle, that of the intestine, or upon a section of it, a muscle which serves, so to speak, as its own tendons and insertions, and is the seat of its own pains, while the tissues next to the muscular, the submucosa and mucosa with the lymph-follicles, become the seats of congestion, inflammation and suppuration. In acute rheumatism, the muscles generate heat without doing any work ; in dysentery there is often febrile heat (although not invariably), and the work of the involuntary muscle is paroxysmal and ineffective. In some such way the parallel suggested by Akenside might be followed out.

After 1762, the next period of epidemic dysentery in England was from about 1779 to 1785, a period when agues also were epidemic, as well as workhouse fevers and typhus under its various names. In London it was prevalent in the autumns of 1779, 1780 and 1781, a strictly autumnal disease like the diarrhoea of children or the cholera nostras of adults. From the list of symptoms, the latter disease must have formed part of the dysenteric epidemic :—"profuse watery evacuations, mucous evacuations mixed with blood, gripings, tenesmus, pain in the back and loins, fever." Some had tormina without flux. Some few old and infirm died ; but usually the malady yielded to treatment[3]. It is heard of also at Liverpool about 1784[4], and its prevalence at Plymouth called forth an essay[5]. It must have been a considerable disease in the dockyard towns ; for a

[1] Hirsch, III. 333 (Eng. transl.) : "As to the influence of an extreme diurnal range of the thermometer (cold nights after very hot days) there is almost complete agreement among the observers in those parts [tropical and subtropical] of the world."
[2] I have enunciated this view of the pathology of acute rheumatism more fully in the Article "Pathology" in the *Encyclopaedia Britannica.*
[3] *Lond. Med. Journal.* Editorial note, II. 211. The parish register of Finchley shows double the average mortality in 1780, and indicates dysentery as a fatal malady. Lysons, *Environs of London.*
[4] Moss, u. s.
[5] Francis Geach, F.R.S., *Some Observations on the present Epidemic Dysentery,* 1781.

body of troops, originally numbering 2800, which arrived at Kingston, Jamaica, in the beginning of August, had been put on board the transports in March with much dysentery and putrid fever among them, so that the diseases with which they put to sea became more violent during the five months' voyage, and caused many deaths. Arriving at Jamaica, four hundred were sent on shore sick, exhausted with flux and fever, of whom scarce the half recovered in the military hospitals[1]. Here we have the singular fact of transports from England bringing dysentery to Jamaica. On the other hand, Clark, of Newcastle, who had seen much of tropical maladies, says that the dysentery which became epidemic there in 1781 was introduced first into a dockyard by some sailors returned from abroad ill of the complaint, and that it soon spread among the workmen, of whom several died. But it was epidemic in London the same year; and in Newcastle itself there were extensive epidemics in 1783 and 1785, for which no foreign source was sought or found. In those years it "attacked great numbers of the poor," as well as some of the richer class, to which Clark's eleven cases from the epidemic of 1785 mostly belong. In the Tables of diseases treated at the Dispensary, the epidemic dysentery of 1783 and 1785 is credited with 329 cases, of which 17 were fatal; but these, of course, were but a fraction of all that occurred in Newcastle and neighbourhood. Every year until 1805 there are a few cases of dysentery in the Dispensary books; but they become fewer to that year (except in 1801 when there were 23 cases), and at length disappear from the list altogether. A remarkable outbreak of dysentery, within narrow limits, occurred in a fishing village or "town" in the neighbourhood of Aberdeen during some months of the spring and summer of 1789: "It has proved fatal to numbers. As such a disease could not be admitted into our hospital, a temporary one has been fitted up for those that are worst, and the faculty here have given their attendance by rotation[2]."

[1] Dennis Ryan, M.D., "Remittent Fever of the West Indies." *Lond. Med. Journ.* II. 253, iii. 63.
[2] Dr Livingston to Dr Lettsom, Aberdeen, 29 June, 1789, in *Memoirs of Lettsom*, III.

Dysentery in the 19th century.

Willan, who was practising in London as early as 1785–6, says that dysentery had not been epidemic there from the autumn of 1780, until the autumn of 1800, his position at the Public Dispensary in Carey Street enabling him to know the prevalent diseases. In the autumn of 1800 the epidemic was extensive. There were, he says, some sporadic cases every autumn, but he never saw a fatal case of it[1]. In Bateman's continuation of the same records from 1804, dysentery first appears in 1805 and remains sporadic every autumn. It was "very prevalent" in the autumn and winter of 1808, but not fatal ; and it was not unusual among the dispensary patients every year until these records end in 1816[2]. The years 1800–02 form one of the more distinct dysenteric periods also for Ireland and Scotland. Old Glasgow practitioners in the severe epidemic of 1827–28 recalled the fact that they had last seen the disease about 1802, and the books of the Glasgow Infirmary bore witness to its prevalence from 1800 to 1803 or 1804. In 1801–2 there was a good deal of it also at Hamilton, among a regiment of dragoons as well as among the people at large[3]. The troops in various parts of Ireland suffered from it in the same years[4]. In 1808, during a somewhat unwholesome season in which agues also were met with, some cases of dysentery were admitted to the General Infirmary of Nottingham[5]. An altogether exceptional outbreak of a dysenteric nature occurred in 1823 among the prisoners in Milbank Penitentiary[6].

The great dysenteric period of the 19th century coincided with, or followed, the two hot summers of 1825 and 1826, the latter of which was probably the hottest and driest summer of the century. Of its prevalence in and near Leeds in 1825, Thackrah says it was "before almost unknown as an epidemic to the

[1] Willan, *Report on the Diseases etc.*, p. 42. The nearest approach to a fatality in dysentery, he says, happened in the case of a lady residing in Spa Fields, at whose window a brown owl, attracted by the solitary light, came flapping and hooting at midnight, to the great aggravation of the patient's symptoms.
[2] Bateman, u. s.
[3] *Glasg. Med. Journ.* IV. (1831), pp. 5, 229.
[4] Cheyne, *Dubl. Hosp. Reports*, III. (1822), p. 3. At Limerick, from June to September, 1821, there were 47 cases among the men of the 79th regiment.
[5] Clarke, *Edin. Med. and Surg. Journ.* IV. 423.
[6] A. C. Hutchinson, *Statement of the extraordinary sickness at the Penitentiary at Milbank*, Lond. 1823 ; P. M. Latham, M.D., *Account of the Disease lately prevalent at the General Penitentiary.* Lond. 1825.

present practitioners of this district." In the same summer it was unusually common in Dublin, and was epidemic the next year in other parts of Ireland as well (*supra*, p. 271). In Glasgow it began about the end of July, 1827, in the flat district to the south of the Clyde, and in the course of the autumn became prevalent in all parts of the city. An outbreak of plague itself could hardly have caused more surprise, so strange was dysentery to that generation. A few deaths by it in one crowded street of the Gorbals were mentioned in a newspaper before the disease had become general, and "gave rise to that groundless fear which pervaded and distracted the public mind during the whole course of the epidemic[1]."

The symptoms were severe and alarming, but the fatalities were few, perhaps not more than one in fifty attacks. The proper dysenteric symptoms usually lasted from ten to fourteen days, and were followed by diarrhoea, it might be, for many weeks. The morbid anatomy showed in the mucous membrane of the great intestine the three degrees of congestion, follicular ulceration and sloughing of the whole mucous coat (in the sigmoid flexure and rectum). The cases were nearly all above the age of puberty, and among the poorer classes. September and October were the worst months. The weather was remarkably close, damp and relaxing. One practitioner saw two cases of genuine ague in natives of Glasgow, having never seen a case of ague before. The ordinary cholera nostras of summer and autumn was much less frequent than for several years before, and it was the general remark that it had given place to the dysentery.

Having declined in the winter of 1827–28, it revived in May, and again reached a great height in the autumn of 1828, while cases of it (probably chronic, or renewals of old attacks) continued to the summer of 1830. The following table shows the number of cases treated by the poor's surgeons in the several seasons, 1827–30; the 435 cases in the autumn of 1827 were nearly a third part of all the cases so treated (1462):

Cases of Dysentery in Glasgow treated by the Surgeons to the Poor.

Quarter	1827	1828	1829	1830
Feb.—April	—	28	29	26
May—July	—	62	35	26
Aug.—Oct.	435	261	50	—
Nov.—Jan.	143	68	22	—

It extended to the villages and country districts all round Glasgow. It was believed to be somewhat general in Scotland in 1827–28, but the only answers to a circular of queries sent out by the editors of the 'Glasgow Medical Journal' came from

[1] James Wilson, *Glasgow Med. Journ.* I. (1828), p. 40.

Hamilton (and Bothwell), Ayr and Callander (including the flooded valley of the Teith and the Braes of Balquhiddar)[1].

In Edinburgh the outbreak of dysentery began about the end of July, 1828, a year later than in Glasgow, just as the epidemic in that city was a year or more later than in Dublin. Attacks of it were numerous among the patients admitted to the Edinburgh Infirmary for other diseases; but it occurred at the same time throughout the city generally and in the country around; "nor has it been confined entirely to the lower orders." In the imperfectly kept register of the Infirmary there were 42 admissions, with 11 deaths, from August to October. Christison, who treated some of these, had never seen dysentery before[2]. The morbid anatomy was the same as at Glasgow—congestions, numerous small ulcerations especially of the transverse colon, or sloughing of considerable portions of the mucous membrane.

In the same years 1827–28 there was much dysentery in the Lunatic Asylum at Wakefield. It is well known that aged paupers in workhouses or asylums are peculiarly subject to the epidemic influences that produce diarrhoeal or choleraic sickness; and there had been much of that disease in the West Riding Asylum from its opening in 1819. Some cases of dysentery had also occurred, but it was not until after the exceptional summer of 1826 that they became common. In 1828 there were 55 cases among 375 inmates, mostly in old and incurable lunatics, the fatalities being at the very high rate of one in four. The morbid anatomy was that of true dysentery—follicular ulceration in the transverse colon, with occasional sloughing of large pieces of the mucous membrane. The whole sewage of the asylum collected in cesspools or "tanks of ordure" within a few feet of the wards[3].

The causes of the rare and surprising outbreak of dysentery in 1827–28 were much debated. In Glasgow it was remarked that the choleraic complaints of the summer and autumn were much less frequent than usual; also that the first season of it, the year 1827, was remarkable for rain every day for some months, and for a close, oppressive, relaxing atmosphere. Brown, of Glasgow, thought the weather might account for it, the labouring class being thereby made peculiarly subject to heats and chills, which, grafted upon the usual bowel-complaints of the season, easily

[1] James Wilson, *Glasgow Med. Journ.* I. 39; James Brown, *ibid.*; Macfarlane, I. 99; Paterson, I. 438; Editors, IV. 1; Hume (Hamilton), IV. 14, and 229; McDerment (Ayr), IV. 19; Macnab (Callander), IV. 241.
[2] Christison, "Notice on the Dysentery which has lately prevailed in the Edinburgh Infirmary." *Edin. Med. Surg. Journ.* XXXI. (Jan. 1829), p. 216, and in *Life of Sir Robert Christison*, "Autobiography," I. 376.
[3] W. H. Gilby, M.D., "On the Dysentery which occurred in the Wakefield Lunatic Asylum in the years 1826, 1827, 1828 and 1829." *North of Eng. Med. and Surg. Journ.* I. (1830–31), 91.

turned them to dysentery. Dr Andrew Buchanan was of opinion
that exhalations from the soil were the chief, if not the sole,
exciting cause of dysentery, reserving the question of contagiousness. Other forms of miasmatic febrile disease, formerly rare,
had, he said, made their appearance of late years and become
epidemic. Christison had already spoken in the same sense for
the Edinburgh outbreak. For five or six weeks, he said, before
the dysentery appeared there in the end of July, 1828, the
tendency to bowel affections during the epidemic fever (which
was chiefly of the relapsing type) was increased in a very marked
degree. The same tendency continued throughout the whole
progress of the dysentery; "nay in some instances true acute
dysentery was formed during the height or towards the termination of continued fever; and now that the dysentery has in great
measure disappeared, or assumed a mild form, the tendency of
low gastro-enteric inflammation to accompany continued fever is
very strongly marked, perhaps is more frequent than ever."
This may relate to a remarkable outbreak of fever among the
richer classes in the New Town of Edinburgh, more talked about
than written on, which seems to have been enteric or typhoid,
according to the clinical history of a case of it that came from
Edinburgh to Hamilton and was recorded by a physician of the
latter place[1]. It was more especially that strange epidemic in
Edinburgh that Dr Andrew Buchanan had in mind when he
wrote that the dysentery of 1827–28 was not the only disease
due to exhalations from the soil with which Scotland had of
late been visited[2]. This is an instructive line to take in seeking

---

[1] Hume, "Case of the Edinburgh New Town Epidemic." *Glasgow Med. Journ.*
IV. 229.

[2] *Ibid.* IV. 7. The following is Buchanan's reference to it: "The only epidemic
fever belonging to the family of diseases we are here considering that occurred in
Scotland during the *dysenteric* years was that of the New Town of Edinburgh, in
1828, of which we have already spoken. As our knowledge of this fever is not
derived from any source on which we can certainly rely, it is possible that we may
have formed an erroneous opinion respecting it; but from all we have heard of its
symptoms and mode of distribution, we are disposed to consider it as totally different
in nature from the common fever of this country. The latter circumstance alone, the
mode of distribution of the disease, is, we think, perfectly sufficient to demonstrate our
proposition. Instead of occupying the Cowgate, the Grassmarket, and the High Street,
the usual haunts of typhus, this fever had its head-quarters in Heriot Row and Great
King Street; and, according to our information, it extended from the last mentioned
street in the direction of the Water of Leith, and from Leith, along the shore, to
Musselburgh. We do not vouch for the accuracy of these minute details, but we believe
the important fact to be beyond doubt that this fever prevailed chiefly, not in the
districts where typhus is invariably to be met with, but in the most fashionable parts
of the New Town."

an explanation of the dysentery of 1827–28, even if we keep something of the old doctrine of heats and chills as affecting those who labour in a damp atmosphere. The ground-water theory of miasmatic infective diseases was not then formulated ; but there has rarely been in our latitudes so signal an instance of extreme drought and heat followed by excessive dampness as in the two years 1825 and 1826, and the year 1827. The second dry year, 1826, was certainly the season when enteric fever was described and figured for the first time in London. It was said, also, that enteric cases occurred among the relapsing fever and dysentery of Dublin in the same year ; and enteric cases are known to have occurred in Edinburgh towards the end of the epidemic of relapsing fever and dysentery, which was one or two years later in that city than in Dublin. In Glasgow, where the dysentery was probably a more extensive outbreak than elsewhere, there appears to have been at that time no enteric fever ; in London, on the other hand, where there was a good deal of the latter, there does not appear to have been any notable prevalence of dysentery.

Along with the cholera nostras which was unusually common in the autumn of 1831, just before the outbreak of Asiatic cholera, there was some dysentery, notably an epidemic at Bolton[1]. At the end of the Asiatic cholera of 1832 a succession of cases of dysentery occurred in the Edinburgh Charity Work-house[2].

The next occasion of dysentery was the autumn of 1836, which was, like that of 1827, a wet season. The outbreak at Glasgow on this occasion is recorded only in a few figures (the medical journal of the city having ceased to appear for a time), according to which there were 144 cases throughout the year treated by the surgeons to the poor, of which 8 were fatal, and 15 cases sent to the Infirmary, of which 4 were fatal[3]. At Dundee also, from October to December, 1836, bowel-complaints were not unusual among the cases of typhus, which occurred in hundreds. "Many of the cases of diarrhoea and dysentery,"

---

[1] James Black, M.D., *Edin. Med. Surg. Journ.* XLV. (1836), p. 63. " As the epidemic was ushered in and was accompanied during the half of its course with cholera, fever of a typhous character followed close in its train among the working and lower classes, and continued more or less during the first months of winter, after dysentery had totally disappeared." The latter had not been seen again down to 1835.

[2] J. Smith, *ibid.* XLII. (1833), p. 342.

[3] Cleland, *Trans. Glasg. and Clydesd. Statist. Soc.* I. 1837.

said Arrott, "occurred in December, and were accompanied by catarrhal and rheumatic symptoms, implying an origin distinct from the bilious diarrhoea and bilious vomiting of summer." Of 22 cases of dysentery at the Infirmary, 2 were fatal[1].

Next year, 1837, there occurred in Somersetshire a remarkable epidemic which was for the most part dysenteric. It was seen first at Bridgewater, and in July it caused two deaths at Taunton, where it afterwards prevailed with high malignancy. Of 223 deaths, 206 were set down to dysentery, 16 to diarrhoea and 1 to cholera; the high ratio of children's deaths in the following table of ages is in accordance with other recent experiences to be given in the sequel:

Ages	0—5	—10	—15	—20	—30	—40	—50	—60	—70	—80	—90	Over 90
Deaths	93	17	11	7	6	3	7	16	26	24	11	2

The monthly mortalities were, 75 in August, 105 in September, 29 in October, 10 in November, 2 in December. The epidemic spread partially amongst the unions around Taunton[2].

In London from the beginning of registration (1837) until 1846, the deaths set down to dysentery averaged fully a hundred in the year—a statistical fact to which there is nothing corresponding in contemporary writings: Watson said it was hardly ever seen in practice except in the chronic form among sailors and soldiers who had contracted it abroad. During the prevalence of the "Irish fever" of 1846–48, the disease was truly epidemic and a cause of many deaths along with typhus itself, especially in Liverpool and mostly among destitute Irish. In 1846 it was in Milbank Penitentiary[3]. A most instructive instance of its connexion with the Irish emigration occurred at Penzance in the summer and autumn of 1848.

The brig 'Sandwich' sailed from Cork for Boston, U.S., in the end of May, carrying a number of Irish farmers and their families. Having met with rough weather and head winds she put in leaky to Penzance on 7 June, sixteen days out from Cork. The provisions had been bad and there was sickness in the ship, with a very filthy state of things. Three of the women passengers died on shore of dysentery. The ship sailed again on 10 July, two more of the emigrants dying of dysentery before she reached Boston, while two of the crew survived the attack. On 16 July, two cases of the same disease occurred among the lower class in Penzance, and thereafter the epidemic spread widely through most parts of the town and the three adjoining parishes of Madron, Galval and Paul, causing a great mortality, as in the following table:

[1] Arrott, *Edin. Med. Surg. Journ.*, Jan. 1839, p. 121.
[2] Farr, in *First Report of the Registrar-General*, 1837-8, p. 103.
[3] Baly, *Pathology and Treatment of Dysentery*. London, 1847.

Deaths from Dysentery in Penzance and three adjoining parishes.

1848

	Deaths from Dysentery in Penzance town	Deaths from Dysentery in 3 other parishes	Total deaths from Dysentery	Deaths from all causes in Penzance and 3 other parishes
July	5	0	5	31
August	37	1	38	71
Sept.	26	12	38	67
Oct.	13	9	22	48
Nov.	1	1	2	31
	82	23	105	248

As many as five hundred cases were under medical treatment in the town. No death occurred there or in the three parishes within the registration district after 10 November, "but very many in the country beyond its limits." Of the 105 deaths in the table, 46 were of young children, 35 of aged persons, and 24 between the ages of five and sixty years[1]. There was no resisting the evidence that an infection had been introduced by the weather-bound Irish emigrants; instances were also known of new foci in the country districts having been created by domestics or others suffering from dysentery who had been sent from Penzance to their homes. At the same time the summer had been exceptionally wet, the rainfall having been as follows :

	Inches of rain			Inches of rain
May	0·777		Sept.	3·042
June	3·287		Oct.	4·425
July	3·277		Nov.	3·981
Aug.	4·972			

A singular epidemic of dysentery occurred between the 14th and 26th September, 1853, among the thirty-six inmates of a row of nine cottages near the village of Hermiston, five miles west of Edinburgh. Seven children were attacked, of whom six died, and six adults, who all recovered. Besides these there were three cases among the four inmates of a cottage about a hundred yards away, and one case in each of two houses in the adjacent village of Hermiston. Christison found that a drain which received the sewage or slops of the hamlet was in a most offensive state, having been choked probably for years, and that the water of a well near it was foetid. These are the conditions that have often caused village epidemics of enteric fever in recent times; but there was no doubt that the disease in this case was dysentery[2]. Another asylum outbreak of dysentery occurred in 1865 in the Cumberland and Westmoreland Asylum[3].

Perhaps the last general prevalence of dysentery was during the Asiatic cholera of 1849, when the house-to-house visitations in Leeds and some other towns brought to light a somewhat surprising number of cases mixed with the more ordinary bowel-complaints of the season.

[1] Moyle, *Lond. Med. Gaz.* N.S. VII. Dec. 29, 1848, p. 1093.
[2] Christison, "On a local Epidemic of Dysentery." *Month. Journ. Med. Sc.* XVII. (Dec. 1853), 508.
[3] T. S. Clouston, *Med. Times and Gaz.* 1865, I. 567.

It is impossible to trace the subsequent history of dysentery in England by the usual statistical means of the Registrar-General's tables of the causes of death, for the reason that dysentery, a rare and curious disease of all ages in this country, is merged with diarrhoea, one of the commonest causes of infantile mortality. However, it is not likely that any such epidemic outbursts, local or general, as those described for certain years of the 18th and 19th centuries could have occurred without their being otherwise known. It may be safely said that there has been little of it in this country for the last thirty or forty years, except among a few soldiers, sailors or others returned from abroad; in Ireland itself, the immemorial "country disease" has now only a small annual total of deaths.

One of the last experiences of dysentery in an English port was instructive for the relation of the disease to typhus fever.

On 16 February, 1861, an Egyptian frigate, the 'Scheah Gehaed,' sent from Alexandria to be fitted with new engines, arrived in the Mersey. The only European on the ship was her commander, an Austrian. She carried 476 men, mostly Arabs, with a small proportion of Nubians and Abyssinians. Some two hundred were convicts, who had been brought on board in chained gangs. The passage had been long and stormy, and attended with much sickness, dysenteric and diarrhoeal; one man died and was thrown overboard two or three days before the ship reached Liverpool. The pilot who boarded her was at once struck by the horrible state of filth of the 'tween decks; he remained two days on board, and on returning home said to his wife, "This frigate will be heard of yet." He sickened in about a week of malignant typhus and died. Two others who boarded the ship took typhus, of whom one recovered. There had been no fever on board during the voyage. Thirty-two of the Arabs or Nubians were admitted to the Southern Hospital suffering, most of them, from dysentery or diarrhoea. Typhus fever attacked 17 of the ordinary patients, 2 nurses, 2 porters, 2 house-surgeons and 2 others in the hospital, of whom several died. The Arabs &c. to the number of 340 were taken in batches of 80 a day to a public bath, in which they remained three hours. Typhus broke out among the bath attendants. The whole number of cases of typhus traced to the ship was 31, of which 8 were fatal. The ship was sunk in the graving dock in order to clean her[1].

This is a classical instance of the breeding of typhus from the effluvia of dysentery, of which other instances, on a greater scale, have been given in connexion with the Jamaica expedition of 1655 (in the former volume), the siege of Londonderry and the camp of Dundalk in 1689, the hospitals after the battle of Dettingen in 1743, and the Irish famine of 1846–48.

[1] W. H. Duncan, M.D., "On the recent Introduction of Fever into Liverpool by the crew of an Egyptian frigate." *Trans. Epidemiol. Soc.* vol. I. pt. 2. p. 246. (1 July, 1861).

CHAPTER IX.

ASIATIC CHOLERA.

THE Indian or Asiatic cholera, which first showed itself on British soil in one or more houses on the Quay of Sunderland in the month of October, 1831, was a " new disease " in a more real sense than anything in this country since the sweating sickness of 1485. The English profession had been hearing a good deal about it for some years before it reached our shores. The outbreak in Lower Bengal in 1817, from which the modern history of cholera dates, had been the subject of reports and essays by Anglo-Indian physicians and surgeons; an extensive prevalence of it in the Madras Presidency shortly after, as well as in Mauritius in 1819 and 1829, had been observed by other medical men in the service of the East India Company or of the British army or navy. Many who had seen cholera in India, and some who had written upon it, returned to England in due course, so that the formidable new pestilence of the East began to be heard of in medical circles at home. Various essays upon it issued from the English press between 1821 and 1830[1]; and in 1825 it appeared for the first time, and at considerable length, in the pages of an English systematic treatise, the new edition of Dr Mason Good's ' Study of Medicine.'

Previous to 1829, Asiatic cholera had obtained no footing in Europe. The first great movement westwards from India

---

[1] James Boyle, surgeon to H. M. S. 'Minden,' *Epidemic Cholera of India*, London, 1821; W. B. Carter, *Cholera Indica vel Spasmodica*, Thesis, Glasgow, 1822; Thomas Brown, of Musselburgh, *On Cholera, more especially as it has appeared in British India*, Edin. 1824; Whitelaw Ainslie, M.D., *The Cholera Morbus of India*, Letter to the Court of Governors, H. E. I. C., Edin. 1825; A. T. Christie, M.D. (of Madras), *Obs. on the Nature and Treatment of Cholera*, Edin. 1828; Charles Searle (of Madras), *Cholera, its Nature, Cause and Treatment*, London, 1830 (dated 1st May, instigated, not by the Orenburg epidemic, but by the deaths of Sir Thomas Monro and others from cholera in Madras).

through Central Asia, which was continuous with the memorable
eruption in Bengal after the rains of 1817, had reached to
Astrakhan, at the mouths of the Volga, and had there caused the
deaths of some 144 persons in September, 1823. Another
progress westwards from India, after an interval of six years,
reached the soil of European Russia in the Government of
Orenburg in August 1829, the mortality in the whole province
during the autumn and winter (to February, 1830) amounting to
about one thousand. A much more severe epidemic of it arose
in the summer of 1830 in the town and province of Astrakhan
(supposed to have been introduced by an infected brig from
Baku), which spread with enormous rapidity, destroying in the
course of a month some four thousand in Astrakhan itself and
upwards of twenty thousand in other parts of the province[1].
Thus established in the basin of the Volga, Asiatic cholera
overran the whole of Russia. Before the spring of 1831 it had
entered Hungary and Poland, and in the end of May had
reached Danzig and other German ports on the Baltic and
North Seas. Lord Heytesbury, the British Ambassador at
St Petersburg, had sent home a despatch upon it early in 1831 ;
in April, the Admiralty issued orders for a strict quarantine of
all arrivals from Russia at British ports, which were afterwards
extended to arrivals from all ports abroad invaded or threatened
by cholera. On 20 June a royal proclamation ordering various
precautions was issued, and next day a Board of Health was
gazetted, composed of leading physicians in London and of the
medical heads of departments, with Sir Henry Halford as
president. Local Boards of Health were formed voluntarily in
many parts of the country during the summer of 1831. Two
medical men were at the same time commissioned by the
Government to proceed to Russia to study the disease there,
their letters to the Board of Health commencing from the 1st of
July. The growing interest in the disease as it came nearer
called forth another crop of writings, some of them based on old
Indian experience, others speculative[2]. The most important of

---

[1] See extract in *Glas. Med. Journ.*, Feb. 1831, p. 105, from *Scottish Mission. and Philan. Reg.*

[2] George Hamilton Bell, *Treatise on Cholera Asphyxia or Epidemic Cholera as it appeared in Asia and more recently in Europe*, Edin. 1831 ; Reginald Orton, *An Essay on the Epidemic Cholera of India*, 2nd. ed. with a supplement, London, 1831 (August); 1st ed. Madras, 1820; H. Young, M.D. (of the Bengal Service), *Remarks on the Cholera Morbus*, 2nd ed. 1831 ; Alex. Smith, M.D. (Calcutta), *Description of*

these was the treatise by Orton, which had been published in its original form at Madras in 1820. Writing from Yorkshire in August, 1831, he surmised (with a proviso that no one could say confidently what might happen) that Asiatic cholera might be expected to be a mild visitation upon Britain at large, falling most upon the large manufacturing towns in which typhus was common, but that it would be " far otherwise" with Ireland owing to its chronic poverty, distress and over-population. By a singular chance the only town which he specially mentioned in England was Sunderland, where, he had been told by Dr Clanny, there had been an unusual number of cases of malignant cholera nostras in the early part of the autumn: "it is greatly to be feared," he said, "that those are but the skirts of the approaching shower[1]."

In other places besides Sunderland there had been perhaps more than the usual amount of summer diarrhoea in 1831. Dr Burne, in his London dispensary reports, entered on the 2nd and 16th July an unusual prevalence of "dysenteric diarrhoea and cholera," and cases of scarlet fever of an "adynamic" type or with a tendency to fatal collapse[2]. (Clanny observed the same type of scarlatina at Sunderland along with some typhus.) Choleraic disorders were uncommonly rife on board the ships of war in the Medway[3]. A succession of twenty-four cases at Port Glasgow, from 2 July to 2 August, chiefly among workers in Riga flax, gave rise to an alarm of the real Asiatic cholera, the more readily that the first case was fatal (the only death)[4]. Similar alarms arose at Leith and Hull.

the Spasmodic Cholera (substance of an old report to the Army Medical Board); W. Macmichael, M.D., *Is the Cholera Spasmodica of India a Contagious Disease?* London, 1831 (Sept.); T. J. Pettigrew, *Obs. on Cholera, comprising a description of the Epidemic Cholera of India*, London, 1831 (13 Nov.); John Austin, *Cholera Morbus, Indian and Russian Cholera*, London, 1831 (July); John Goss, late H. E. I. C. S., *Practical Remarks on the Disease called Cholera*, London, 1831 (Nov.); Whitelaw Ainslie, *Letters on the Cholera*, London, 1832 (from Edinburgh, Dec. 1831); Henry Penneck, M.D., *Nature and Treatment of the Indian Pestilence commonly called Cholera*, London, 1831 (Penzance, 24 Nov.); A. P. Wilson Philip, *Nature of Malignant Cholera*, London, 1832; *Official Reports made to Government by Drs Russell and Barry on Cholera Spasmodica observed during the Mission to Russia in 1831*, London, 1832; John V. Thompson, Dep. Insp. Gen. of Hosps. *The Pestilential Cholera unmasked*, Cork, 1832 (January).

   [1] *Op. cit.* p. 469.
   [2] *Lond. Med. Gaz.* 1831.
   [3] James Hall, "Narrative of an Epidemic English Cholera that appeared on board ships of war lying in ordinary in the River Medway during the Summer and Autumn of 1831." *Edin. Med. Surg. Journ.*, Feb. 1832, p. 295.
   [4] John Marshall, M.D., *Obs. on Cholera as it appeared at Port Glasgow in July and August, 1831. Illustrated by numerous cases.* 1831.

Asiatic Cholera at Sunderland in October, 1831.

In the end of July and in August, Sunderland and the adjoining villages and farms in the valley of the Wear were visited with "a very general prevalence of the indigenous cholera of the country, bearing in most instances its usual leading feature—that of excessive bilious discharges[1]." Few, who were not attacked with actual cholera nostras, were altogether free, it was said, from diarrhoea or disordered digestion. Many of the choleraic cases were unusually malignant, of which the following are instances:

Allison, aged fifty, a painter of earthenware residing in a low situation on the bank of the Wear two miles above the town, was attacked at 4 a.m. on the 5th of August with vomiting and purging of a watery whitish fluid, like oatmeal and water. His hands and feet were cold, his skin covered with clammy sweat, his face livid and the expression anxious, his eyes sunken, his lips blue, thirst excessive, his breath cold, his voice weak and husky, and his pulse almost imperceptible. He passed into a stage of reactive fever and got well. Arnott, a farm-labourer on the opposite bank of the Wear from the man Allison, was seized at 2 a.m. on the 8th August with precisely the same symptoms, and died in twelve hours. Neither he nor Allison had any intercourse or relation with seamen or the shipping of Sunderland[2]. Another case on the 8th of August came to light afterwards. A woman in the village of West Bolden, four miles from Sunderland, on the Newcastle road, was found by a surgeon from the town to be suffering from choleraic sickness, of which she died twelve hours from its onset[3].

A week after these cases in the country not far from Sunderland, there occurred the death, on 14 August, of one of the Wear pilots named Henry. He had been troubled with diarrhoea for some time before, but not so as to keep him from his occupation. Having gone down in the direction of Flamborough Head to look for ships, he picked up a vessel between that and the Wear, piloted her in, and, a few days after, piloted her out again. The identity of the vessel was never traced, but it was alleged that she had come from an infected port abroad. The last time Henry was in his boat he was seized with violent vomiting and purging, and died at his house after an illness of twenty hours. A brother pilot, who looked in at the house on the day of his death, fell into a similar choleraic disorder, but recovered[4]. On the 28th of August a shipwright died of the same; also about the end of August two persons at a distance of four or five miles from Sunderland. In September, it is said, there were other cases and fatalities. Early in October the authentic particulars of cholera in Sunderland begin. Dixon attended one case, which was fatal on the 9th October. Another case, which came to light three months after, was that of a girl of twelve, named Hazard, residing on the Fish Quay, who was well enough on Sunday the 16th October to have been twice at church. She was seized in the middle of the night following with the sudden and appalling symptoms of

[1] William Dixon, *Lond. Med. Gaz.* 4 Feb. 1832, IX. 668.
[2] Dixon, u. s.
[3] Kell, p. 22.
[4] Kell, Dixon, and others; the statements about Henry's case are contradictory.

choleraic disease and died on the Monday afternoon[1]. A few doors off on the same quay lived a keelman named Sproat, aged sixty ; he occupied a large, clean, well-ventilated room on the first-floor of a house in the most open part of the quay, opposite to a crowded part of the anchorage. He was in failing health, and had been troubled with diarrhoea for a week or ten days previous to the 19th October, on which day he had to give up work. Next day, Thursday, the 20th, a surgeon who had been sent for found him vomiting and purging, but not at all collapsed, with no thirst, and in good spirits. He improved so much that on Friday he had toasted cheese for supper and on Saturday a mutton chop for dinner, after which he went out to his keel on the river for a few minutes. On his return he was seized with rigor, cramps, vomiting and purging. Medical aid was not sent for until seven on Sunday morning, when he was found in a sinking state, pulseless, speaking in a husky whisper, his face livid and pinched, his limbs cramped, the purgings like "meal washings." He continued like that for three days, and died on Wednesday, the 26th October, at noon.

This came to be reckoned the first death from Asiatic cholera in England.

His grandchild, a girl of eleven, while moving about the room an hour after the death, was suddenly seized with faintness, pains in the stomach-region, vomiting and purging of watery matters ; she was taken to the Infirmary and soon got well. The day after his father's death, Thursday, the 27th October, William Sproat, junior, a fine athletic young keelman, who had attended on his parent during his illness, was found lying in a low damp cellar near to the Fish Quay, suffering from choleraic symptoms ; he had been ill only a few hours, and was removed (with his daughter as above) to the Infirmary the same evening. He became gradually worse: on the 30th he was continually throwing himself about, moaning and biting the bedclothes ; on the 31st he was lying on his back comatose, his eyes open, the pupils wide and insensible, and the breathing stertorous, in which state he died the same day. An old nurse at the Infirmary (Turnbull) helped to place the body in the coffin, went to bed in a state of considerable fear, and was seized at one in the morning with symptoms of cholera, of which she died after a few hours.

Meanwhile there had been two other fatal cases unconnected with the Sproats or the Fish Quay. On the quay of Monk Wearmouth, across the river, lived a shoemaker named Rodenburg, aged thirty-five. He occupied a poor hovel and had a large family, but he was in good work and wages. On Sunday, the 30th October, he had pork for dinner, and what was left of it for supper. In the middle of the night he was seized with vomiting, and with purging of a fluid like water-gruel in vast quantities ; when visited by the medical men, he spoke in a husky whisper, his nails were blue, his skin livid, covered by cold sweat, his limbs cramped. The spasms ceased about nine o'clock on Monday morning ; about noon he asked to be raised in bed, and died as they were raising him. On the very same night, between Sunday and Monday, a keelman named Wilson, who lived with his wife in a decent room in the High Street, and had attended the Methodist chapel on Sunday, was seized with cholera at 4 a.m. on Monday, and died the same afternoon at three.

These six cases within a few days, all fatal but that of the girl of eleven, looked like the real Asiatic disease. Kell, an

[1] Clanny, p. 19.

army assistant-surgeon stationed at Sunderland with the reserve companies of the 82nd Regiment, had suspected that the earlier case of the pilot Henry was true Asiatic cholera (which he had seen in Mauritius in 1829), and had written to the Board of Health. At a meeting of the faculty at the Infirmary on the morning after the admission of Sproat junior and his child (28th October), Kell urged upon them that the disease was Asiatic cholera, but all the twelve present, save Dr Clanny, who was in the chair, maintained that it was common indigenous cholera. However, when the younger Sproat died, and the nurse after him, and two others in different parts of the town, a full meeting of medical men at the Exchange came unanimously to the opinion that these were cases of "spasmodic cholera." A meeting of the Board of Health and leading citizens was at once held, who were informed that, in the unanimous opinion of the medical gentlemen of the town, "spasmodic cholera prevailed in Sunderland." The authorities in London having been kept informed (principally by Kell), a surgeon of Indian experience was sent down by the Board of Health on the 5th November, and a colonel by the lords of the Council on the 6th, to act as commissioners.

It happened that no more cases occurred for three days after the death of the nurse at the Infirmary; so that the doctors, like Pharaoh in the intervals between the plagues of Egypt, were beginning to repent of their diagnosis. The shipping trade of Sunderland was threatened by these newspaper alarms, and by the presence of two Government commissioners in the town; while Kell was demanding a ship of war off the mouth of the Wear, and a battery on shore, to make the quarantine respected. The Marquis of Londonderry, interested in the coal-trade, wrote to the *Standard* that the alarm was false. The magistrates, shipowners and leading residents, who had met on the 9th November to raise money for a cholera hospital, assembled again in various public meetings or caucuses on the 10th and 11th, and passed resolutions that there was no Indian or other foreign imported cholera in Sunderland, that it was a wicked and malicious falsehood to say there was, and that there was no need of quarantine on the Wear. One of these meetings was attended by fifteen medical men (most of them from the residential suburb of Bishop Wearmouth), who severally expressed the opinion in various terms, that the recent fatal cases were aggravated cases of English cholera, not contagious or infectious, while three more sent letters backing up Lord Londonderry and the shipowners. On the 12th of November, twenty-seven medical men signed a declaration to the same effect. Some of these remained unconvinced by the progress of events, Dixon arguing as late as 23 January, 1832, that the epidemic in Sunderland, which was by that time over, had been one of "spontaneous malignant cholera."

Two new seizures occurred on the 7th November, none on the 8th, seven on the 9th, one on the 10th, and so on for fully six weeks longer until Christmas, when the cases became very occasional, so that on the 9th of January, 1832, Sunderland was declared by the Board of Health to be free of cholera. The largest number of seizures reported on one day was nineteen on the 8th of December; on the 10th of that month there were sixty-three cases under treatment at once; the whole number of cases from 23rd October to 31st December was 418, of which 202 were fatal; the whole deaths at Sunderland by the cholera of 1831–32 are given at 215, so that the epidemic exhausted itself there before it had well begun elsewhere in the country. The effect of it upon the death-rate is shown in a comparison of the burials for November and December in three successive years[1]:

Burials in the parish of Sunderland.

	November	December
1829	29	44
1830	39	76
1831	122	127

The way by which the virus entered Sunderland was never traced. It was known, however, that deaths from cholera had occurred among the crews of Sunderland ships lying at Cronstadt and Riga; and as it was the practice for vessels owned in Sunderland to come home from their summer trading towards the end of the season, so as to lay up during the winter, it was suspected that the clothes of some of the dead men had been brought over and sent ashore. The quarantine in the Wear was far from effective: the station was higher up the river than the loading moorings, so that suspected ships had to pass through a crowd of ordinary shipping to get to it. It appears that hardly any ships were quarantined, except some from Dutch ports where no cholera then existed.

This first experience of Asiatic cholera on British soil brought out very clearly one character of the infection which was seen to attend it everywhere during the following year, and has always attended it in every subsequent invasion of the disease. The virus, for all its opportunities, showed a marked preference for, an almost exclusive selection of the lowest and least cleanly localities, and a considerable preference for persons

---

[1] A table of the daily course of the cholera at Sunderland, which I must omit for want of space, is given in the essay by Haslewood and Morbey, *History and Medical Treatment of Cholera as it appeared in Sunderland in* 1831, London, 1832, p. 151.

of drunken or negligent habits. Sunderland consisted of three parts—the parish so named, the parish of Bishop Wearmouth, which was the west end of Sunderland or the residential quarter of the wealthier class, and across the river the parish of Monk Wearmouth, with the adjoining Shore. The cholera was almost wholly confined to Sunderland proper; Ainsworth says that no cases occurred, to his knowledge, in the parish of Bishop Wearmouth, and not above six in Monk Wearmouth; another gave six or eight cases in each of these parishes, but increased the estimate to eighteen or twenty in each according to later information. Bishop Wearmouth stood about seventy feet higher than the highest part of Sunderland; it was well built, and its population of 14,462 (with 363 more in the Pans), included the whole of the wealthier class with the trades dependent on them. Monk Wearmouth, with a population of 1498, and the adjoining Shore with a population of 6051, were irregularly built on the north bank, and occupied by the same class (keelmen, sailors, labourers and workmen in the coal, iron and shipping trades) as Sunderland itself; but for some reason, connected perhaps with its soil and elevation, it escaped with a very few cases of cholera[1]. The parish of Sunderland, with a population of 18,916, was not all visited equally. The focus of the cholera, says Ainsworth, was the town moor, a large piece of pasture-land stretching to the sea-shore at the south-east end of the town, having a subsoil tenacious of water, marshy in the winter months, and its roads almost impassable. Upon this open space was deposited, and left to accumulate for weeks together, the filth from the narrow lanes and passages of the low-lying and crowded quarter at the seaward end of the parish, to the south of the High Street. Some of the streets occupied by the poorer class consisted of old residences of the well-to-do, now divided into tenements. Certain streets had as many as a dozen or twenty common middens, "let in" to the street fronts of houses and covered by trap-doors, in which the domestic refuse and sweepings of the street were collected as a source of profit, and sold at stated times to farmers for manure. Most of the attacks happened in this low-lying part of Sunderland, with a soil and foundations sodden with filth, houses overcrowded and badly ventilated, and its residents subject to the alternations

---

[1] Kell, however, suspected that there were many malignant cases in Monk Wearmouth after the 31st of October, which were not reported. l. c. p. 73.

of excess and want (with much pawning of clothes, &c.) peculiar to a port from which one or two hundred sail would leave with a fair wind or arrive in the river together[1]. About four hundred were attacked in a population of eighteen thousand during a space of two months. The cases among the wealthier classes were nearly all in the households of medical men :—the mother of one doctor, living with him, died of Asiatic cholera, the wife of another came safely through an attack, one or more medical men had the symptoms in one degree or another. In the end of November, five old people in the poor's house were fatally attacked all at once, in different parts of the building. A cholera hospital had been provided at an early stage of the outbreak, but the relatives of those attacked seldom permitted their removal to it, a prejudice against it having been aroused by the post-mortem examination of the first victims. Most of the cases were accordingly treated at their homes, which were "always crowded to excess by the immediate attendants or relatives, and by others from mere curiosity." A fund of two thousand pounds was raised for the distressed families, to which the Government gave one hundred. Sunderland became for two or three weeks a centre of interest to medical men, who came to see the cholera from various parts of England, Ireland and Scotland, while MM. Magendie and Guillot came from Paris, and M. Dubuc from Rouen.

The symptoms and morbid anatomy of cholera as it was known in India were seen without ambiguity in the Sunderland epidemic. In a few cases death followed very quickly without the distinctive intestinal symptoms; but usually the unmistakeable thing was a sudden seizure, often in the night after a hearty supper, marked by profuse "meal-and-water" or "rice-and-water" purging, by vomiting, faintness or sinking at the pit of the stomach, thirst, pulselessness, cramps of the limbs, restless tossing, coldness, blueness and clamminess of the surface, and shrunken features. The *facies Hippocratica* had not been seen on so extensive a scale in England since the sweating sickness of

---

[1] Clanny says (p. 42), "At first our epidemic appeared only in certain streets or lanes, namely, the Fish Landing, Long Bank, Silver Street, High Street, Burleigh Street, Mill Hill, Sailors' Alley, Love Lane, Wood Street, Warren Street; as also in several lanes in Bishopwearmouth, the New Town, Ayre's Quay, and on the north side of the river in Monkwearmouth, in several of the byelanes near the river... Generally speaking the disease fixed its residence in such places as medical men could have pointed out *à priori*."

three hundred years before. The end was sometimes in deep coma, at other times in delirium with convulsive or spasmodic movements. The chief point in the morbid anatomy was the engorgement of the lungs, great veins, and right side of the heart, from which the disease was named "cholera asphyxia." The blood was thick and tarry[1].

Extension of Cholera to the Tyne, December, 1831.

Before Sunderland had been declared by the Board of Health to be free of cholera, on the 7th of January, 1832, the infection had gained a footing in Newcastle, Gateshead, North Shields, Houghton-le-Spring, and some places on the road to Edinburgh. The mildness of that winter was somewhat favourable to its diffusion; in November there had been some days of severe frost in the midst of generally mild weather, December was warmer than usual, the pastures being green and spring-like, while January was warm and dry almost beyond precedent. The first cases in new centres were usually tramps or others who had come from Sunderland[2]; but there were some puzzling attacks. Thus Dixon says that on 12th December, 1831, he visited a woman of fifty who died of cholera after twelve hours, "in a lonely district unconnected in situation with any previously infected place," and where there had been no personal liability to contagion; a young man lodging in the house died three days after with the same symptoms.

At Newcastle, as at Sunderland, fatal cases of choleraic disease were discovered from the beginning of autumn; one such, on 4 August, at the village of Team, two miles to the south-west of Newcastle, was said to have been as little of the nature of bilious cholera, and as truly spasmodic cholera, as those in the subsequent great epidemic. Another suspicious death occurred a little below Newcastle on the 26th October, the same day as the first acknowledged death from the Asiatic disease in Sunderland. A month passed before the next death, marked by spasmodic and non-bilious symptoms, occurred at Newcastle—on the 26th November.

---

[1] Besides the essay of Haslewood and Morbey, and the paper by Dixon, *supra*, the following were written on the Sunderland cholera: W. Ainsworth, *Obs. on the Pestilential Cholera at Sunderland*, London, 1832; John Butler Kell, surgeon to the 82nd Regt., *Cholera at Sunderland in* 1831, Edin. 1834; W. Reid Clanny, M.D., (chairman of the Local Board of Health), *Hyperanthraxis, or the Cholera of Sunderland*, Lond. 1832; Emile Dubuc, *Rapport sur le Cholera Morbus à Sunderland, Newcastle, etc.* Rouen, 1832.

[2] Ainsworth, p. 164, u. s., says: "Dennis Mc Gwin, who took the disease to North Shields, came from Sunderland. The first case in South Shields was a boy from Gateshead. A pedler woman took it to Houghton, a traveller to Morpeth, and I have no doubt its arrival could similarly be traced to Durham, Haddington and Tranent, all towns on the same high road. A wanderer also perished of the disease at Doncaster; but luckily there were no other cases."

At length, on the 7th of December, 1831, the Asiatic cholera was declared to be in the town. The earliest cases of it were found in low-lying poor houses along the river[1]. Gateshead, on the south bank of the Tyne, had only two cases until a day or two before Christmas; at length, on Christmas-day, there was a sudden explosion of the infection simultaneously at many points.

"On the 25th [December, 1831] about one o'clock," wrote Brady[2], "we were assailed by a third and fourth example of the disease, and before the next morning at ten o'clock, very considerable numbers had fallen sacrifices to its pestilential ravages. Within a space of twelve hours it spread itself over a diameter of two miles, and appeared to pay but very little distinction to altitude of situation, for the higher parts of the town were laid under its stroke in an equal degree, or nearly so, with the lower. Pipewellgate, Hillgate, the banks above Pipewellgate, Oakwellgate, the lanes leading from it, Jackson's chare, Nun's Lane, Wreckington, Gateshead Low Fell, Low Team—situations as different in their external character as can well be conceived—were all indiscriminately exposed to its fury."

Greenhow's summary of this remarkable explosion on the afternoon and night of Christmas-day is that "at nearly fifty different points cases occurred almost at the same instant." The attack at Gateshead was short and severe; at Newcastle it was less concentrated and of longer duration, affecting the population in the low and dissolute localities along the river, such as Sandgate and the Close, while there were two or three fatalities about the 6th January among the wealthier residents. The hospital cases in Newcastle and Gateshead to the 9th of February were:

	Cases	Deaths
Sandgate Hospital	55	23
Castle Hospital	12	8
St John's and St Andrew's	15	8
Gateshead Hospital	36	21
	118	60

As at Sunderland, the bulk of the cases were treated at their homes—1330 cases, with 437 deaths, to the 9th of February. As the whole number of deaths at Newcastle and Gateshead, while the cholera of 1832 lasted, was 801 in the returns to the Board of Health, it would appear that the epidemic had

---

[1] T. M. Greenhow, M.D., *Cholera as it has recently appeared in the Towns of Newcastle and Gateshead, including Cases,* London, 1832; Thomas Mollison, M.D., *Remarks on the epidemic Disease called Cholera, as it occurred in Newcastle,* Edin. 1832. (He arrived at Newcastle from Edinburgh on the 21st Dec. and remained eleven days.)

[2] In Greenhow, u.s.

dragged on through the spring and perhaps the summer, which were its seasons elsewhere.

The colliers' villages on both sides of the Tyne for two or three miles above and below Newcastle and Gateshead were sharply visited at the same time. Below Newcastle, on the north bank, it invaded Dent's Hole, a dirty narrow lane along the margin of the river, overhung by its banks, filled with mud and filth rising in heaps above the thresholds of the houses; also on the same side, Walker, Howden-Pans, and so on to North Shields; on the south side below Gateshead it visited Felling and other villages. South Shields and Westoe escaped for several weeks, but at length about the 20th of February the epidemic began there and caused 147 deaths before it ceased.

Some of the worst village outbreaks occurred above Newcastle on both sides of the river. Swalwel, a low dirty village of iron-workers, near the confluence of the Derwent with the Tyne had a very virulent attack. Dunston, another low-lying village on the south bank, two miles above Gateshead, subject to inundation from the small tributary stream running through it, had twenty-three deaths among the 400 inhabitants in about a fortnight, most of the victims being old, dissipated and debilitated. On the other hand, Whickam Fell, standing on the hill between Dunston and Swalwel, escaped with only one case, while Bensham, another elevated village between Gateshead and Dunston, escaped altogether; just as Byker, a high-lying village on the north bank, only half a mile from Dent's Hole, had but a single mild case.

On the north bank above Newcastle the disease was most severe in the villages of Bell's Close, Lemington and Newburn. The epidemic in the last of these was indeed unparalleled. As in all the other villages attacked, the epidemic was soon over, but not before two-thirds of the inhabitants had suffered either from choleraic diarrhoea or cholera proper. Newburn was a village of some 131 houses, built in the face of the high north bank of the river five miles above Newcastle, its population being 550. The houses stood in two rows, one above the other, the church and churchyard standing in open ground midway between the lower and upper streets of the village; a small stream ran through it to the Tyne. The inhabitants were mostly wherry-men, coal labourers, or glassworkers; they were a healthy community, above indigence, housed in clean, neat, comfortably furnished clay-floored cottages. The first case of cholera, in a man who lived close to the brook, proved fatal on the 4th of January, 1832. There was no new case until the 10th, after which there were several deaths every day. From the night of the 15th until noon of the 16th fifty were attacked, twelve or thirteen of them with the worst kind of spasmodic cholera, the rest with diarrhoea. By the 2nd of February the epidemic was over. Three hundred and twenty had either cholera or cholerine, of whom fifty-seven died (the Board of Health return gives 274 cases and 65 deaths to 25 January), the daily deaths having been as follows[1]:

Cholera in Newburn, near Newcastle, 1832.

	Deaths			Deaths
Jan. 4	1		Jan. 20	3
11	4		21	2
12	3		22	3
13	4		23	2
14	6		24	2
15	5		25	1
16	6		26	2
17	3		27	1
18	5		28 ⎫	1
19	3		29 ⎭	

The other chief centres of cholera in the northern coal district, besides those mentioned, were Houghton-le-Spring and Hetton (which had together 311 cases and 66 deaths to the 28 of January), the colliery village of Earsden, and the port of Tynemouth.

The Cholera of 1832 in Scotland.

It was not until April that the infection began to show itself on the same scale in other parts of England. The next parts of the kingdom to be invaded after the Wear and the Tyne were the coal and iron districts of East Lothian and Lanarkshire, the cities of Edinburgh and Glasgow becoming infected soon after. A fatal case, in a destitute tramping sailor occurred at Doncaster, in the beginning of January, but led to no outbreak; two fatal cases occurred at Morpeth about the same time, the second of the two in a bagman who had just spent three days making his rounds in Newcastle and the infected villages near

[1] Craigie, *Edin Med. Surg. Journ.* XXXVII. 337.

it. It was on the high road to Edinburgh, at Haddington, Tranent and Musselburgh, that the next focus of cholera was established. Previous to the 14th of January there had been 47 cases, with 18 deaths, in and near Haddington, among the miners and others of the labouring class. At Tranent, seven miles nearer Edinburgh on the main road, with a population of 1700 miners and labourers, a boy died of cholera on the 18th January, the infection spreading so rapidly that before the 25th there had been 61 attacks with 26 deaths, which rose to 205 attacks and 60 deaths by the 8th of February. A few cases occurred also at North Berwick and a good many at Preston Pans ; while Musselburgh became the scene of one of the most deadly outbreaks in the whole history.

Musselburgh, with Fisherrow, was not then the place of villas which it afterwards became, but was occupied by a working class, who combined the three industries of coal-mining, weaving or other factory work, and fishing. To add to the ordinary insanitary risks of such a combination, some fifteen hundred hands had been out of work for two months, and were in " a state of great misery." The first case of cholera appeared there on Wednesday, the 18th January, three days after the first death at Tranent. The virulence and certainty of the infection will appear from the following by D. M. Moir, the distinguished author of *Mansie Waugh* and other writings in prose or verse, who practised his profession at Musselburgh :

" A girl at Musselburgh, whose mother kept a lodging-house, was found in a state of complete collapse on the morning of Thursday, the 19th January —the day after the first appearance of the pestilence. She died on that afternoon, between five and six, and was buried by moonlight the same evening....The mother during the night of Saturday was also similarly seized, and fell a victim on the following noon. Her sister, who had walked from Leith on the same morning to condole with her in her family distress, was immediately affected on entering the house ; but her symptoms being over-looked in the misery around her, medical assistance was not called in, until, on the return of the nieces from the interment, their aunt was discovered dead on the floor of the dwelling. Her husband, Baxter, a man of intem-perate habits, came out to enquire into her fate ; and immediately on his return home to Leith was seized with the distemper and died."

In three weeks there were more deaths from cholera than from all causes in the whole of an ordinary year. To the 22nd of February, just over a month from its outbreak, the disease had attacked 435, of whom 193 died. The medical profession (the senior of whom was a man of original talent, Thomas Brown, author of an essay on smallpox, in 1808, and one on the Indian cholera in 1824), were greatly taxed by the numerous calls upon them: Moir met one night a young colleague who complained of feeling ill, and was advised by the former to go home at once; he continued his rounds for an hour longer, and died of cholera next morning. Edinburgh, only five miles distant, was in constant communication with Musselburgh; and at length three or four cases appeared in the city in persons who had been at the infected place. The Edinburgh cases, however, did not multiply rapidly; to the 8th of February, there had been 8 cases with four deaths; to the 28th of February, 35 cases, with 18 deaths; to the 20th of March, 39 cases, with 20 deaths. On the other hand, the suburb of Water of Leith, had 48 cases, with 23 deaths at the same date. On the 6th April, 1832, the figures for Edinburgh and certain of its suburbs respectively were:

	Cases	Deaths
Portobello	44	24
Water of Leith	58	30
Canonmills	18	12
Duddingston	10	3
Edinburgh	62	38

Of the border towns, Hawick was infected on the 14th January, probably from Morpeth, and had a not very extensive epidemic, of somewhat mild type[1]. Coldstream, on the Tweed, a few miles above Berwick, had 109 cases and 37 deaths to the 20th of March.

Meanwhile the infection had sought out the weak spots in the west of Scotland—the mining and weaving villages in Lanarkshire, the city of Glasgow and the manufacturing town of Paisley. On Sunday, the 22nd January, a boy was taken ill in church at Kirkintilloch (a village on the Forth and Clyde canal, seven miles north-east of Glasgow), and died next morning: that was the first case in the west of Scotland. Cases multiplied in Kirkintilloch, so that by the 6th of March there had been thirty-two deaths, but no more for the rest of the season. A few days after the boy was seized in church there, a first case occurred in the mining village of Coatbridge, six or seven miles to the south-east, in an old man living in a "back land" in very poor circumstances, who had not been

[1] John Douglas, M.D., "History of the Epidemic Cholera of Hawick," in *Cholera Gazette*, no. 6, April 7, p. 234.

in Kirkintilloch nor had communication with such as had been there ; other cases followed slowly, and at length there was a more severe outbreak.

Glasgow at once took precautions. A Board of Health had been formed there early in the summer of 1831. In February, it had command of £8000 raised by voluntary subscriptions, and it made provision of 236 cholera beds in five hospitals. The theatres were closed, and "evening sermons" discouraged ; while all the passenger boats (for a time also the goods barges) on the Forth and Clyde canal, and on the Monkland canal (near to which was Coatbridge) were stopped. District committees were formed in all parts of the city.

The first victim was Janet Lindsay, a drunken old woman who lodged with widow Proudfoot and her daughter in Todd's Close, Goosedubs ; she was asthmatic, and had not been beyond the Goosedubs for weeks. Her seizure, with vomiting and purging, was on the afternoon of Thursday, 9th February, and her death on Saturday morning. Also on the 9th February, in the suburb of Woodside, remote from Goosedubs, the infant of one McGie was attacked with cholera, suffered much from cramps on the 10th and died on the 11th, the father, mother and others of the family afterwards suffering from cholera. The third case, fatal in a few hours, appeared early in the morning of Friday the 10th in a boy living in Millroad Street, a mile east of the Goosedubs, who had been subject to diarrhoea for some weeks. The fourth victim was a gardener in Macalpine Street, a locality also remote from the Goosedubs and in the opposite direction from Millroad Street, who had walked three miles to Pollokshaws on the 9th, and had partaken of tea with friends at Crossmyloof on his way back, in excellent health : he was seized at midnight with purging, and died on the afternoon of the second day. The fifth case was in Partick on the 11th, the sixth in Bridgegate on the 12th, not far from the close in the Goosedubs where the first case had occurred. On the 17th the first of many cases occurred in Paisley, and on the same day there was a case at Maryhill (population of some 500), followed by six more before the next afternoon. Thus there were, besides the case of cholera in the very heart of old Glasgow, half-a-dozen other cases the same day or in the next day or two, at scattered points all round the city. About fifty of the neighbours had visited Janet Lindsay in Todd's Close, and some had helped to lay her out. The next case in the close was of a woman who had stopped in the street to talk with the widow Proudfoot shortly after the body had been removed ; this woman was seized at seven next morning (Sunday, the 12th Feb.), and died in the hospital after twenty-four hours. Three days passed, and then there occurred two other cases, both fatal, in Todd's Close, one of them being the widow Proudfoot herself, who refused to be taken to the hospital, and would receive no other medicine or cordial but whisky. No other cases occurred in the close for several weeks ; but within a range of two hundred yards of it there were 46 cases from the 13th to the 29th of February. It was, indeed to this region of Glasgow, the Goosedubs and the Wynds, that the infection was chiefly confined for the first few weeks ; it was especially severe in Francis's Close, Broomielaw, a collection of small wretched hovels, in which some twenty died of cholera[1]. The state of the

---

[1] Chiefly from the paper by Professor George Watt, *Glas. Med. Journ.* v. 298, 384 ; see also Bryce, *ibid.* 262.

three old Wynds of Glasgow and of other the like localities has been already referred to under a date a year or two before the outbreak of cholera (supra p. 598).

No better instance could be given of the inscrutable ways in which the infection of cholera found out the weak places and the likely subjects than the explosion in the Glasgow Town's Hospital or pauper infirmary on the 22nd of February, some twelve days after the first cases in various parts of the city and suburbs.

The infirmary, built in two blocks on the north bank of the Clyde, contained 395 inmates occupying 296 beds, some 60 or 70 of whom were insane or fatuous. The fatuous lived in ground-floor cells of the north block, from seven to eleven feet square, with a stone vaulted roof, a stone floor, no fireplace, damp from situation and want of sun, but all the more damp from being often washed owing to the uncleanly habits of the inmates. At eight on the morning of the 22nd February two fatuous paupers in adjoining cells were found cold and pulseless; they had vomited and purged during the night, although they had been well the evening before; each of the two cells had three beds with five occupants. One of the two seized died next day, the other recovered in a week, having had severe spasms and a degree of collapse. Cases appeared almost at the same time in various parts of the building, most of them in scattered individuals, but in one instance in as many as five together in a garret holding twenty-two. From the 22nd February to the 9th of March there were 64 attacks of cholera in this pauper institution[1]. Besides the five deaths in the Sunderland Workhouse, this was the first of many instances of the remarkable invasion of such institutions.

Until July the infection had been limited in Glasgow to certain of the lowest localities, and even in these it had declined almost to extinction in the last week of May. As the summer advanced it increased somewhat again, and in the first days of August it took a sudden start, reaching a maximum of 181 attacks in one day, and 817 in a week. It was no longer confined to the poorest districts, but became diffused all over Glasgow, so that "there was scarcely a street where one or more cases did not occur." From this enormous prevalence in August, it declined again in September, but once more took a start in the last few days of that month and in the first week or two of October. The last outburst was ascribed to the effects of the Glasgow public holiday on 28 September, to celebrate the passing of the Reform Bill for Scotland, but the course of the epidemic clearly followed the season, being precisely parallel in Edinburgh, in Dumfries and in the coast towns of Fife. From

[1] W. Auchincloss, M.D., "Report of the Epidemic Cholera as it appeared in the Town's Hospital of Glasgow in February and March, 1832," *Glas. Med. Journ.* v. 113.

the middle of October, the disease declined rapidly and was extinct before the middle of November. The following table shows week by week the number of new cases reported daily to the Board of Health, and the deaths in each week [1].

Cholera in Glasgow, 1832 (*population* 202,426).

Week ending	New cases	Deaths	Week ending	New cases	Deaths	Week ending	New cases	Deaths
Feb. 19	62	21	May 20	41	31	Aug. 19	483	228
26	113	46	27	21	11	26	419	178
Mar. 4	68	39	June 3	6	7	Sept. 2	231	122
11	85	60	10	45	17	9	117	50
18	94	50	17	72	39	16	60	31
25	150	61	24	168	70	23	84	33
April 1	138	74	July 1	127	72	30	165	90
8	112	57	8	131	62	Oct. 7	310	140
15	99	50	15	143	68	14	173	95
22	120	60	22	229	101	21	95	58
29	71	40	29	218	113	28	47	29
May 6	71	39	Aug. 5	817	356	Nov. 4	41	18
13	73	39	12	699	339	11	10	11
						Total	6208	3005

The effect of the epidemic upon the general mortality of Glasgow is shown in the table of deaths from all causes and from cholera month by month, compiled from the burial registers, which make the cholera deaths 161 more than the returns to the Board of Health.

Glasgow Mortality in 1832.

	All deaths	Cholera deaths		All deaths	Cholera deaths
Jan.	824	—	July	990	441
Feb.	874	87	Aug.	1755	1222
March	955	264	Sept.	749	243
April	816	229	Oct.	755	334
May	677	125	Nov.	529	25
June	783	196	Dec.	571	—
				10,278	3166

While the cholera lasted (12 Feb.–11 Nov.) the burials from all other or ordinary causes were 4958; in the corresponding nine months of 1831 they were 4862, having been excessive in that year owing to fever. The baptisms from 15 December, 1831, to 14 December, 1832, were 3388; so that the cholera alone destroyed nearly as many lives, chiefly adult, as there were children born in the year.

[1] James Cleland, LL.D., and James Corkindale, M.D., *Edin. Med. Surg. Journ.* XXXIX. 503.

Upwards of a thousand of the cases were treated at the Albion Street Hospital, under the direction of Dr Lawrie, who had had a large experience of cholera in India. His statistics are as follows[1]:

Albion Street Cholera Hospital, Glasgow, Feb.—Sept. 1832.

Males		Females		Both sexes		Percentages
Cases	Deaths	Cases	Deaths	Cases	Deaths	of deaths
370	251	662	419	1032	670	64·9

Ages	Cases	Deaths	Percentage of deaths
0—7	43	25	58·1
7—20	93	47	50·5
20—30	231	112	48·8
30—40	211	137	64·9
40—50	204	136	66·1
50—60	116	95	81·0
Over 60	134	120	89·5

Monthly Cases and Deaths.

	Cases	Deaths	Percentages of deaths
Feb.	40	33	82·5
March	97	69	71·1
April	122	81	66·3
May	56	40	71·4
June	126	94	74·5
July	240	143	59·5
Aug.	273	176	64·4
Sept.	64	33	51·5

The noteworthy points are: first, the great excess of women admitted, which was observed also at Edinburgh; secondly, the higher rate of fatality at the two extremes of life, which is the rule in some other infections; and thirdly, the lower ratio of deaths to cases during the height of the epidemic in the end of summer, which is explained, as Craigie remarked for Edinburgh, simply by the fact that the infection was no longer in the worst localities, but was attacking "a greater number of persons, and consequently much better constitutions."

The Glasgow cholera of 1832 was far more destructive than that of Edinburgh per head of the population, according to the following:

	Glasgow	Edinburgh
Population	202,426	136,301
Attacks of Cholera	6208	1886
Deaths by Cholera	3005	1065

---

[1] J. Adair Lawrie, M.D., "Report of the Albion Street Cholera Hospital." *Glas. Med. Journ.* v. 309, 416.

The fluctuations of the epidemic in the two cities were closely parallel. In Edinburgh from the middle of February to the middle of June the new cases usually ranged from five to ten or fifteen a day, with an occasional excess, as on the 29th of April when there were twenty-six persons seized. As in Glasgow, there was a marked lull in the end of May and beginning of June, after which the seizures became more common and remained somewhat steady to the end of July, some days having as many as twenty attacks. The largest number in one day in August was nineteen, the September maximum sixteen (on the 28th). Edinburgh thus missed the enormous outburst that Glasgow had in August, while the September experiences were much the same in the two cities. The first week of October, which was the time of a second maximum in Glasgow (far below that of August), was the worst time of the whole epidemic in Edinburgh, the cases coming from all parts of the city, as in Glasgow they had done in August.

Successive days of most extensive Cholera in Edinburgh, 1832.

		New cases			New cases
Oct.	1	22	Oct.	6	30
	2	23		7	27
	3	44		8	18
	4	45		9	13
	5	23		10	26

This gives 214 cases in the week ending 7th October, as compared with Glasgow's 310 in the same week.

At the Castle Hill Cholera Hospital, 318 were admitted and 187 died. The ages, with the rates of fatality at each age-period, agree closely with those already given for the chief hospital in Glasgow. The smaller ratio of hospital fatality in the second half of the epidemic was perhaps more marked in Edinburgh: 119 cases, with 85 deaths, from the opening of the hospital to 5 July; 199 cases, with 97 deaths, from 5 July to the closing of the hospital. That larger proportion of recoveries may have been due in part, Craigie thinks, to better methods of treatment; but, in his opinion, it was mainly owing to the greater number of strong constitutions among those attacked over a wider area of the city.

Beyond the statistics and other particulars for Glasgow and Edinburgh, and the minute accounts of the first outbreaks in the beginning of the year, there is little exactly recorded of the cholera of 1832 in the rest of Scotland; but the following table, compiled according to counties from the alphabetical list of the London Board of Health, will serve to show the epidemic in outline.

Deaths by Asiatic Cholera in Scotland, 1832.

Counties	Deaths	No. of places attacked	Places with highest mortalities in each county
Caithness	96	iii	Wick 69, Thurso 26, Latheron 1
Sutherland	—	—	
Ross and Cromarty	102	vii	Tain 55, Dingwall 17, Avoch 12, Cromarty 11, Several villages no return
Inverness-shire	191	iii	Inverness 177
Nairnshire	5	i	Nairn 5
Moray	—	—	
Banffshire	15	i	Rathven (Buckie) 15
Aberdeenshire	108	ii	Aberdeen and Footdee 99, Collieston 9
Kincardine	—	—	
Forfarshire	552	iv	Dundee 512, Cupar Angus 17, Arbroath 13, Liff and Benvie 10
Perthshire	81	v	Perth 66, Auchterarder 7, Kenmore 4, Tulliallan 3
Fife and Kinross	301	xii	Cupar and district 108, Kirkaldy and Dunnikier 104, Dysart 39, Wester Wemyss 17, Kinghorn 15, Burntisland 13, Anstruther 10, Leven 14, St Andrews 5
East Lothian	213	vii	Tranent 78, Haddington 65, Dunbar etc. 38, Prestonpans 28
Berwickshire	41		Coldstream 41
Midlothian	1780	xiii	Edinburgh 1065, Suburbs of, 146, Leith 267, Musselburgh and Fisherrow 202, Newhaven 52, Portobello 33
Linlithgowshire	—	—	
Clackmannanshire	75	i	Clackmannan 75
Stirlingshire	247	x	Alloa 72, Stirling 35, Falkirk 36, Larbert 31, Balfron 28, St Ninian's 15, Bothkenner 10, Carriden 13, Grangemouth 8
Lanarkshire	3575	xii	Glasgow 3005, Pollokshaws 143, Govan 77, Old Monkland 125, Rutherglen 65
Renfrewshire	1001	xi	Paisley 444, Greenock 436, Port Glasgow 69
Dumbartonshire	86	iii	Dumbarton 67, Bonhill 13, Helensburgh 6
Bute	14	i	Rothesay 14
Argyle	35	ii	Inverary 25, Campbelltown 10
Ayrshire	466	x	Kilmarnock 205, Ayr 190, Dalry 22, Irvine 19
Kirkcudbrightshire	133	iv	Troqueer (Maxwelltown) 125, Kirkcudbright 3
Dumfriesshire	441	v	Dumfries 418, Caerlaverock 15
Roxburghshire	34	i	Hawick 34 (second outbreak only).

Near Glasgow numerous centres of cholera were established, among which Paisley, Greenock and Dumbarton suffered heavily during the same space as Glasgow, from February to November. Rothesay, Campbelltown and Inverary had epidemics in spring or early summer. In June and July the infection was carried effectually into Ayrshire (an earlier importation to Doura, near Kilwinning, in March, having proved abortive) and caused great mortalities at Kilmarnock[1] and Ayr[2], as well as much alarm and a good many deaths at Dalry, Irvine and Loudoun.   In the latter half of September a most disastrous outbreak began in Dumfries and in the neighbouring Maxwelltown[3].

The epidemic in Leith and Newhaven proceeded at the same time as in Edinburgh.   Another important centre was the midland coal-field of Stirlingshire and Lanarkshire, where the mortality was mostly autumnal.   Perth had been reached early in March, Dundee at the end of April, the latter having a visitation on the same scale as Glasgow, Edinburgh, Paisley and Greenock. From Dundee, Cupar Fife was infected about the middle of August, and had a severe epidemic almost confined to paupers[4]. In the autumn there was much cholera among the fishing population from Thurso to Dunbar and Berwick.   Inverness had been infected early in May, and was probably the centre from which the disease spread in the end of summer, during the herring fishery, to the coast towns and fishing villages, as well as to Tain and Dingwall.   Only a few of these places made returns to the Board of Health; but it is probable from what Hugh Miller relates of the villages near Cromarty that the disease had been more widely spread.   That author has described the condition of things in his native town.   Its landlocked bay had been made a quarantine station, and was full of shipping flying the yellow flag.   Cholera had "more than decimated" the villages of Portmahomak and Inver, and was prevalent in the parishes of Nigg and Urquhart, with the towns of Inverness, Nairn, Avoch, Dingwall and Rosemarkie.   The numerous dead at Inver were buried in the sand, infected cottages had been burned down, the infected hamlets of Hilton and Balintore had been shut off from the neighbouring country by a cordon[5].   The citizens of Cromarty, hitherto untouched, followed the advice of Miller at a public meeting and took the law into their own hands, guarding all the approaches to their peninsula and subjecting

---

[1] *Month. Journ. Med. Sc.* March, 1850, p. 302.
[2] Wood, *Glas. Med. Journ.* VI. 1833.
[3] Grieve, *Month. Journ. Med. Sc.* IX. 1849, p. 777.
[4] Scott, *Edin. Med. and Surg. Journ.* XXXIX. 276.   For a whole month it was confined to one suburb.   All the earlier cases were without exception fatal.   There were 130 cases and 65 deaths.
[5] It is probably to Portmahomak or Inver that Howison refers in the following (*Lancet*, 10 Nov. 1832, p. 203): Cholera broke out in a small village several miles from Tain, and in a few days it carried off 41 out of a population of 120 to 140. Coffins could not be made fast enough.   Many were buried in sailcloth.   The people fled from their houses to the fields.

all arrivals to fumigation with sulphur and to some undescribed application of chloride of lime. The infection, however, got in by an unguarded channel. A Cromarty fisherman had died of cholera at Wick; his clothes had been ordered to be burned, but a brother of the dead man, who was in Wick at the time, secured some of them and brought them home. He kept them in his chest for a month before he ventured to open it. Next day he was seized with cholera and died in two days. Thereafter the disease crept about the streets and lanes for weeks, striking down both the hale and the worn-out. Pitch and tar were kept burning during the night at the openings of the infected lanes; the clothes of the dead were burned; many of the fishers left their cottages and lived in the caves on the hill until the danger was past[1].

Among the numerous fishing villages of the Moray Firth, Buckie is the only one given as severely touched by the infection (fifteen deaths). Only one small village of the Aberdeenshire coast, Collieston, is known to have had cholera (nine deaths)[2]. The Aberdeen epidemic was not severe, and appears to have been mostly in the fishers' quarter. The Montrose district escaped altogether in 1832; but in June, 1833, the true Asiatic cholera broke out in the fishing villages of Ferryden and Boddin, on the opposite shore of the South Esk from Montrose. Arbroath had a few deaths in August, 1832, while several of the small towns on the coast of Fife had from that time to the end of the year visitations which were only less alarming than those on the south side of the Firth of Forth at the beginning of the year. To sum up the epidemic in Scotland, it caused nearly ten thousand deaths, of which Glasgow and its suburbs had about one-third, Edinburgh, Leith, Dundee, Greenock, Paisley and Dumfries, another third, while a large part of the remainder occurred among the mining and fishing populations[3].

---

[1] Hugh Miller, *My Schools and Schoolmasters*, Chap. XXII.

[2] The good account by Paterson, "Observations on Cholera as it appeared at Collieston and Footdee," *Edin. Med. and Surg. Journ.* XLIX. (1838), p. 408, shows how much panic a mortality of nine stood for.

[3] Sir J. Y. Simpson gave to Dr Graves of Dublin a list of some places in Scotland where cholera had appeared, which contains the additional names of Helmsdale (23 July), Fort William (24 Sept.), Fort George (7 May), Islay (23 Oct.), Portpatrick (7 Aug.), Crieff (2 Oct.), and Kelso (29 Oct.).

The Cholera of 1832 in Ireland.

The forecast of Orton in the summer of 1831, that Ireland
would be the chosen soil of the Asiatic pestilence owing to the
state of misery, at that time, of the mass of its people, was
realized in a measure.   But the cholera in Ireland, as elsewhere
in Europe, showed itself chiefly as an urban disease, falling
disastrously upon the poorest quarters of Dublin, Limerick,
Cork, Galway, Sligo, Drogheda and other towns, but by no
means seriously upon the immense population who occupied
the country cabins.   Scotland, indeed, had a higher ratio of
cholera deaths than Ireland per head of the population; whereas
Dublin had nearly twice as many deaths as Glasgow, their
populations being almost exactly equal (about 200,000), and
Cork had nearly the same number as Liverpool.   The following
table gives the comparison of the three divisions of the United
Kingdom, including the cholera deaths of 1831 in England, but
not those of 1833, which were more numerous in Ireland than
elsewhere.

	Population in 1831	Cholera deaths
England and Wales	13,897,187	21,882
Ireland	7,784,539	20,070
Scotland	2,365,114	9592

The first undoubted case of Asiatic cholera was found in
Dublin on 22 March, 1832.   On the 25th of that month, Harty,
who was physician to all the Dublin prisons, notified to the
Board of Health cases in the Richmond Bridewell which he
believed to be true spasmodic or malignant cholera[1].   It was
reported from Cork on the 12th of April, from Belfast on the
14th, Tralee on the 28th, Galway on the 12th of May, Limerick
on the 14th, Tuam the 4th of June, Waterford the 1st of July,
but not until 21 August from Wexford and about the same
time from Londonderry.   Doubtless remoteness from the ordinary routes of vagrants was the reason why the infection was
later in some places, such as Wexford.   The old Liberties of
Dublin, which harboured crowds of beggars in dilapidated
tenement-houses, became a focus of virulent infection.   As the
summer advanced whole families in some of the most wretched
lanes were cut off; news from Dublin on 29 June says that the
pestilence was worst in Sycamore Alley, in a single house of

[1] *Dubl. Journ. Med. Sc.* III. 74.

which twenty persons had died in the course of four or five days[1]. Certain streets sent fifty patients to the Cholera Hospital for one sent by other streets that were seemingly no better off[2]. The great hospital in Grange Gorman Lane, capable of holding 700 and sometimes occupied by 500, would on some nights or early mornings (from midnight to 7 a.m.) receive forty or fifty new cases, and within a week would be having at the same hours only two applications. During four successive days it admitted a total of 285 cases, during the next four days 497 cases, and during four days a fortnight later only 134 cases. The worst time was from the 10th to the 14th of July, when 615 were admitted. A day or two of rain seemed always to send up the number of cases carried to the hospital[3]. Until the beginning of June hardly anyone under fifteen was attacked; but in July the attacks of children were about one in thirteen or fourteen of adults, a case of pure cholera having been observed in an infant three weeks old. As at Glasgow and Edinburgh, more women than men were taken to the hospital (138·17 females to 100 males)[4].

As the infection spread in Dublin during the early summer a panic arose in the city, and alarm over the whole province of Leinster. Runners, as in the old times of the torch of war, were to be seen hurrying everywhere through the neighbouring counties carrying a smouldering peat, of which they left a small portion at every cabin in their direct line, with a sacred obligation upon the inmates to carry the charm to seven other houses, and the following exhortation: "The plague has broken out; take this, and while it burns offer up seven paters, three aves, and a credo in the name of God and the holy St John that the plague may be stopped"! Men, women and children scoured the country with the charmed turf in every direction, "each endeavouring to be foremost in finding unserved houses." One man in the Bog of Allen had to run thirty miles before he had discharged the obligation laid upon him[5]. It does not appear, however, that the infection was at all general among the

---

[1] *Times*, 1 July, 1832.

[2] Simon McCoy, "Notes on Malignant Cholera as it appeared in Dublin," *Dub. Journ. Med. Sc.* II. 357, and III. 1.

[3] Compare Grimshaw's observations on the admissions for fever to the Cork Street Hospital in the summer of 1864, *supra*, p. 298.

[4] Wilde, *Census of Ireland* 1841. Table of Deaths, p. xxi.

[5] *Gent. Magaz.* 1832, June, p. 555; *Annual Register*, 1832, Chronicle (June), p. 71.

scattered cabins, hamlets or even considerable villages. In the rural parts of Wicklow there were only eight deaths from it, in Fermanagh four, in county Derry three, in Armagh thirteen, in Carlow none until the next year. In Clare the deaths in country districts were more than twice as many as in Ennis and other towns of the county. In Sligo county, again, there were only 62 deaths among the peasantry to 698 in the towns, nearly the whole of the latter total belonging to the county town and seaport. The epidemic in Sligo town was one of the worst in Ireland. It was reported that forty or fifty were buried in one day in a trench, one-half of them without coffins but wrapped in tarred sailcloth. It is said, also, that seven of the medical men died of cholera in the course of three months [1]. Thousands of the population, which numbered about 14,000, fled from the town, the wealthier paying large sums for a room or two in a country cottage, the poorer living in tents or sleeping under the hedges. In August the guard of the mail coach which ran from Sligo by way of Strabane to Londonderry was taken with cholera on the road and died at the latter town, no case having occurred in Londonderry up to that time [2].

The outbreak at Drogheda was as sudden and disastrous as at Sligo. At Belfast also the disease began with enormous fatality, but, according to the table, the deaths eventually were few in proportion to the attacks. The other towns which had highest mortalities were Cork, Limerick, Galway and Kilkenny —all seaports except the last. In Waterford the great outbreak was delayed until 1833.

Many of the counties had more deaths among the peasantry in 1833 than in 1832, Limerick county in particular. The following instance is related of a small hamlet about a mile to the south-east of Armagh:

The hamlet consisted of five or six dwellings on both sides of the road. On the 19th July, 1833, a man in delicate health, who had received a jar of sea-water two days before, and had drunk three or four pints of it, was seized with cramps, and blueness and collapse, after the purging induced by the sea-water; he died on the 20th and was buried on the 21st. His brother, who lived next door under the same roof, was seized with cholera on the evening of the 21st, having attended the funeral, and died comatose after five or six days' illness. A man who lived across the road, and had also been

[1] Graves, *Dubl. Quart. Journ. Med. Sc.* Feb. 1849, p. 31, from information by Dr Little of Sligo.
[2] W. Howison, M.D., of Edinburgh, *Lancet*, 10 Nov. 1832, p. 203. He was at Londonderry in August, and had probably heard the reports of the Sligo cholera there.

at the funeral of No. 1, was seized with cholera the same evening (21st), and died in forty-eight hours. On the night of his burial his son aged thirteen and a married daughter who lived in the house were seized, the boy dying the same night "very black," and the daughter after a lingering illness of five or six days. The only other attacked was a girl, who recovered under treatment by bleeding &c.[1]

In 1833 the whole number of deaths assigned to cholera in country places was 2,756, while 2,552 deaths were reported from the towns. It appears to be accepted (by Wilde) that true Asiatic cholera lingered in Ireland until 1834, and that it had caused a considerable part of the 4,419 deaths assigned to "cholera" under that year in the Census of 1841. There is one reference to undoubted cases of the Asiatic type in 1834 in Ross, Nenagh and other places in the same district[2].

Assuming that all the deaths so called in the three years 1832, 1833 and 1834 were true Asiatic cholera, that imported infection accounted for 1 in 5·68 deaths from all causes in Munster, 1 in 5·98 in Leinster, 1 in 9·86 in Connaught and 1 in 15·15 in Ulster. The proportion of attacks to fatalities in eight of the principal towns in the following table varies much, Belfast having comparatively few deaths for all its many cases, and Kilkenny three deaths to about five cases: these differences must have depended upon the number of cases of "cholerine" or diarrhoea which attended the true "spasmodic" or collapse-cholera, and may or may not have been counted in the returns.

Deaths from Asiatic Cholera in Ireland, 1832-33.

	1832		1833		
	Country deaths	Town deaths	Country deaths	Town deaths	No. of places with Cholera
LEINSTER					
Carlow	—	—	64	116	vi
Dublin	460	187	32	17	xxiv
Dublin City	—	5632	—	166	
Kildare	108	72	55	104	xi
Kilkenny	91	14	130	29	ix
Kilkenny City	—	296	—	144	
King's	40	288	10	—	v
Longford	22	63	—	—	iii
Louth	115	189	—	—	viii
Meath	61	105	81	113	vii
Drogheda Town	—	491	—	—	
Queen's	17	111	16	—	iv
Westmeath	18	121	84	5	iv
Wexford	126	362	24	150	v
Wicklow	8	40	—	23	iv

[1] John Colvan, M.D., *Dubl. Journ. Med. Sc.* IV. 186. These five deaths in Armagh County in 1833 do not appear in the table.

[2] Graves, u.s. 1849, VII. 246.

	1832		1833		No. of places with Cholera
	Country deaths	Town deaths	Country deaths	Town deaths	
MUNSTER					
Clare	453	281	166	8	xiii
Cork	325	1028	466	240	xxxv
Cork City	—	1385	—	234	
Kerry	87	440	109	181	viii
Limerick	82	4	668	173	xvi
Limerick City	—	1105	—	—	
Tipperary	198	910	224	208	xii
Waterford	52	52	48	79	ix
Waterford City	—	24	—	245	
ULSTER					
Antrim	70	66	—	75	v
Belfast Town	—	418	—	—	
Armagh	13	57	2	—	vi
Cavan	21	11	70	51	vi
Donegal	37	139	141	—	vii
Down	110	423	65	37	xiv
Fermanagh	4	50	—	9	iv
Londonderry	3	222	—	—	iv
Monaghan	64	50	13	43	iv
Tyrone	100	193	17	9	ix
CONNAUGHT					
Galway	141	430	82	—	xii
Galway Town	—	596	—	—	
Leitrim	1	—	101	—	vi
Mayo	151	325	12	68	xi
Roscommon	47	105	38	25	vii
Sligo	62	698	25	—	iv

The Cholera of 1832 in England.

The certainty that Asiatic cholera was at Sunderland in November and at Newcastle in December, 1831, led to quarantine of ships arriving in the Thames from the Wear and the Tyne. The early numbers of the 'Cholera Gazette' published lists of vessels from these northern coal ports detained at Stangate Creek on the Medway[1]. At length about the middle of February, 1832, three suspicious cases occurred together in Rotherhithe, one of them being of a man who had been scraping the bottom of a Sunderland vessel. Other cases came close upon these in the parishes on both sides of the Thames from Rotherhithe and Limehouse to Lambeth and Chelsea, especially in the Southwark parishes.

[1] Roupell, *Croomian Lectures on Cholera*, Lond. 1833, p. 33, gives the suspicious case of a man named Webster, who sailed from Sunderland on 20 Jan. and arrived in the Thames about the 30th. "The vessel immediately obtained *pratique*; but a few days after, this man was seized with extreme pain in the epigastrium" &c. and died suddenly after symptoms in part those of cholera. Postmortem, 20 oz. of blood were found in the peritoneum, and some blood in the lower part of the bowel.

The diagnosis of Asiatic cholera was vehemently contested for several weeks by a section of the profession, who frequented the Westminster Medical Society and had for their organ the 'London Medical and Surgical Journal.' The slow progres of the disease at first, and the apparent extinction of it for a week or two at the end of May (as at Glasgow and elsewhere in Scotland in the same weeks) encouraged these doubts, although the 994 fatalities in 1848 cases from 14 February to 15 May were quite unlike any experience of cholera nostras. After the river-side parishes, cases were reported most from other crowded parts, such as St Giles's in the Fields. From the middle of June the infection became more severe and widely spread, still making the river-side parishes its chief seat, but extending beyond Southwark on one side, and on the north side to such localities as Fetter Lane, Field Lane and parts of the City. From the 15th of June to the 31st October the cases in London were 9142 and the deaths 4266 ; in November and December only thirty more cases were known, of which one half were fatal. The total for the year in London came to 11,020 cases with 5275 deaths. This was admitted to have been for Asiatic cholera a slight and partial visitation of the metropolis. London with a population of a million and a half had actually fewer deaths than Dublin with its two hundred thousand inhabitants. Paris had more cholera deaths in one week of April (5523 deaths, April 8—14) than London had in all the year.

The Asiatic Cholera of 1831–32 *in England.*

	Deaths	No. of places attacked	Places with highest mortalities in each county
London	5275		
Surrey, part of	—	—	
Kent	135	xi	Minster (Sheerness) 38
Sussex	—	—	
Hampshire	91	ii	Portsmouth 86, *Southampton no return*
Berkshire	52	iv	Wantage 27
Middlesex, part of	62	iv	Uxbridge 34, Edmonton 11
Buckinghamshire	105	iv	Aylesbury 60, Olney 22
Oxfordshire	219	xii	Oxford 86, Bicester 64
Northamptonshire	—	—	
Huntingdonshire	45	iii	Fenstanton 21, Ramsey 20, St Ives 4
Bedfordshire	40	ii	Bedford 36
Cambridgeshire	208	iv	Whittlesea 97, Ely 61, Wisbech 41
Essex	38	iv	Barking 18, Chelmsford 10
Suffolk	1	i	Woodbridge 1
Norfolk	232	vi	Norwich 129, Lynn 49, Denver 27, *Yarmouth no return*

	Deaths	No. of places attacked	Places with highest mortalities in each county
Wiltshire	14	ii	Chippenham 9, Farley 5, *Salisbury no return*
Dorset	19	ii	Bridport 16, Charmouth 3
Devon	1901	xxvii	Plymouth 702, Devonport 228, East Stonehouse 133, Exeter 386
Cornwall	308	xi	St Paul 81, Penzance 64
Somerset	142	v	Paulton 66, Bath 49, Tiverton 23
Gloucestershire	932	viii	Bristol 630, Clifton 64, Gloucester 123, Tewkesbury 76, Upton 34
Herefordshire	—	—	
Shropshire	158	vii	Shrewsbury 75, Oldbury 37, Madeley 27
Staffordshire	1870	xiv	Bilston 693, Tipton 281, Sedgley 231, Wolverhampton 193, King's Winsford 83, Wednesbury 78, Walsall 77, Newcastle-u.-Lyme 60, W. Bromwich 59, Darlaston 57, Stoke 46
Worcestershire	579	xi	Dudley 77, Worcester 79, Kidderminster 67, Droitwich 63, Redditch 38
Warwickshire	188	xii	Nuneaton 56, Coleshill 32, Birmingham 21
Leicestershire	5	i	Castle Donington 5
Rutland	—	—	
Lincolnshire	80	viii	Gainsborough 41, Owston 17
Nottinghamshire	352	vii	Nottingham and suburbs 322, Newark 25
Derbyshire	16	i	Derby 16
Cheshire	111	vi	Northwich 30, Stockport 29, Runcorn 18, Nantwich 14, Chester 14, Brimmington 6
Lancashire	2835	xiv	Liverpool 1523, Manchester 706, Salford 216, Warrington 168, Lancaster 114, Wigan 30
West Riding, York	1416	xxvii	Leeds 702, Sheffield 402, Hull 300, York 185,
East Riding, York	507	iiii	Wakefield 62, Rotherham 34, Selby 32,
North Riding, York	47	ii	Goole 36, Bradford 30, Whitby 27, Doncaster 26
Durham	850	viii	Sunderland 215, Gateshead 148, S. Shields 147, Stockton 126, Jarrow and Hebburn 70, Hetton &c. 97
Northumberland	1394	xiv	Newcastle 801, Villages near 259, N. Shields &c. 98, Berwick 84, Tweedmouth 72, Blyth 42
Cumberland	702	vii	Carlisle 265, Whitehaven 244, Workington 119, Maryport 42, Cockermouth 25, Allonby 4
Westmoreland	68	i	Kendal 68
Monmouth	15	ii	Newport 13, Abergavenny 2
South Wales	343	vii	Merthyr Tydvil 160, Swansea 152, Haverfordwest 16
North Wales	140	viii	Denbigh 47, Carnarvon 30, Flint 18, Newtown 17
Isle of Man	146	i	Douglas 146

It will appear from the annexed table (here compiled according to counties for the first time) that the cholera of 1832 visited most parts of England. The dates of outbreak at each place (omitted in the table) show that its great seasons everywhere, except at Sunderland, Newcastle and Musselburgh, were the summer and autumn. New centres or foci of infection were made in all directions, and in a good many small places there were epidemics which produced much alarm although the figures look insignificant in the statistical table. Some counties, such as Leicestershire, Herefordshire, Derbyshire, Northamptonshire,

Lincolnshire, Suffolk, Sussex, Dorset, Wiltshire, and several of the Welsh counties, escaped with a few cases at perhaps one village or town. Some towns, such as Birmingham, Cheltenham, Cambridge and Hereford, had only a few cases (or none) in 1832 as in the later epidemics in England. Most of the towns which now head the list of high death-rates by common summer diarrhoea, chiefly infantile (as in the preceding chapter), had only a few imported cases but no real epidemic extension; these were Preston, Blackburn, Bury, Rochdale, Oldham, Bolton, Halifax, Leicester and Coventry; while Bradford, Stockport and Wigan had comparatively few. The greater epidemics, besides those which started the disease at Sunderland and Newcastle, were, in order of time, at Hull and Goole, Liverpool, Manchester, Warrington, Leeds, Sheffield, Nottingham, Bristol, Plymouth, with Devonport and Stonehouse, Southampton, Portsmouth, Exeter, Salisbury, various towns of the Black Country in South Staffordshire, Dudley, Merthyr Tydvil, Carlisle, Whitehaven, with other ports of the Cumberland coal-fields, and Douglas in the Isle of Man. Devonshire, Cornwall, the West Riding of Yorkshire, Worcestershire and Warwickshire had each a large number of minor centres, besides the greater foci at Plymouth and Exeter, and at Leeds and Sheffield. The severity of the disease in some parts of England called forth a few special accounts, from which certain representative details may be taken.

The most disastrous outbreak in all England was at Bilston, in the centre of the Black Country, near Wolverhampton[1]. The first cases in that part of England were at Dudley early in June, in some travelling German broom-sellers. In the end of June a canal boatman from Manchester died of cholera in his boat four miles from Wolverhampton; the boat was sunk. In the first week of July another canal boatman died of cholera at Tipton, after returning from Liverpool. The infection became established during July in the parish of Tipton, thickly peopled with miners and iron-workers[2]. At length on the 4th of August a case occurred in the adjoining town of Bilston, about two and a half miles to the south-east of Wolverhampton.

---

[1] The populous parishes of the Black Country around Wolverhampton came under notice in another way in 1832 as a crucial instance in the redistribution of seats by the Reform Act.

[2] T. Ogier Ward, "Cholera in Wolverhampton in Aug.–Oct. 1832," *Trans. Prov. Med. and Surg.* Assoc. II. 368.

Bilston was a town of 14,492 inhabitants, nearly all of the working class. It was irregularly built on high ground, full of forges and surrounded by mines. Its soil was perfectly dry "from the water having been drawn off for the purpose of getting the mines[1]." The streets were for the most part wide and open; many houses stood in courts and back yards, but the town was so irregularly built as not to be densely crowded. The Birmingham and Staffordshire Canal passed through the whole length of the township, and there was one small brook traversing the town. The people usually earned good wages, but trade had been depressed since March, 1832. There was a good deal of drunkenness among them, and a peculiar addiction to the sports for which the Black Country is still celebrated, including at that time bull-baiting. The public health was in general good, the deaths having been 23 in May, 31 in June, and 25 in July. The churchyard of the original chapel was full; a new chapel had been built, and a burial-ground consecrated, in 1831. Bilston wake had been held on 29th July, 1832, with the usual orgies notwithstanding the depression of trade. On the night of Friday the 3rd of August a married woman in Temple Street, occupying a poor and filthy house, who had supped heartily on pig's fry and had drunk freely of small beer, was seized with purging, which turned to fatal spasmodic cholera. Within an hour medical aid was sought for two more cases of the same in poor and filthy houses in Bridge Street and Hall Street, about four hundred yards from each other and from the house in Temple Street. At the back of the latter was a most offensive pigsty, and beyond the pigsty a poor cottage in which lived a widow and four children; cholera attacked them, two of the children dying on the 6th August and another on the 7th. The night of the 9th of August was most oppressively hot. In the week ending the 10th August there had been 150 cases and 36 deaths from cholera. On the 10th the disease appeared in a new quarter to the west, called Wynn's Fold; the 12th was again an oppressively hot day, followed by rain over-night. On the 14th the disease began its ravages in Etlingshall Lane, at the western end of the township, a mile from the scene of the first outbreak. The attacks in the week ending 17 August had risen to 616 and the deaths to 133. On the 16th it was remarked that the flies had disappeared and the swallows with them; both came back together when the epidemic was declining. Whole families were now being cut off, father, mother and perhaps three children. Mr Leigh, the curate of the parish, went on the 18th to Birmingham to secure a supply of coffins and medical aid, the medical men of the town being worn out (two of them died a few days after). The deaths between the 19th and 26th of August numbered 309. On the latter date a dispensary was opened, after which the proportion of fatalities to attacks became less. On the 18th of September, the last death occurred, and the epidemic was over, having attacked 3568 in a population of 14,492, and destroyed 742, of whom 594 were over ten years of age. The following is the complete bill:

Cholera at Bilston, 1832.

Week ending		Attacks	Deaths	Deaths under ten years
Aug.	10	150	36	5
	17	616	133	23
	24	924	298	58
	31	832	184	34
Sept.	7	694	62	18
	14	250	23	6
	21	102	6	4
		3568	742	148

[1] Rev. W. Leigh, *An authentic narrative of the awful visitation of Bilston by Cholera in Aug.–Sept.* 1832. Wolverhampton, 1833.

No fewer than 450 Bilston children under the age of twelve were left orphans by the cholera ; for them a national subscription was made to the amount of £8536. 8s. 7d., and applied to the building and support of a Cholera Orphan School, which was opened on the 3rd of August, 1833, the first anniversary of the outbreak of cholera in the town.

In the adjoining parish of Sedgley, although the deaths were only 290 in a larger population (20,577), the infection was as severe in certain places. "Sometimes a whole hamlet seemed to be smitten all at once, so that, in some of the streets, or rather rows of tenements, there was scarcely a house without one sick, or dying, or dead." At Tipton, in one family of 14 no fewer than 12 died ; and in eight different tenements every inhabitant was swept off. At Dudley one had a narrow escape of being buried alive. In twelve parishes or townships, with a population of 160,000, cholera attacked about 10,000 and cut off about 2000. The effects of the pestilence were all the more terrible from its swiftness, for in each parish it was in full vigour not above a month. The population of miners and iron-workers, a rough set addicted to brutal sports and to drunkenness, could not believe that brandy was not a specific, and made it circulate at funerals to fortify against infection. A reformation of morals and revival of religion is said to have followed the scourge[1]. The following is the list of chief centres in the Black Country :

	Cholera deaths		Cholera deaths
Bilston	693	Wednesbury	78
Tipton	281	Walsall	77
Sedgley	231	Newcastle-under-Lyme	60
Dudley	277	West Bromwich	59
Wolverhampton	193	Darlaston	57
King's Winford	83	Stoke-on-Trent	46

Wolverhampton, which was one of the chief Staffordshire centres of the next cholera in 1849, got off somewhat easily in 1832 with 576 attacks (193 deaths), or one in forty of the population.

It was most common and fatal in a lane called Caribee Island, a narrow filthy cul-de-sac with an open stagnant ditch down the middle, inhabited chiefly by poor Irish. The influence of ground soaked with sewage was shown also in the frequency of cases of cholera among persons in easy circumstances in the residential locality of Darlington Street—"a wide airy street consisting of two rows of houses at its upper end, nearest the centre of the town, but of only one at the lower part, where it is a raised causeway, open on one side to the gardens and meadows beyond. The lower rooms of the houses, being below the level of the street, are consequently very damp ; and within a few yards of the backs of these houses runs a wide ditch, the main sewer of that side of the town, which is dammed up and diverted into several large cesspools, or receptacles for the mud and filth which it deposits. These, in warm weather, emit such offensive exhalations as to be almost intolerable to the persons who live near them....It is singular that this was the only part of the town in which persons in easy circumstances took the disease[2]."

[1] Rev. C. Girdlestone, *Seven Sermons preached during the prevalence of the Cholera in the parish of Sedgley, with a narrative of that visitation.* London, 1833.
[2] T. Ogier Ward, u.s., p. 376.

The cholera had reached Liverpool in the end of April (perhaps from Hull and York), and attacked 4912 in a population of 230,000, causing 1523 deaths before the end of autumn. The very large number of cellar-dwellings and back-to-back houses in the town at that time favoured the infection; but Liverpool was on all subsequent occasions one of the worst centres. Two incidents in 1832 are connected with ships.

On 18 May, 1832, the 'Brutus,' of 384 tons, sailed from Liverpool for Quebec, with a crew of 19, and 330 emigrants who were pauper families from agricultural districts sent to Canada at the cost of their respective poor-law Unions. The emigrants were ill-provided with bedding and clothes, and the ship was under-provisioned. Two days after sailing, or seven days, or nine days (accounts differing), a case of cholera occurred in an adult, who recovered. Other cases quickly followed, with enormous fatality, until the deaths reached 24 in a day. On the 3rd of June the captain put back for Liverpool, his provisions having run short, and his drugs (laudanum) being exhausted. By the time the ship reached Liverpool there had been 117 cases of cholera (of which four were among the crew) and 81 deaths, seven cases remaining at her arrival, of which two ended fatally, making the deaths 83[1].

Another Liverpool incident is noteworthy :

" One morning a mate and one or two men, who had gone to bed the preceding evening in good health on a vessel lying in one of the Liverpool docks, were found suffering from cholera. The men were immediately removed to a hospital and the vessel ordered into the river ; when another vessel, with a healthy crew took its situation in the dock : the next morning all the hands on board the second vessel fell sick of the cholera. Upon examining the dock in this part, a large sewer was found to empty itself immediately under the spot where these vessels had been placed[2]."

One of the ablest accounts of the cholera of 1832 was that by Dr Gaulter, of Manchester. The deaths there were 706, and 216 in Salford ; but it appeared surprising that, being so many and widely spread, they should not have been many more.

An inspection by the local Board of Health two months before the first case appeared " disclosed in the quarters of the poor—a name that might be almost taken [at that time] as a synonym with that of the working classes—such scenes of filth and crowding and dilapidation, such habits of intemperance and low sensuality, and in some districts such unmitigated want and wretchedness," that the picture correctly drawn seemed to many a malicious libel. From that picture, "it was certainly to have been expected that nearly the whole mass of the working population would have been swept away by the disease." There were few good sewers, and it would have required £300,000 to sewer Manchester thoroughly. As it was, the infection

---

[1] James Collins, M.D., *Lond. Med. Gaz.* 30 June, 1832, p. 412; and report by Thompson, surgeon of the ' Brutus,' in the *Cholera Gazette*, s.d.

[2] Henry Gaulter, M.D., *The Origin and Progress of the Malignant Cholera in Manchester*. London, 1833, p. 113.

progressed slowly from the first case on 17th May until the end of July[1]. It was the same in Salford, where it "crept about slowly for three or four weeks attacking solitary individuals or single families in streets and situations the most distant and unconnected, and then suddenly fixing itself in the lower and most populous part of the town." It was in the end of July and beginning of August that the sharp outburst took place in Manchester also. An old soldier well known in the streets as a seller of matches, who "could take a pint of rum without winking," died of cholera in Allen's Court. His body was allowed to lie in the house two days and a half. In four houses of Allen's Court, 17 cases occurred within forty-eight hours, of which 14 were fatal; this court was afterwards known as Cholera Court. In the same few days the infection was most deadly in Back Hart Street, "infamous as a nest of vagabonds and harlots," and in a street behind it, in which nearly the whole of fourteen attacks ended fatally. Blakely Street, a bad fever locality in the time of Ferriar (*supra*, p. 150), had the most malignant kind of cholera in its lodging-houses. It was remarked that few of the factory hands took it: of 1520 employed in Birley and Kirk's mill, only 4 were attacked during the epidemic; more women than men took cholera, and generally those that were employed about dwelling-houses were the victims[2].

The whole cholera bill at Manchester was as follows:

Progress of the Epidemic.

	Attacks		Attacks		Attacks
May	4	August	650	Nov.	33
June	37	Sept.	261	Dec.	2
July	108	Oct.	172	Jan.	2

[1] The first case was of a coach-painter, who had had frequent attacks of painter's colic. Opposite his house was a large stable dunghill in a very foetid state. On the evening of the 16th May he had eaten a heavy supper of lambs' fry, and had been ill thereafter, the symptoms becoming those of Asiatic cholera on the night of the 18th, death ensuing at 2 p.m. 20th.

[2] In the hamlet adjoining a cotton-mill at Hinds, near Bury, consisting of thirty cottages in a row between the mill lade and the canal, wretchedly built, without chimneys, with windows that would not open, the inmates sleeping four or five in a bed, there were 32 cases of cholera with 7 deaths, but none of these were in persons who worked in the mill. Gaulter, u.s. citing Goodlad. He cites also Flint, of Stockport, for the rarity of attacks among the mill workers in that town. See also Samuel Gaskell, "Malignant Cholera in Manchester," *Edin. Med. and Surg. Journ.* XL. 52. The microbic theory, or, as it was then called by Sir Henry Holland and others, the "hypothesis of insect life," was happily thought of by a working cotton-spinner in Manchester to explain the immunity of the mill-workers in 1832. Gaulter (u.s. p. 120) gives in correct English what would probably have been said in the vernacular as follows: "I've been thinkin', Maister," said a spinner to Mr Sowden, a millowner, "as how th' cholery comes o' hinsecks that smo' as we corn'd see 'em, an' they corn'd live i' factories for th' 'eät and th' ile. Me an' my mates wor speakin' o't last neet, an' we o' on us thowt th' saäm thing." Hahnemann, cited by the *Times*, 17 July, 1831, believed that the cholera insect escaped from the eye, and fastened upon the hair, skin, clothes, &c. of other persons. The common microscopic objects uniformly found in the choleraic discharges by later observers have been vibrios, of which half-a-dozen, or perhaps a dozen, varieties have been distinguished. One of these was somewhat audaciously named the "cholera germ" or "comma bacillus of cholera" by Dr R. Koch, who went to Calcutta in 1884. All vibrios, which have a corkscrew form when in motion, are apt to assume the comma form when at rest.

Ages of the patients.

	Attacks	Deaths		Attacks	Deaths
1—15	199	101	45—55	197	116
15—25	153	53	55—65	120	85
25—35	264	98	65—80	85	68
35—45	192	93 p			

Three cholera hospitals were provided in Manchester, at which about one-half of all the cases were received:

	Cases	Deaths
Swan Street Hospital	443	234
Knott Mill Hospital	242	122
Chorlton on Medlock Hospital	29	17
At their homes	697	335

In Salford all the patients were treated at their homes— 644 with 197 deaths; there were also 60 cases among the prisoners in the New Bailey, with 19 deaths.

The Swan Street Hospital was the occasion of a remarkable cholera riot on the 2nd of September. A mob numbering several thousand persons filled the streets near the hospital; in the thick of it was carried a small coffin, from which the headless trunk of a child was taken at intervals and shown to the crowd. The child had died of cholera in the hospital and the body had been examined *post mortem*. Some rumours of this had gone abroad, the body was exhumed, and was found unaccountably mangled. This was the time when intense feeling had been roused all over the country by the procuring of bodies for anatomical dissection, the prejudice extending to the ordinary pathological inspection also. At Sunderland the holding of two or three necropsies had turned the people against the Cholera Hospital. At Dublin there was a rigid rule that no body was to be examined after death in the great cholera hospital of some 700 beds. The body of the child exhumed at Manchester had been found with the head severed, and the rioters declared that it had been murdered. They broke into the hospital, carried off the patients to their homes, and wrecked the furniture and fittings of the wards. The military was at length called out to clear the streets[1].

The epidemic of cholera at Bristol reproduced most of the incidents at other places. There had been numerous suspicious cases of choleraic disease in the early summer, including an outbreak in the gaol in the first week of July.

The first unequivocal cases occurred on the 11th July in a filthy court, in strangers from Bath where there was then no cholera. About the same time the infection showed itself at several places apart, especially in the destitute suburb of St Philip, in the south-east of the city. One of the worst centres was the city Poorhouse, in which 268 cases with 94 deaths occurred from the 24th July to the 20th August. The largest number of seizures on one day was 79 on the 17th August, the largest number of deaths 33 on the 15th. After that it gradually declined, and was over by the middle of November. The attacks reported were 1612, the deaths 626; but these figures came short of the truth, as many cases were not reported, and the burials from all causes were in excess of the average for the season after deducting the reported cholera deaths. Although it fell at Bristol, as elsewhere, upon the

[1] *Times*, Sept. 5, 1832.

poorest quarters and the most abandoned or destitute class, yet it showed caprices among these. Marsh Street, the abode of the lower Irish, and one of the most thickly peopled parts of the city, was the last place visited. Lewin's Mead, a low and crowded quarter, had only a few scattered cases[1].

Little is known of the great epidemic in Plymouth, Devonport, and East Stonehouse, beyond the gross result that it caused 1063 deaths in the town and the two dockyards[2]. Of the outbreak at Southampton not even the figures are known, the only important omission, besides the epidemic at Salisbury, in the whole of the cholera of 1832. On the other hand the Exeter cholera has been related at greater length than any[3].

It was mainly an autumnal outbreak, the largest number of attacks on one day being 89 on the 13th August, and the maximum daily burials 30 a few days before. The total attacks were 1135, the deaths 345 ; they were chiefly in the south-western suburb of the city, among the poorer class, the two St Mary parishes having 3·65 and 3·26 per cent. of their population attacked, the parish of St George 3·41, St John 2·73, and Trinity 1·54, while two whole parishes had no cases.

Somewhat late in the autumn the infection spread through Cornwall. Its general prevalence was also late in the South Wales mining district (insignificant compared with its enormous ravages there in the next cholera of 1849) and in Carlisle, in Whitehaven and the other seaports of Cumberland. Hartlepool, for all its nearness to the original centre of cholera infection in Sunderland, was one of the last places to be infected, in the autumn of 1832[4].

The Central Board of Health made no report upon the cholera of 1832, unless a document sent to the king (William IV.) may have consisted of something more than the alphabetical list of infected places, with dates and numbers, which Sir James

---

[1] John Addington Symonds, "Progress and Causes of Cholera in Bristol, 1832." *Trans. Prov. Med. Surg. Assoc.* III. 170.
[2] Some cases were detailed by Edward Blackman, M.D., *Lond. Med. Gaz.* 1832, pp. 473, 546.
[3] Thomas Shapter, M.D., *The History of the Cholera in Exeter in* 1832. London, 1849, pp. 297.
[4] Besides the papers or books already cited, accounts were published for the following places : Warrington, by Mr Glazebrook, secretary to the Local Board of Health ; Oxford, by Rev. V. Thomas; Hull, by James Alderson, M.D. ; Kendal, by Thomas Proudfoot, M.D. (*Edin. Med. and Surg. J.* XXXIX. 85); various places by J. Y. Simpson, M.D. (*ibid.* XLIX. 358); Tynemouth, by E. H. Greenhow, M.D. (*Trans. Epid. Soc.* 1861); London, by Halma-Grand (*Relation* etc. Paris, 1832), and by Gaselee and Tweedie (Lond. 1832). There are also various minor notices : for Whittlesea (*Lond. Med. Gaz.* I. 1832, p. 448), Hutton, Yorkshire (*ibid.* II. 1832, p. 316), York (*Lancet*, 13 Oct. 1832, p. 72), Cheltenham, showing how it was kept free (*ibid.* Nov. 10, p. 210), St Heliers, Jersey (*Lond. Med. Surg. J.* II. 359), Derby (*ibid.* II. 383).

Clark found some years after in a drawer of the royal library. But some lessons of the epidemic were obvious without the aid of an official report. The late summer and autumn was undoubtedly its chief season—except in places where the poison had, as it were, spent itself in the winter or early spring, such as Sunderland and Musselburgh. A subsidence and seeming extinction of the epidemic in spring and early summer was observed at Glasgow and Edinburgh as well as in London; but it was far otherwise in Paris, where sixteen thousand deaths occurred in the single month of April[1]. As to locality, the infection seemed to prefer low grounds, such as the shore quarters of seaports and the banks of rivers. The town moor of Sunderland, around which the infection found its first habitat in Britain, appeared to be a typical cholera soil—a wet bottom of tenacious clay, almost impassable in winter from the water standing in it, the surface covered with heaps of excremental and other refuse from the crowded lanes near it. But the greatest centre of cholera in England in 1832, the town of Bilston, seemed to be the reverse of this—a rising ground from which the water had been drained away by the numerous mines of coal, iron and limestone all round it. Again, in towns or villages built upon a slope or on heights and hollows, such as Gateshead, Newburn and Collieston (most of all in Quebec on the steep bank of the St Lawrence), the infection did not confine itself to the lower part only. But it was remarked that among the Tyneside villages several on high ground escaped altogether, although within a mile or two of others severely visited. This question of elevation comes up more definitely in the cholera of 1849.

Another obvious thing in the epidemic of 1832 was that many of the first victims were among the destitute, drunken or

---

[1] The daily mortality in Paris at the beginning of the epidemic was as follows (*Annual Register*, 1832, p. 318):

Days	Cholera deaths	Days	Cholera deaths	Days	Cholera deaths
March 27–31	98	April 6	416	April 12	768
April 1	79	7	582	13	816
2	168	8	769	14	692
3	212	9	861	15	567
4	242	10	848	16	572
5	351	11	769		

To the 16th of April the deaths were about 8700; before the end of the month the total was nearly doubled. As the whole cholera mortality of Paris in 1832 was about 19,000, April must have had much the greater part of it.

reckless class.   But there were innumerable exceptions, notably in Paris, where the multitude of victims included several peers, deputies, diplomatic personages and the prime minister.

One of the most striking things in the habits or preferences of cholera in 1832 was the early and unaccountable selection of the inmates of lunatic asylums, the fatuous paupers of workhouses, prisoners, or other immured persons badly housed and ill-fed.   In most of these cases it was a mystery how the poison of cholera had got inside the walls.   The earliest important instance was that of the Town Hospital or pauper infirmary of Glasgow. Other instances were the lunatic wards of Haslar Hospital, Hanwell asylum, Bethnal Green lunatic asylum, Lancaster county asylum, the Manchester New Bailey, situated in Salford, Coldbath Fields Prison, London, Clerkenwell workhouse (65 deaths), Bristol poorhouse (94 deaths).   In the remote Westmoreland village of Hawkshead, thirteen miles from Kendal, cholera appeared unaccountably among the sixteen inmates of the poorhouse, attacking eight of them with sudden and severe symptoms so that four died ; it was impossible to trace the introduction of the virus, but the poorhouse was nearly surrounded with stagnant water[1].

Hardly anything was more keenly debated than the question as to how cholera spread.   It was not difficult to find some instances of infection seemingly got from contact with living or dead cholera bodies : cases suggestive of that occurred at Sunderland at the outset, and later in Ireland more especially[2]. In the Swan Street cholera hospital at Manchester, eight nurses took the infection, of whom four died.   But on the whole the immunity of nurses (as in the Great Gorman Lane hospital of Dublin) and of medical men was remarkable.   Although constantly in the presence of cholera patients, sometimes lingering over them, as in the operation of blood-letting, very few took the disease.   In Manchester only one medical practitioner was known to have had an attack, a mild one. Gaulter says that Dr Alsop, of Birmingham, and Mr Keane, of Warrington, were the only two medical men known to him to have died of cholera in England ; but two of the Bilston doctors died in the height of the epidemic there, one died at Musselburgh, seven at Sligo, and two at Enniskillen.   The truth of the matter in cholera appeared to be the same as in plague and yellow fever, the two great infections that resembled cholera most closely as soil-poisons : namely, that contagion from the persons of the sick was a contingency, as Rush, of Philadelphia, had taught for yellow fever in the end of last century, and Blane

[1] Proudfoot, *Edin. Med. and Surg. Journ.* XXXIX. 99.
[2] Graves, who was a strong contagionist (l.c. 1848–49), cites the instances of nuns, nurses and porters at Tuam, and of medical men at Sligo.

had taught after him. A London writer stated this very fairly in 1832[1]:

"I believe that this disease, like many other epidemic diseases, although communicable by miasma in the atmosphere, and originating or being producible from a peculiar state of that acting upon the earth, is sometimes contagious (or communicable from person to person) and sometimes not contagious. I believe the contagious nature of the disease depends : first, upon the number accumulated in one place, and the unhealthiness or ill-ventilated state of that place ; or, in other words, upon the degree in which the miasma is condensed ; secondly, upon the length of time a person remains exposed to the poison ; third, upon the debility, or morbid irritability, and consequent susceptibility of the person's frame, especially of the abdominal viscera." The miasmata of an apartment, to be strong enough to become contagious, must arrive at a certain degree of concentration.

Cholera was, at all events, very different from typhus fever in the point of contagiousness : for in the epidemics of the latter many medical men fell victims, and the susceptibility to contagion was greater in proportion to the health and vigour of those who mixed with the sick.

It was well understood in 1832 that foul linen, bedding and clothes were a most certain means of carrying the poison, especially if they had been kept concealed for a time, or packed away in a chest or bundle. This was precisely the old experience of plague. The theory that the poison of cholera was conveyed in the drinking-water, of which illustrations were collected in 1849 and 1854, was not applied to any of the particular outbreaks in 1832. But one writer made a guess at it, assuming, as Snow did in 1849 and 1854, that the stomach and bowels were the organs by which the virus entered the system :

"From an attentive observation of the course this epidemic has taken in those places and countries which it has hitherto visited, I have been induced to draw the conclusion that a noxious matter or poison, being generated in the earth, has been diffused in the different springs in such situations [therefore he suggests the filtering of water through charcoal], and that this matter, being conveyed into the stomach with the fluid in question, produces that train of symptoms which, commencing in this organ, afterwards extends with more or less rapidity to the rest of the body[2]."

In the treatment of cholera in 1832 many things were tried. The view taken of the pathology naturally determined the means of cure. To check the premonitory diarrhoea was seen to be of the first importance, and to that end laudanum or other form of opium was the familiar means. Lawrie, at Glasgow, found it most satisfactory, at a time when the profession in London were, as he says, denouncing it as a pernicious error. Towards the end of the epidemic in Dublin, Graves combined with the opium acetate of lead in large doses (a scruple of acetate of lead with a grain of opium,

---

[1] G. D. Dermott, lecturer in Anatomy and Surgery, *Lond. Med. and Surg. Journ.* 1832, p. 274.
[2] John Parkin, surgeon H.E.I.C.S., "Cause, Nature and Treatment of Cholera." *Lond. Med. and Surg. Journ.* 1 Sept. 1832.

divided into twelve pills, one to be given every half-hour until the rice-water evacuations from the stomach and bowels began to diminish)[1]. Some professed to find great benefit from blood-letting at a sufficiently early stage in the attack[2]. The enormous drain of the fluids, leaving the blood thick or tarry, suggested to some that saline substances would be beneficial. The saline treatment was indeed the principal subject of writing during the year 1832. One way was to give saline drugs by the mouth; another way was to inject into a vein a large quantity of distilled water with some common salt and bicarbonate of soda dissolved in it, the vein at the bend of the elbow being usually chosen to operate on. Some were confident that they had saved lives in this manner, others were equally clear that salines were useless. One writer had abandoned salines by the mouth as a "most useless remedy," while he had not lost faith in their intravenous injection, four having recovered out of twenty-three in which he had tried it. At length, however, the intravenous use of salines was abandoned also[3].

It is well known that the greatest of all the lessons taught by cholera was the need of sanitary reform. The disease in its successive visitations so obviously sought out the spots of ground most befouled with excremental and other filth as to bring home to everyone the dangers of the casual disposal of town refuse. It was not until some years after the first visit of cholera that much was done in the way of extending the main drainage of towns, connecting the house-drainage systematically therewith, getting rid of open nuisances in back yards, and protecting the water-supplies from contamination. The Report of the Health of Towns Commission, 1844, was "the great magazine from which sanitary reformers drew their weapons[4]." In the next few years an active school of sanitarians arose, including

[1] Graves, *Clinical Medicine*, 1843, p. 700: "I could bring forward the names of many medical men in Dublin whose lives, I am happy to say, were saved by the use of this remedy."

[2] Paterson, u.s. for the fishing village of Collieston, Aberdeenshire: "In most instances where the lancet was used at the proper period little else was required. The patient, although in an apparently hopeless state at the time of my visit, was in these instances not unfrequently in the course of twenty-four hours out of danger."

[3] A correspondent of the *Lond. Med. Gaz.* Sept. 1832, p. 731, dating from Warrington, proved by a statistical arrangement of 103 cases of cholera, that the saline treatment was nearly certain recovery, that the same combined with blood-letting was certain recovery, that blood-letting alone was certain death, and that opium with stimulants, and Morison's pill, were each uniformly followed by a fatal result.

	Cases	Deaths	Percentage of recoveries
Aged, neglected or seen too late	30	30	o
Obstinately refused medicine	4	4	o
Treated by opium and stimulants	23	23	o
,, by Morison's pill	3	3	o
,, by blood-letting	13	13	o
,, by blood-letting and salines	7	o	100
,, by salines alone	23	2	92·3
	103	75	27 per cent.

Quarterly Review, CXVIII. 256.

Sutherland of Liverpool, Grainger of London, and others. In 1848 was passed the first Public Health Act, administered by a Board of Health, of which Lord Shaftesbury was chairman, Chadwick and Southwood Smith members. London was excepted from the scope of the Act; but the City had a most vigorous medical officer in the person of John Simon, whose reports dealt with public sanitation on broad principles applicable to the capital and the whole kingdom. The movement in favour of sanitation, thus begun, received an irresistible impulse from the cholera of 1849, the lessons of which were as obvious as those of 1832.

The cholera which reached Orenburg in 1829 and Astrakhan in 1830 lingered in one part of Europe or another until 1837, Portugal and Spain having been its chief theatre in 1833, the south of France in 1834, Italy in 1835 and 1836, Austria, the Tyrol, Bavaria and (for the second time) Poland and the Baltic ports in 1837. In England, there was some revival of the seeds of it in 1833, as many as 1454 deaths being put down to Asiatic cholera in London from the 1st of August to the 7th of September. There was an undoubted epidemic of it at the fishing village of Ferryden, near Montrose, in June, 1833 (27 deaths during four weeks in a population of 700), the infection having been brought by one or more of the crew of the smack 'Eagle' from the Thames[1]. In Glasgow a case occurred in Boar Head Close, High Street, on 30 May, 1833, which had the blueness, pinched face, whispering voice and cold clammy skin of Asiatic cholera[2]. In Ireland there were a good many outbreaks in 1833, especially in villages or hamlets, and it is believed that these were renewed in 1834. But the most singular reappearance of cholera in the British Isles was in the month of December, 1837, some two months after it is believed to have ceased elsewhere in Europe. Outbreaks of true cholera in that month were observed at several places in the south of Ireland—around Bere Haven[3], at Youghal, at Waterford, and at

---

[1] Reported by Brewster to J. Y. Simpson, *Edin. Med. Surg. Journ.* XLIX. (1838), p. 368.

[2] *Glas. Med. Journ.* VI. (1833), p. 366. Stark says, perhaps for Edinburgh, that cholera recurred in the end of 1833 and beginning of 1834, with a high degree of fatality.

[3] Edmond Sharkey, M.B., *Dubl. J. Med. Sc.* XVI. 13. Of 28 houses or cabins (nearly all in three hamlets) which together had 76 cases, 16 cabins had each two cases, 8 had each three, 1 had four, 2 had each five, and 1 had six. The type of sickness was the same as in 1832–33.

Dungarvan, where they went so far as to form a board of health[1]. It was suspected to have been in Limehouse, on the Thames, in November. The most remarkable explosion of it was in the month of January following (1838) among the inmates of the Coventry House of Industry, of whom no fewer than 55 died in the course of four weeks—a mortality from choleraic disease that could hardly be explained on the hypothesis of cholera nostras even if the season had been the proper one[2].

The Cholera of 1848–49 in Scotland.

The invasion of cholera from India, which reached Britain in the autumn of 1848, had progressed as far as Peshawur and Cabul from 1842 to 1844, and thereafter step by step continuously through Herat, Samarkand, Bokhara, Astrabad and Teheran by the caravan routes. In the beginning of 1847 it entered Russia by the two great interior waterways of the Volga and the Don. Next year, 1848, it reached the German shores of the Baltic and North Seas, and within a few weeks of its appearance at Hamburg, it was found established on British soil at Edinburgh and Leith in the beginning of October. The severe outburst which followed in the south of Scotland was purely a winter epidemic, like that of Durham, Northumberland and East Lothian on the last occasion in the winter of 1831–32. It will not be necessary to give the details of the cholera of 1848–49 so fully as has been done for 1831–32, but merely to notice special points.

The cholera of 1848 broke out almost simultaneously at Newhaven and Edinburgh, on the 1st and 2nd of October, and

---

[1] R. Green, M.D., *Lancet,* 14 April, 1838, p. 83: true Asiatic cholera began at Youghal in the second week of December, 1837, and lasted two months, about 200 having been attacked: "two of my relatives, Miss A. —— and Mrs K. ——, died in December of cholera, one in fourteen hours, the other in ten hours."

[2] Deaths from Cholera in the Coventry House of Industry:

1838.

Jan. 7—11	Jan. 12—16	Jan. 17—21	Jan. 22—26	Jan. 27—31	Feb. 1—5	Total
7	4	15	20	7	2	55

Twenty-seven were males and twenty-eight females. The ages were as follow :

under one	1—5	5—10	10—20	20—40	40—60	60—80	80—90	Total
1	6	4	4	3	8	20	9	55

—*Second Report of the Registrar-General,* p. 98.

53—2

at Leith on the 9th. At Newhaven nearly the whole population was suffering from diarrhoea, in the midst of which epidemic the true cholera raged for four weeks only, to the 28th October, attacking 30, of whom 20 died. In Leith the deaths were 185 (males 75, females 110). The Edinburgh outbreak lasted until the 18th of January, 1849, causing 801 attacks, with 448 deaths (or 478 deaths, of which 196 were males and 282 females). A cholera hospital was opened in Surgeons' Square on the 28th of October, the admissions and fatalities to 14th December being as follows:

	Females	Males	Total
Admitted	152	96	248
Died	90	64	154

Of the whole 248 cases, the Grassmarket sent 42, the Cowgate 37, the Canongate 33, College Wynd 16, High Street 14, and numerous scattered localities of the New and Old towns one or more cases each. Severe outbreaks took place also at Niddry, Restalrig and Loanhead, villages close to Edinburgh[1]. While this limited epidemic was proceeding in and around the capital, the infection appeared in the mining region of Carron at the head of the Firth of Forth, where there were some 400 cases after the 6th of December, and in some other mining villages of the Scotch midlands.

Glasgow was infected on the night of the 11th November, in the suburban district of Springburn, on the north-west of the city close to the Forth and Clyde Canal. The choice of this spot to begin upon was intelligible enough in one way, but singular in another. Springburn had come into existence as a poor village of weavers about the year 1820; before the cholera year of 1832 it had grown to a population of 600, and was thought a likely spot for cholera inasmuch as it was one of the most wretched communities in Scotland. It occupied the site of a half-drained bog below the level of the canal, from which the water percolated into its subsoil; its houses were low, always damp, and full of filth. During all the cholera in Glasgow in 1832 there had not been a case in Springburn until the 6th of September, when a girl of the village came home with it and died; during her brief illness she was visited by the greater

[1] Stark, *Ed. Med. and Surg. Journ.* LXXI. (1849), p. 388; W. Robertson, *Month. Journ. Med. Sc.* IX. (1849). The other outbreaks reported in that part of Scotland (*ibid.*) were slight—at Dalkeith, Haddington, Borrowstowness.

part of the villagers, but no other case occurred until six weeks after, on the 15th of October[1].   At this spot, where the cholera of 1832 may be said to have left off, it began in 1848 with a sudden explosion of numerous attacks scattered all over the locality ; a doctor attended twenty-one cases before he found two together in the same house or even in the same lane.   There had been forty cases there in November, before any case was discovered in Glasgow ; at length it seemed to spread from Springburn all round as if from a centre, while it also lingered there longer than anywhere else in the city and suburbs[2].   On the 5th of December a case was reported on the south bank of the Clyde, and another on the 9th in the west end.   Within a few days the disease fell upon all parts of the city with the suddenness of a thunder shower ; it reached a height in the Christmas week, one day, the 30th December, having 158 burials from cholera.   After the orgies of the New Year there was a fresh outburst, 235 cases having been reported on the 5th of January.   The proportion of fatalities was as high as 60 per cent. at the beginning of the epidemic, 50 per cent. about Christmas and the New Year, and thereafter from 30 to 40 per cent.   The epidemic was short and sharp, declining irregularly after the first or second week of January, and ceasing, but for a few dropping cases, about the 8th of March.

The deaths in Glasgow, which included many among the wealthier class and made the festival season of 1848–49 to be long remembered, were about 3800, or 1·06 per cent. of the population (355,800), a higher total but a lower ratio than in 1832, when the deaths, distributed over many more weeks of the year and largely due to two revivals in August and October, were 1·4 per cent. of the population.   At Paisley there were 68 deaths from 26 December to 24 February, and at Charlestown 115 deaths all in some five weeks from 15 January to 19 February.

It was in the same season of midwinter that the cholera burst suddenly upon many mining villages of Lanarkshire and Ayrshire.

In that unlikely season there was an almost universal prevalence of diarrhoea.   At the mining village of Carnbroe, near Coatbridge, there were five sudden attacks on the last night of the old year, one of them fatal.   On New Year's day there were forty attacks, thirteen of them fatal in a few

---

[1] Easton, *Glas. Med. Journ.* v. 444.
[2] Sutherland, *Report of the Board of Health.*

hours. Terror seized the whole place : one man cut his throat in sheer fright. Diarrhoea attacked 1100 of the 1200 inhabitants, and turned to spasmodic or rice-water cholera in 240 of them, of whom 94 died, the rate of fatality being excessive only in the first few days. By the end of February the epidemic was over.

In the town of Coatbridge, with a population of 4000, the various grades of sickness were classified as follows :

Diarrhoea	Vomiting, purging and cramp	Rice-water purging	Cholera	Deaths by Cholera
2659	480	175	107	61

In the town of Hamilton, population 9000, the infection was most malignant, 440 cases yielding 251 deaths from the 24th of December to the 7th of March. The same ravages of winter cholera occurred at some of the Ayrshire ironworks, such as Glengarnock, among a very rough and drunken class, who were made more than ordinarily reckless and drunken by this unaccountable visitation. It was also severe in Riccarton and other mining villages round Kilmarnock, but less prevalent in that town itself. Dumfries and Maxwelltown, which had been among the last places visited by the cholera of 1832, were infected in the middle of November, 1848, about the same time as Springburn near Glasgow. One of the Dumfries doctors died of rapid cholera on the 10th December, the parochial board fell into disputes with the faculty, and the infection proceeded amidst great confusion in the poorest parts of the town, causing about 250 deaths before Christmas. After that it subsided quickly [1].

The other centres in the south of Scotland were Selkirk (13 deaths), Kelso (Dec. to end of Jan., maximum of 12 attacks in a day) and Jedburgh, which last had escaped in 1832 but had now a very rapid and extensive epidemic in its lower parts among drunken people especially. A few cases occurred at Moffat, in December ; a man who was seized in crossing the hills died in a shepherd's hut eight miles from Moffat after twenty-one hours illness [2].

The only recorded epidemic in the north of Scotland in the proper cholera season, the summer of 1849, was at Dundee. But there was a small outbreak in March and April at Campbelton (41 cases, 14 deaths) and Inverness (23 cases, 12 deaths) [3].

The infection began in Dundee on the 29th of May, 1849, in Fish Street, the filthiest part of the town. It prevailed in high and low situations, but usually in the old localities of typhus fever. One group of houses, said to have had a population of 100, had 40 deaths. Dudhope Crescent, consisting of seventeen large five-storied tenement houses occupied by clean and respectable people, had 57 deaths. In about a fourth part of all the fatalities, death was from sudden collapse ; this was a feature of the 1849 cholera also in Ireland ; but in Dundee, as elsewhere, there was usually premonitory

[1] Sutherland, *Report*, u.s.; Grieve, *Month. J. Med. Sc.* IX. 777. Barker, *ibid.* 940 (gives good account of the stormy weather).
[2] *Month. Journ. Med. Sc.* IX. 783, 857, 1011, X. 403.
[3] *Ibid.* IX. 1009.

diarrhoea, and a very general prevalence of diarrhoea which never came to true cholera[1].

The Cholera of 1849 in Ireland.

The cholera of 1849 found Ireland in a state of exhaustion and confusion. The fever and dysentery that followed the great potato famines of 1845 and 1846 were still far from extinct; the workhouses, which had not existed in 1832, were full of paupers. The mortality of nearly half a million in the famine years, and the emigration of perhaps three times as many, had reduced greatly the population of the scattered cabins, hamlets and villages; but the towns were more populous than ever from the immense number of destitute persons that had gravitated to them. In these circumstances it was not surprising that the cholera of 1849 should have been more disastrous than that of 1832. The infection appeared first in Belfast in November, 1848, in a man who had come with his family from Edinburgh and had been admitted into the workhouse. Some thirty cases of cholera among the inmates followed his death, and at length the infection was started at large in the town, probably by a man who had been discharged from the workhouse[2]. The cholera of 1849 in the capital of Ulster was more fatal than that of 1832, causing 969 deaths in 2705 attacks. Over Ireland generally its great season appears to have been, as in England, the summer, and in part also the spring. Excepting Belfast, the principal cities and towns had fewer deaths than in 1832; Dublin having only 1664 as compared with 5632, Cork 1329, or nearly the same number as in 1832, Limerick 746, which was about a fourth less, Galway less, Waterford about the same as in 1832 and 1833 together, and Drogheda as severe an epidemic as last time. But

[1] Sutherland, *Report*, u.s. The year 1847, in which there was no cholera, had been much more fatal in the chief towns of Scotland, than either 1848 or 1849, owing to the great prevalence of typhus (Stark):

Deaths from all causes.

	1846	1847	1848	1849
Edinburgh	4594	6706	5475	4807
Glasgow	10854	18071	12475	12231
Dundee	1531	2520	2146	2312
Paisley	1429	2068	1552	1712
Leith	801	955	1212	1066
Greenock	1087	2214	1289	2344
Aberdeen	1315	1466	2366	

[2] H. MacCormac to Graves, *Dub. Journ. Med. Sc.* N.S. VII. 245.

the smaller towns and the rural districts generally suffered more. The deaths for all Ireland returned to the Board of Health were 19,325, nearly the same total as in 1832; but there were no returns included from Wicklow, Cavan, Fermanagh and Donegal, and it is probable that the returns were otherwise incomplete, the census taken in 1851 giving 30,156 cholera deaths under the year 1849, and 35,989 in the whole decennial period from 1841. The larger total was distributed as follows:

Urban	Rural	In hospitals	In workhouses
10,653	10,656	7964	6716

The number of rural deaths is much larger than in 1832. There were only a few towns with over 2000 inhabitants that escaped—one in Connaught, six in Munster, one out of forty-one in Leinster, while seventeen towns were visited in Ulster. The counties of Dublin, Carlow, Clare and Galway suffered most; of the smaller towns, Tralee and Dingle lost heavily, both among the poor and the rich. The town of Ballinasloe, near the confluence of the Suck with the Shannon, had 756 deaths from 23 April to 19 August, a great part of them in the workhouse. In clinical characters, the cholera of 1849 was noted in Ireland, as in Scotland and England, for the high proportion of sudden fatalities, about one-third, without the warnings of diarrhoea or the usual choleraic symptoms. It was remarked also that many children under the age of seven died of cholera, about one in ten of all ages. There was a second season in 1850, with 1768 deaths (according to the census), but hardly comparable to the return of cholera in 1833 in the country districts more particularly.

The Cholera of 1849 in England.

The brief but very severe epidemic of cholera in the south of Scotland in midwinter was all over and done with for good before the disease really began in England. Hull, which had a few cases on board ship in the end of 1848, about the same time as the infection began to rage in Edinburgh and Leith, was spared its great visitation, the greatest in all England, until the late summer and autumn[1]. The progress of the infection in

---

[1] Most of the information on the cholera of 1849 in England comes from two sources: (1) the *Report of the General Board of Health on the Epidemic Cholera of 1848 and 1849* (Parl. papers, 1850), containing the detailed reports of Mr R. D. Grainger for London, and of Dr John Sutherland for various other towns; and (2) the *Quarterly Reports of the Registrar-General for the year* 1849. See also note 3, p. 846.

London also was strangely different from that in Scotland. There were undoubted cases in Bethnal Green and other out-parishes in the autumn of 1848, and there seemed no reason why the infection should not run through the population and exhaust itself at once, as in Glasgow. But it will appear from the following table of the deaths in London that the real outburst was delayed until the summer and autumn of 1849:

1848	Cholera deaths	1849	Cholera deaths
Sept.	11	April	9
Oct.	122	May	13
Nov.	215	June	246
Dec.	131	July	1952
1849		Aug.	4251
Jan.	262	Sept.	6644
Feb.	181	Oct.	464
March	73	Nov.	27

Although a certain number of deaths were returned in October and November, 1848, they came in twos or threes from many parishes of the metropolis and made no great impression upon any one locality. It was not until the beginning of December that the presence of cholera was fully realized, owing to an extraordinary explosion of the disease in a huge pauper institution at Tooting. The school contained about a thousand children, of whom some three hundred took Asiatic cholera, with one hundred and eighty deaths, in the course of three or four weeks: this was the whole cholera mortality that the parish of Streatham had from first to last. In the spring months the cases declined all over London in a very remarkable way, so that it looked for a time as if the infection were extinct, just as in 1832. But in June there was a revival, and thereafter a steady increase to the maximum of 6644 deaths in September. The table given under the year 1866 shows upon what parishes the mortality fell most—those of Southwark, Bermondsey, Rotherhithe, Greenwich, Newington, Lambeth and Battersea on the south side, of Westminster, the City and Liberties, Shoreditch, Bethnal Green and Whitechapel on the north side of the Thames. It was a more severe visitation per head of the inhabitants than that of 1832, cutting off many beyond the limits of the destitute and reckless class who were its most usual victims on the first occasion. Many of the respectable class of workmen and small shopkeepers were among the victims. Several medical men died of it, including one well-known surgeon, Mr Aston Key, at his house in St Helen's Place, Bishopsgate, on 23 August, after a few hours' illness. As in Ireland, and at Dundee, an unusually large proportion of the London deaths, perhaps a fourth part, were from sudden collapse and blueness, without premonitory diarrhoea or predominant intestinal symptoms. Opinion was strongly against contagiousness in this epidemic. There were 478 cases treated in St Bartholomew's Hospital, but not one of the nurses took cholera.

The infection seemed to find out the insanitary spots and to act miasmatically upon the residents. The common remark in all parts of England, Scotland and Ireland was that the localities that suffered most from the typhus fever of 1847–48 suffered most also from cholera. The one black spot in Kensington was a poor district on the north side of the parish known as the Potteries, where an immense number of pigs were kept.

One of the most remarkable features of the cholera-seasons of 1848–49 was the extensive prevalence of common bowel-complaints. Evidence of this has been given for the south of Scotland just before or during the cholera of midwinter, a season when diarrhoea is not usual. It was equally remarked in England in the course of 1849. In the Taunton workhouse, where true Asiatic cholera broke out in November, there had been many cases of bowel-complaint, as well as of fever, in the spring (7 deaths from dysentery and diarrhoea, 5 from fever). In the Exeter workhouse there were eighteen deaths from dysentery in the end of the year, although there is nothing said of cholera, which caused only 44 deaths in the whole city. The efforts of the inspectors sent by the Board of Health were in great part directed to finding out the cases of "premonitory" diarrhoea, by house-to-house visitation, and insisting upon the importance of checking it before it could turn to true cholera. Leeds will serve as an example of English towns. In an incomplete survey after the month of July there were found 5129 cases of simple diarrhoea, 1484 cases of dysentery, 1273 cases of choleraic diarrhoea, and 1090 cases of true cholera[1]. It was something of a paradox that, with such excessive prevalence of

---

[1] Sutherland, *Report*, u.s. p. 121. At Sheffield (*ibid.* p. 108) a sudden outbreak of diarrhoea occurred on 26 August over the whole town; 5319 cases of it were known, with only 76 cases of cholera and 46 deaths.

ordinary bowel-complaints, an unusual proportion of the cases of true cholera proved quickly fatal with symptoms of collapse and asphyxia only.

Just as the first startling indication of the presence of Asiatic cholera in London was the enormous fatality in the pauper school at Tooting in the winter, so in some other towns the infection seemed to pick out workhouses or prisons to begin upon. At Belfast there were forty cases in the workhouse before there was one in the town. At Liverpool there were 28 cholera deaths in the first quarter of 1849, of which 8 were in the workhouse. At Wakefield, 19 died of cholera in January, 16 of these in the House of Correction. Among the people at large the infection made little progress until the summer. In the first and second quarters of the year it is heard of, but to a moderate extent, in the towns and colliery districts of Durham and Northumberland, which were the scene of its earliest outbreak in the winter of 1831–32. It was also beginning in the poorest and filthiest parts of Liverpool, Bristol and Plymouth. Its great season all over England was July, August and September, the incidence of the disease according to counties being shown in the table. The right-hand column, showing the number of deaths at the principal centres in each county, must serve for a conspectus of the epidemic.

Cholera Mortality in England and Wales in 1849.

	Deaths	Death-rate per 1000 inhab.	Principal centres in each county
England and Wales	53293	3·0	
London	14137	6·2	Lambeth 1618, Newington 907, Bermondsey 734, Southwark 1704
Surrey, part of	255	1·3	
Kent, part of	1208	2·5	Gravesend, Milton, Rochester, Chatham, Margate, Ramsgate, Maidstone
Sussex	346	1·1	Hastings
Hampshire	1245	3·2	Portsmouth 568, Southampton 240
Berkshire	148	·8	
Middlesex	406	2·7	Edmonton, Barnet
Hertfordshire	323	1·9	Hitchin 127, Hertford 81, Watford 45
Buckinghamshire	175	1·2	Marlow, Wycombe 100
Oxfordshire	117	·7	Oxford 44, Witney 33
Northamptonshire	141	·7	Northampton 49, Peterborough 49
Huntingdonshire	14	·2	
Bedfordshire	72	·6	Bedford 37, Biggleswade 28
Cambridgeshire	269	1·4	Wisbech 138, North Witchford 85
Essex	580	1·7	West Ham 134, Romford 163, Rochford 105, Harwich
Suffolk	79	·2	Ipswich 18, Mutford 27
Norfolk	223	·5	Yarmouth 87, Norwich 38

	Deaths	Death-rate per 1000 inhab.	Principal centres in each county
Wiltshire	320	1·3	Salisbury 165, Devizes 67
Dorset	122	·7	Weymouth 59, Poole 31
Devon	2366	4·2	Plymouth 830, Stonehouse 171, Stoke Damerel 721, Plympton St Mary 151, Tavistock 140, Totnes 107
Cornwall	835	2·4	St Germans 236, Liskeard 132, St Austell 135, Redruth 133
Somerset	923	2	Bridgewater 235, Keynsham 77, Bath 90, Bedminster 281
Gloucestershire	1465	3·5	Bristol 591, Tewkesbury 59, Gloucester 119, Clifton 563, Dursley 58
Herefordshire	1	·01	
Shropshire	316	1·3	Bridgnorth 75, Shrewsbury 116
Staffordshire	2672	4·4	Newcastle-under-Lyme 241, Wolverhampton (incl. Bilston, Tipton, Sedgley) 1365, Stoke 103, W. Bromwich 250, Dudley 412, Walsall 186
Worcestershire	432	1·7	Stourbridge 314
Warwickshire	293	·6	Coventry 202, Birmingham 29, Warwick 20
Leicestershire	8	·08	Loughborough 7, Leicester 2
Rutlandshire	7	·4	
Lincolnshire	372	·9	Gainsborough 246, Boston 35, Grimsby 29
Nottinghamshire	137	·5	East Retford 21, Basford 42, Nottingham 18
Derbyshire	50	·06	Derby 18
Cheshire	653	1·6	Nantwich 181, Runcorn 82, Stockport 72, Birkenhead 139
Lancashire	8184	4·1	Liverpool and W. Derby 5308, Wigan 503, Manchester 878, Chorlton 280, Salford 237
West Riding	4151	3·2	Huddersfield 52, Bradford 426, Hunslet 884, Dewsbury 224, Wakefield 241, Pontefract &c. 238, Leeds 1439
East Riding	2140	8·7	Hull and Sculcoates 1834, York 174, Pocklington 37, Howden 58
North Riding	47	·2	Whitby 10
Durham	1642	4·2	Darlington 4, Stockton 248, Durham 192, Hartlepool, Chester-le-Street 134, Sunderland 363, Gateshead 257, S. Shields 201
Northumberland	1417	4·8	Newcastle 295, Tynemouth 815, Alnwick 142
Cumberland	419	2·2	Carlisle 51, Cockermouth 282, Whitehaven 79
Westmoreland	1	·02	
Monmouth	775	4·1	Newport 246, Pontypool 69, Abergavenny 438
S. Wales	3544	6·1	Merthyr Tydvil 1682, Cardiff 396, Neath 738, Llanelly 45, Swansea 262, Carmarthen 142, Crickhowell 95
N. Wales	245	·6	Holywell 86, Montgomery 37, Carnarvon 21

The highest rates in the table are for the East Riding, owing to Hull (24·1), for South Wales, owing to Merthyr Tydvil (23·4), for Northumberland and Durham, for Staffordshire, owing to the iron district round Wolverhampton, for Devonshire, owing to Plymouth, for Lancashire, owing to Liverpool, and for Monmouth, owing to a few mining places. The miners suffered most, the lower class in the seaports next most severely. The Black Country in the south of Staffordshire, which had been the worst centre of the 1832 cholera, was again one of its chief centres in 1849, the mortality falling most, as before, upon the town of Bilston, and next to it upon Willenhall and Wolverhampton. But a great rival to the Staffordshire coal and iron mining had sprung up since 1832 in Glamorgan; and it was in this comparatively new region of miners that cholera in 1849 reproduced the Black Country horrors of 1832 and, indeed, surpassed them.

Merthyr Tydvil had sprung up more like a vast miners' camp than like a well-ordered municipality. Along the eastern side of the Taff valley, on the slopes and in bottoms of the hills, but everywhere at an elevation of some four or five hundred feet above the level of Cardiff docks, were numerous groups of mean-looking miners' cottages, with their attendant ale-houses, small retail shops, schools and meeting-houses. This peculiar township had drawn to itself the special notice of the Health of Towns Commission in 1844: "From the poorer inhabitants (who constitute the mass of the population) throwing all slops and refuse into the nearest open gutter before their houses, from the impeded course of such channels, and the scarcity of privies, some parts of the town are complete networks of filth emitting noxious exhalations... During the rapid increase of the town no attention seems to have been paid to its drainage."

In this district the registrar had returned 162 deaths from "cholera" in the year 1841, which must have been from an unusually severe type of cholera nostras or British cholera. A first case of Asiatic cholera occurred at Cardiff in a sailor on the 13th of May, 1849, a week after there was a case at Lower Merthyr, and a week after that another at Upper Merthyr. In the course of the summer the ravages of the disease were enormous in the hilly mining regions of the interior of Glamorgan and Monmouth, as well as severe in the seaports:

Merthyr Tydvil	1682	Abergavenny district	438
Cardiff	396	Pontypool	69
Neath	738	Newport	246
Swansea	262		

The peculiar selection of the mining townships was well shown in the district of Abergavenny: of 378 deaths from cholera in the third quarter of 1849, only 9 occurred in Abergavenny town, while 157 were at the iron-works of Tredegar and 210 at those of Aberystruth, just as, in the winter preceding, the villages of the iron-works all round Kilmarnock had been ravaged by cholera while there was little of it in that town itself.

Another chief centre of cholera in 1849 was the port of Hull. Including the district of Sculcoates, it had the following enormous mortalities from cholera in four weeks of September: 398, 507, 524 and 171, the whole epidemic from July to the 18th of October producing 2534 deaths[1]. Its neglect of scavenging became a classical instance of the favouring conditions of cholera. An open space at Witham called the "muckgarths," from the refuse deposited upon it, was one of the worst centres,

---

[1] Henry Cooper, "On the Cholera Mortality in Hull during the epidemic of 1849," *Journ. Statist. Soc.* XVI. 347. The total is higher than that in the Table.

just as the town moor of Sunderland, used for the same purpose, had been in 1831[1]. In the other ports, Liverpool, with West Derby, Bristol with Clifton, and Plymouth with East Stonehouse and Devonport, the infection was most severe (see Table), and was observed to choose the poorest streets, lanes and houses, where there had been most typhus for a year or two before[2]. On the Tyne, the greatest centre on this occasion was not Newcastle, but Tynemouth. The city of Durham, which escaped the cholera of 1832, had a severe visitation. The chief inland centres, besides the mining districts of Staffordshire and Glamorgan, were Manchester and the cloth-making towns of Airedale,—Leeds, Hunslet, Bradford, Dewsbury, and some others in the West Riding. Most of the Lancashire towns occupied with the cotton industry again escaped with little cholera— Preston, Clitheroe, Oldham, Bury, Rochdale, Bolton, Blackburn, Ashton and Chorley. Wigan had nearly twenty times as many deaths as in 1832; on the other hand Sheffield had only a quarter of its former cholera mortality, while Nottingham and Norwich had this time very little. Birmingham, Leicester, Cheltenham, Hereford, Stafford, Ipswich, Cambridge and Colchester were again almost or altogether free from infection. The agricultural counties, notably the Eastern counties, escaped once more with few centres of infection, and these unimportant. Cumberland as a whole had fewer deaths than in 1832, while Cockermouth had more. Exeter, which was severely visited on the former occasion, escaped almost wholly, while Totnes and Tavistock, with the surrounding Dartmoor country and other towns in Devon, had epidemics of the first degree for their size. In England as a whole the cholera of 1849 was more severe relatively to the numbers living than that of 1832, its great centres having been the same, or of the same kind, on both occasions[3].

[1] Sutherland, *Report*, u.s., with map.

[2] For Bristol, Sutherland (p. 126) cites Goldney: "In a certain lodging-house there were 35 attacks and 33 deaths during the epidemic of 1832....Out of the same house in 1849, 64 people were turned, of whom 49 were sent to the House of Refuge." Not one case of cholera occurred among these, but many attacks of diarrhoea, which was general all through the epidemic, especially along the Frome.

[3] The epidemic in the small Devonshire fishing village of Noss Mayo near Plympton St Mary, was very fully investigated by A. C. Maclaren, *Journ. Statist. Soc.* XIII. (1850), p. 103. The Oxford epidemic (75 deaths) was described by Greenhill and Allen in the *Ashmolean Society Reports.* For Tynemouth, see Greenhow, *Trans. Epid. Soc.* The volume by Baly and Gull, *Reports on Epidemic Cholera drawn up at the desire of the Cholera Committee Roy. Col. Phys.* London, 1854, is in great part a review of the epidemic of 1849, in the form of a general discussion of the

The cholera of 1849 reproduced very closely the former characteristics. The attacks were often in the night, especially in persons who had supped heartily on the coarser kinds of savoury meat. With the same undoubted preference for the poorer and more filthy quarters of towns, the infection showed also a certain apparent caprice in fixing on some places and avoiding others.

Thus at Leeds it was most malignant in the locality of York Street and Marsh Lane (an old centre of plague and typhus), which had lately been drained at a cost of some thousands of pounds, "whilst in the adjoining district, which lies nearly level with the river, and will scarcely admit of any sewerage, I have not heard," writes the registrar, "of a single case of cholera"—an experience similar to that of a low-lying district of Bristol in 1832. At Liverpool, where much had been undertaken for sanitation since the disastrous Irish fever of 1847-48, the cholera appeared to Dr Duncan, the medical officer of health, to attack sewered and unsewered streets impartially. Another singular thing, which used to be noticed in the plague and is observed in the malarial fevers of towns abroad, was the choice of one side of a street only : thus, at Rotherhithe, in a street where numerous deaths occurred, they were nearly all one side of the street, in houses occupied by respectable private families, only one house having been infected on the other side ; at Bedford, two streets showed the same thing.

In London, the least elevated parishes on both sides of the Thames were again its chief seats. Dr Farr, the superintendent of statistics, deduced the law that the death-rate from cholera in London was inversely as the altitude of the parish, and he showed, by a somewhat rough grouping of the cholera deaths, that the law applied to all England[1]. An empirical generality such as that may have some value ; but it is the exceptions to it that show the inward meaning of the fact.

Merthyr Tydvil, which was the worst cholera-spot in England with the possible exception of Hull, was five hundred feet above the level of Cardiff, its seaport, where the death-rate was much lower. Neath, also, had much more cholera than Swansea. Newcastle-under-Lyme, situated near the source of the Trent, and the highest town in the course of that river, had a far more severe visitation of cholera than any other town upon it all the way to its mouth. At Tavistock among the Dartmoor hills, cholera "sat for many a week," as Kingsley says, "amid the dull brown haze, and sunburnt bents and dried-up watercourses, of white dusty granite." But the poorer and more populous part of Tavistock was a somewhat peculiarly shut-in basin, which was "very often involved in fog during the night." The town had escaped cholera in 1832, but one of its physicians, writing in 1841, and recalling its dreadful plague of 1626, did not feel sure that it would escape if cholera came back[2]. Again, one thinks of Salisbury as standing among high

whole problem of Asiatic cholera. A subcommittee of the College also published a *Report on the nature of the microscopic bodies found in the intestinal discharges of Cholera,* London, 1849.

[1] Farr, "Influence of elevation on the mortality of Cholera." *Journ. Statist. Soc.* XV. (1852), p. 155, and in the Reports of the Registrar-General.

[2] C. Barham, M.B., "Tavistock Parish Register," *Journ. Statist. Soc.* IV. 37.

downs ; but it had a wet subsoil, bad sewerage, and bad water supply, and in 1849 it had 200 deaths from cholera among all classes in two months[1].

In the not very extensive outbreak at Sheffield, one of its chosen seats was an elevated district called the Park, inhabited by colliers. At Bedlington colliery, near Morpeth, the cholera deaths in November were in the miners' houses on the hill side. The elevated, airy and clean village of Loanhead, near Edinburgh, had 46 deaths in its population of 1200, during a few weeks of midwinter. In Dundee, built upon a steep slope at the waterside, there were bad centres of cholera in the higher parts as well as in the lower.

The determining thing appears to have been not so much the elevation as the configuration of the ground ; any basin, or cup, or shelving terrace, any natural collecting-ground of moisture and organic refuse in the soil, may become a seat of cholera, whether it be at the sea-level or several hundred feet above it, provided it have a sufficient number of human occupants and a mode of drainage inadequate to its peculiar needs. Such was the situation of Merthyr Tydvil, of Neath, of Newcastle-under-Lyme, of Tavistock, of some colliery villages, and of certain localities in towns such as Dundee. Such, of course, was also the situation of the London parishes next the river on the south and east, of Hull, of Plymouth, of Liverpool, and of other seaports on estuaries. Neither altitude nor configuration means anything for cholera unless the ground itself be full of rotting filth. In all England and Scotland the cholera chose, as if by an unerring instinct, those not very extensive mining parts of the counties of Stafford, Glamorgan, Durham, Lanark and Ayr, which had as many hundreds of inhabitants to the square mile, and as little provision for the safe disposal of their excrements, as those village communities of Lower Bengal in which the infection had become established since 1817 as if it were an annual product of the soil.

The Report of the Board of Health brought to light many instances in which it seemed probable that cholera had been favoured, if not induced, by the water of wells contaminated with organic filth soaking through the ground or entering with the surface water. This was especially the case at Merthyr Tydvil. It was during the next cholera, that of 1854, that the question of contaminated water came into great prominence, in connexion both with wells and with the vast volumes of water supplied through the mains of water companies.

[1] Middleton, " Sanitary Statistics of Salisbury," *ibid.* XXVII. (1864), p. 541.

The Cholera of 1853 at Newcastle and Gateshead.

The third visitation of Great Britain and Ireland by Asiatic Cholera was in 1853–54. There had been none of it in any part of the kingdom since 1850; but it is not so clear that all other European countries, especially Poland, were equally free from it. Whether due to a new approach from Asia, or to a rekindling of smouldering fires, cholera appeared in the Baltic ports in the summer of 1853, and soon after reached the Tyne. For the third time a severe but localized epidemic was the prelude—this time at Newcastle and Gateshead, just as in 1848 at Edinburgh, Glasgow and the south of Scotland, and in 1831 at Sunderland and Newcastle.

In the cholera of 1849, which was the most general and the most severe visitation that England has had, Newcastle escaped with a light visitation and Gateshead with a moderate or average one, while Tynemouth (with North Shields) had about twice as many deaths as Newcastle and Gateshead together (12·9 deaths per 1000 inhabitants). In 1853 it was the turn of Newcastle— for no better reason, perhaps, than its escape last time. The very thorough and masterly inquiry by Messrs Simon, Bateman and Hume did, indeed, reveal a most unwholesome state of things; but the town was no worse or only a little worse than in 1849, when the cholera had dealt lightly with it, and it was probably an average sample of the insanitary condition of the greater English industrial towns in the time of their rapid growth and before the period of well-ordered local government had arrived. In some parts, such as Sandgate, the dwellings of the labouring class were "not fit to live in"; in the newer mean suburbs, it was found, as in Glasgow twenty years before, that cellars had become the dwelling-places of a class who in former times lived above ground. Those who had been dispossessed by the railways and other public structures had not been provided for elsewhere; so that, with more trade and better wages, the working class were worse housed than before. Overcrowding, for which the ports on the Tyne and Wear are still pre-eminent, was then most excessive. Only the better-class houses had the water laid on. Excremental offences to sight and smell were everywhere. There was a system of main sewers, passably good; but house-drainage or connexions with the main drains were quite casual. The scavenging of the town was greatly neglected. Piggeries, slaughter-houses and other such nuisances, were uncontrolled. The burial-grounds were over-full. With all this the death-rate of Newcastle could be low enough in a good year, such as 1844, when it was 20·9 per 1000; in the year of the Irish fever, 1847, it rose to 32·8; and in other years it fluctuated between those extremes, according to the nature of the seasons[1].

The cholera of 1853 was a sudden explosion in the heavy stagnant atmosphere of the month of September. No one knew where the infection came from; there were, of course, ships arriving from the Baltic, but no particular source was ever traced. On the 30th or 31st of August, a case occurred of the rapidly fatal kind; before a week there were about a hundred attacks daily all over the town. From the 13th of September the deaths in Newcastle mounted up rapidly as follows :

		Cholera deaths			Cholera deaths
Sept.	13	59	Sept.	19	111
	14	90		20	85
	15	106		21	68
	16	114		22	82
	17	103		23	60
	18	103		24	56

In the thirty days of September there were 1371 deaths, and some one or two hundreds more in the first part of October, when the infection ceased almost abruptly, the total of deaths to the 4th of November having been 1533. During the same time Gateshead with a population of 26,000, had 433 deaths, or in a ratio nearly equal to that of Newcastle. On the other hand Tynemouth, with a population of 30,000, had only twelve deaths, several of them in vagrants or other arrivals from Newcastle, the rest in a cluster of pitmen's cottages on the outskirts of North Shields.

It was freely rumoured at the time, and was even repeated with much unction in so dry and deliberate a work as the report of the Registrar-General, that the cholera at Newcastle and Gateshead in September, 1853, was owing to the sudden contamination of the town's water with sewage. The facts about the water-supply are as follows: Previous to 1848, Newcastle was supplied with Tyne water pumped up at Elswick, and passed through the settling tanks and filtering beds. In 1848 the Whittle Dean Water

---

[1] *Report of the Commissioners appointed to inquire into the late outbreak of Cholera in Newcastle, Gateshead and Tynemouth.* Parl. papers, 1854, pp. xl and 580.

Company, incorporated in 1845, had their new supply ready, and the old company, with its pumping station at Elswick, was superseded. The new supply was collected from landward sources, and was apt to be peaty. There was a great demand upon it, especially for public works (it was supplied to comparatively few houses), so that the distribution in 1853 had increased 2½ times since the company began in 1848. They had extended their collecting area to meet this demand; but, owing probably to the drought, they found it necessary on the 6th of July, 1853, to resort to the old pumping-station at Elswick for about a third part of all the water that flowed daily through the mains. This had gone on for eight weeks before the epidemic began, and was promptly discontinued on 15 September, as soon as the possible danger from Tyne water was realized. The pumping-station was higher up the river than the only one of the Newcastle sewers that discharged in its vicinity. There were complaints about the water, but these appear to have been chiefly of the peaty colour or flavour, which came from the Whittle Dean part of the mixture. The water from the mains was not equally bad at all points, as if the suspected contamination might have occurred in its transit through the town. Also the water of some wells was complained of as offensive at the same time, which was the season of the year when the springs are lowest. Gateshead was also supplied by the mains of the Whittle Dean Company. It is clear from the report of the Commissioners that they considered the water of Newcastle and Gateshead to have been a very subordinate factor, if a factor at all, in the epidemic of cholera.

The Cholera of 1854 in England.

The great epidemic at Newcastle and Gateshead was over by November, 1853, those towns having no share in the general epidemic in England in 1854, although it visited their near neighbour Tynemouth. The interest of the cholera of 1854 centres chiefly in London[1]. Few of the great foci of infection in 1849 were visited severely. Liverpool, which never escaped, had a moderate epidemic, Merthyr Tydvil also had about a fourth part of its 1849 mortality, Dudley had the disease somewhat severely, while some towns, such as Norwich, Wisbech and Sheffield, had more than usual. But Plymouth, Hull, Bristol, Manchester, Leeds, the towns of the Black Country and nearly all the populous places that had suffered heavily either in 1832 or in 1849, or on both occasions, escaped in 1854 with little cholera or none[2]. The table shows the incidence of the epidemic (as well as that of 1866) according to counties.

[1] The most elaborate and minute account of an epidemic on this occasion was that for Oxford, *Memoir on the Cholera at Oxford in the year* 1854. By H. W. Acland, M.D., in which all the points in the problem of cholera are illustrated from the easily surveyed local circumstances.
[2] The registration district of Bideford had 46 deaths in 1854, the only large total in the West country. Kingsley's graphic picture of the cholera of 1854 in *Two Years Ago* may have corresponded to these naked figures in the registration tables; but no place in Cornwall, in which county the scene appears to be laid, could have furnished so considerable an epidemic as the novelist describes, a few places in it having had each some half-dozen deaths.

Cholera Mortality in England and Wales in 1854 and 1866.

	1854 Deaths	1854 Rate per 1000	1866 Deaths	1866 Rate per 1000	Principal centres in each county 1854	1866
England and Wales	20097		14378			
London	10738	4·3	5596	·19	South of Thames, Eastern parishes	Eastern parishes 3691
Surrey, part of	252	1·2	82			
Kent, part of	1056	2·1	284			
Sussex	94	·3	79			
Hampshire	130	·3	417	·9	Portsea Island 20, Southampton 48	Portsea Island 129, Southampton 41
Berkshire	49	·2	3			
Middlesex, part of	380	2·4	51		Brentford 196	
Hertfordshire	97	·5	9			
Buckinghamshire	68	·5	10			
Oxfordshire	183	1·0	4			
Northamptonshire	152	·7	7		Towcester 86	
Huntingdonshire	18	·3	1			
Bedfordshire	61	·4	22			
Cambridgeshire	270	1·3	7		Wisbech 176, Ely 46	
Essex	513	1·4	471	1·0	West Ham 124, Romford 113, Maldon 102	West Ham 389
Suffolk	67	·2	15			
Norfolk	381	·8	15		Norwich 193, Yarmouth 41	
Wiltshire	60	·2	11			
Dorset	45	·2	6			
Devon	188	·3	525	·9	Plymouth 59, Stonehouse 15, Devonport 2, Bideford 46	Exeter and St Thomas 247, Newton Abbot 57, Totnes 146
Cornwall	24	·06	21			
Somerset	21	·04	68			
Gloucestershire	260	·6	39		Bristol 76, Clifton 92, Gloucester 48	
Herefordshire	1	·01	2			
Shropshire	13	·05	17			
Staffordshire	426	·6	30		Dudley 256, Wolverhampton 80	
Worcestershire	103	·4	36		Worcester 45	
Warwickshire	89	·2	15			
Leicestershire	14	·06	3			
Rutlandshire	9	·08	—			
Lincolnshire	134	·3	48		Great Grimsby 68	
Nottinghamshire	80	·3	12		Worksop 27, Nottingham 16	
Derbyshire	17	·06	20			
Cheshire	141	·3	391			Chester
Lancashire	1775	·8	2600	1·0	Liverpool 1084, W. Derby 206, Wigan 158	Liverpool and W. Derby 2122, Wigan 137
West Riding	470	·3	283		Sheffield 126, Dewsbury 66, Leeds 48	
East Riding	70	·3	54		Hull 27	
North Riding	84	·4	21		Whitby 33, Guisboro' 30	

	1854 Deaths	1854 Rate per 1000	1866 Deaths	1866 Rate per 1000	Principal centres in each county 1854	1866
Durham[1]		2·9	352	·6	Stockton, Auckland, Durham	
Northumberland[2]		5·7	224		Newcastle 1431, Gateshead 525, Tynemouth 203	
Cumberland	35	·2	32			
Westmoreland	1	·02	1			
Monmouth	18	·1	204			
South Wales	887	1·4	2033	2·9	Merthyr Tydvil 455, Cardiff 255, Neath 54, Brecon 54	Swansea 521, Neath 520, Llanelly 232, Merthyr Tydvil 229
North Wales	34	·08	256			

The London cholera of 1854, like that of 1832 and of 1849, fell most upon the southern (Southwark etc.), eastern and south-eastern parishes (Table, p. 858). But it fell somewhat unequally upon these; and for Southwark and Lambeth the water supply was seized upon as the thing that made the difference. There were two water companies in South London, the Lambeth company and the Southwark and Vauxhall company. The parish of Christ Church, Lambeth, chiefly supplied by the Lambeth company, had a death-rate from cholera in 1854 of only 0·43 per 1000 inhabitants; whereas the parish of St Saviour, supplied by the Southwark and Vauxhall company, had a death-rate of 2·27 per 1000. In 1849 there had been no such disparity between them, the death-rate of Christ Church being if anything the higher of the two. Now it happened that in the interval of the two epidemics of cholera the Lambeth company had removed their intake works from opposite Hungerford Market to Thames Ditton, whilst the Southwark and Vauxhall company still continued to draw their supply from the Thames near Vauxhall. Here was a fine instance of the logical method of difference. Farther, within the parish of Christ Church itself, it was sought to show that the cholera followed the lines of old water supplies, and did not follow the mains from Thames Ditton. After 1854 the Southwark and Vauxhall company also made their intake at Thames Ditton. According to the water-hypothesis of cholera, it is not surprising, as we shall duly find, that the whole of the South London parishes, which had been the chief seats of the cholera in 1832, 1849, and 1854, escaped in 1866 with a

[1] More than half in the end of 1853.
[2] Nearly all in the end of 1853.

very slight visitation. Newcastle was another chosen instance of cholera distributed by the water mains; but, as we have seen, that was improbable. Another instance was Exeter: its water supply in 1832, when part of it had a disastrous epidemic of cholera, was taken from the Exe, and was impure; in 1849, when it had only a tenth part of its last cholera mortality, its water supply had been greatly improved; in 1854 it had 10 deaths; but in 1866, Exeter with the registration district of St Thomas had 247 deaths, and Totnes had 146,—for their size about the most severely visited towns in England.

In the London cholera of 1854 a very sudden and simultaneous explosion in the district of Soho attracted much notice[1]. The district stands high, which did not save it from being the scene of the first outbreak in the great plague of 1665. In the subdistricts of St Anne, Golden Square and Berwick Street, with a population of 42,000, many of them well-to-do families, there were 537 deaths from cholera, a rate of 12·8 per 1000, contrasting with the rate of 6 per 1000 for all London. The attacks and fatalities were remarkably numerous for one or two days, falling at once thereafter to about a half. There was a pump in Broad Street, in the centre of this district, which was supposed to have dispersed cholera broadcast in its contaminated water; a death had occurred in Swain's Lane, at the foot of Highgate Hill, of a person who had drank the water of the Broad Street pump. The whole incident was seized upon and worked up by Dr Snow, who had written a speculative essay in 1849 upon the probability of cholera being conveyed by water, according to the similar theory of Parkin in 1832[2]. The Board of Health, having very full data before them of the Soho outbreak in all its aspects (including a whole biological treatise upon the organisms found in water), did not adopt Snow's conclusion, although he had enthusiastic followers at the time, and has probably more now[3]:

" In explanation of the remarkable intensity of this outbreak within very definite limits, it has been suggested by Dr Snow that the real cause of whatever was peculiar in the case lay in the general use of one particular well, situate at Broad Street in the middle of the district, and having (it was

[1] It was reported on by three commissioners, Dr Donald Fraser and Messrs Thomas Hughes and J. M. Ludlow, in the *Report of the Committee for Scientific Inquiries, Cholera Epidemic of* 1854. Appendix.
[2] John Snow, M.D., *On the mode of communication of Cholera.* London, 1849, 2nd ed. 1855.
[3] *General Board of Health, Report on Scientific Inquiries,* 1854, p. 52.

imagined) its waters contaminated by the rice-water evacuations of cholera patients. After careful inquiry we see no reason to adopt this belief. We do not find it established that the water was contaminated in the manner alleged ; nor is there before us any sufficient evidence to show whether inhabitants of the district, drinking from that well, suffered in proportion more than other inhabitants of the district who drank from other sources."

The Cholera of 1853–54 in Scotland and Ireland.

The cholera of 1853–54 in Scotland has not been so fully recorded as either of the two preceding epidemics. It is said to have caused about six thousand deaths, of which 3892 were in Glasgow alone, and a considerable part of the remainder in Edinburgh and Dundee. The infection began to appear in the end of September, having been derived probably from the dreadful explosion at Newcastle. A few early cases occurred at Dunse, in Berwickshire. On the 16th September, 1853, the old Cholera Hospital at Edinburgh, in Surgeons' Square, was opened, but received only 45 cases until the beginning of June, 1854, when it was closed. In the autumn of 1854 the real epidemic began, the hospital being re-opened on 24th August, from which date until the 30th November the admissions were 198. These hospital figures indicate for Edinburgh a milder epidemic than that of the winter of 1848, which was itself milder than that of 1832. The cases came mostly from the very same localities of the old town as in 1848. There were 145 females to 97 males ; the deaths were 117 in 243 cases admitted[1].

The epidemic at Dundee was a late autumnal or winter one, in the end of 1853, and of great severity, the mortality having probably exceeded 500. The Glasgow epidemic had a course very nearly parallel to that of 1832, and quite unlike the extraordinary winter explosion of 1848–9. It began, indeed, in winter—about the 15th of December, 1853, and had caused 849 deaths to the 27th of February ; there was a sharp rise of the mortality from the 13th to the 24th of March, the total deaths to that date being 1306. As in 1832, the infection appeared to die out in the late spring and early summer ; but in June it revived and increased in virulence until August, after which it subsided gradually until November, the whole mortality having been 3892, or ·98 per cent. of the population, nearly the same ratio as in 1848–9, (1·06) and a lower ratio than in 1832 (1·4).

[1] J. W. Begbie, *Ed. Med. and Surg. Journ.* April, 1855, p. 250.

The first part of the epidemic fell chiefly on the north and east of the city, the second part, in summer and autumn, was all over the city, as in 1832, and among all classes, as in the winter of 1848–49, but perhaps less disastrously in the best quarters of the city than the last had been. The cholera hospital received a comparatively small part of all the cases—600 of cholera, 253 of diarrhoea, the deaths being 306, or less than a tenth part of the whole mortality[1].

It is probable that the mortalities in Scotland on this occasion, besides those in Glasgow, Edinburgh and Dundee, were neither so general nor so great as in 1832. One remarkable outbreak happened at the village of Symington, in Ayrshire: in a population of 240 there were 110 attacks and 30 deaths; nearly all the cases were in houses on one side of the village street, which got their water from a public well; the houses on the other side, having private wells (and differing, doubtless, in other respects), were notably free from the infection[2].

The cholera of 1854 was unimportant in Ireland. Cases appeared among emigrants on board ships in Belfast Lough and at Queenstown in the end of 1853, but no diffusion took place until 1854, and then only to a moderate extent. It is supposed that some 1706 persons died of it in Ireland in that year, according to the retrospective figures of the census of 1861; but a good many deaths from "cholera" were returned for every year of the decennium, so that it is improbable that the whole 1706 in 1854 were of the true Asiatic type. Ulster had 895 of these, Leinster 453, Munster 324, and the whole of Connaught only 34[3].

The Cholera of 1865–66.

Asiatic cholera reached Europe by a new route in 1865—by the way of Egypt with the pilgrims returning from the Hâj at Mecca. In the course of the autumn it appeared at Southampton and caused 35 deaths from 24 September to 4 November. A

---

[1] *Glas. Med. Journ.* N.S. II. 127; III. 116, 500; John Crawford, M.D., "Report of Cases in the Cholera Hosp." *ibid.* III. 48.

[2] W. Alexander, M.D., *Edin. Med. Journ.* II. 86. The *Edin. Med. Journ.* I. July, 1855, p. 81, contains a few lines of abstract of a paper by W. T. Gairdner on the diffusion of cholera in the remote districts of Scotland. Information on the subject is invited, but it does not appear that any full account of the cholera of 1854 in Scotland was published. It is known to have been in Aberdeen.

[3] *Census of Ireland* 1861, Part III. vol. 2, p. 23.

strange extension from Southampton (or from Weymouth) took place to the village of Theydon Bois in Epping Forest, where nine deaths were traced to one house from 28 September to 31 October, unhappily including the death of a most estimable medical gentleman who tasted the water of a well into which the evacuations of the sick had probably percolated.

The cholera having become established on the continent of Europe in the end of 1865, was brought into England by emigrants passing from Hull and Grimsby to Liverpool on their way to America. On board one of the emigrant steamships, the 'England,' a very severe epidemic arose in mid-Atlantic in April. Liverpool had once more a severe epidemic (2122 deaths); but the only other important centres in England, besides London, were Swansea, Neath, Llanelly and Merthyr Tydvil, Chester and Northwich, a group of towns on the Exe in Devonshire, and Portsmouth with other places in Hampshire. Still, the deaths in all England made the large total of 14,378, no county excepting Rutland being absolutely free. That means that the infection, although widely diffused, now wanted the conditions favourable to its development and effectiveness; and that, again, seems to mean that a vast improvement had been made in the sewering of towns, in scavenging, and in all other matters of municipal police by which the soil of inhabited spots is preserved from saturation with excremental and other filth.

The interest of the cholera of 1866 centres in London, and chiefly in the fact that three-fourths of the deaths, to the number of 3696, took place in the eastern parishes, Whitechapel, Bethnal Green, Poplar, Stepney, Mile End, St George's in the East, and Greenwich. These had in former epidemics a fair share; but hitherto they had been surpassed by the Southwark parishes and others on the south of the Thames from Battersea to Rotherhithe, and nearly equalled by Shoreditch and the Liberties of the City. The comparative table of the four great choleras of London shows how remarkably the infection in 1866 had left its old principal seats, remaining, as if a residue, only in the East End, with death-rates comparable to those of 1849.

Comparative view of the Four Epidemics of Cholera in the several parishes of London[1].

	1832		1849		1854 (17 wks. end. 4 Nov.)		1866	
	Rate per 10,000	Deaths	Rate per 10,000	Deaths	Rate per 10,000	Deaths	Rate per 10,000	Deaths
Kensington	10	52	24	260	35	490	3'7	85
Chelsea	80	272	46	247	47	300	3'3	22
St George, Hanover Sq.	10	74	18	131	38	295	1'7	18
Westminster	50	450	68	437	60	423	6'2	43
St Martin in the Fields	—	—	37	91	24	58	4'2	10
St James, Westminster	—	—	16	57	152	485	3'5	13
Marylebone	30	355	17	261	16	347	3'0	54
Hampstead	—	—	8	9	11	14	'8	2
Pancras	20	230	22	360	13	248	6'0	138
Islington	10	39	22	187	8	97	4'3	120
Hackney	2	8	25	139	11	73	10'6	103
St Giles	50	280	53	285	21	115	9'2	49
Strand	1	26	35	156	24	111	6'6	29
Holborn	10	46	35	161	5	25	5'2	22
Clerkenwell	10	65	19	121	9	59	7'0	45
St Luke	30	118	34	183	9	52	8'1	46
East City			45	182	23	85	15'7	59
West City	50	605	96	429	10	126	18'8	60
City			38	207	14	71	5'0	20
Shoreditch	10	57	76	789	20	237	10'7	139
Bethnal Green	50	345	90	789	20	192	60'4	611
Whitechapel	110	736	64	506	40	330	84'2	909
St George in the East	30	123	42	199	30	154	87'9	385
Stepney	50	358	47	501	32	388	107'6	559
Mile End Old Town	—	—	—	—	—	—	67'7	501
Poplar	40	101	71	313	38	208	90'8	837
St Saviour	120	1128	153	539	134	495	7'4	32
St Olave			181	349	162	315	8'5	21
Bermondsey	70	210	161	734	158	845	5'3	35
St George, Southwark	—	—	164	836	101	546	6'6	38
Newington	40	200	144	907	101	696	2'8	26
Lambeth	40	337	120	1618	63	941	6'5	114
Wandsworth	10	46	100	484	77	422	4'8	40
Camberwell	30	107	97	504	91	553	5'6	46
Rotherhithe	10	19	205	352	147	285	8'7	25
Greenwich	20	149	75	718	53	576	19'5	284
Lewisham	—	—	30	96	20	81	6'1	56
Stratford	—	—	—	—	—	—	77'6	—
West Ham	—	—	—	—	—	—	49'3	—
Leyton	—	—	—	—	—	—	13'1	—

There was one significant thing associated with the peculiar incidence of the cholera of 1866 upon the East End. The main drainage of London, consisting of a high level and a low level sewer on each side of the Thames, was commenced in 1859, and

[1] Compiled from Grainger's report for 1849, the Registrar-General's Reports for 1854 and 1866, a table in *Lancet*, I. 1867, p. 125, and, for 1866, a table by Radcliffe, in *Rep. Med. Off. Priv. Council for* 1866, p. 339.

was formally opened on 4 April, 1865.   The two levels on each side of the river made together a length of eighty-two miles ; the cost, with pumping station, was £4,200,000.   When the cholera of 1866 broke out, only one part of the system was incomplete and not yet in working, namely, the low level main drainage on the northern side, which served the whole of the cholera-stricken parishes from Aldgate to Bow.   However, the official mind in this country has somehow become prejudiced against the well-known and usually accepted generalities of von Pettenkofer, which make more of a foul soil in the causation of miasmatic infections, than of contaminated surface water or contaminated water from reservoirs.   Accordingly, the somewhat remarkable fact that the East End of London alone retained its old proclivity for choleraic infection was not joined to the fact of its being the only great division of the capital still unsewered, but to the fact that it was supplied by water taken in from the river Lea in Hertfordshire and (it was alleged) insufficiently filtered or otherwise purified at the Old Ford waterworks[1].

The extension to Scotland in 1866 was late in the season and insignificant compared with former epidemics.   It was heard of about the end of summer in Fraserburgh and one or two other ports or fishing places on the East Coast, but it was not until October and November that it attracted notice in the eight principal towns, the whole mortality from it in Glasgow being 53, in Edinburgh 154, in Dundee 105, in Aberdeen 62, in Paisley 2, in Greenock 14, in Leith 95, and in Perth 15.   Besides these deaths there were 435 more in smaller towns or villages. The year was a very healthy one, the death-rates of Glasgow, Greenock and Perth having been below the mean of the previous ten years.

In Ireland the cholera of 1866 was even slighter than in Scotland, the only considerable epidemic having been at Belfast.

Cholera has never obtained a footing in London since the epidemic of 1866.   In 1873, while the disease was unusually active in some parts of Europe, a few cases occurred in Wapping among Scandinavian emigrants on their way to America, who had been landed for a few days.   But the infection did not spread.   In 1884, when cholera came from Cochin China to Toulon and Marseilles, two or three cases occurred on board

[1] Radcliffe, *Rep. Med. Off. Privy Council for* 1866, p. 294.

steamships arriving at Cardiff and Liverpool. In 1893, when the disease raged in Hamburg, a number of choleraic cases occurred at Grimsby in August, which were considered certainly Asiatic owing to their high degree of fatality. In August–October, the deaths from cholera, whether cholera nostras or the Asiatic type, or both together, were about thirty in Grimsby, eighteen in Hull, and about fifty more in various other places, chiefly in the south of Yorkshire. The autumn of that year was favourable to bowel-complaints and to enteric fever.

The Antecedents of Epidemic Cholera in India.

The antecedents and circumstances that made the year 1817 so critical for cholera in India, and for its diffusiveness far beyond India, constitute one of the greatest problems in epidemiology. A full and minute examination of them cannot be attempted here; but the chapter would be incomplete without some statement on the subject, which, if summary, need not be dogmatic. Cholera with the same symptoms and a similar degree of fatality was certainly not new to India about the year 1817; it can be traced from the earliest records of the Portuguese and other Europeans in India, if not also in other countries in ancient times[1]. The mortalities among troops during the military operations in the Northern Circars in 1781 and 1790, and the deaths of some 20,000 pilgrims in eight days during the Hurdwar festival of 1783, were undoubtedly from the same epidemic infective cholera that was seen fifty years after in Europe. But these were occasional great explosions, which arose suddenly and ceased abruptly; whereas from about 1817 onwards the infection became, as it were, a seasonal product of the soil of Lower Bengal year after year, and at the same time began to range widely beyond its "endemic area" to other provinces of India, beyond the North-Western frontier to Central Asia and to Europe, and across the ocean to America. It was not by any sudden change in the year 1817, we may be sure, that cholera began to be endemic at various places far apart in the valley of the Ganges. Things must have been tending towards that

---

[1] Scoutetten, *Histoire médicale et topographique du Cholera Morbus*, Metz, 1831; and *Histoire chronologique du Cholera*, Paris, 1870. David Craigie, M.D., "Remarks on the History and Etiology of Cholera," *Edin. Med. and Surg. Journ.* XXXIX. (1833), 332. John Macpherson, M.D., *Annals of Cholera*, London, 1872 and 1884. N. C. Macnamara, *A History of Asiatic Cholera*, London, 1876.

manifestation for some time before, and those things must have been of the same kind that made the great explosion at Hurdwar in 1783 and have made many other great explosions at the Indian religious festivals in later times. Briefly the opinion may be hazarded, that it was the permeation with excremental matters of the soil at large in and around Bengali villages that gave rise to the endemic miasmatic infection of cholera. The *odor stercoreus* of those innumerable village communities is, or used to be, a familiar fact, just as it is well known to be the custom there to dispense with latrines or other systematic provision for the disposal of faecal matters. But it may seem improbable that personal habits of the peasantry, not unknown in other countries, and immemorial in Lower Bengal itself, should have led to a definite disease-effect in a certain year of the 19th century and perennially thereafter. As to the special risk of engendering such a soil-poison in the valley of the Ganges, it has to be said that the region is peculiar in its alternations from extreme saturation to extreme dryness, within a stratum of alluvial or other porous soil which has a bed of impervious blue clay beneath it at a depth seldom more than 10 feet. It is just where such extreme fluctuations of the ground-water within a limited range occur from season to season, that organic matters in the soil are most apt to develop a miasmatic infective property. But why should the year 1817 have been, by the general consent of Anglo-Indian observers, the beginning of a new era in the history of cholera? The guiding principle in all such cases is, that things must have been moving that way before, and that in the particular season there had been reached at length such a degree of aggravation as to make a specific result manifest or the cumulative causes effective. Two things may be indicated as relevant to this assumed aggravation, or integration of accumulating causes. One was a certain gradual change in the beds of rivers, especially in the province of Behar, which entirely altered the relative amount of water flowing above ground and under ground, and must have made a difference in kind and in degree to the decomposition-processes in the soil. (In Burdwan these changes in the ground-water have caused much miasmatic fever since about thirty years ago.) The other thing was the increase of the number of cultivators per square mile under British rule. The latter cannot be stated with even approximate exactness for periods before the census of 1872 ; but there can be no reasonable doubt that the increase was great and progressive from the end of last century, owing to the cessation of intertribal wars, and of famines which were chiefly caused by the overflow of rivers now no longer subject to floods, and of wilful and barbarous checks to population. Among the cholera localities of 1817 were some that have now the greatest pressure of inhabitants on the soil, not in cities, but in uniformly dispersed rural communities—such as the division of Patna with 637 inhabitants per square mile, the district of Jessore with 693, and of Dacca with 756. This is of course a very general account of the matter, which a minute study of localities and seasons might show to be highly inadequate ; but in seeking for some circumstances of aggravation at the particular juncture, the two things that have been mentioned, both of them coincident historical matters of fact, will appear to be not irrelevant according to the received teaching on the favouring conditions of cholera.

NOTE ON CEREBRO-SPINAL FEVER.

British experience, or the records of it, afford so little material for the history of epidemic cerebro-spinal fever (very abundant for France, Germany and the United States of America, see Hirsch, III. 547) that it has not seemed desirable to interpolate the subject in the chapter on Typhus and other Continued Fevers. Although our experience of it has fallen perhaps wholly within the period of exact statistics of the causes of death (saving some doubtful identifications in the 18th century), yet the registration tables contain so few deaths from it that it hardly seems as if a new and remarkable type of fever of the typhus kind had really been in our midst. There are, however, two periods when a good many papers were written upon it in Ireland and England, the years 1865–67 and the year 1876. When the first cases were seen in London in 1865 Murchison pronounced the new fever to be closely allied to typhus (*Lancet*, 1865, p. 1417). At the same time in Ireland it was sometimes called "the black death," from the dark or livid vibices of the skin, or purpura maligna, or purpuric fever (J. T. Banks, *Dubl. Quart. Journ. Med. Sc.* XLIII. 98 ; E. W. Collins, *ibid.* XLVI. 170 ; Cogan, *ibid.* XLIV. 172 ; Gordon, *ibid.* XLIV. 408 ; H. Wilson, *ibid.* XLIII. ; Haverty, *ibid.* ; T. W. Belcher, *Med. Press*, N. S. III. 167 ; J. H. Benson, *ibid.* III. 387 ; editor, *ibid.* 506. For England, S. Wilks, *Lancet*, 1865, I. 388, *Brit. Med. Journ.* 1868, I. 427 ; F. J. Brown, *Trans. Epid. Soc.* II. (1865), 391 ; J. N. Radcliffe in Reynolds' *System of Medicine*, 1st ed. II. 676 ; H. Day, *Lancet*, 1867, I. 731). In the second period, 1876, there were many cases in England, especially in the Midlands, but it is said that they were usually diagnosed as typhoid fever (Sir Walter Foster, *Brit. Med. Journ.* 1892, II. 278, and *Lancet*, 1876, I. 849 ; Neville Hart (for Birmingham), *St Barth. Hosp. Rep.* XII. (1876), 105 ; H. Thompson, *Lancet*, 1876, I. 849. The Irish papers in the second period are by T. W. Grimshaw, *Dub. Journ. Med. Sc.* LXI. 520, and LVII. 375 ; E. H. Bennett, *ibid.* LIX. ; Brabazon, *Brit. Med. Journ.* 1876, I. 509). An epidemic of cerebro-spinal fever, resembling typhoid, was described for a Shropshire village in May, 1891 (Monk, *Brit. Med. Journ.* 1892, II. 278). A case which came under my notice on 19 March, 1894, in an eastern parish of London, has led me to doubt whether the half-dozen or so of deaths annually certified in London as from cerebro-spinal fever (contrasting with as many hundreds in New York), are of the slightest statistical value.

A young woman, aged 16, an artificial flower maker, became ill with pains in the limbs and was taken as an out-patient to a hospital. Thereafter she became light-headed. A private practitioner (M.R.C.S.) was called in, who found her with a temperature of 103°, excited, and inclined to clutch spasmodically at his arms ; her coarse black hair was full of pediculi and nits. She died next day, having had sent her by the practitioner a draught of chlorodyne on account of her extreme restlessness. An inquest was appointed, and the practitioner ordered to make a post-mortem examination. He attended the inquest and gave evidence that death was due to "congestion of the brain." The jury were dissatisfied, and the coroner adjourned the inquest for a second examination by a skilled pathologist.

After spending two hours looking for the cause of death (there was no congestion of the brain), I discovered that the base of the brain had been left in the skull intact, the hemispheres having been sliced off by a horizontal section in the plane of the saw-draught round the cranium. On raising the frontal lobes I saw green flaky lymph lying on the orbital plates and on the corresponding surfaces of the arachnoid ; the same was found on the optic commissure, the surface of the pons, the medulla and over a small area of the under convexities of the lateral lobes of the cerebellum, where it amounted to little more than whitish opacity. The lymph was purely basal, solely on the arachnoid, not in the fissures or sulci. The examination having already lasted over two hours, it was found impracticable to expose the spinal cord. The facts previously found were : an extensive blood-shot state of the left conjunctiva with oedema of the upper lid (there was no obvious intra-orbital disease) ; round dusky-red spots on the outer sides of the thighs and on the shoulders ; both lungs in a state of solid purple congestion at the bases, crepitant at the apices, the costal pleura dark red or livid ; the tongue large and flabby, congested around the broad papillae ; the stomach at the cardiac end, exactly corresponding to the pressure of a mass of hard undigested food, dotted with numerous small round ecchymoses under the serosa ; six inches of the lower end of the jejunum, corresponding to a mass of hard impacted faeces, dotted with the same subserous ecchymoses ; a narrow belt of deep congestion round the broad ends of the kidney pyramids ; the mucosa of the fundus uteri haemorrhagic. There was no herpetic eruption. At the adjourned inquest the cause of death was found to be cerebro-spinal fever, and was so certified by the coroner to the Registrar-General. The practitioner who attended the deceased was unable to say whether the most distinctive of all the symptoms, the violent retraction of the occiput upon the shoulders, was present or absent. It is improbable that this was a solitary case of epidemic cerebro-spinal meningitis in the East End of London in the spring of 1894, (the early spring being the distinctive season of the infection). Even if it were the only case, it narrowly missed being returned as a death from "congestion of the brain," and that, too, after post-mortem inquisition. The practitioner's statutory fees were three guineas. There has lately been collected much evidence upon certificates of death, and upon diagnosis under the Notification Act, which makes it doubtful whether our mortality statistics are as correct in substance as they are methodical and exhaustive in form.

INDEX.

Aberdeen, famine of 1622 30, relapsing fever of 1818 175, typhus of 1838–40 189, 192, relapsing of 1843 204, ratio of enteric in 1864 210, influenza of 1831 379 *note*, smallpox in 1610 434, measles of 1808 651–2, putrid sorethroat in 1790 718, dysentery near 784, cholera in 1832 815

Aberystruth, cholera in 1849 845

Ackworth bill of mortality 528 *note*

Acland, Sir H. W., cholera at Oxford in 1854 851 *note*

Adams, Joseph, cowpox 559, liberty for inoculators 609

Adynamic fever 182

Ague, etymology of, 225, 301, name of typhus in Ireland 301

Agues, epidemic, joined with influenzas 300, summary of in 16th and 17th cent. 306–14, of 1678–80 329, in Scotland after the union 341, of 1727–29 341, of 1780–85 366, table of, at Kelso Dispensary 370, of 1826–28 378, of 1827 in Ireland 273, in 1846 47 391, in a Somerset village 393, no record of, during the influenzas of 1890–94 397

Aikin, John, Warrington smallpox 553

Akenside, Mark, dysentery in London 1762 778, theory of dysentery and rheumatic fever 782

Alderson, John, contagion of typhus 153

Alison, William P., no enteric cases in 1827 187

Althaus, Julius, nervous sequelae of influenza 397 *note*

Amyand, sergeant-surgeon, inoculations by, 469–70

Andrew, John, formal inoculation 497

Anstruther, enteric fever 1835–39 199

Arbuthnot, John, malignant fever in London 67, pestilent air of cities 84, influenza of 1733 347, theory of influenza 402–5

Armagh, smallpox burials at in 1818 572, cholera in a hamlet near 818

Arnot, Hugh, inoculation a complete remedy 516

Arrott, James, fever at Dundee 192–3

Astruc, Jean, history of whooping-cough 666

Asylums, cholera in 809, 831, dysentery in 787, 791

Aubrey, T., miasmata of Guinea Coast the cause of dengue 424

Aylesbury, gaol typhus 153

Aynho, statistics of smallpox in 1723 520

Ayr, dysentery 787, cholera of 1832 814

Ayrshire, cholera at iron-works 837

Baillou, G. de, first to mention whooping-cough 666

Baker, Sir George, history of cinchona bark 320 *note*, merits of Talbor 322, epidemic agues of 1780–85 366–7. failure of bark in ditto 368, merits of Jurin 479, Sutton's inoculation 498, cowpox 558, dysentery of 1762 778

Ballard, Edward, occupation of mothers as a cause of infantile diarrhoea 766 *note*, "healthy" infants have due share of same 768, slight fatality of diarrhoea in adults 769

Banff, inoculation not general 510

Bangor, enteric fever in 1882 220

Barbone, Nicholas, builder in London after the Fire 86

Barcelona, sickness at among the troops in 1705 106

Bard, Samuel, throat-disease in New York 690

Bark, cinchona, use and abuse of in fevers 318–25, failure of in epidemic agues 368

Barker, John, of Sarum, epidemic typhus of 1741 79, 80, 83 ; Sydenham as phlebotomist 450

Barker, John, of Coleshill, type of fever in 1794 157, agues in 1781 367, influenzas of 1788 and fol. years 370, smallpox a bugbear 517

C. II.   55

866 *Index.*

Bartholin, Thomas, transplantation of disease 474

Bateman, Thomas, decline of fever 1804–16 163, epidemic fever of 1816–19 168, cause of differences of type 169, ratio of relapsing cases 172, fatal smallpox in Shoe Lane 547, 568, measles of 1807 650, dysentery rare 785

Bath, rumour of plague &c. in 1675 34, 458, influenza of 1782 364 *note*, of 1788 372, of 1803 375, smallpox of 1837 604, age-incidence of same 624

Beddoes, Thomas, influenza of 1803 375

Belfast, mortality in military hospital 1689–90 234, fatality of fever and dysentery 1846 294, recent enteric fever 299, cholera in 1832 818, in 1849 839, in 1853–4 856

Bent, Thomas, crystalline smallpox at Derby in 1818 577

Berkeley, Bishop, queries on Irish economics 239, dysentery and fever at Cloyne, &c. 1740–41 241–2, tar water in smallpox 546

Berkeley, relapsing fever in 1794–5 156

Berkhamstead, general inoculation at 509

Bernoulli, saving of life by inoculation 629

Bilge-water a cause of ship-fever 105, 106 *note*

Bideford, incidence of influenza in 1803 376, cholera in 1854 851 *note*

Bilston, cholera in 1832 824, in 1849 845

Birmingham, scarlatina in 1778 710

Black, William, safety of inoculation 608

Black Assizes at Taunton in 1730 92, alleged at Launceston in 1742 93, at the Old Bailey in 1750 93, at Dublin in 1776 98

"**Black Death,**" Irish name of cerebro-spinal fever 863

Black Fever, Irish name of relapsing fever 289

Blackmore, Sir Richard, hysteric or little fever 68, against inoculation 479

Blagden, Charles, materies of influenza 406

Blakiston, Peyton, influenza of 1837 387

Blandford, effects of inoculation on small-pox at 513

Bloodletting in fevers, Sydenham's practice in 3, attack on in 1741 83, in ship-fevers 104, from the jugular by Freind 107, of doubtful use in low fever 122, revival of in 1817 170, 172, in relapsing fever 174, 175 *note*, 176, unsuitable in the fevers of 1830–40 189, unsuitable in the relapsing fever of 1842 203, in case of Charles II. 325, in influenza of 1743 350, failure of in influenza of 1833 381, Whitmore op-

posed to in influenza of 1658 381 *note*, history of in smallpox 445–50, in whooping-cough 667, 668, injurious in epidemic angina 701, in the cholera of 1832 833

Boate, Gerard, fluxes and fevers of Ireland, 226

Boerhaave, Hermann, antidotes to small-pox 494

Bolton, dysentery in 1832 789

Boringdon, Lord, Vaccination Bills in 1813 and 1814 609

Borlase, Edmund, dysentery of Ireland 228

Boston, U. S., inoculation 483, 485, smallpox epidemic of 1721 485, tar-water in smallpox 546, adult cases in the smallpox of 1721 and 1752 626, throat-distemper of 1735–6 688

Boston, Eng., agues in 1780 367, 368, statistics of smallpox 18th cent. 525, 540, 557

Boufflers, Madame de, smallpox after inoculation 495, 500

Bowel-hive, meaning of 758 *note*

Boyle, Robert, influenza not due to the weather 399, hypothesis of subterrane-ous miasmata 400–2, 408, agues rare in Scotland 341

Boylston, Zabdiel, inoculations at Boston 483, 485

Brest, malignant typhus in 1757 113

Bridgenorth, epidemic agues in 1784 368

Bright, Richard, enteric fever in London in 1825–6 186

Bristol, fever in 1696 46, types of the fever of 1817–19 173, fever-cases in general wards 179, type of fever in 1834 201, cholera of 1832 828, of 1849 846 *note*

Bromfeild, William, against Sutton's inoculations 499, abandons inoculation 515

Bromley, malignant sore-throat in 1746 696

Brown, Andrew, fevers of the seven ill years in Scotland 48

Browne, Sir Thomas, urn-burial **and** Norwich churchyards 38

Brownrigg, William, nature of Leyden fever of 1669 19 *note*, contagion of **fever** in ships of war 114

Buchanan, Andrew, state of the poor **in** Glasgow 1830 598, Edinburgh **New** Town epidemic of 1828 788 *note*

Buchanan, Sir G., desires definition **of** "influenza proper" 397 *note*

Buckie, cholera of 1832 815

Budd, William, epidemic fever of 1839 **at** North Tawton 196

Burial in relation to plague 36–39

Burke, Edmund, dearth of 1795 158 *note*

sources of miasmata of influenza in 1693 420, epidemic of 1688 and the earthquake of Lima 421, possible sources of S. American epidemic in 1720, direction in which the true theory lies 425, outbreaks at sea 425–431, strangers' colds 431–433. See also Horses.

Inoculation of smallpox, a Greek practice 463, begun in London 467, popular origins of 471, Voltaire's legend of Circassian 472 *note*, probably grew out of transplantation of disease 474, religious symbolism of inoculation 475, etymology of 476, not an antidote 477, controversy on in England 477, reality of as practised by Nettleton 482, at Boston, New England 485, cases of failure 487, cases of death from 489, revival of in 1741 489, at Charleston in 1738 490, as practised by Frewen 492, by Kirkpatrick 493, the blister method of 494, Gatti's practice in 495, Sutton's practice in 498, opposition to Sutton's method of 499, Watson's experiment in 500, Mudge's experiment in 501, tests of its validity 502, extent of in England in 18th cent. 504–9, in Scotland 509, value of 511, at Blandford 513, at the Foundling Hospital 514, known failures of 515, testimonies to value of 516, advocates of in 19th cent. 586, Lipscomb's poem on 587, preference of populace for 589, practised by Walker as vaccination 590, extent of 590–2, made penal 606, history of the doctrine that it was a nuisance 607–10, did not contain the principle of re-vaccination 610

Intermittent Fevers, Sydenham's view of 11, in Ireland after the relapsing fever of 1826 273, and of 1847–9 297. See also **Ague.**

Inverness, typhus at 110, cholera of 1832 814, of 1849 838

Ipswich, ship typhus at 110, scarlatina in 1771 708

Jamaica, sickness after earthquake 416

Jenner, Edward, relapsing fever in his house 156, inoculates with crude matter 502, collects failures of inoculation 515, inoculates with swinepox 558, proposes to inoculate with cowpox 558, indicates ulcerous characters of cowpox 560, his opinion on origin of smallpox and cowpox 562, calls cowpox *variolae vaccinae* 563, tests the virtue of cowpox 565, makes interest with the great 566, demands prohibition of inoculation 609, opposes Watt's doctrine of measles 657

Jenner, J. C., epidemic ague in 1784 369,

general inoculation 509, why smallpox malignant 550

Jenner, Sir William, diagnosis of continued fevers 4, 183, diphtheria 739 *note*, rickets a diathesis 767

Jesty, Benjamin, inoculates with cowpox 558

Johnstone, James, Kidderminster fevers 1752–56 124, sequelae of measles 660 *note*, sore-throat and fever 702, 704, the scarlet eruption, 710

Johnstone, James, junior, dies of gaol fever 153, writes on the scarlatina of 1778 710

Jolly rant, name of influenza in 1675 327 *note*, 328

Jones, John, fevers of the Greeks not in our climate 301, agues of 1558 307

Jones, John, dysentery in Wales 777

Jurin, James, arguments for inoculation 479, his authority 480, biographical sketch of 481 *note*

Kanturk, incidents at in famine of 1818 265

Katharine, Queen of Charles II., her fever in 1663 13

Kell, John Butler, cholera at Sunderland 1831 798

Kellwaye, Simon, measles and smallpox 633

Kelso, agues in 18th cent. 369, cholera in 1848–9 838

Kendal, vaccination 1819–21 584

Kendall, Henry, type of Dublin fever in 1847 289, in 1862 298

Kennedy, Peter, inoculation at Constantinople 464, procuring smallpox in Scotland 471

Kerr, George, fever in Aberdeen 176

Kidderminster, fevers in 1727–29 124 *note*, in 1751–56 124, sequelae of measles 660, sore-throat and fever in 1748 701, 704, in 1778 710

Kilgour, Alexander, typhus one of the exanthemata 189, ratio of spotted cases 193

Kilkenny, sickness in 1846 282

Kilmarnock, 18th cent. smallpox 526, cholera of 1832 814, of 1849 838

Kiltearn, paupers in 1697 51 *note*, smallpox in 18th cent. 541

Kingsley, Charles, cholera of 1854 851 *note*

Kink, old name of whooping-cough 666

Kirkmaiden, smallpox and fever in 18th cent. 528

Kirkpatrick, or Kilpatrick, J., inoculates at Charleston 90, in London 491, 493

Kite, Charles, second inoculations 503, failures of inoculation 515